Data Mining and Medical Knowledge Management: Cases and Applications

Petr Berka
University of Economics, Prague, Czech Republic

Jan Rauch
University of Economics, Prague, Czech Republic

Djamel Abdelkader Zighed
University of Lumiere Lyon 2, France

MEDICAL INFORMATION SCIENCE REFERENCE
Hershey · New York

Director of Editorial Content: Kristin Klinger
Managing Editor: Jamie Snavely
Assistant Managing Editor: Carole Coulson
Typesetter: Sean Woznicki
Cover Design: Lisa Tosheff
Printed at: Yurchak Printing Inc.

Published in the United States of America by
Information Science Reference (an imprint of IGI Global)
701 E. Chocolate Avenue, Suite 200
Hershey PA 17033
Tel: 717-533-8845
Fax: 717-533-8661
E-mail: cust@igi-global.com
Web site: http://www.igi-global.com/reference

and in the United Kingdom by
Information Science Reference (an imprint of IGI Global)
3 Henrietta Street
Covent Garden
London WC2E 8LU
Tel: 44 20 7240 0856
Fax: 44 20 7379 0609
Web site: http://www.eurospanbookstore.com

Library of Congress Cataloging-in-Publication Data

Data mining and medical knowledge management : cases and applications / Petr Berka, Jan Rauch, and Djamel Abdelkader Zighed, editors.
p. ; cm.
Includes bibliographical references and index.
Summary: "This book presents 20 case studies on applications of various modern data mining methods in several important areas of medicine, covering classical data mining methods, elaborated approaches related to mining in EEG and ECG data, and methods related to mining in genetic data"--Provided by publisher.
ISBN 978-1-60566-218-3 (hardcover)
1. Medicine--Data processing--Case studies. 2. Data mining--Case studies. I. Berka, Petr. II. Rauch, Jan. III. Zighed, Djamel A., 1955-
[DNLM: 1. Medical Informatics--methods--Case Reports. 2. Computational Biology--methods--Case Reports. 3. Information Storage and Retrieval--methods--Case Reports. 4. Risk Assessment--Case Reports. W 26.5 D2314 2009]
R858.D33 2009
610.0285--dc22

2008028366

British Cataloguing in Publication Data
A Cataloguing in Publication record for this book is available from the British Library.

Editorial Advisory Board

List of Reviewers

Table of Contents

Section II
General Applications

Section III
Specific Cases

Detailed Table of Contents

Section I
Theoretical Aspects

This section provides a theoretical and methodological background for the remaining parts of the book. It defines and explains basic notions of data mining and knowledge management, and discusses some general methods.

Jana Zvárová, Institute of Computer Science of the Academy of Sciences of the Czech Republic v.v.i., Czech Republic; Center of Biomedical Informatics, Czech Republic
Arnošt Veselý, Institute of Computer Science of the Academy of Sciences of the Czech Republic v.v.i., Czech Republic; Czech University of Life Sciences, Czech Republic
Igor Vajda, Institutes of Computer Science and Information Theory and Automation of the Academy of Sciences of the Czech Republic v.v.i., Czech Republic

This chapter introduces the basic concepts of medical informatics: data, information, and knowledge. It shows how these concepts are interrelated and can be used for decision support in medicine. All discussed approaches are illustrated on one simple medical example.

Michel Simonet, Laboratoire TIMC-IMAG, Institut de l'Ingénierie et de l'Information de Santé, France
Radja Messai, Laboratoire TIMC-IMAG, Institut de l'Ingénierie et de l'Information de Santé, France
Gayo Diallo, Laboratoire TIMC-IMAG, Institut de l'Ingénierie et de l'Information de Santé, France
Ana Simonet, Laboratoire TIMC-IMAG, Institut de l'Ingénierie et de l'Information de Santé, France

In this chapter, biomedical image registration and fusion, which is an effective mechanism to assist medical knowledge discovery by integrating and simultaneously representing relevant information from diverse imaging resources, is introduced. This chapter covers fundamental knowledge and major methodologies of biomedical image registration, and major applications of image registration in biomedicine.

This chapter describes methods for preprocessing, analysis, feature extraction, visualization, and classification of electrocardiogram (ECG) signals. First, preprocessing methods mainly based on the discrete wavelet transform are introduced. Then classification methods such as fuzzy rule-based decision trees and neural networks are presented. Two examples - visualization and feature extraction from Body Surface Potential Mapping (BSPM) signals and classification of Holter ECGs – illustrate how these methods are used.

This chapter deals with the application of principal components analysis (PCA) to the field of data mining in electroencephalogram (EEG) processing. Possible applications of this approach include separation of different signal components for feature extraction in the field of EEG signal processing, adaptive segmentation, epileptic spike detection, and long-term EEG monitoring evaluation of patients in a coma.

In this chapter, existing clinical risk prediction models are examined and matched to the patient data to which they may be applied using classification and data mining techniques, such as neural Nets. Novel risk prediction models are derived using unsupervised cluster analysis algorithms. All existing and derived models are verified as to their usefulness in medical decision support on the basis of their effectiveness on patient data from two UK sites.

Foreword

Current research directions are looking at Data Mining (DM) and Knowledge Management (KM) as complementary and interrelated fields, aimed at supporting, with algorithms and tools, the lifecycle of knowledge, including its discovery, formalization, retrieval, reuse, and update. While DM focuses on the extraction of patterns, information, and ultimately knowledge from data (Giudici, 2003; Fayyad et al., 1996; Bellazzi, Zupan, 2008), KM deals with eliciting, representing, and storing explicit knowledge, as well as keeping and externalizing tacit knowledge (Abidi, 2001; Van der Spek, Spijkervet, 1997). Although DM and KM have stemmed from different cultural backgrounds and their methods and tools are different, too, it is now clear that they are dealing with the same fundamental issues, and that they must be combined to effectively support humans in decision making.

The capacity of DM to analyze data and to extract models, which may be meaningfully interpreted and transformed into knowledge, is a key feature for a KM system. Moreover, DM can be a very useful instrument to transform the tacit knowledge contained in transactional data into explicit knowledge, by making experts' behavior and decision-making activities emerge.

On the other hand, DM is greatly empowered by KM. The available, or background knowledge, (BK) is exploited to drive data gathering and experimental planning, and to structure the databases and data warehouses. BK is used to properly select the data, choose the data mining strategies, improve the data mining algorithms, and finally evaluates the data mining results (Bellazzi, Zupan, 2008; Bellazzi, Zupan, 2008). The output of the data analysis process is an update of the domain knowledge itself, which may lead to new experiments and new data gathering (see Figure 1).

If the interaction and integration of DM and KM is important in all application areas, in medical applications it is essential (Cios, Moore, 2002). Data analysis in medicine is typically part of a complex reasoning process which largely depends on BK. Diagnosis, therapy, monitoring, and molecular research are always guided by the existing knowledge of the problem domain, on the population of patients or on the specific patient under consideration. Since medicine is a safety critical context (Fox, Das, 2000),

Figure 1. Role of the background knowledge in the data mining process

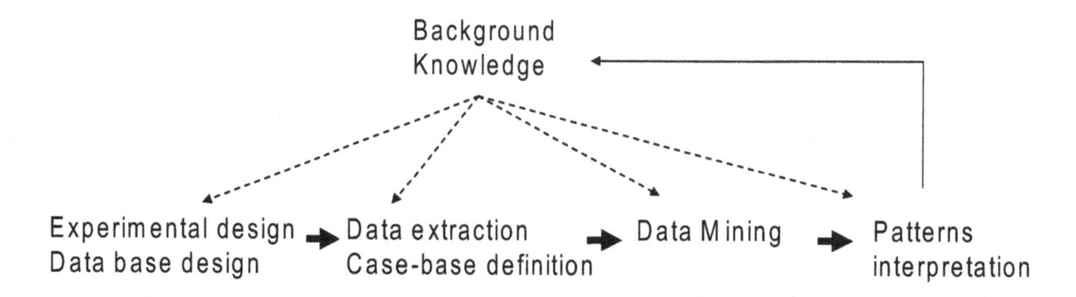

decisions must always be supported by arguments, and the explanation of decisions and predictions should be mandatory for an effective deployment of DM models. DM and KM are thus becoming of great interest and importance for both clinical practice and research.

As far as clinical practice is concerned, KM can be a key player in the current transformation of healthcare organizations (HCO). HCOs have currently evolved into complex enterprises in which managing knowledge and information is a crucial success factor in order to improve efficiency, (i.e. the capability of optimizing the use of resources, and efficacy, i.e. the capability to reach the clinical treatment outcome) (Stefanelli, 2004). The current emphasis on Evidence-based Medicine (EBM) is one of the main reasons to utilize KM in clinical practice. EBM proposes strategies to apply evidence gained from scientific studies for the care of individual patients (*Sackett, 2004)*. Such strategies are usually provided as clinical practice guidelines or individualized decision making rules and may be considered as an example of explicit knowledge. Of course, HCO must also manage the empirical and experiential (or tacit) knowledge mirrored by the day-by-day actions of healthcare providers. An important research effort is therefore to augment the use of the so-called "process data" in order to improve the quality of care (Montani et al., 2006; Bellazzi et al. 2005). These process data include patients' clinical records, healthcare provider actions (e.g. exams, drug administration, surgeries) and administrative data (admissions, discharge, exams request). DM may be the natural instrument to deal with this problem, providing the tools for highlighting patterns of actions and regularities in the data, including the temporal relationships between the different events occurring during the HCO activities (Bellazzi et al. 2005).

Biomedical research is another driving force that is currently pushing towards the integration of KM and DM. The discovery of the genetic factors underlying the most common diseases, including for example cancer and diabetes, is enabled by the concurrence of two main factors: the availability of data at the genomic and proteomic scale and the construction of biological data repositories and ontologies, which accumulate and organize the considerable quantity of research results (Lang, 2006). If we represent the current research process as a reasoning cycle including inference from data, ranking of the hypothesis and experimental planning, we can easily understand the crucial role of DM and KM (see Figure 2).

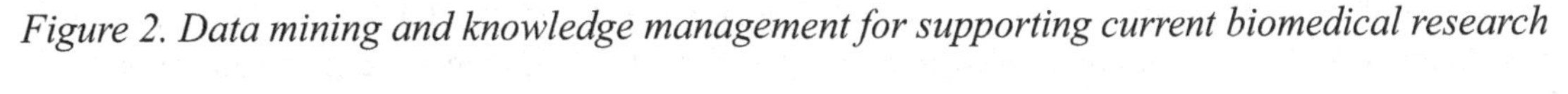

Figure 2. Data mining and knowledge management for supporting current biomedical research

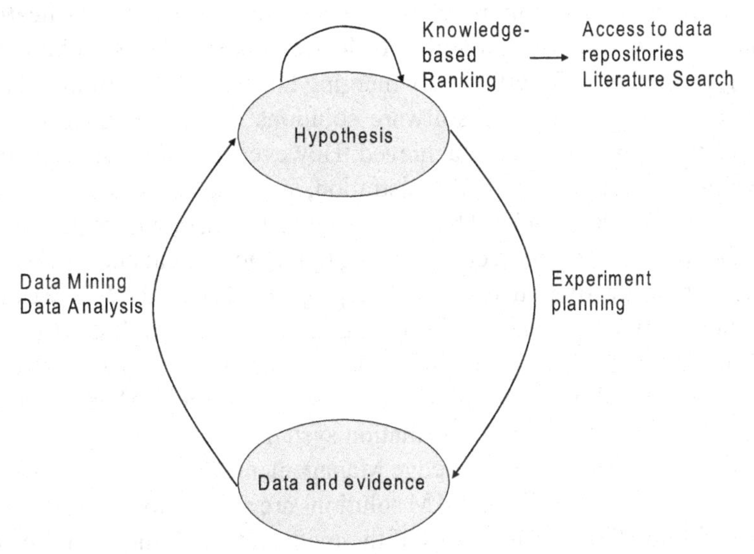

In recent years, new enabling technologies have been made available to facilitate a coherent integration of DM and KM in medicine and biomedical research.

Firstly, the growth of Natural Language Processing (NLP) and text mining techniques is allowing the extraction of information and knowledge from medical notes, discharge summaries, and narrative patients' reports. Rather interestingly, this process is however, always dependent on already formalized knowledge, often represented as medical terminologies (Savova et al., 2008; Cimiano et al., 2005).

Indeed, medical ontologies and terminologies themselves may be learned (or at least improved or complemented) by resorting to Web mining and ontology learning techniques. Thanks to the large amount of information available on the Web in digital format, this ambitious goal is now at hand (Cimiano et al., 2005).

The interaction between KM and DM is also shown by the current efforts on the construction of automated systems for filtering association rules learned from medical transaction databases. The availability of a formal ontology allows the ranking of association rules by clarifying what are the rules confirming available medical knowledge, what are surprising but plausible, and finally, the ones to be filtered out (Raj et al., 2008).

Another area where DM and KM are jointly exploited is Case-Based Reasoning (CBR). CBR is a problem solving paradigm that utilizes the specific knowledge of previously experienced situations, called cases. It basically consists in retrieving past cases that are similar to the current one and in reusing (by, if necessary, adapting) solutions used successfully in the past; the current case can be retained and put into the case library. In medicine, CBR can be seen as a suitable instrument to build decision support tools able to use tacit knowledge (Schmidt et al., 2001). The algorithms for computing the case similarity are typically derived from the DM field. However, case retrieval and situation assessment can be successfully guided by the available formalized background knowledge (Montani, 2008).

Within the different technologies, some methods seem particularly suitable for fostering DM and KM integration. One of those is represented by Bayesian Networks (BN), which have now reached maturity and have been adopted in different biomedical application areas (Hamilton et al., 1995; Galan et al., 2002; Luciani et al., 2003). BNs allow to explicitly represent the knowledge available in terms of a directed acyclic graph structure and a collection of conditional probability tables, and to perform probabilistic inference (Spiegelhalter, Lauritzen, 1990). Moreover, several algorithms are available to learn both the graph structure and the underlying probabilistic model from the data (Cooper, Herskovits, 1992; Ramoni, Sebastiani, 2001). BNs can thus be considered at the conjunction of knowledge representation, automated reasoning, and machine learning. Other approaches, such as association and classification rules, joining the declarative nature of rules, and the availability of learning mechanisms including inductive logic programming, are of great potential for effectively merging DM and KM (Amini et al., 2007).

At present, the widespread adoption of software solutions that may effectively implement KM strategies in the clinical settings is still to be achieved. However, the increasing abundance of data in bioinformatics, in health care insurance and administration, and in the clinics, is forcing the emergence of clinical data warehouses and data banks. The use of such data banks will require an integrated KM-DM approach. A number of important projects are trying to merge clinical and research objectives with a knowledge management perspective, such as the I2B2 project at Harvard (Heinze et al. 2008), or, on a smaller scale, the Hemostat (Bellazzi et al. 2005) and the Rhene systems in Italy (Montani et al., 2006). Moreover, several commercial solutions for the joint management of information, data, and knowledge are available on the market. It is almost inevitable that in the near future, DM and KM technologies will be an essential part of hospital and research information systems.

The book "Data Mining and Medical Knowledge Management: Cases and Applications" is a collection of case studies in which advanced DM and KM solutions are applied to concrete cases in biomedical research. The reader will find all the peculiarities of the medical field, which require specific solutions to complex problems. The tools and methods applied are therefore much more than a simple adaptation of general purpose solutions: often they are brand-new strategies and always integrate data with knowledge. The DM and KM researchers are trying to cope with very interesting challenges, including the integration of background knowledge, the discovery of interesting and non-trivial relationships, the construction and discovery of models that can be easily understood by experts, the marriage of model discovery and decision support. KM and DM are taking shape and even more than today they will be in the future part of the set of basic instruments at the core of medical informatics.

Riccardo Bellazzi
Dipartimento di Informatica e Sistemistica, Università di Pavia

REFERENCES

Abidi, S. S. (2001). Knowledge management in healthcare: towards 'knowledge-driven' decision-support services. *Int J Med Inf,* 63, 5-18.

Amini, A., Muggleton, S. H., Lodhi, H., & Sternberg, M.J. (2007). A novel logic-based approach for quantitative toxicology prediction. *J Chem Inf Model*, 47(3), 998-1006.

Bellazzi, R., Larizza, C., Magni, P., & Bellazzi, R. (2005). Temporal data mining for the quality assessment of hemodialysis services. *Artif Intell Med*, 34(1), 25-39.

Bellazzi, R., & Zupan, B. (2007). Towards knowledge-based gene expression data mining. *J Biomed Inform*, 40(6), 787-802.

Bellazzi, R, & Zupan, B. (2008). Predictive data mining in clinical medicine: current issues and guidelines. *Int J Med Inform*, 77(2), 81-97.

Cimiano, A., Hoto, A., & Staab, S. (2005). Learning concept hierarchies from text corpora using formal concept analysis. *Journal of Artificial Intelligence Research*, 24, 305-339.

Cios, K. J., & Moore, G. W. (2002). Uniqueness of medical data mining. *Artif Intell Med,* 26, 1-24.

Cooper, G. F, & Herskovits, E. (1992). A Bayesian method for the induction of probabilistic networks from data. *Machine Learning*, 9, 309-347.

Dudley, J., & Butte, A. J. (2008). Enabling integrative genomic analysis of high-impact human diseases through text mining. *Pac Symp Biocomput,* 580-591.

Fayyad, U., Piatetsky-Shapiro, G., & Smyth, P. (1996). Data mining and knowledge discovery in databases. *Communications of the ACM*, 39, 24-26.

Fox, J., & Das, S. K. (2000). *Safe and sound: artificial intelligence in hazardous applications*. Cambridge, MA: MIT Press.

Galan, S. F., Aguado, F., Diez, F. J., & Mira, J. (2002). NasoNet, modeling the spread of nasopharyngeal cancer with networks of probabilistic events in discrete time. *Artif Intell Med*, 25(3), 247-264.

Giudici, P. (2003). *Applied Data Mining, Statistical Methods for Business and Industry*. Wiley & Sons.

Hamilton, P. W., Montironi, R., Abmayr, W., et al. (1995). Clinical applications of Bayesian belief networks in pathology. *Pathologica*, 87(3), 237-245.

Heinze, D. T., Morsch, M. L., Potter, B. C., & Sheffer, R.E Jr. (2008). Medical i2b2 NLP smoking challenge: the A-Life system architecture and methodology. *J Am Med Inform Assoc*, 15(1), 40-3.

Lang, E. (2006). Bioinformatics and its impact on clinical research methods. Findings from the Section on Bioinformatics. *Yearb Med Inform*, 104-6.

Luciani, D., Marchesi, M., & Bertolini, G. (2003). The role of Bayesian Networks in the diagnosis of pulmonary embolism. *J Thromb Haemost*, 1(4), 698-707.

Montani, S. (2008). Exploring new roles for case-based reasoning in heterogeneous AI systems for medical decision support. *Applied Intelligence*, 28(3), 275-285.

Montani, S., Portinale, L., Leonardi, G., & Bellazzi, R. (2006). Case-based retrieval to support the treatment of end stage renal failure patients. *Artif Intell Med*, 37(1), 31-42.

Raj, R., O'Connor, M. J., & Das, A. K. (2008). An Ontology-Driven Method for Hierarchical Mining of Temporal Patterns: Application to HIV Drug Resistance Research. *AMIA Symp.*

Ramoni, M., & Sebastiani, P. (2001). Robust learning with Missing Data. *Machine Learning*, 45, 147-170.

Sackett, D. L., Rosenberg, W. M., Gray, J. A., Haynes, R B., & Richardson, W. S. (2004). Evidence based medicine: what it is and what it isn't. BMJ, 312 (7023), 71-2.

Savova, G. K., Ogren, P. V., Duffy, P. H., Buntrock, J. D., & Chute, C. G. (2008). Mayo clinic NLP system for patient smoking status identification. *J Am Med Inform Assoc,* 15(1), 25-8.

Schmidt, R., Montani, S., Bellazzi, R., Portinale, L., & Gierl, L. (2001). Case-based reasoning for medical knowledge-based systems. *Int J Med Inform*, 64(2-3), 355-367.

Spiegelhalter, D. J., & Lauritzen, S. L. (1990). Sequential updating of conditional probabilities on directed graphical structures. *Networks*, 20, 579-605.

Stefanelli, M. (2004). Knowledge and process management in health care organizations. *Methods Inf Med*, 43(5), 525-35.

Van der Spek, R, & Spijkervet, A. (1997). Knowledge management: dealing intelligently with knowledge. In J. Liebowitz & L.C. Wilcox (Eds.), *Knowledge Management and its Integrative Elements*. CRC Press, Boca Raton, FL, 1997.

Ricardo Bellazzi *is associate professor of medical informatics at the Dipartimento di Informatica e Sistemistica, University of Pavia, Italy. He teaches medical informatics and machine learning at the Faculty of Biomedical Engineering and bioinformatics at the Faculty of Biotechnology of the University of Pavia. He is a member of the board of the PhD in bioengineering and bioinformatics of the University of Pavia. Dr. Bellazzi is past-chairman of the IMIA working group of intelligent data analysis and data mining, program chair of the AIME 2007 conference and member of the program committee of several international conferences in medical informatics and artificial intelligence. He is member of the editorial board of Methods of Information in Medicine and of the Journal of Diabetes Science and Technology. He is affiliated with the American Medical Informatics Association and with the Italian Bioinformatics Society. His research interests are related to biomedical informatics, comprising data mining, IT-based management of chronic patients, mathematical modeling of biological systems, bioinformatics. Riccardo Bellazzi is author of more than 200 publications on peer-reviewed journals and international conferences.*

Preface

The basic notion of the book "*Data Mining and Medical Knowledge Management: Cases and Applications*" is knowledge. A number of definitions of this notion can be found in the literature:

- Knowledge is the sum of what is known: the body of truth, information, and principles acquired by mankind.
- Knowledge is human expertise stored in a person's mind, gained through experience, and interaction with the person's environment.
- Knowledge is information evaluated and organized by the human mind so that it can be used purposefully, e.g., conclusions or explanations.
- Knowledge is information about the world that allows an expert to make decisions.

There are also various classifications of knowledge. A key distinction made by the majority of knowledge management practitioners is Nonaka's reformulation of Polanyi's distinction between tacit and explicit knowledge. By definition, *tacit knowledge* is knowledge that people carry in their minds and is, therefore, difficult to access. Often, people are not aware of the knowledge they possess or how it can be valuable to others. Tacit knowledge is considered more valuable because it provides context for people, places, ideas, and experiences. Effective transfer of tacit knowledge generally requires extensive personal contact and trust. *Explicit knowledge* is knowledge that has been or can be articulated, codified, and stored in certain media. It can be readily transmitted to others. The most common forms of explicit knowledge are manuals, documents, and procedures. We can add a third type of knowledge to this list, the *implicit knowledge*. This knowledge is hidden in a large amount of data stored in various databases but can be made explicit using some algorithmic approach. Knowledge can be further classified into procedural knowledge and declarative knowledge. *Procedural knowledge* is often referred to as knowing how to do something. *Declarative knowledge* refers to knowing that something is true or false.

In this book we are interested in knowledge expressed in some language (formal, semi-formal) as a kind of model that can be used to support the decision making process. The book tackles the notion of knowledge (in the domain of medicine) from two different points of view: data mining and knowledge management.

Knowledge Management (KM) comprises a range of practices used by organizations to identify, create, represent, and distribute knowledge. Knowledge Management may be viewed from each of the following perspectives:

- **Techno-centric:** A focus on technology, ideally those that enhance knowledge sharing/growth.
- **Organizational:** How does the organization need to be designed to facilitate knowledge processes? Which organizations work best with what processes?

- **Ecological:** Seeing the interaction of people, identity, knowledge, and environmental factors as a complex adaptive system.

Keeping this in mind, the content of the book fits into the first, technological perspective. Historically, there have been a number of technologies "enabling" or facilitating knowledge management practices in the organization, including expert systems, knowledge bases, various types of Information Management, software help desk tools, document management systems, and other IT systems supporting organizational knowledge flows.

Knowledge Discovery or Data Mining is the partially automated process of extracting patterns from usually large databases. It has proven to be a promising approach for enhancing the intelligence of systems and services. Knowledge discovery in real-world databases requires a broad scope of techniques and forms of knowledge. Both the knowledge and the applied methods should fit the discovery tasks and should adapt to knowledge hidden in the data. Knowledge discovery has been successfully used in various application areas: business and finance, insurance, telecommunication, chemistry, sociology, or medicine. Data mining in biology and medicine is an important part of biomedical informatics, and one of the first intensive applications of computer science to this field, whether at the clinic, the laboratory, or the research center.

The healthcare industry produces a constantly growing amount of data. There is however a growing awareness of potential hidden in these data. It becomes widely accepted that health care organizations can benefit in various ways from deep analysis of data stored in their databases. It results into numerous applications of various data mining tools and techniques. The analyzed data are in different forms covering simple data matrices, complex relational databases, pictorial material, time series, and so forth. Efficient analysis requires knowledge not only of data analysis techniques but also involvement of medical knowledge and close cooperation between data analysis experts and physicians. The mined knowledge can be used in various areas of healthcare covering research, diagnosis, and treatment. It can be used both by physicians and as a part of AI-based devices, such as expert systems. Raw medical data are by nature heterogeneous. Medical data are collected in the form of images (e.g. X-ray), signals (e.g. EEG, ECG), laboratory data, structural data (e.g. molecules), and textual data (e.g. interviews with patients, physician's notes). Thus there is a need for efficient mining in images, graphs, and text, which is more difficult than mining in "classical" relational databases containing only numeric or categorical attributes. Another important issue in mining medical data is privacy and security; medical data are collected on patients, misuse of these data or abuse of patients must be prevented.

The goal of the book is to present a wide spectrum of applications of data mining and knowledge management in medical area.

The book is divided into 3 sections. The first section entitled "*Theoretical Aspects*" discusses some basic notions of data mining and knowledge management with respect to the medical area. This section presents a theoretical background for the rest of the book.

Chapter I introduces the basic concepts of medical informatics: data, information, and knowledge. It shows how these concepts are interrelated and how they can be used for decision support in medicine. All discussed approaches are illustrated on one simple medical example.

Chapter II introduces the basic notions about ontologies, presents a survey of their use in medicine and explores some related issues: knowledge bases, terminology, and information retrieval. It also addresses the issues of ontology design, ontology representation, and the possible interaction between data mining and ontologies.

Health managers and clinicians often need models that try to minimize several types of costs associated with healthcare, including attribute costs (e.g. the cost of a specific diagnostic test) and misclassification costs (e.g. the cost of a false negative test). Chapter III presents some concepts related to cost-sensitive learning and cost-sensitive classification in medicine and reviews research in this area.

There are a number of machine learning methods used in data mining. Among them, artificial neural networks gain a lot of popularity although the built models are not as understandable as, for example, decision trees. These networks are presented in two subsequent chapters. Chapter IV describes the theoretical background of artificial neural networks (architectures, methods of learning) and shows how these networks can be used in medical domain to solve various classification and regression problems. Chapter V introduces classification networks composed of preprocessing layers and classification networks and compares them with "classical" multilayer perceptions on three medical case studies.

The second section, "*General Applications*," presents work that is general in the sense of a variety of methods or variety of problems described in each of the chapters.

In chapter VI, biomedical image registration and fusion, which is an effective mechanism to assist medical knowledge discovery by integrating and simultaneously representing relevant information from diverse imaging resources, is introduced. This chapter covers fundamental knowledge and major methodologies of biomedical image registration, and major applications of image registration in biomedicine.

The next two chapters describe methods of biomedical signal processing. Chapter VII describes methods for preprocessing, analysis, feature extraction, visualization, and classification of electrocardiogram (ECG) signals. First, preprocessing methods mainly based on the discrete wavelet transform are introduced. Then classification methods such as fuzzy rule-based decision trees and neural networks are presented. Two examples, visualization and feature extraction from body surface potential mapping (BSPM) signals and classification of Holter ECGs, illustrate how these methods are used. Chapter VIII deals with the application of principal components analysis (PCA) to the field of data mining in electroencephalogram (EEG) processing. Possible applications of this approach include separation of different signal components for feature extraction in the field of EEG signal processing, adaptive segmentation, epileptic spike detection, and long-term EEG monitoring evaluation of patients in a coma.

In chapter IX, existing clinical risk prediction models are examined and matched to the patient data to which they may be applied, using classification and data mining techniques, such as neural Nets. Novel risk prediction models are derived using unsupervised cluster analysis algorithms. All existing and derived models are verified as to their usefulness in medical decision support on the basis of their effectiveness on patient data from two UK sites.

Chapter X deals with the problem of quality assessment of medical Web sites. The so called "quality labeling" process can benefit from employment of Web mining and information extraction techniques, in combination with flexible methods of Web-based information management developed within the Semantic Web initiative.

In medicine, doctors are often confronted with exceptions both in medical practice or in medical research; a proper method of how to deal with exceptions are case-based systems. Chapter XI presents two such systems. The first one is a knowledge-based system for therapy support. The second one is designed for medical studies or research. It helps to explain cases that contradict a theoretical hypothesis.

The third section, "*Specific Cases*," shows results of several case studies of (mostly) data mining, applied to various specific medical problems. The problems covered by this part range from discovery of biologically interpretable knowledge from gene expression data, over human embryo selection for the purpose of human in-vitro fertilization treatments, to diagnosis of various diseases based on machine learning techniques.

Discovery of biologically interpretable knowledge from gene expression data is a crucial issue. Current gene data analysis is often based on global approaches such as clustering. An alternative way is to utilize local pattern mining techniques for global modeling and knowledge discovery. The next two chapters deal with this problem from two points of view: using data only, and combining data with domain knowledge. Chapter XII proposes three data mining methods to deal with the use of local patterns, and chapter XIII points out the role of genomic background knowledge in gene expression data mining. Its application is demonstrated in several tasks such as relational descriptive analysis, constraint-based knowledge discovery, feature selection, and construction or quantitative association rule mining.

Chapter XIV describes the process used to mine a database containing data related to patient visits during Tinnitus Retraining Therapy.

Chapter XV describes a new multi-classification system using Gaussian networks to combine the outputs (probability distributions) of standard machine learning classification algorithms. This multi-classification technique has been applied to the selection of the most promising embryo-batch for human in-vitro fertilization treatments.

Chapter XVI reviews current policies of tuberculosis control programs for the diagnosis of tuberculosis. A data mining project that uses WHO's Direct Observation of Therapy data to analyze the relationship among different variables and the tuberculosis diagnostic category registered for each patient is then presented.

Chapter XVII describes how to integrate medical knowledge with purely inductive (data-driven) methods for the creation of clinical prediction rules. The described framework has been applied to the creation of clinical prediction rules for the diagnosis of obstructive sleep apnea.

Chapter XVIII describes goals, current results, and further plans of long time activity concerning application of data mining and machine learning methods to the complex medical data set. The analyzed data set concerns longitudinal study of atherosclerosis risk factors.

The book can be used as a textbook of advanced data mining applications in medicine. The book addresses not only researchers and students in the field of computer science or medicine but it will be of great interest also for physicians and managers of healthcare industry. It should help physicians and epidemiologists to add value to their collected data.

Petr Berka, Jan Rauch, and Djamel Abdelkader Zighed
Editors

Acknowledgment

The editors would like to acknowledge the help of all involved in the collation and review process of the book, without whose support the project could not have been satisfactorily completed.

Most of the authors of chapters included in this book also served as referees for chapters written by other authors. Thanks go to all those who provided constructive and comprehensive reviews. However, some of the reviewers must be mentioned as their reviews set the benchmark. Reviewers who provided the most comprehensive, critical and constructive comments include: Ricardo Bellazzi of University Pavia, Italy; Lenka Lhotská of Czech Technical University, Prague; and Ján Paralič of Technical University Košice, Slovakia. Support of the department of information and knowledge engineering, University of Economics, Prague, is acknowledged for archival server space in the completely virtual online review process.

Special thanks also go to the publishing team at IGI Global, whose contributions throughout the whole process from inception of the initial idea to final publication have been invaluable. In particular to Deborah Yahnke and to Rebecca Beistline who assisted us throughout the development process of the manuscript.

Last, but not least, thanks go to our families for their support and patience during the months it took to give birth to this book.

In closing, we wish to thank all of the authors for their insights and excellent contributions to this book.

Petr Berka & Jan Rauch, Prague, Czech Republic
Djamel Abdelkader Zighed, Lyon, France
June 2008

Section I
Theoretical Aspects

Chapter I
Data, Information and Knowledge

Jana Zvárová
Institute of Computer Science of the Academy of Sciences of the Czech Republic v.v.i., Czech Republic; Center of Biomedical Informatics, Czech Republic

Arnošt Veselý
Institute of Computer Science of the Academy of Sciences of the Czech Republic v.v.i., Czech Republic; Czech University of Life Sciences, Czech Republic

Igor Vajda
Institutes of Computer Science and Information Theory and Automation of the Academy of Sciences of the Czech Republic v.v.i., Czech Republic

ABSTRACT

This chapter introduces the basic concepts of medical informatics: data, information, and knowledge. Data are classified into various types and illustrated by concrete medical examples. The concept of knowledge is formalized in the framework of a language related to objects, properties, and relations within ontology. Various aspects of knowledge are studied and illustrated on examples dealing with symptoms and diseases. Several approaches to the concept of information are systematically studied, namely the Shannon information, the discrimination information, and the decision information. Moreover, information content of theoretical knowledge is introduced. All these approaches to information are illustrated on one simple medical example.

INTRODUCTION

Healthcare is an information-intensive sector. The need to develop and organize new ways of providing health information, data and knowledge has been accompanied by major advances in information and communication technologies. These new technologies are speeding an exchange and use of data, information and knowledge and are eliminating geographical and time barriers. These processes highly accelerated medical informatics development. Opinion that medical informatics is just a computer application in healthcare, an applied discipline that has not acquired its own theory is slowly disappearing. Nowadays medical informatics shows its significance as a multidisciplinary science developed on the basis of interaction of information sciences with medicine and health care in accordance with the attained level of information technology. Today's healthcare environments use electronic health records that are shared between computer systems and which may be distributed over many locations and between organizations, in order to provide information to internal users, to payers and to respond to external requests. With increasing mobility of populations, patient data is accumulating in different places, but it needs to be accessible in an organized manner on a national and even global scale. Large amounts of information may be accessed via remote workstations and complex networks supporting one or more organizations, and potentially this may happen within a national information infrastructure.

Medical informatics now exists more then 40 years and it has been rapidly growing in the last decade. Despite of major advantages in the science and technology of health care it seems that medical informatics discipline has the potential to improve and facilitate the ever-changing and ever-broadening mass of information concerning the etiology, prevention and treatment of diseases as well as the maintenance of health. Its very broad field of interest is covering many multidisciplinary research topics with consequences for patient care and education. There have been different views on informatics. One definition of informatics declares informatics as the discipline that deals with information (Gremy, 1989). However, there are also other approaches. We should remind that the term of informatics was adopted in the sixties in some European countries (e.g. Germany and France) to denote what in other countries (e.g. in USA) was known as computer science (Moehr, 1989). In the sixties the term informatics was also used in Russia for the discipline concerned with bibliographic information processing (Russian origins of this concept are also mentioned in (Colens, 1986)). These different views on informatics led to different views on medical informatics. In 1997 the paper (Haux, 1997) initiated the broad discussion on the medical informatics discipline. The paper (Zvárová, 1997) the view on medical informatics structure is based on the structuring of informatics into four information rings and their intersections with the field of medicine, comprising also healthcare. These information rings are displayed on Figure 1.

Basic Information Ring displays different forms of information derived from data and knowledge. *Information Methodology Ring* covers methodological tools for information processing (e.g. theory of measurement, statistics, linguistics, logic, artificial intelligence, decision theory). *Information Technology Ring* covers technical and biological tools for information processing, transmitting and storing in practice. *Information Interface Ring* covers interface methodologies developed for effective use of nowadays information technologies. For better storing and searching information, theories of databases and knowledge bases have been developed. Development of information transmission (*telematics*) is closely connected with methodologies like coding theory, data protection, networking and standardization. Better information processing using computers strongly relies on computer science disciplines, e.g. theory of computing, programming languages, parallel computing, numerical methods. In medical informatics all information rings are connected with medicine and health care. Which parts of medical informatics are in the centre of scientific attention can be seen from IMIA Yearbooks that have been published since 1992 (Bemmel, McCray, 1995), in the last years published as a special issue of the international journal "Methods of Information in Medicine".

Figure 1. Structure of informatics

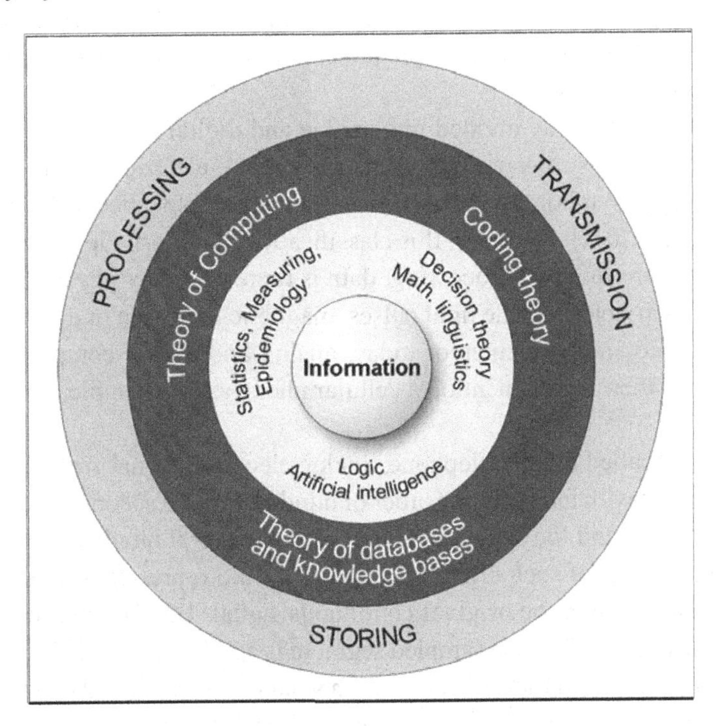

At the end of this introduction, the authors would like to emphasize that this chapter deals with medical informatics – applications of computers and information theory in medicine – and not with the medicine itself. The chapter explains and illustrates new methods and ideas of medical informatics with the help of some classical as well as number of models and situations related to medicine and using medical concepts. However, all these situations and corresponding medical statements are usually oversimplified in order to provide easy and transparent explanations and illustrations. They are in no case to be interpreted in the framework of the medicine itself as demonstrations of a new medical knowledge. Nevertheless, the authors believe that the methods and ideas presented in this chapter facilitate creation of such a new medical knowledge.

DATA

Data represents images of the real world in abstract sets. With the aid of symbols taken from such sets, data reflects different aspects of real objects or processes taking place in the real world. Mostly data are defined as facts or observations. Formally taken, we consider symbols $x \in \mathsf{X}$, or sequences of symbols $(x_1, x_2, \ldots, x_k) \in \mathsf{X}^k$ from a certain set X, which can be defined mathematically. These symbols may be numerals, letters of a natural alphabet, vectors, matrices, texts written in a natural or artificial language, signals or images.

Data results from a process of measurement or observation. Often it is obtained as output from devices converting physical variables into abstract symbols. Such data is further processed by humans or machines.

Human data processing embraces a large range of options, from the simplest instinctive response to applications of most complex inductive or deductive scientific methods. Data-processing machines also represent a wide variety of options, from simple punching or magnetic-recording devices to the most sophisticated computers or robots.

These machines are traditionally divided into analog and digital ones. Analog machines represent abstract data in the form of physical variables, such as voltage or electric current, while the digital ones represent data as strings of symbols taken from fixed numerical alphabets. The most frequently used is the binary alphabet, $X = \{0, 1\}$. However, this classification is not principal, because within the processes of recording, transmitting and processing, data is represented by physical variables even in the digital machines – such variables include light pulses, magnetic induction or quantum states. Moreover, in most information-processing machines of today, analog and digital components are intertwined, complementary to each other. Let us mention a cellular phone as an example.

Example 1. In the so-called digital telephone, analog electrical signal from the microphone is segmented into short intervals with length in the order of hundredths of a second. Each segment is sampled with a very high frequency, and the signal is quantized into several hundreds of levels. This way, the speech is digitalized. Transfer of such digitalized speech would represent a substantially smaller load on the transmission channel than the original continuous signal. But for practical purposes, this load would still be too high. That is why each sampled segment is approximated with a linear autoregression model with a small number of parameters, and a much smaller number of bits go through the transmission channel; into these bits, the model's parameters are encoded with the aid of a certain sophisticated method. In the receiver's phone, these bits are used to synthesize signal generated by the given model. Within the prescribed time interval, measured in milliseconds, this replacement synthesized signal is played in the phone instead of the original speech. Digital data compression of this type, called *linear adaptive prediction*, is successfully used not only for digital transmission of sound, but also of images – it makes it possible for several TV programs to be sent via a single transmission channel.

In order to be able to interpret the data, we have to know where it comes from. We may not understand symbols of whose origin we know nothing. The more we know about the process of obtaining the data and the real objects or processes generating the data, the better we can understand such data and the more qualified we are to interpret, explain and utilize such data.

Example 2. Without further explanations we are unlikely to understand the following abstract symbol: خ. Part of the readers may guess that it is a derivative of an unknown function denoted by a Greek letter ح, which we usually read as *tau*. After specification that it is a letter of the Arabic alphabet, this first guess will be corrected and the reader will easily look it up as a letter corresponding to Czech "*ch*".

Example 3. A lexical symbol *list* and a string of binary digits 111000 are also examples of data. Interpreting *list* as a Czech word, we will understand it as *plant leaf* or *sheet of paper*. In English it will be *narrow strip* or *a series of words or numerals*. The sequence 111000 cannot be understood at all until we learn more about its origin. If we are told that it is a record of measurements taken on a certain patient, its meaning will get a little clearer. As soon as it turns out that the digits describe results of measurements of the patient's brain activity taken in hourly intervals, and 1 describes activity above the threshold characterizing the condition *patient is alive*, while 0 describes activity below this threshold, we begin to understand the data. Namely, the interpretation is that the patient died after the third measurement.

Example 4. A graphical image translated into bytes is another example of data. Using a browser, we are able to see the image and get closer to its interpretation. In order to interpret it fully, we need more information about the real object or process depicted, and the method of obtaining this image.

Example 5. A computer program is a set of data interpreted as instructions. Most programming languages distinguish between programs and other data, to be processed with the aid of the instructions. An interpretation of this "other data" may, or may not, be available. In certain programming languages, for example, Lisp, the data cannot be recognized as different from the instructions. We can see that situation about data and its interpretation can be rather complex and requires sensitive judgment.

Data can be viewed as *source* and *derived.* Source or raw data is the data immediately recorded during measurements or observations of the sources, i.e., the above-mentioned objects or processes of the real world. For the purposes of transmission to another location (an addressee, which may be a remote person or machine) or in time (recording on a memory medium for later use), the source data is modified, encoded or otherwise transformed in different ways. In some cases, such transformations are reversible and admit full reconstruction of the original source data. The usual reason for such transformations is, however, compression of the data to simplify the transmission or reduce the load of the media (information channels or memory space). Compression of data is usually irreversible – it produces derived data. Even a more frequent reason for using derived data instead of the source one is the limited interest or capacity of the addressee, with the consequent possibility, or even necessity, to simplify data for subsequent handling, processing and utilization.

Example 6. The string of numerals (1, 1, 1, 0, 0, 0) in Example 3 is an obvious instance of derived data. The source data from which it comes might have looked like $(y, m, d, h, s_1, s_2, s_3, s_4, s_5, s_6)$. Here y stands for year, m for month, d for day, and h for hour at which the patient's monitoring was started, and $s_1, s_2, s_3, s_4, s_5, s_6$ denote the EEG signal of his brain activity recorded in six consecutive hours. On the basis of these signals, the conclusion (1, 1, 1, 0, 0, 0) concerning the patient's clinical life, or rather death, was based. It is clear that for certain addressees, such as a surgeon who removes organs for transplantation, the raw signals $s_1, s_2, s_3, s_4, s_5, s_6$ are not interesting and even incomprehensible. What is necessary, or useful, for the surgeon it is just the conclusion concerning the patient's life or death issue. If the addressee has an online connection, the time-stamp source (y, m, d, h) is also irrelevant. Such an addressee would therefore be fully satisfied with the derived data, (1, 1, 1, 0, 0, 0). Should this data be replaced with the original source data $(y, m, d, h, s_1, s_2, s_3, s_4, s_5, s_6)$, such a replacement would be a superficial complication and nuisance.

Example 7. Source data concerning occurrence of influenza in a certain time and region may be important for operative planning of medicine supplies and/or hospital beds. If such planning is only based on data taken from several selected healthcare centers, it will be derived data strictly speaking, and such data may not reflect properly occurrence of the influenza in the entire region. We often speak that these derived data are *selective.* Then a decision-making based on selective data may cause a financial loss measured in millions of crowns. However, in case that the derived data will have the same structure as original source data, we will call them *representative.* Decision-making based on representative data can lead to good results.

Example 8. The source vector of data in Example 6, or at least its coordinate h, as a complement to the derived vector (1, 1, 1, 0, 0, 0) of Example 3, will become very important if and when a dispute arises about the respective patient's life insurance, effective at a given time described by vector (y, m, d, h_0). Inequalities $h > h_0$ or $h < h_0$ can be decisive with respect to considerable amounts of money then. The derived data vector itself, as defined in Example 1.3, will not make such decision-making possible, and a loss of source data might cause a costly lawsuit.

The last three examples show that *sufficiency* or *insufficiency* of derived data depends on the source and on the actual decision-making problem to be resolved on the basis of the given source. In Example 6, a situation was mentioned in which the derived data of Example 3, (1, 1, 1, 0, 0, 0), was sufficient. On the other hand, Example 8 refers to a situation in which only extended derived data, (h, 1, 1 ,1, 0, 0, 0), was sufficient. All these examples indicate that, when seeking optimal solutions, we sometimes have to return to the original source data, whether completely or at least partly.

Due to the importance of data and processing thereof in the information age we live in, as well as the attention both theory and practice of handling data receives, we can say that a new field is being born, called *data engineering.* One of the essential notions of data engineering is metadata. It is "data about data", i.e., a data description of other data. As an example we can mention a library catalog, containing information on books in a library.

INFORMATION

The word *information* is often used without carefully distinguishing between different meanings it has taken on during its history. Generally, it refers to a finding or findings concerning facts, events, things, people, thoughts or notions, that is, a certain reflection of real or abstract objects or processes. It usually consists of its syntactic (structure), semantic (meaning), and pragmatic (goal) components. Therefore information can be defined as data that has been transformed into a meaningful and useful form for specific human beings.

Communications from which we learn about the information can be called *messages.* The latter are usually represented by texts (text messages) or, strings of numerals (data messages), i.e., by data in the general sense introduced above.

Data whose origin is completely unknown to us can hardly bring any information. We have to "understand" the data, i.e., only data we can interpret are deemed messages. An idea of where and under what conditions the data was generated is an important context of each message, and it has to be taken into account when we establish the information content of a message. Data sources thus become important components of what we are going to call information sources below.

An amount of information contained in a message delivered to us (or to an information-processing system) is related to the set of prior admissible realizations the message might take on under the given circumstances. For example, if the message can only have one outcome we know in advance, it brings zero information. In other words, establishing the information amount in message x requires prior knowledge of the respective information source, represented by set X of possible realizations of that message.

The cornerstone of an information source model, built to enable us to express an amount of information contained in a message, is thus the range of possible realizations, or values, of the message.

In this sense, obtaining information is modeled by finding out which of the prior possible values of the information source was actually taken on. This principal viewpoint was first formulated by the founder of cybernetics, Norbert Wiener (Wiener, 1948). Below, ranges of possible values taken by messages x, y, z from three different sources will be denoted by symbols X, Y, Z, etc.

Example 9. Message $x = (1, 1, 1, 0, 0, 0)$ introduced at the beginning of Example 3 cannot be assessed from the point of view of its information content at all. The same message in the context of the end of Example 3 already admits such assessment because we can establish the set of its possible realizations, $\mathsf{X} = \{0,1\}^6$.

Apart from the prior possible realizations, the information content in a message also obviously depends on all additional information we have about the respective data source under the given conditions. If we have at our disposal an online "message daemon", whose knowledge of the source enables it to reliably predict the generated messages, the information content in a message received is reduced to zero, as explained above.

Example 10. Consider the situation of a potential organ donor after a heavy car accident. Let message $x = (x_1, x_2, \ldots, x_6)$ describe results of measurements of a donor's brain activity, taken hourly, and $x_i =$ 1 means that the donor is alive at the v i-th hour, while $x_i = 0$ means the contrary. The space of admissible realizations of message x, regardless of interpretation, is $\mathsf{X} = \{0, 1\}^6$ (cf. Example 9). If moreover message $x \in \mathsf{X}$ was generated under a condition that the probability of the donor's death in each hour exactly equals $p \in (0, 1)$, then the probability value of the particular message $x = (1, 1, 1, 0, 0, 0)$ of Example 1.3 will be given as:

$$P(x) = p(1-p)^3$$

For example, probability value $p = 1/2$ implies $1 - p = 1/2$, hence:

$$P(x) = \left(\frac{1}{2}\right)^4 = \frac{1}{16} = 0.0625$$

while $p = 3/4$ provides an approximately five times smaller chance in the same message x:

$$P(x) = \frac{3}{4}\left(\frac{1}{4}\right)^3 = \frac{3}{256} = 0.010547$$

The probability $P(x)$ of the donor's death after exactly three hours grows for p growing in interval (0, 1/10) and decreases for p growing in interval (2/10, 1). The maximum of this probability value is taken on $p \in (1/10, 2/10)$ which solves the equation $(1-p)^3 = 3p$.

Detailed analysis of mechanisms that would enable us to exactly predict messages generated by data source is often unfeasible for scientific, economic or time reasons. Additional insight into data sources is usually based on summary, empiric knowledge of certain categories of data sources; such additional description is of a stochastic nature. This means that, for individual admissible messages:

$$x \in \mathsf{X} = \{x_1, x_2, \ldots, x_n\} \tag{1}$$

there are probability values $P(x)$, that is, a probability distribution:

$$P = (p_1 \equiv P(x_1), p_2 \equiv P(x_2), \ldots, p_n \equiv P(x_n)) \tag{2}$$

The pair of set X and distribution P, dented by (X, P), is called probability space in mathematics. Equivalently, instead of a probability space we can speak about random variable X given by its sample space (X, P). Elements $x_1, x_2, \ldots, x_n$ of set X are particular messages, representing possible realizations of random variable X, and $p_i = P(x_i) = \mathrm{P}(X = x_i)$ are probability values of such realizations. Interchangeability between random message X and its sample space (X, P) is denoted by symbol $X \sim$ (X, P). A stochastic model of an information source represented by random message $X \sim$ (X, P) therefore consists of set of messages X and probability distribution P on this set. This model was introduced by the founder of information theory, Claude Shannon, in his fundamental work (Shannon, 1948).

Let us denote by $p \in [0,1]$ the probability $P(x)$ of a message $x \in$ X from information source $X \sim$ (X, P). As we have already mentioned, $p = P(x) = 1$ implies zero information content, $I(x) = 0$, in message x, while positive values $I(x) > 0$ should correspond to values $p < 1$. Let $f(p)$ be a function of variable $p \in [0, 1]$ for which $f(1) = 0$, and $f(p) > 0$ for $p \in (0, 1)$; we are aiming at taking this function for the rate of information content in ea message with probability value p, i.e.:

$$I(x) = f(P(x)), \quad x \in \mathsf{X} \tag{3}$$

is the information content in each message x.

It is natural to request that, for small changes of probability value p, information $f(p)$ should not change in a large step. This requirement leads to the following condition.

Condition 1. Function $f(p)$ is positive and continuous on interval $p \in (0,1]$; we further define:

$$f(0) = \lim_{p \downarrow 0} f(p)$$

Intuitive understanding of information and stochastic independence fully corresponds to the following condition.

Condition 2. Let a source $X \sim$ (X, P) consist of two mutually independent components $Y \sim$ (Y, Q) and $Z \sim$ (Z, W), that is:

$$(\mathsf{X}, P) = (\mathsf{Y} \otimes \mathsf{Z}, Q \otimes W)$$

Then, for all $x = (y, z) \in \mathsf{Y} \otimes \mathsf{Z}$, it holds:

$$I(x) = I(y) + I(z)$$

A reasonable requirement, fully in line with the natural understanding of probability and information, is that information $f(p)$ does not grow for growing p, i.e., the following condition should hold.

Condition 3. If $0 \leq p_1 < p_2 \leq 1$, then $f(p_1) \geq f(p_2)$.

Under the above-mentioned conditions, an explicit formula is implied for information (3); this formula is specified in the following Theorem.

Theorem 1. If Conditions 1 through 3 hold, the only function f compliant with formula (3) is $f(p) = -\log p$, and equation (3) takes on the form:

$$I(x) = -\log P(x), \quad x \in \mathsf{X} \qquad (4)$$

Here $-\log 0 = \infty$, and log is logarithm with an arbitrary base $z > 1$.

Proof. Using (3), we get from Condition 2 the Cauchy equation:

$$f(qw) = f(q) + f(w)$$

for all $q, w \in (0, 1)$. This and Condition 1 imply the statement because it is known that logarithmic function is the only continuous solution of the Cauchy equation.

Theorem 1 says that the more surprising occurrence of a message is, the more information this message contains. If probability value $P(x)$ of message $x \in \mathsf{X}$ approaches zero, the corresponding information content $I(x)$ grows beyond all limits.

We should also mention the fact that the numerical expression of information according to formula (4) depends on selection of a particular logarithmic function. The base of the logarithm implies the units in which the information content is measured. For base $z = 2$ the unit is a *bit*, for natural base $z = e$ the unit is a *nat*, and for $z = 256$ it is a *byte*. Hence:

$$1\ bit = \log_e 2 \equiv 0.693\ nat = \log_{256} 2 \equiv 1/8\ byte,$$
$$1\ nat = \log_2 e \equiv 1.4427\ bits = \log_{256} e \equiv 0.180\ byte$$

and

$$1\ byte = \log_e 258 \equiv 5.545\ nats = \log_2 256 \equiv 8\ bits$$

Example 11. In the situation of Example 10, we get information as follows:

$$I(x) = 3\log \frac{1}{1-p} + \log \frac{1}{p}$$

Specifically, at $p = 1/2$ we get $I(x) = 4\log_2 2 = 4$ bits $= 1/2$ byte, while at $p = 3/4$ we get $I(x) = 3\log_2 4 + \log_2 (4/3) = 6.4143$ bits $\cong 4/5$ byte. In this instance, the information content is increased by about one-half.

Apart from the information content $I(x)$ in individual messages $x \in \mathsf{X}$ from a general information source $X \sim (\mathsf{X}, P)$, quantity of information $I(X)$ generated by the source as such is also important. It is given as information contained in one message from this source whose particular value is not known in advance, but the range X of such values is given together with a probability distribution on this range.

So, it is information contained in a random message X representing information source (X, P). and simultaneously represented by this source. Instead of $I(X)$ we could as well use $I(\mathsf{X}, P)$; but the former variant is preferred to the latter because it is simpler.

Shannon (1948) defined the information in random message X by the formula:

$$I(X) = \sum_{x \in \mathsf{X}} P(x) I(x) = -\sum_{x \in \mathsf{X}} P(x) \log P(x) \qquad (5)$$

According to this definition, $I(X)$ is the mean value of information content $I(x)$ in individual admissible realizations $x \in \mathsf{X}$ of this message. Definition (5) formally coincides with that of Boltzman entropy:

$$H(x) = -\sum_{x \in \mathsf{X}} P(x) \log P(x) \qquad (6)$$

of a random physical system X, which takes on states $x \in \mathsf{X}$ with probabilities $P(x)$.

Theorem 2. Information $I(X)$ is a measure of uncertainty of message $X \sim (\mathsf{X}, P)$, i.e., a measure of difficulty with which its actual realization can be predicted in the sense that the range of values is given by inequalities:

$$0 \leq I(X) \leq \log|\mathsf{X}| \qquad (7)$$

where $|\mathsf{X}|$ is the number of admissible realizations and the smallest value:

$$I(X) = 0 \qquad (8)$$

is taken on if and only if only one realization is admissible, $x_0 \in \mathsf{X}$, that is:

$$P(x_0) = 1 \text{ and } P(x) = 0 \quad \text{for all } x \in \mathsf{X}, x \neq x_0 \qquad (9)$$

while the largest value:

$$I(X) = \log|\mathsf{X}| \qquad (10)$$

is taken on if and only if all realizations $x \in \mathsf{X}$ are equally admissible, i.e.:

$$P(x) = 1/|\mathsf{X}| \quad \text{for all } x \in \mathsf{X} \qquad (11)$$

Proof of this Theorem will be given later on. Let us only note now that a distribution P which fulfills Condition (9) for a certain $x_0 \in \mathsf{X}$ is called *Dirac* distribution; and the distribution fulfilling (11) is called *uniform*. It is obvious that the number of all different Dirac distributions is $|\mathsf{X}|$, while the uniform distribution is unique. Dirac distributions represent the utmost form of non-uniformness. Theorem 2 therefore indicates that $I(X)$ is also a measure of uniformness of probability distribution P of source X. Uncertainty of message X in the sense reflected by the information measure, $I(X)$ is directly proportionate to uniformness of probability values $P(x)$ of the respective realizations $x \in \mathsf{X}$.

Example 12. Information source (X, P)= ({0, 1}^{6} , P) of Example 10 generates seven practically feasible messages $\{x^{(i)}: 1 \leq i \leq 7\}$ with i-1 representing the number of measurements at which the donor was clinically alive, with the following probability values:

$$P(x^{(1)}) = P(0, 0, 0, 0, 0, 0) = p$$
$$P(x^{(2)}) = P(1, 0, 0, 0, 0, 0) = p(1 - \mathrm{p})$$
$$P(x^{(3)}) = P(1, 1, 0, 0, 0, 0) = p(1 - p)^2$$
$$P(x^{(4)}) = P(1, 1, 1, 0, 0, 0) = p(1 - p)^3$$
$$P(x^{(5)}) = P(1, 1, 1, 1, 0, 0) = p(1 - p)^4$$
$$P(x^{(6)}) = P(1, 1, 1, 1, 1, 0) = p(1 - p)^5$$
$$P(x^{(7)}) = P(1, 1, 1, 1, 1, 1) = p\sum_{i=6}^{\infty}(1-p)^i = (1 - p)^6$$

for a certain value $p \in (0, 1)$. Message X of whether and when the donor's clinical death occurred, therefore contains the information:

$$I(X) = -\sum_{i=1}^{7} P(x^{(i)}) \log P(x^{(i)}) = \sum_{i=0}^{5} p(1-p)^i \left[\log\frac{1}{p} + i\log\frac{1}{1-p}\right] + 6\,(1 - p)^6\, log\frac{1}{1-p}$$

At p = 1/2 and log = $\log_2$, we get the following information content somewhat smaller than two bits:

$$I(X) = \sum_{i=0}^{5}\left(\frac{1}{2}\right)^{i+1}(1+i) + \frac{6}{64} = 1 + \frac{31}{32} = 1.96815 \text{ bits}$$

Message $x^{(4)}$ alone in Example 11 brings four bits of information, but its probability is as small as 0.0625 according to Example 10. That is why it only contributes to the overall information balance with 4 × 0.0625 = 1/4 bits. The more likely message $x^{(1)}$ contributes much more; namely:

$$p \log\frac{1}{p} = \frac{1}{2}\log 2 = 1/2 \text{ bits}$$

even though the message itself only gives $I(x^{(1)}) = \log 1/p = 1$ bit. On the contrary, a much smaller value:

$$6\,(1 - p)^6 \log = 6/64 = 1/8 \text{ bits}$$

is contributed to $I(X)$ by message $x^{(6)}$, despite that the fact that this message by itself gives as much as:

$$I(x^{(6)}) = 6 \log (1/(1 - p)) = 6 \text{ bits}$$

Information $I(X)$ defined by Formula (5) has the following additivity property, which is in a very good compliance with intuitive perceptions.

Theorem 3. If message $X \sim$ (X, P) consists of independent components:

$X_1 \sim (\mathrm{X}_1, P_1), \ldots, X_k \sim (\mathrm{X}_k, P_k)$, then

$$I(X) = I(X_1) + \ldots + I(X_k) \tag{12}$$

Proof. Partition $X = (X_1, \ldots, X_k)$ into independent components $X_1, \ldots, X_k$ means that values $x \in \mathsf{X}$ of message X are vectors $(x_1, \ldots, x_k)$ of values $x_i \in \mathsf{X}_i$ for messages X_i, that is:

$$x = (x_1, \ldots, x_k) \in \mathsf{X}_1 \otimes \ldots \otimes \mathsf{X}_k$$

and the multiplication rule is valid:

$$P(x_1, \ldots, x_k) = P_1(x_1) \ldots P_k(x_k) \qquad (13)$$

Logarithm of a product is a sum of logarithms, hence:

$$I(x) = I(x_1, \ldots, x_k) = I(x_1) + \ldots + I(x_k)$$

According to (3.5) it follows:

$$I(X) = \sum_{x \in \mathsf{X}} P(x) I(x) = \sum_{x_1, \ldots x_k \in \mathsf{X}_1 \otimes \ldots \otimes \mathsf{X}_k} P(x_1) \ldots P(x_k)[I(x_1) + \ldots + I(x_k)]$$
$$= \sum_{x_1 \in \mathsf{X}_1} P(x_1) I(x_1) + \ldots + = I(X_1) + \ldots + I(X_k) \qquad \text{(Q.E.D.)}$$

Additivity (12) is a characteristic property of Shannon information (5). This means that there does not exist any other information measure based on probability values of the respective messages, and reasonable and additive in the above-mentioned sense. This claim can be proven in a mathematically rigorous way – the first one who put forth such a proof was Russian mathematician Fadeev, see (Feinstein, 1958).

An instructive instance of information content $I(X)$ is the case of a binary message, $Y \sim (\mathsf{Y} = \{y_1, y_2\}, Q)$, as we call a message which can only take on two values y_1, y_2. Let us denote the respective probability values as follows:

$$Q(y_1) = q, \; Q(y_2) = 1 - q$$

According to definition (5):

$$I(Y) = -q \log - (1 - q) \log (1 - q) \equiv h(q) \qquad (14)$$

where $h(q)$ is an abbreviated form of $I(Y)$, written as a function of variable $q \in [0, 1]$ (cf. Table 1). The shape of this function for $\log = \log_2$ is seen in Figure 2, which shows that information content $I(Y)$ can be zero bits, and this is the case if Q is one of the two Dirac distributions this binary case admits, in other words, the value of Y is given in advance with probability 1. On the other hand, the maximum information content $I(Y) = 1$ bit is achieved when both options, $Y = y_1$ and $Y = y_2$ are equally probable.

This fact enables us to define 1 bit as the quantity of information contained in a message X which can take on two values and both are equally probable. Similarly we can define 1 byte as the quantity of information contained in a message $X = (X_1, \ldots, X_8)$ with independent components taking on two equiprobable values.

Table 1. Information function I(Y) from (14) in bits

q	$-q\log_2 q$	$-(1-q)\log_2(1-q)$	$h(q)$ (*bits*)
0	0	0	0
0.05	0.216	0.070	0.286
0.10	0.332	0.137	0.469
0.11	0.350	0.150	0.500
0.15	0.411	0.199	0.610
0.20	0.464	0.258	0.722
0.25	0.500	0.311	0.811
0.30	0.521	0.360	0.881
1/3	0.528	0.390	0.918
0.35	0.530	0.404	0.934
0.40	0.529	0.442	0.971
0.45	0.518	0.474	0.993
0.50	1/2	1/2	1

Figure 2. Information function I(Y) from (14) in bits

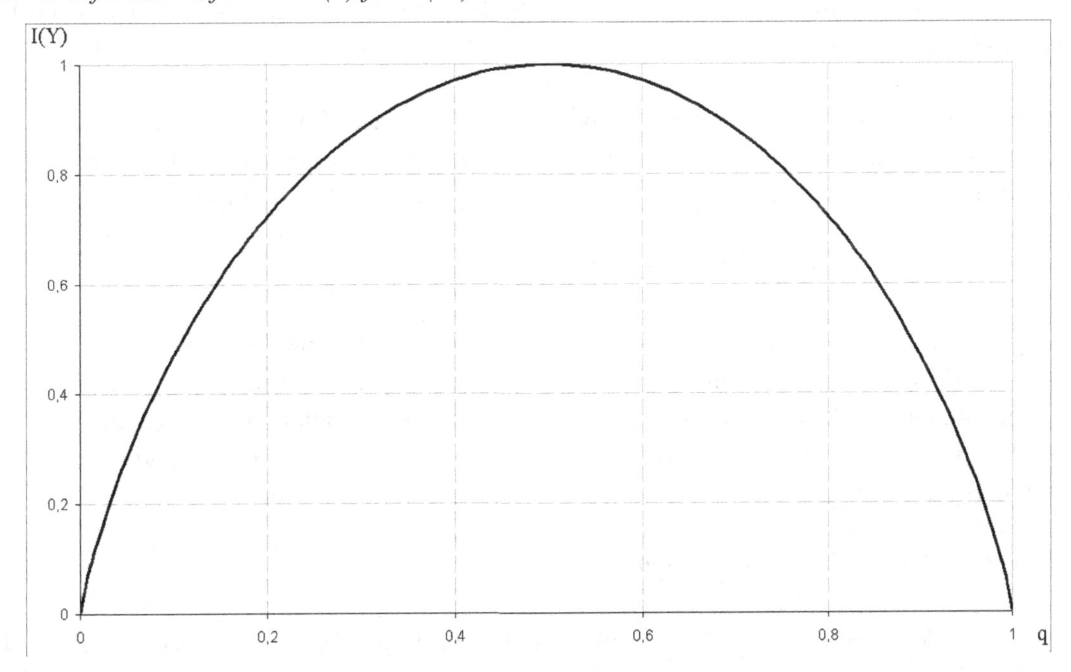

Example 13. In Example 12, there is message $X = (X_1, \dots, X_6) \sim (\mathrm{X}, P)$, where components $X_i \sim (\mathrm{X}_i, P_i) = (\{0,1\}, P_i)$ are not independent. Instead of message $X \sim (\mathrm{X}, P)$, let us consider a reduced message Y saying whether $X_6 = 1$, i.e. whether the donor was or was not clinically alive at the time of the last 6-th measurement. This message would, for example, be relevant for a surgeon who wants to remove a transplant organ from the donor. Here the information source is binary, $Y \sim (\mathrm{Y}, Q)$, and:

$Y = y_1$ if $X \in \{x^{(1)}, x^{(2)}, x^{(3)}, x^{(4)}, x^{(5)}, x^{(6)}\}$

and $Y = y_2$, if $X = x^{(7)}$ (ef definition of $x^{(i)}$ in Example 12).

This implies $Q(y_1) = q = (1 - p)^6$, and therefore $Q(y_2) = 1 - q = 1 - (1 - p)^6$. Hence:

$$I(Y) = h((1-p)^6) = (1-p)^6 \log \frac{1}{(1-p)^6} + [(1-(1-p)^6] \log \frac{1}{1-(1-p)^6}$$

For $p = 1/2$ we get a special value:

$$I(Y) = \frac{3}{32} + \frac{63}{64} \log_2 \frac{64}{63} = 0.116 \text{ bits}$$

Message $Y = y_2$ (donor is still alive) has a small probability value, $q = 1/64$, so that the information content of this message $I(y_2) = -\log_2 q = 6$ bits (cf. (4)). The contrary message $Y = y_1$ is near to certainty, and as such it bears much smaller information content $I(y_1) = -\log_2 (1-q) = \log_2 (64/63) = 0.023$ bits. The average information $I(Y) = 0.116$ bits is between these extremes.

Information $I(X)$ in message X from information source (X, P) defined by (5) can be viewed as a *communication information* because it characterizes the memory capacity or channel capacity needed for recording or transmitting this message. We will not study this fact in detail here, and only illustrate it in the two following Examples.

Example 14. Approximately 6.5 billion people live in the world, 6.5×10^9. Let message $X \sim$ (X, P) identify one of them. If any inhabitant of our planet is chosen with the same likelihood, $x \in$ X, then $P(x) = 1/(6.5 \times 10^9)$, and the maximum achievable information in message X will be equal to:

$$I(X) = \log |\mathrm{X}| = \log_2 (6.5 \times 10^9) = 32.60 \leq 33 \text{ bits}$$

In other words, a citizen of the Earth can be uniquely registered by means of 33 binary digits, i. e. by means of 33/8 < 5 bytes of information. If distribution P is restricted to subset $\mathrm{Y} \subset \mathrm{X}$ of inhabitants of the Czech Republic, which has about 10 million elements, identification of one inhabitant will be a message $Y \sim (\mathrm{Y}, Q)$ from a different source, where $Q(y) = 1/10^7$ for all $y \in \mathrm{Y}$. Consequently, the information content is reduced to:

$$I(Y) = \log_2 10^7 = 7 \log_2 10 \leq 24 \text{ bits} = 3 \text{ bytes}$$

Let us have a look at birth registration numbers in the Czech Republic, with 10 decimal digits. If all birth registration numbers were equally probable, information content in birth registration number Y of a citizen chosen in random would be:

$$I(Y) = \log_2 10^{10} = 10 \log_2 10 = 33.22 \text{ bits}$$

which significantly exceeds the 24 bits mentioned above. The actual information content of birth registration numbers is lower, however, because certain combinations are principially excluded, and not all of the remaining ones actually occur.

Example 15. Our task is to provide a complete recording of the measurement described in Example 12 for a databank of 1024 donors, for whom we expect $p = 1/2$. Result of measurements for each donor consists of six binary digits:

$$x = (x_1, x_2, x_3, x_4, x_5, x_6) \in \mathsf{X} \text{ where } \mathsf{X} = \{0, 1\}\otimes \ldots \otimes\{0, 1\} \text{ (6 times)} = \{0, 1\}^6$$

hence the data space for the entire recording is $\mathsf{Y} = \mathsf{X}\otimes \ldots \otimes\mathsf{X}$ (1024 times) $= \mathsf{X}^{1024} = \{0, 1\}^{6144}$. In order to make such a recording we need $\log_2 |\mathsf{Y}| = \log_2 2^{6144} = 6144$ binary digits, i.e. the memory capacity of more than 6 kilobits. Having in mind the fact that transitions $x_i \rightarrow x_{i+1}$ of type $0 \rightarrow 1$ are impossible, the basic data space X is reduced to seven admissible messages $x^{(1)}, \ldots, x^{(7)}$, written down in Example 12. In fact the capacity necessary for the required recording will be less than one-half of the above-mentioned value, namely, $1024 \times \log_2 7 = 2869$ bits < 3 kilobits. From Example 12 we see that if $p=1/2$ then all seven admissible messages $x^{(1)}, x^{(2)}, x^{(3)}, x^{(4)}, x^{(5)}, x^{(6)}, x^{(7)} \in \mathsf{X}$ will not have the uniform probability $P(x) = 1/7$, but:

$$P(x^{(1)}) = 1/2,\ P(x^{(2)}) = 1/4,\ P(x^{(3)}) = 1/8,\ P(x^{(4)}) = 1/16,\ P(x^{(5)}) = 1/32,\ P(x^{(6)}) = 1/64 = P(x^{(7)})$$

Numbers of the messages in our set will be expected to follow Table 2.

If measurement results x taken in donors of our set are rewritten in binary digits $\beta(x)$ according to the Table 2, the flow of this binary data can be stored in the memory without additional requirements for separators between records (automatically separated by each sixth one or zero). The expected number of binary digits in the complete recording of the measurements therefore will be:

$$512 \times 1 + 256 \times 2 + 128 \times 3 + 64 \times 4 + 32 \times 5 + 32 \times 6 = 2016 = 1024 \times I(X)$$

where, similar to Example 12, symbol $I(X) = 1.96875$ denotes the information content in result X of a measurement taken in one of the donors within the respective set. If the required record is compressed according to the last table, the memory need is expected to amount to 2016 bits $\approx$ 2 kilobits which is well below the non-compressed memory capacity evaluated above at more than 6 kilobits.

In addition to the communication information in the message $X \sim (\mathsf{X}, P)$, which we have considered up to now, another type of information to be studied is *discrimination information.* It is the quantity of information provided by message X enabling us to discriminate its probability distribution from another

Table 2. Messages, their probabilities, expected numbers and binary records

message x	$P(x)$	expected number	binary record $\beta(x)$
$x^{(1)}$	½	1024/2 = 512	1
$x^{(2)}$	¼	1024/4 = 256	01
$x^{(3)}$	1/8	1024/8 = 128	001
$x^{(4)}$	1/16	1024/16 = 64	000 1
$x^{(5)}$	1/32	1024/32 = 32	000 01
$x^{(6)}$	1/64	1024/64 = 16	000 001
$x^{(7)}$	1/64	1024/64 = 16	000 000

distribution, say Q, on the set of all admissible values X. This type of information will be denoted by $I(P,Q)$. Kullback and Leibler (1951) defined this information by the formula:

$$I(P,Q) = \sum_{x \in X} P(x) \log \frac{P(x)}{Q(x)} \tag{15}$$

where, for $Q(x) = 0$, the respective term is zero if $P(x) = 0$ and infinity if $P(x)$ is strictly positive. In fact, if a value $X = x$ is admissible, it will occur in a finite number of independent realizations of random variable X, and thus distribution P of X is distinguished with certainty from distribution Q under which value x is not admitted. On the other hand, if $Q(x)$ is strictly positive for all $x \in X$ and there is $P(x) = 0$ for a certain $x \in X$, then the discrimination value of information $I(P, Q)$ remains finite – no number of realizations of X will enable us to conclude with certainty that distribution Q. is the underlying on. This is also a reasoning of the fact that discrimination information (15) is not symmetric.

Let us mention fundamental properties of the discrimination information.

Theorem 4. Discrimination information $I(P, Q)$ is nonnegative; its value is zero if and only if distributions P, Q are identical.

Proof. For $P=Q$, the definition implies $I(P, Q) = 0$. If there exists $x \in X$ such that $P(x) > 0$ and $Q(x) = 0$, then the value of $I(P, Q)$ is infinite, so the proof is finished. It is therefore sufficient to assume that $Q(x) > 0$ for all $x \in X$ such that $P(x) > 0$, ant to prove under this assumption that $I(P, Q) \geq 0$, with $I(P, Q) = 0$ implying $P = Q$. Let $X_0 \subset X$ be the subset of messages $x \in X$ for which $P(x) > 0$. According to (15), it holds:

$$I(P,Q) = \sum_{x \in X_0} \Phi\left(\frac{P(x)}{Q(x)}\right) Q(x)$$

where $\Phi(t) = t \log t$ is a strictly convex function of variable $t > 0$. The Jensen inequality now implies:

$$I(P,Q) \geq \Phi\left(\sum_{x \in X_0} Q(x) \frac{P(x)}{Q(x)}\right) = \Phi\,(1) = 0$$

with equality if and only if $P\,(x)=Q\,(x)$ for all $x \in X$. However:

$$\sum_{x \in X_0} P(x) = 1$$

and equality $P(x) = Q(x)$ in X_0 implies that this equality holds everywhere in X. (Q.E.D.)

Proof of Theorem 2. Since $P(x) \in [0, 1]$, $\log P(x) \leq 0$ and definition (5) implies $I(x) \geq 0$; moreover, this inequality is strict as soon as $P(x) \notin \{0, 1\}$ holds for at least one $x \in X$. Hence $I(X) = 0$ is true just for Dirac distributions P. For the uniform distribution we have:

$Q(x) = 1/|X|$ for all $x \in X$

Hence (3.15) implies:

$$0 \leq I(P, Q) = \sum_{x \in X} P(x) \log P(x) + \log|X|$$

and consequently:

$$-\sum_{x\in X} P(x)\log P(x) \le \log|X|$$

with $I(X) \le \log|X|$. Theorem 4 further implies that the equality only holds for uniform P, which completes the proof.

Theorem 5. Discrimination information is additive in the sense:

$$I(P_1 \otimes P_2, Q_1 \otimes Q_2) = I(P_1, Q_1) + I(P_2, Q_2)$$

Proof. Since the logarithmic function is additive, it holds:

$$I(P_1 \otimes P_2, Q_1 \otimes Q_2) = \sum_{x_1\in X_1}\sum_{x_2\in X_2} P_1(x_1)P_2(x_2)\log\frac{P_1(x_1)P_2(x_2)}{Q_1(x_1)Q_2(x_2)} =$$

$$\sum_{x_1\in X_1}\sum_{x_2\in X_2} P_1(x_1)P_2(x_2)\left[\log\frac{P_1(x_1)}{Q_1(x_1)} + \log\frac{P_2(x_2)}{Q_2(x_2)}\right]$$

$$\sum_{x_1\in X_1} P_1(x_1)\log\frac{P_1(x_1)}{Q_1(x_1)} + \sum_{x_2\in X_2} P_2(x_2)\log\frac{P_2(x_2)}{Q_2(x_2)} = I(P_1, Q_1) + (P_2, Q_2)\,. \qquad \text{(Q.E.D.)}$$

Example 16. Consider formally the same situation as in Example 12 with p=1/2 and X describing survival of the victims of bomb attacks in the Middle East. Then $P(x^{(i)})$ is the probability that a victim of the Middle East bomb attack was observed the last time alive at the (i-1)-st measurement for $1 \le i \le 7$ (as the last is the 6-th measurement). The probabilities $P(x)$ were for all $x \in \{x^{(1)}, \ldots, x^{(7)}\}$ given in Table 2. The hypothesis is that in Baghdad, where the bomb attacks seem to be more violent, the victims will not survive the second measurement, i.e. that $P_B(x) = 0$ for all $x \in \{x^{(4)}, \ldots, x^{(7)}\}$. Under this hypothesis we get the conditional Baghdad probability distribution P_B with nonzero probabilities only for $1 \le i \le 3$, namely:

$$P_B(x^{(i)}) = \frac{P(x^{(i)})}{\sum_{j=1}^{3} P(x^{(i)})} = \frac{P(x^{(i)})}{1 - p\sum_{j=4}^{\infty}(1-p)^{i-1}} = \frac{P(x^{(i)})}{1-\left(\frac{1}{2}\right)^3} = \frac{8P(x^{(i)})}{7}$$

The numerical values of $P_B(x)$ are given together with those of $P(x)$ for all $x \in \{x^{(1)}, \ldots, x^{(7)}\}$ in Table 3. It is easy to verify from the definition (15) and Table 3 that the discrimination information $I(P_B, P)$ between the hypothetic Baghdad distribution P_B and the universal Middle East distribution P satisfies the relation:

$$I(P_B, P) = \tfrac{4}{7}\log\tfrac{8}{7} + \tfrac{2}{7}\log\tfrac{8}{7} + \tfrac{1}{7}\log\tfrac{8}{7} = (\tfrac{4}{7} + \tfrac{2}{7} + \tfrac{1}{7})\log\tfrac{8}{7} = \log\tfrac{8}{7} = 0.1335 \text{ nat} = 0.1926 \text{ bit}$$

This information is rather small and thus discrimination between P_B and P on the basis of observation X is not easy.

Table 3. Hypothetic Baghdad probabilities $P_B(x)$ and the Middle East probabilities $P(x)$

value x of X	$P_B(x)$	$P(x)$
$x^{(1)}$	$\frac{8}{7}\cdot\frac{1}{2}=\frac{4}{7}$	$\frac{1}{2}$
$x^{(2)}$	$\frac{8}{7}\cdot\frac{1}{4}=\frac{2}{7}$	$\frac{1}{4}$
$x^{(3)}$	$\frac{8}{7}\cdot\frac{1}{8}=\frac{1}{7}$	$\frac{1}{8}$
$x^{(4)}$	0	$\frac{1}{16}$
$x^{(5)}$	0	$\frac{1}{32}$
$x^{(6)}$	0	$\frac{1}{64}$
$x^{(7)}$	0	$\frac{1}{64}$

In mathematical statistics, we consider a problem of estimating by $Q = (Q(x_1), Q(x_2), \ldots, Q(x_k))$ an unknown distribution $P_0 = (P_0(x_1), P_0(x_2), \ldots, P_0(x_k))$ of data source (X, P_0) on the basis of independent realizations $X_1, X_2, \ldots, X_N$ of variable (message) $X \sim (\mathsf{X}, P_0)$, where $\mathsf{X} = \{x_1, x_2, \ldots, x_k\}$. Let us begin with absolute frequencies:

$$N_i = \text{Number}\ \{\ 1 \leq j \leq N: X_j = x_i\}$$

of $x_i \in \mathsf{X}$ data occurrence, from which empirical distribution:

$$P = (P_1 \equiv N_1 / N,\ P_2 \equiv N_2 / N,\ \ldots\ P_k \equiv N_k / N)$$

is derived on X, that is, a vector of relative frequencies for individual data $x_i \in \mathsf{X}$ in the sequence of realizations $X_1, X_2, \ldots, X_N$.

The best estimate will be given by distribution $\hat{Q} = (\hat{Q}_1, \hat{Q}_2, \ldots, \hat{Q}_k)$ "least discernible" from the observed empirical distribution. In other words, we seek arguments of minima or maxima:

$$\hat{Q} = \arg\min_Q I(P, Q) = \arg\min_Q \sum_{i=1}^{k} P_i \log \frac{P_i}{Q_i}$$

$$= \arg\max_Q \sum_{i=1}^{k} \frac{N_i}{N} \log Q_i = \arg\max_Q \sum_{j=1}^{N} \log Q(X_j) \qquad (16)$$

If the unknown probability $P_0(x_j)$ is sought in a restricted class $Q_\theta(x_j)$ dependent on a scalar or vector parameter $\theta \in \Theta$, , then the least discernible (in the sense of the discrimination information) will be the estimate $Q_{\hat{\theta}} = (Q_{\hat{\theta}}(x_1), Q_{\hat{\theta}}(x_2), \ldots, Q_{\hat{\theta}}(x_k))$ for parameter value θ, obtained from:

$$\hat{\theta} = \arg\max_\theta \sum_{j=1}^{N} \log Q_\theta(X_j) \qquad (17)$$

It is easy to see that (16) and (17) are general nonparametric and parametric *maximum likelihood estimates* well-known in mathematical statistics.

We have just proven that the known statistical principle of maximum-likelihood estimation is identical with estimating on the basis of minimum discrimination between the theoretical and empirical pictures of reality.

Example 17. Let us find the maximum likelihood estimate $\hat{p}$ of the parameter p in Example 12. In this situation $k = 7$ and $\hat{p}$ is estimated on the basis of the observed frequencies $N_1, \ldots, N_7$ of the realizations $x^{(1)}, \ldots, x^{(7)}$. By (16), for $Q_i = P(x^{(i)})$ given in Example 12:

$$\hat{p} = \arg\max \sum_{i=1}^{7} N_i \log P(x^{(i)}) = \arg\max \left[\sum_{i=1}^{6} N_i \log p(1-p)^{i-1} + N_7 \log(1-p)^6 \right] =$$

$$= \arg\max \left[(N - N_7) \log p + \sum_{i=1}^{7} (i-1) N_i \log(1-p) \right]$$

Therefore $\hat{p}$ is solution of the equation:

$$\frac{N - N_7}{p} - \frac{1}{1-p} \sum_{i=2}^{7} (i-1) N_i$$

i.e.:

$$\hat{p} = \frac{N - N_7}{N - N_7 + \sum_{i=2}^{7} (i-1) N_i}$$

We see that if $N_1 = N$ then $\hat{p} = 1$ and if $N_2 = N$ then $\hat{p} = 1/2$. The value $\hat{p} = 1/2$ used in the previous examples is obtained also when $N_i = N/2^i$ for $1 \leq i \leq 6$, for example when $N = 64$ and:

$$N_1 = 32, N_2 = 16, N_3 = 8, N_4 = 4, N_5 = 2, N_6 = 1$$

Now we can show that the discrimination information makes it possible to extend the notion of communication information, and that the latter is a special instance of the former. To this end, let us consider a situation in which message $Y \sim (\mathsf{Y}, P_Y)$ is observed instead of $X \sim (\mathsf{X}, P_X)$. A general model for a pair of random messages, (X, Y), is random message:

$$Z = (X, Y) \sim (\mathsf{Z} = \mathsf{X} \otimes \mathsf{Y}, P_{XY})$$

where:

$$P_{XY}(z) = P_{XY}(x, y) \text{ for } z = (x, y)$$

are probability values for simultaneous occurrence of components $(x, y) \in \mathsf{X} \otimes \mathsf{Y}$ in composite messages $z \in \mathsf{Z}$. A special instance is the product:

$$P_{XY}(x, y) = P_X(x)\, P_Y(y) \text{ for } (x, y) \in \mathsf{X} \otimes \mathsf{Y}$$

This means that messages X and Y are independent, $P_{XY} \equiv P_X \otimes P_Y$.

The discrimination information:

$$I(X;Y) = I(P_{XY}, P_X \otimes P_Y) \tag{18}$$

between the joint distribution P_{XY} of messages X, Y and the product distribution $P_X \otimes P_Y$, which would describe pair X, Y if X and Y were independent, is a measure of association between messages X and Y, called *communication information* about message X contained in message Y. Basic properties of information $I(X;Y)$ are summed up in the following theorem.

Theorem 6. Information $I(X;Y)$ is symmetric in its variables X, Y, and the following inequalities:

$$0 \leq I(X;Y) \leq \max \{I(X), I(Y)\} \tag{19}$$

hold, with $I(X;Y) = 0$ if and only if messages X and Y are independent, and:

$$I(X;Y) = I(X) \text{ or } I(X;Y) = I(Y) \tag{20}$$

if and only if there exists a function Φ: $\mathsf{X} \to \mathsf{Y}$ or Ψ: $\mathsf{Y} \to \mathsf{X}$ for which:

$$Y = \Phi(X) \text{ or } X = \Psi(Y) \tag{21}$$

Proof. The symmetry is a direct consequence of (15) and (18). The nonnegative values, plus the condition for the zero value, follow from (18) and Theorem 3. Further, (8) implies:

$$I(X;Y) = \sum_{(x,y)\in \mathsf{X}\otimes\mathsf{Y}} P_{XY}(x,y) \left[\log \frac{1}{P_X(x)} + \log P_{X|Y=y}(x) \right] = I(X) - \sum_{y\in\mathsf{Y}} I(X \mid Y=y) P_Y(y) \tag{22}$$

where:

$$I(X \mid Y=y) = -\sum_{x\in\mathsf{X}} P_{X|Y=y}(x) \log P_{X/Y=y}(x) \tag{23}$$

is information contained in X on the condition that $Y=y$. From Theorem 1 se know that this information content is nonnegative, with the zero value if and only if $P_{X|Y=y}$ is Dirac distribution with the unit mass of a certain point $x = \Psi(y) \in \mathbf{X}$. Consequently:

$$I(X;Y) \leq I(X)$$

and equality occurs if and only if $X = \Psi(Y)$. This statement and the symmetry, $I(X;Y) = I(Y;X)$, imply the remaining claims (19) – (21).

A special instance of mapping $\Phi : \mathsf{X} \to \mathsf{Y}$ is the identity if $\mathsf{Y} = \mathsf{X}$. Then it is $\Phi(X) = X$, and consequently, for all message pairs X, Y, it holds:

$$I(X;Y) \leq I(X) = I(X;X) \tag{24}$$

In other words, the largest amount of the communication information about message X is obtained when $Y = X$, i.e. when this message is directly observed. In this case the value of this amount is specified by the above-given formula (5). Another point is that the particular communication information $I(X)$ is a special instance of the discrimination information because:

$$I(X) = I(P_{XX}, P_X \otimes P_X)$$

Example 18. In Example 12 we considered message $X \sim (\mathsf{X}, P)$ whether and when the donor's clinical death occurred and for $p = ½$ we calculated the Shannon information $I(X)$=1.96875 bits. In Example 13, a reduction of this message was studied, $Y \sim (\mathsf{Y}, Q)$, only whether the donor's clinical death occurred, and for $p = ½$ we calculated its Shannon information $I(X;Y) = I(Y) = 0.116$ bits. Here $Y = \Phi(X)$, i.e. Y functionally depends on X. Therefore Theorem 6 implies that the Shannon information $I(X;Y)$ coincides with $I(Y)$. In other words, the Shannon information in Y about X is $I(X;Y) = 0.116$ bits. This means, that in this instance the prevailing proportion of information content in X regards the time of the death (if any), while only a smaller part is concerned with the mere fact of tits occurrence. It is so because, under the given conditions, the occurrence of clinical death is highly probable, $Q(y_1) = 63/64$.

Denote by:

$$I(X \mid Y) = \sum_{y \in \mathsf{Y}} I(X \mid Y = y) P_Y(y) \qquad \text{(cf. (23))}$$

the variable used in (22). It represents the conditional Shannon information in X given Y. Relations (22) and (23) imply the next theorem and the next formula (25).

Theorem 7. Communication (Shannon) information $I(X;Y)$ in message Y about message X equals the amount by which the prior communication information carried by message X decreases when message Y is conveyed.

Since information $I(X)$ equals entropy $H(X)$ in (6), and entropy is interpreted as a measure of uncertainty, Theorem 7 can be viewed as a statement that information $I(X;Y)$ equals the difference between prior and posterior uncertainties $H(X)$ and $H(X \mid Y)$ of message X, in symbols:

$$I(X,Y) = H(X) - H(X \mid Y) \qquad (25)$$

The last type of information considered in this paper is a *decision information* in message $X \sim (\mathsf{X}, \pi P + (1 - \pi) Q)$, providing the possibility to quantize reduction of decision-making risks.

For the sake of simplicity, let us consider a situation with two decisions, r and s, out of which the one is *correct*, leading to a zero loss, and the other one is *incorrect*, with a unit loss. Let H be correct with a prior probability $\pi \in (0, 1)$, and A be correct with the complementary prior probability $1 - \pi$. The posterior information about which of the decisions is the correct one is conveyed by a random observation X distributed by P if H is correct and by Q if A is correct. Under these conditions, we get a *prior Bayes risk:*

$$R(\pi) = \min\{\pi, 1 - \pi\}$$

and a *posterior Bayes risk:*

$$R(\pi \mid P, Q) = \sum_{x \in X} \min\{\pi P(x), (1-\pi)Q(x)\} \leq R(\pi) \tag{26}$$

where the "risk" means in fact the probability of an incorrect decision. Bayes decision risk is therefore reduced by:

$$I_\pi(P, Q) = R(\pi) - R(\pi \mid P, Q) \tag{27}$$

on the basis of observation X; we will call $I_\pi(P, Q)$ *decision information* contained in X.

Decision information was first introduced by De Groot (De Groot, 1962) with a slightly different terminology. In (Liese, Vajda, 2006) one can find a proof that the above introduced discrimination information $I(P, Q)$ is the mean decision information $I_\pi(P, Q)$ if the mean is taken over the set of prior probabilities π with weight function:

$$W(\pi) = \frac{1}{\pi^2(1-\pi)}, \; 0 < \pi < 1 \tag{28}$$

Theorem 8. Discrimination information is the mean decision information in the sense of formula:

$$I(P, Q) = \int_0^1 I_\pi(P, Q) w(\pi) d\pi \tag{29}$$

where $w(\pi)$ is the density of non-symmetric beta distribution (28).

The range of values of decision information (27) is characterized by the following Theorem.

Theorem 9. Decision information (27) is a bounded function and takes on values within interval:

$$0 \leq I_\pi(P, Q) \leq R(\pi)$$

where the left-hand inequality turns to equality for $P = Q$, while the right -hand inequality turns to equality if support of distributions P and Q are disjoint sets; the last fact is denoted by a symbol $P \perp Q$.

Proof. The inequalities follow from the definition (23) and from the inequality (26). The conditions for equalities can be deduced from the definition of $R(\pi|P,Q)$ in (26).

Example 19. Let us consider the situation of Example 16. In this situation we shall test the hypothesis H that the Baghdad probability distribution is P_B against the alternative that this distribution coincides with the Middle East average P. In other words, we shall decide between H: P_B and A: P for P_B and P given in Table 3.

i. If we have no observation X then we must decide on the basis of an a priori given probability π that H holds. The Bayes decision δ leading to the prior Bayes risk $R(\pi)$ is:

$$\delta = H \quad \text{if} \quad \pi \geq 1-\pi, \quad \text{i.e.} \quad \pi \geq \frac{1}{2} \tag{30}$$

while:

$$\delta = A \quad \text{if} \quad \pi < 1-\pi \quad \text{i.e.} \quad \pi < \frac{1}{2} \tag{31}$$

This risk takes values between $R(\pi) = 0$ (when $\pi = 0$ or $\pi = 1$) and $R(\pi) = 1/2$ (when $\pi = 1/2$).

ii. If the decision $\delta = \delta(x)$ is based on an observation $X = x \in \{x^{(1)}, \ldots, x^{(7)}\}$ then:

$$\delta(x) = H \quad \text{if} \quad \pi P_B(x) \geq (1-\pi)P(x) \tag{32}$$

and:

$$\delta(x) = A \quad \text{if} \quad \pi P_B(x) < (1-\pi)P(x) \tag{33}$$

From here and from the concrete values of $P_B(x)$, $P(x)$ in Table 3 we see that if $x \in \{x^{(4)}, \ldots, x^{(7)}\}$ then:

$$\delta(x) = A \text{ for all } \pi$$

and:

$$\sum_{i=4}^{7} \min\{\pi P_B(x^{(i)}), (1-\pi)P(x^{(i)})\} = \sum_{i=4}^{7} \pi P_B(x^{(i)}) = 0 \tag{34}$$

On the other hand, if $x \in \{x^{(1)}, x^{(2)}, x^{(3)}\}$ then the Bayes decision $\delta(x)$ depends on π. Similarly as above, we see from (32), (33) and Table 3 that:

$$\delta(x) = H \quad \text{if} \quad \frac{8\pi}{7} \geq 1-\pi, \quad \text{i.e.} \quad \pi \geq \frac{7}{15} \tag{35}$$

and:

$$\delta(x) = A \quad \text{if} \quad \pi < \frac{7}{15} \tag{36}$$

From (35) and (34) we see that if $\pi \geq 7/15$ then:

$$R(\pi \mid P, Q) = (1-\pi)\sum_{i=1}^{3} P(x^{(i)}) + \pi \sum_{i=4}^{7} P_B(x^{(i)}) =$$

$$(1-\pi)(\tfrac{1}{2} + \tfrac{1}{4} + \tfrac{1}{8}) = \tfrac{7(1-\pi)}{8} \leq \tfrac{7}{15} \tag{37}$$

Similarly, if $\pi < 7/15$ then:

$$R(\pi \mid P, Q) = \pi \sum_{i=1}^{7} P(x^{(i)}) = \pi \tag{38}$$

We see that in the both cases (37), (38) it holds $R(\pi|P,Q) \leq R(\pi) = \min\{\pi, 1-\pi\}$.

iii. By (27) the decision information is:

$$I_\pi(P_B,P) = \pi - \pi = 0 \quad \text{if} \quad \pi < \frac{7}{15} \tag{39}$$

$$I_\pi(P_B,P) = \pi - \frac{7(1-\pi)}{8} = \frac{15\pi - 7}{8} \quad \text{if} \quad \frac{7}{15} \le \pi < \frac{1}{2} \tag{40}$$

and:

$$I_\pi(P_B,P) = (1-\pi) - \frac{7(1-\pi)}{8} = \frac{1-\pi}{8} \quad \text{if} \quad \pi \ge \frac{1}{2} \tag{41}$$

The graph of $I_\pi(P_B,P)$ is in Figure 3.

iv. The last step of this example will be the illustration of Theorem 8 by verifying the formula (29):

$$\int_0^1 \frac{I_\pi(P,Q)}{\pi^2(1-\pi)} d\pi = \frac{1}{8}\int_{\frac{7}{15}}^{\frac{1}{2}} \frac{15\pi - 7}{\pi^2(1-\pi)} d\pi + \frac{1}{8}\int_{\frac{1}{2}}^{1} \frac{1-\pi}{\pi^2(1-\pi)} d\pi =$$

$$= -\frac{7}{8}\int_{\frac{7}{15}}^{\frac{1}{2}} \frac{d\pi}{\pi^2} + \int_{\frac{7}{15}}^{\frac{1}{2}} \frac{d\pi}{\pi(1-\pi)} + \frac{1}{8}\int_{\frac{1}{2}}^{1} \frac{d\pi}{\pi^2} = \int_{\frac{7}{15}}^{\frac{1}{2}} \frac{d\pi}{\pi(1-\pi)} =$$

$$= \int_{\frac{7}{15}}^{\frac{1}{2}} \left(\frac{1}{\pi} + \frac{1}{1-\pi}\right) d\pi = \left[\log_e \frac{\pi}{1-\pi}\right]_{\frac{7}{15}}^{\frac{1}{2}} = \log_e \frac{8}{7} = 0.1335 \text{ nat}$$

This result coincides with the value $I(P_B, P)$ found by a direct calculation in Example 16 which confirms the validity of Theorem 8.

With nowadays information technology physicians and other health researchers can store large database of observations where many features on patients and diseases are recorded. To reveal features that will bring quickly sufficient information for medical decision-making at the minimal costs is very important task of medical research. In fact, it is a special case of a general problem of choice of a relevant piece of

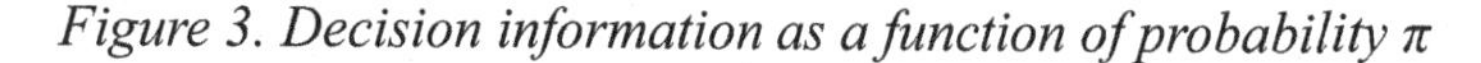

Figure 3. Decision information as a function of probability π

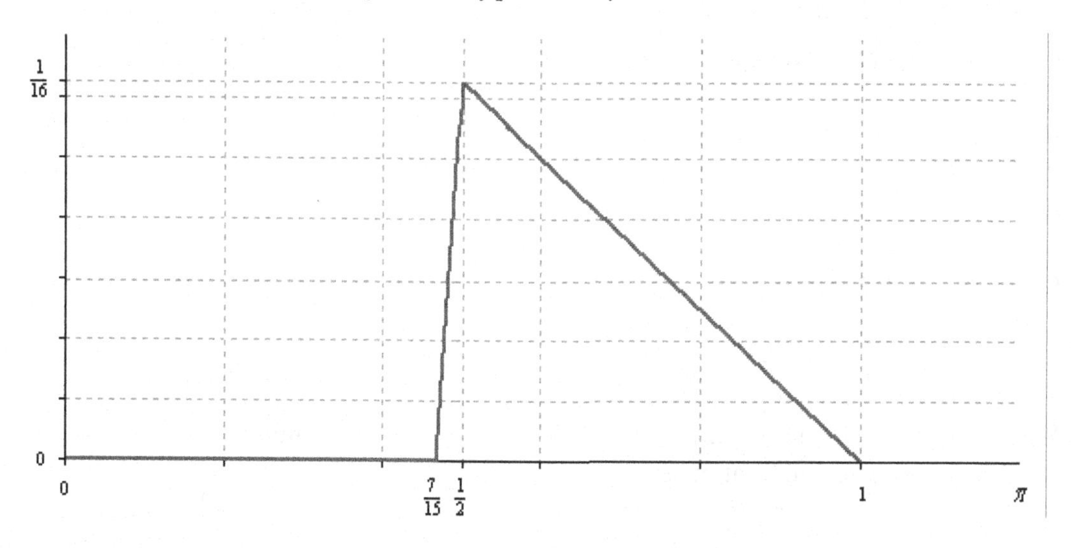

information for decision- making. This general problem has appeared also in information theory, where some tools for its solving were developed. We have in mind various information theoretical measures of mutual information, information measures of statistical dependence or conditional statistical dependence. We can concentrate on two problems. The first problem is the *constitution of data* that solves the question whether the given medical database contains sufficient information for decision-making. The second problem is the *reduction of data* that offers solutions how to remove redundant piece of information, which is sometimes caused by mutual dependence among features. General approach to data constitution and reduction was presented in (Zvárová, Studený, 1997).

KNOWLEDGE

The notion of *knowledge* is related to that of language-ontology; within this model, the notion of knowledge can be treated in a more specific sense. This model is based on an assumption that there exists the universe (ontology) consisting of objects which have certain properties and among which certain relations take place. Further we assume that there exists language in which ontology can be described. A universal language for describing ontology is the predicate calculus; hence, when we mention a language below, it will always mean the predicate calculus. The language has names for objects, properties and relations within ontology. Objects are denoted by individual constants, while properties and relations are denoted by predicates. The language further contains individual variables and logical operators. The latter include, first of all, the universal and existential quantifiers; together with individual variables, the quantifiers make it possible to set up general statements like: for all x it holds true that they have property $P(x)$, in symbols $\forall x\ P(x)$, or: there exists x such that $Q(x)$ holds true, in symbols $\exists x\ Q(x)$, etc. Other logical operators include the so-called logical connectives, non ($\neg$), and ($\wedge$), or ($\vee$), imply ($\supset$), etc., with the aid of which composite statements are put together from simpler ones. For example, a statement that object a has properties P and Q is expressed as $P(a) \wedge Q(a)$, etc.

Assignment of predicates to properties and relations as well as individual constants to objects is called interpretation of the language. Behavior of ontological objects can be described by a theory. A theory consists of a certain number of statements deemed true and called axioms, and propositions, whose validity can be derived from axioms purely with the aid of logical means.

Scientific theories in experimental sciences are formulated on the basis of experiments carried out. Results of experiments, written as logical formulas, and called either atomic formulas (Russell) or protocol propositions (Carnap), form a basis for formulating hypothetical statements, whose validity must be verified by more experiments. Protocol propositions only contain constants referring to particular real objects used in the experiment. On the other hand, hypothetical statements of scientific theories also refer to objects that do not directly appear in the protocol propositions. For example, in physics they include an electron, photon, electromagnetic field, etc. Logists and philosophers dealing with methodology of science tried hard, for several decades, to answer the question whether theoretical terms can or cannot be defined on the basis of protocol propositions. Discussions on these issues drew a modern parallel to those between realists and nominalists in classical philosophy. Carnap himself tried, for many years, to prove that this reduction of theoretical terms was possible. However, his effort was in vain and eventually Carnap accepted the opinion, which prevails today, namely, that this reduction is impossible (Carnap, 1937, Carnap, 1950). A prevailing majority of experts, who deal with methodology of science nowadays, think that properties of theoretical terms can be defined with the aid of the so-called semantic postulates. Semantic postulates of the theoretical terms used by a theory can then be included in this theory's axioms.

The notion of knowledge is mainly used intuitively. Within the above-mentioned model of language-ontology, its meaning can be defined in a more specific way. Knowledge will be understood as a true proposition concerning the ontology, formulated in the underlying language.

There are different kinds of knowledge. *Analytical knowledge* comprises those true propositions the validity of which can be derived from semantic postulates using purely logical means. It does not depend on the ontology, i.e., is valid in each and every one. Statements put forth within mathematical theories are examples of analytical knowledge. E.g., statements of the theory of sets can be derived from its axioms, which can be viewed as semantic postulates specifying the properties of a theoretical notion of a set. On this example we can see that propositions in analytical knowledge need not be just trivial logical consequences of semantic postulates; on the contrary, obtaining such propositions may be very difficult.

Analytical knowledge also includes statements whose validity can be derived by purely logical means without using semantic postulates. We call such statements tautologies. They are not interesting from the scientific point of view.

Synthetic knowledge is knowledge, which is not true in every ontology and its validity must be decided on the basis of an experiment. Basic examples of synthetic knowledge include statements whose validity has been confirmed by direct observations, such as statement $P(a)$ saying that object a has property P. Such items of synthetic knowledge are called facts.

Experimental sciences derive from facts general statements with the aid of a process called induction. For example, if ontology has established that all rooks $a, b, c, \ldots$, observed so far have been black, we formulate a general statement that all rooks are black. In a symbolic way, induction can be depicted as follows ($C(x)$ denotes predicate "x is a rook" and $B(x)$ denotes "x is black"):

Facts: $C(a)\wedge B(a),\ C(b)\wedge B(b),\ C(c)\wedge B(c), \ldots$

A general statement: $\forall x(C(x) \supset B(x))$

From valid formulas, theories can be created by accepting certain statements as axioms of a theory. Such statements must be consistent; otherwise any statements of the resulting theory could be derived and the theory would be useless. Other statements are then derived from the axioms. It has already been mentioned that such statements are valid in each ontology in which these axioms are true.

If the theory should be interesting for practical use, its axioms must include general statements. If it were not true, the theory would not be able to derive any factual statements of the objects of the respective ontology, which are not already contained in the axioms. E.g. if the axioms of our theory were just statements that particular rooks $a, b, c, \ldots$ are black, the theory would not be able to derive that rook z, not explicitly referred to in the axioms, is also black. A theory whose axioms are only facts is just reduced to a mere database of established facts.

Because axioms must be established with the aid of induction, we cannot ever be sure that the resulting theory is correct. This correctness can be confirmed through observations and experiments (Moehr, 1989). This confirmation, or validation, is based on deriving logical consequences of axioms and checking compliance of these consequences with practice. Oftentimes, consequences are identified whose validity is intuitively difficult to accept. This effort is called an attempt at rejection or refutation of a theory. If an invalid consequence is found, the theory is refuted and a new one is sought. In physics, new theories usually modify the original ones to make them more accurate. Even a refuted theory approximately may describe the reality. And the old theory is often simpler to be applied than the new one, so the old theory is successfully used for practical purposes. For example, most technical applications utilize classical mechanics, even though it was refuted due to its invalid consequences. An exact description of the reality is provided by relativistic mechanics, which has not been refuted yet.

Information is a notion whose meaning is double, depending on the context:

1. A concrete collection of data and knowledge.
2. An abstract measure of amount by which a particular piece of information reduces uncertainty contained in our image of reality.

It is not unusual in science that a meaning of a certain notion depends on the context. Let us consider the notion of mass as used in physics. In the concrete sense it includes real objects such as electrons, photons, water, electric conductor, etc. In the abstract sense, it is a measure of a body to accelerate its movement when force is applied to it. It could be suggested that the two meanings of "information" should be distinguished by using different words for each of them. For the abstract meaning, something like "informativeness" could be used. However, an approach of this kind has not been proposed in the literature and the meaning of "information" does depend on the context.

Shannon introduced information as a measure of uncertainty reduction upon receiving a certain message. As such it was a basis for many important applications in practice. The basic idea goes as follows. The ontology states are deemed realizations of random variable X. If the underlying probability distribution P_X is known, entropy $H(X) \geq 0$ can be calculated as the average measure of uncertainty of saying which of the ontology states has occurred or will occur. It can further be assumed that a message is available, characterized by random variable Y. If the conditional probability distribution, $P_{X|Y}$, is known, conditional entropy $H(X|Y)$ can be calculated. This value of conditional entropy equals zero if the message realization uniquely determines the ontology state; it equals $H(X)$ if random variables X and Y are independent. Information content in the message is then given by Theorem 6:

$$I(X;Y) = H(X) - H(X|Y)$$

and expresses a reduction of uncertainty in our image of the real world after receiving the given message.

Ontology X may, for example, be a set of patient's diseased conditions, with message Y expressing results of examinations. If probability distributions P_X and $P_{X|Y}$ are known, information $I(X;Y)$ enables us to assess to what extent individual examinations are adequate.

Not only Shannon-like messages reduce uncertainty in our image of an ontology. This uncertainty is also modified by knowledge, which reduces the scope of the admissible states within the given ontology. Moreover, it is obvious that some items of knowledge say more about the ontology than others. Analytic knowledge, to give an example, is valid in every ontology and that is why it does not affect our idea of the ontology, i.e., it has a zero value of informativeness. A question naturally arises whether this reduction of uncertainty by knowledge can be measured in a Shannon-like manner. In other words, a reasonable measure of uncertainty reduction by obtaining a piece of knowledge should be proposed. We will propose such a measure below, and call it *information content in knowledge* (Vajda, Veselý, Zvárová, 2005).

Let us suppose that language J describes ontology Ω and contains predicates $\pi_1, \ldots, \pi_r$ describing properties of objects within ontology Ω, as well as individual constants $\omega_1, \ldots, \omega_s$ representing individual objects Ω. States of ontology Ω can be described by conjunctions α:

$$\alpha = \alpha(\omega_1) \wedge \ldots \wedge \alpha(\omega_j) \wedge \ldots \wedge \alpha(\omega_s), \qquad (42)$$
$$\alpha(\omega_j) = l_1(\omega_j) \wedge \ldots \wedge l_i(\omega_j) \wedge \ldots \wedge l_r(\omega_j), j = 1, \ldots s, \text{ where}$$
$$l_i(\omega_j) = \pi_i(\omega_j) \text{ if } \pi_i(\omega_j) \text{ holds, and}$$
$$l_i(\omega_j) = \neg\pi_i(\omega_j) \text{ if } \pi_i(\omega_j) \text{ does not hold in } \Omega$$

Let us introduce an ordering of states Ω, and denote by $\alpha_1, \ldots, \alpha_M$, $M = 2^{rs}$ the conjunctions which describe such states according to (42).

In the predicate calculus, it holds (cf. e.g. (Mendelsson, 1997)) that each formula β in language J describing finite ontology Ω can be equivalently expressed by formula:

$$\beta \equiv \bigvee_{i \in I_\beta} \alpha_i, \text{ where}$$

$$I_\beta = \{ i \in \{1, \ldots, M\}: \beta \text{ holds in state } \alpha_i \text{ of ontology } \Omega \}$$

It means that I_β is the set of indices $i = 1, \ldots$ M of all states α_i in which formula β holds true. It can therefore be understood as a state representation (or state spectrum) of formula β.

Example 20. Let us study relation between the symptom fever F and disease D. Suppose that 1000 patients were examined with the results summarized in Table 4.

Using formalization described above we may proceed as follows. Ontology Ω might consist of one element ω only interpreted as generic patient. The statement $\pi_1(\omega)$ or simply π_1 may denote the fact that the generic patient has symptom F and the statement $\pi_2(\omega)$ or simply π_2 the fact that the generic patient has disease D. The ontology can be in 2^2=4 different states as is evident from Table 5. In the table π_i = 0 means that π_i does not hold and π_i = 1 means that π_i does hold in the corresponding ontology state.

Table 4. Distribution of 1000 examined patients

	Disease	
Fever	yes	no
yes	200	0
no	100	700

Table 5. Truth values an probabilities of ontology states α_i

i	ontology states α_i	π_1	π_2	$\pi_1 \supset \pi_2$	p_i
1	$\neg\pi_1 \wedge \neg\pi_2$	0	0	1	0.7
2	$\neg\pi_1 \wedge \pi_2$	0	1	1	0.1
3	$\pi_1 \wedge \neg\pi_2$	1	0	0	0
4	$\pi_1 \wedge \pi_2$	1	1	1	0.2

1000 examined patients form 1000 independent realizations of ontology states and therefore we can calculate an estimate of probability distribution of ontology states. This estimate is given in the last column of Table 5.

From Table 4 we see that the formula $\pi_1 \supset \pi_2$ holds in all considered realizations of ontology states. From the Table 5 we can see that the formula $\beta = \pi_1 \supset \pi_2$ can be equivalently written as:

$$\beta \equiv (\neg\pi_1 \wedge \neg\pi_2) \vee (\neg\pi_1 \wedge \neg\pi_2) \vee (\neg\pi_1 \wedge \neg\pi_2)$$

and therefore that the spectrum (state representation) of β is $\boldsymbol{I}_\beta = \{1, 2, 4\}$.

Example 21. Let us study relationships between three symptoms in a patient and a particular disease he may suffer from. The ontology here consists of one element (generic patient) and his four properties. Language J describing this ontology contains individual constant ω denoting the generic patient and predicates π_1, π_2, π_3 representing his symptoms and predicate π_4 representing the disease he might suffer from. For the sake of simplicity, we will write:

$$\pi_1(\omega) = s_1,\ \pi_2(\omega) = s_2,\ \pi_3(\omega) = s_3,\ ,\ \pi_4(\omega) = d$$

Since $s = 1$ and $r = 4$, this ontology may be in one of $2^{rs} = 16$ states. Ontology states can be easily ordered as follows from Table 6. From this table we see that for example formula $\beta = ((s_1 \wedge s_2) \supset d) \wedge (d \supset (s_1 \wedge s_2))$ holds in ontology states $\alpha_1, \alpha_3, \alpha_5, \alpha_7, \alpha_9, \alpha_{11}, \alpha_{14}, \alpha_{16.}$ Therefore the spectrum of β is $\boldsymbol{I}_\beta = \{1, 3, 5, 7, 9, 11, 14, 16\}$ and:

Table 6. Truth table of the formula $\beta = ((s_1 \wedge s_2) \supset d) \wedge (d \supset (s_1 \wedge s_2))$

ontology states α_i	s_1	s_2	s_3	d	β
$\alpha_1 \equiv \neg s_1 \wedge \neg s_2 \wedge \neg s_3 \wedge \neg d$	0	0	0	0	1
$\alpha_2 \equiv \neg s_1 \wedge \neg s_2 \wedge \neg s_3 \wedge d$	0	0	0	1	0
$\alpha_3 \equiv \neg s_1 \wedge \neg s_2 \wedge s_3 \wedge \neg d$	0	0	1	0	1
$\alpha_4 \equiv \neg s_1 \wedge \neg s_2 \wedge s_3 \wedge d$	0	0	1	1	0
$\alpha_5 \equiv \neg s_1 \wedge s_2 \wedge \neg s_3 \wedge \neg d$	0	1	0	0	1
$\alpha_6 \equiv \neg s_1 \wedge s_2 \wedge \neg s_3 \wedge d$	0	1	0	1	0
$\alpha_7 \equiv \neg s_1 \wedge s_2 \wedge s_3 \wedge \neg d$	0	1	1	0	1
$\alpha_8 \equiv \neg s_1 \wedge s_2 \wedge s_3 \wedge d$	0	1	1	1	0
$\alpha_9 \equiv s_1 \wedge \neg s_2 \wedge \neg s_3 \wedge \neg d$	1	0	0	0	1
$\alpha_{10} \equiv s_1 \wedge \neg s_2 \wedge \neg s_3 \wedge d$	1	0	0	1	0
$\alpha_{11} \equiv s_1 \wedge \neg s_2 \wedge s_3 \wedge \neg d$	1	0	1	0	1
$\alpha_{12} \equiv s_1 \wedge \neg s_2 \wedge s_3 \wedge d$	1	0	1	1	0
$\alpha_{13} \equiv s_1 \wedge s_2 \wedge \neg s_3 \wedge \neg d$	1	1	0	0	0
$\alpha_{14} \equiv s_1 \wedge s_2 \wedge \neg s_3 \wedge d$	1	1	0	1	1
$\alpha_{15} \equiv s_1 \wedge s_2 \wedge s_3 \wedge \neg d$	1	1	1	0	0
$\alpha_{16} \equiv s_1 \wedge s_2 \wedge s_3 \wedge d$	1	1	1	1	1

$\beta \equiv \vee_{i \in I_\beta} \alpha_i$, $I_\beta = \{1, 3, 5, 7, 9, 11, 14, 16\}$

Let us suppose that $T(\beta_1, \ldots, \beta_m)$ is a theory with axioms $\beta_1, \ldots, \beta_m$ and that our current knowledge of the probability distribution governing the states of ontology Ω is $Q = \{q_i : i \in N\}$. Assume that $T(\beta_1, \ldots, \beta_m)$ truthfully describes ontology Ω, i.e. that all axioms $\beta_1, \ldots, \beta_m$ are true in Ω. Information $\mathtt{I}(T)$ contained in theory $T(\beta_1, \ldots, \beta_m)$ is defined as follows:

$$\mathtt{I}(T) = -\log \sum_{i \in I_T} q_i, \text{ where } I_T = I_{\beta 1} \cap \ldots \cap I_{\beta m} \tag{43}$$

Here $I_{\beta 1}, \ldots, I_{\beta m}$ are state representations (spectrums) of axioms in theory T, and their intersection I_T is a state representation (spectrum) of the theory itself.

For information $\mathtt{I}(T)$, the following Theorem 10 holds. In this theorem a T-normalization $\tilde{Q} = \varphi(Q, T)$ of probability distribution $Q = \{q_i : i \in N\}$ is used:

$$\tilde{q}_i = 0 \qquad \text{if } i \notin I_T \tag{44}$$

$$\tilde{q}_i = \frac{q_i}{\sum_{i \in I_T} q_i} \qquad \text{if } i \in I_T \tag{45}$$

where I_T is defined in formula (43). Formulas (44) and (45) indicate that it is a natural adjustment (normalization) of probability distribution Q after certain ontology states α_i, $i \in N - I_T$ are excluded by theory T.

Theorem 10. Information $\mathtt{I}(T)$ contained in a theory $T(\beta_1, \ldots, \beta_m)$ that truthfully describes ontology Q has the following properties:

1. $\mathtt{I}(T) > 0$.
2. If theory T_1 is an extension of theory T_2 (i.e. $T_1 \supseteq T_2$), then $\mathtt{I}(T_1) \geq \mathtt{I}(T_2)$.
3. $\mathtt{I}(T_1) > \mathtt{I}(T_2)$ if and only if $I(P, \varphi(Q, T_1)) < I(P, \varphi(Q, T_2))$
   where P is the actual probability distribution of the ontology states and the expression:

$$I(P, Q) = \sum_i p_i \log \frac{p_i}{q_i} \tag{46}$$

in which it is specified that $p \log p/q = 0$ for $p=0$, $q \geq 0$ and $p \log p/q = \infty$ for $p > 0$, $q = 0$, denotes the discrimination information corresponding to distributions P and Q (cf. Section 3).

Proof. Properties under 1 and 2 are directly implied by definition of information (43). Let us denote $A = \sum_{i \in I_T} q_i$. Since $i \notin I_T$ implies $p_i = 0$ and consequently $p_i \log p_i/q = 0$, we get:

$$I(P, Q) - I(P, \varphi(Q, T)) = \sum_i p_i \log \frac{p_i}{q_i} - \sum_i p_i \log \frac{p_i}{\tilde{q}_i} = \sum_{i \in I_T} p_i \log \frac{p_i}{q_i} - \sum_{i \in I_T} p_i \log \frac{p_i}{\tilde{q}_i}$$

$$= \sum_{i \in I_T} p_i \log \frac{p_i}{q_i} - \sum_{i \in I_T} p_i \log \left(\frac{p_i}{q_i} A \right) = -\sum_{i \in I_T} p_i \log A = -\log A = -\log \sum_{i \in I_T} q_i = \mathtt{I}(T)$$

Hence:

$\mathtt{I}(T_1) = I(P, Q) - I(P, \varphi(Q, T_1))$
$\mathtt{I}(T_2) = I(P, Q) - I(P, \varphi(Q, T_2))$.

therefore:

$\mathtt{I}(T_1) - \mathtt{I}(T_2) = I(P, \varphi(Q, T_2)) - I(P, \varphi(Q, T_1))$

We see from here that $\mathtt{I}(T_1) > \mathtt{I}(T_2)$ if and only if:

$I(P, \varphi(Q, T_1)) < I(P, \varphi(Q, T_2))$ (Q.E.D.)

Information content $\mathtt{I}(T)$ in theory T is defined above. Properties of this measure of information can be simply described as follows: if T_1 and T_2 are two theories with $\mathtt{I}(T_1) > \mathtt{I}(T_2)$, and our knowledge of the ontology is given by an estimate of the probability distribution Q which governs the states of the given ontology, then axioms of theory T_1, containing a higher amount of information, admit a natural transformation (namely, T_1-normalization) of distribution Q to $\tilde{Q} = \varphi(Q, T)$ and the latter is closer to the unknown actual distribution P of the ontology states than the result of T_2-normalization applied on distribution Q with the aid of axioms of theory T_2, containing a lower amount of information. If we have no estimate of the actual distribution governing the ontology states, we take uniform distribution as its initial estimate Q.

Theories containing more information therefore admit more accurate approximations of the actual probability distribution governing the ontology states. Optimum decision-making within a given ontology requires knowledge of the actual probability distribution governing the ontology states. Hence theories with higher information content potentially improve the decision-making processes.

Example 22. Let us consider the ontology Ω consisting of one element ω interpreted as a generic victim in the Middle East bomb attacks. Let $B = \pi_1(\omega)$ means that a victim is from Baghdad and $D = \pi_2(\omega)$ means that the victim will survive the second measurement as described in Example 16. Assume that the true distribution of the states of ontology Ω is $P=\{p_i\}$ and that the current knowledge concerning the distribution of the ontology states is represented by the distribution $Q=\{q_i\}$ (see Table 6). We see that the statement $\beta \equiv B \supset \neg D$ represents a theory true in this ontology with the spectrum $\{1, 2, 3\}$. This statement is nothing but the hypothesis about the Baghdad bomb victims considered previously in Example 19. Therefore the information contribution of the theory $T(\beta)$ to the current knowledge is:

$$\mathtt{I}(T(\beta)) = -\log \sum_{i \in I_T} q_i = -\log 0.8 = 0.32 \text{ bit}$$

We see that in the situation described by the distribution Q is the information content of the theory β quite small.

Example 23. Let us continue Example 21, the study of relationships between three symptoms in a patient and a particular disease he may suffer from. Suppose there is a large set of patients at our disposal with verified diagnoses, and we want to establish, and express in the form of logical formulas, laws

Table 7. Truth values and probabilities of ontology states

i	ontology states α_i	B	D	$\neg D$	$B \supset \neg D$	p_i	q_i
1	$\neg B \wedge \neg D$	0	0	1	1	0.7	0.6
2	$\neg B \wedge D$	0	1	0	1	0.1	0.1
3	$B \wedge \neg D$	1	0	1	1	0	0.1
4	$B \wedge D$	1	1	0	0	0.2	0.2

governing relationships between the symptoms and disease. In such a situation, data-mining methods are utilized to generate IF THEN rules. Let us further suppose that the ontology may be only in 3 states described with the conjunctions:

$$\alpha_1 \equiv \neg s_1 \wedge \neg s_2 \wedge \neg s_3 \wedge \neg d$$
$$\alpha_{12} \equiv s_1 \wedge \neg s_2 \wedge s_3 \wedge d$$
$$\alpha_{16} \equiv s_1 \wedge s_2 \wedge s_3 \wedge d$$

Under these circumstances, the data-mining methods may generate the following IF THEN rules:

$\beta_1 \equiv s_1 \wedge s_2 \supset d$ (i.e., IF s_1 AND s_2 THEN d)
$\beta_2 \equiv s_1 \wedge s_3 \supset d$
$\beta_3 \equiv \neg s_1 \wedge \neg s_3 \supset \neg d$
$\beta_4 \equiv s_1 \supset d$
$\beta_5 \equiv s_2 \supset d$
$\beta_6 \equiv \neg s_3 \supset \neg d$,
$\beta_7 \equiv s_1 \vee s_2 \vee \vee s_3 \supset d$
$\beta_8 \equiv \neg s_1 \vee \neg s_3 \supset \neg d$

On the basis of these IF THEN rules one can formulate three theories:

$T_1 = \{\beta_1, \beta_2, \beta_3\}$, $T_2 = \{\beta_4, \beta_6\}$, $T_3 = \{\beta_4, \beta_5, \beta_6\}$, $T_4 = \{\beta_7, \beta_8\}$

A question arises which of these theories is the most informative one. Let us apply the above-introduced measure $\mathtt{I}(T)$ and establish information content in these theories. Since we have no initial estimate of the probability distribution governing the ontology states, we will suppose it is uniform.

Spectra of axioms $\beta_1, \ldots, \beta_8$ are established using their truth tables given in the Table 8.

The resulting spectra are given in the Table 9. Spectra of theories T_1, T_2, T_3, T_4 are:

$$I_{T1} = I_{\beta 1} \cap I_{\beta 2} \cap I_{\beta 3} = \{1, 3, 5, 6, 7, 8, 9, 10, 12, 14, 16\}$$
$$I_{T2} = I_{\beta 4} \cap I_{\beta 6} = \{1, 3, 4, 5, 7, 8, 12, 16\}$$
$$I_{T3} = I_{\beta 4} \cap I_{\beta 5} \cap I_{\beta 6} = \{1, 3, 4, 8, 12, 16\}$$
$$I_{T4} = I_{\beta 7} \cap I_{\beta 8} = \{1, 12, 16\}$$

Table 8. Truth tables of axioms $\beta_1, \beta_2, \beta_3, \beta_4, \beta_5, \beta_6, \beta_7, \beta_8$

state of Ω	s_1	s_2	s_3	d	β_1	β_2	β_3	β_4	β_5	β_6	β_7	β_8
α_1	0	0	0	0	1	1	1	1	1	1	1	1
α_2	0	0	0	1	1	1	0	1	1	0	1	0
α_3	0	0	1	0	1	1	1	1	1	1	0	1
α_4	0	0	1	1	1	1	0	1	1	1	1	0
α_5	0	1	0	0	1	1	1	1	0	1	0	1
α_6	0	1	0	1	1	1	1	1	1	0	1	0
α_7	0	1	1	0	1	1	1	1	0	1	0	1
α_8	0	1	1	1	1	1	1	1	1	1	1	0
α_9	1	0	0	0	1	1	1	0	1	1	0	1
α_{10}	1	0	0	1	1	1	1	1	1	0	1	0
α_{11}	1	0	1	0	1	0	1	0	1	1	0	1
α_{12}	1	0	1	1	1	1	1	1	1	1	1	1
α_{13}	1	1	0	0	0	1	1	0	0	1	0	1
α_{14}	1	1	0	1	1	1	1	1	1	0	1	0
α_{15}	1	1	1	0	0	0	1	0	0	1	0	1
α_{16}	1	1	1	1	1	1	1	1	1	1	1	1

Table 9. Spectra of axioms $\beta_1, \beta_2, \beta_3, \beta_4, \beta_5, \beta_6, \beta_7, \beta_8$

axiom	**spectrum of axiom β_i**
β_1	{1, 2, 3, 4, 5, 6, 7, 8, 9, 10, 11, 12, 14, 16}
β_2,	{1, 2, 3, 4, 5, 6, 7, 8, 9, 10, 12, 13, 14, 16}
β_3	{1, 3, 5, 6, 7, 8, 9, 10, 11, 12, 13, 14, 15, 16}
β_4	{1, 2, 3, 4, 5, 6, 7, 8, 10, 12, 14, 16}
β_5	{1, 2, 3, 4, 6, 8, 9, 10, 11, 12, 14, 16}
β_6	{1, 3, 4, 5, 7, 8, 9, 11, 12, 13, 15, 16}
β_7	{1, 2, 4, 6, 8, 10, 12, 14, 16}
β_8	{1, 3, 5, 7, 9, 11, 12, 13, 15, 16}

For uniform Q calculations of $\mathtt{I}(T)$ provide:

$$\mathtt{I}(T_1) = -\log \sum_{i \in I_{T1}} q_i = \log(16/11) = 0.541 \text{ bit}$$

$$\mathtt{I}(T_2) = -\log \sum_{i \in I_{T2}} q_i = \log(16/8) = 1 \text{ bit}$$

$$\mathtt{I}(T_3) = -\log \sum_{i \in I_{T3}} q_i = \log(16/6) = 1.415 \text{ bit}$$

$$\mathtt{I}(T_4) = -\log \sum_{i \in I_{T4}} q_i = \log(16/3) = 2.415 \text{ bits}$$

As the axioms of the theory T_4 hold only in admissible ontology states α_1, α_{12}, α_{16}, the theory T_4 and theories equivalent to T_4 are the strongest theories about the ontology possible. Their information content reaches maximal possible value 2.415 bits.

A natural question arises. How we can utilize in practice the proposed information measure? In these days, knowledge bases are created in addition to traditional databases and data stores. Together with the traditional systems supporting decision-making, which need extensive data sets, knowledge-based systems supporting decision-making find an ever-growing scope of applications. The range of knowledge items that can be obtained by dialogues with experts or by automated methods is very wide. This is also seen if we realize that an infinite number of equivalent knowledge items (valid formulas) exist on a finite ontology. This underlines importance of methods to be used for assessment relevance of individual items of knowledge for practical utilization in decision-making models.

Methods assessing the relevance of knowledge represented by a logical formula can obviously be based on logical consequences. Let us define relation $\supseteq$ on the set of all formulas: $\alpha \supseteq \beta$ holds, if validity of α logically implies validity of β. Relation $\supseteq$ complies with the axioms of partial ordering on the set of all formulas. If $\alpha \supseteq \beta$ holds, we deem α "more relevant" than β. We thus come to a conclusion, which is rather natural from the methodological point of view: namely, knowledge items that can be derived from other items are not interesting. However, applications of this simplest method of comparison are rather limited. Firstly, this ordering is only partial, and most items of knowledge cannot be compared with each other. Secondly, no quantitative expression of relevance is available for individual items.

The above-defined measure resolves both these disadvantages. It defines a complete ordering and fully quantifies relevance ("*informativeness*") of an item or more items of knowledge. Moreover, this quantification complies with an intuitive requirement that an item of knowledge that is more relevant according to this criterion also enables higher quality of decision-making.

ACKNOWLEDGMENT

The work was supported by the research institutional plan AV0Z10300504 of the ICS AS CR and by the projects MSMT CR 1M0572 and 1M06014.

REFERENCES

Carnap, R. (1937). *The Logical Syntax of Language.* New York: Harcourt.

Carnap, R. (1950). *Logical Foundation of Probability.* Chicago: University of Chicago Press.

Colens, M. F. (1986). Origins of medical informatics. *Western Journal of Medicine,* 145, 778-785.

De Groot, M. H. (1962). Uncertainty, information and sequential experiments. *Annals of Mathematical Statistics,* 33, 404-419.

Feinstein, A. (1958). *Foundation of Information Theory.* Mc Graw Hill, New York.

Gremy, F. (1989). Crisis of meaning and medical informatics education: A burden and/or a relief? *Methods of Information in Medicine,* 28,189-195.

Haux, R. (1997). Aims and tasks of medical informatics. *International Journal of Medical Informatics,* 44, 3-10.

Kullback, S., & Leibler, R. (1951). On information and sufficiency. *Annals of Mathematical Statistics,* 22, 79-86.

Liese, F., Vajda, I. (2006). On divergences and information in statistics and information theory. *IEEE Transactions on Information Theory,* 52, 4394-4412.

Mendelsson, E. (1997). *Introduction to Mathematical Logic.* London: Chapman & Hall.

Moehr, J. R. (1989). Teaching medical informatics: Teaching on the seams of disciplines, cultures, traditions. *Methods of Information in Medicine,* 28, 273-280.

Shannon, C. (1948). A mathematical theory of communication. *Bell System Technical Journal,* 27, 397-423 and 623-656.

Vajda, I., Veselý, A., & Zvárová, J. (2005). On the amount of information resulting from empirical and theoretical knowledge. *Revista Matematica Complutense,* 18, 275-283.

van Bemmel, J. H., & McCray, A. T. *eds.* (1995). *Yearbook of Medical Informatics.* Stuttgart: Schattauer Verlagsgesellschaft.

Wiener, N. (1948). *Cybernetics: On the Control and Communication in the Animal and the Machine.* Cambridge, MA: MIT Press.

Zvárová, J. (1997). On the medical informatics structure. *International Journal of Medical Informatics,* 44, 75-82.

Zvárová, J., & Studený, M. (1997). Information theoretical approach to constitution and reduction of medical data. *International Journal of Medical Informatics,* 44, 65-74.

KEY TERMS

Analytical Knowledge: True propositions about ontology verifiable by logical means.

Communication Information: It characterizes capacities needed for recording and transmitting of data.

Medical Informatics: Informatics focused to the field of medicine and health care.

Data: Images of the real word in abstract sense.

Decision Information: It characterizes a possibility to reduce decision-making risk.

Discrimination Information: It characterizes a possibility to discriminate among various data sources.

Information Content: It characterizes an uncertainty reduction by obtaining a piece of knowledge.

Knowledge: True propositions about ontology in a language system.

Synthetic Knowledge: True propositions about ontology verifiable empirically.

Chapter II
Ontologies in the Health Field

Michel Simonet
Laboratoire TIMC-IMAG, Institut de l'Ingénierie et de l'Information de Santé, France

Radja Messai
Laboratoire TIMC-IMAG, Institut de l'Ingénierie et de l'Information de Santé, France

Gayo Diallo
Laboratoire TIMC-IMAG, Institut de l'Ingénierie et de l'Information de Santé, France

Ana Simonet
Laboratoire TIMC-IMAG, Institut de l'Ingénierie et de l'Information de Santé, France

ABSTRACT

Health data and knowledge had been structured through medical classifications and taxonomies long before ontologies had acquired their pivot status of the Semantic Web. Although there is no consensus on a common definition of an ontology, it is necessary to understand their main features to be able to use them in a pertinent and efficient manner for data mining purposes. This chapter introduces the basic notions about ontologies, presents a survey of their use in medicine and explores some related issues: knowledge bases, terminology, and information retrieval. It also addresses the issues of ontology design, ontology representation, and the possible interaction between data mining and ontologies.

INTRODUCTION

Ontologies have become a privileged and almost unavoidable means to represent and exploit knowledge and data. This is true in many domains, and particularly in the health field. Health data and knowledge had been structured through medical classifications and taxonomies long before ontologies had acquired their pivot status of the semantic web. In the health field, there are still more than one hundred classifications (e.g., ICD10, MeSH, SNOMED), which makes it very difficult to exploit data coded according to one or the other, or several of these classifications. The UMLS (Unified Medical Language System) initiative tries to provide a unified access to these classifications, in the absence of an ontology of the whole medical domain - still to come.

In order to apprehend the interest of ontologies in data mining, especially in the health domain, it is necessary to have a clear view of what an ontology is. Unfortunately, there is no consensus within the scientific community on a common definition of an ontology, which is somewhat paradoxical, as one of the characteristics of an ontology is to represent a consensus of a community on a given domain. However, one does not need to enter the specialists' debate on ontologies to understand their main characteristics and therefore be able to use them in a pertinent and efficient manner for data mining purposes.

On a first level, one can think of an ontology as a means to name and structure the content of a domain. Among the numerous definitions that have been given, there is some kind of agreement that an ontology represents the concepts of a domain, the relationships between these concepts (IS-A and other relationships), the vocabulary used to designate them, and their definition (informal and/or formal). The IS-A relationship plays a central role, as it provides the (tree-like) skeleton of an ontology. This structure need not be a tree, as a concept may specialize several upper concepts, contrary to a taxonomy. Compared with a thesaurus, an ontology is freed from a particular language: an ontology deals with concepts, independently from the (natural) language that is used to designate them, while a thesaurus deals with terms that are expressed in a particular language. Moreover, a thesaurus does not enable the creation of new relationships between terms, whereas ontologies do.

There is no strict boundary between taxonomies, thesauri and ontologies, and a taxonomy may be considered as a particular case of an ontology. In practice, most ontologies rely on a taxonomic skeleton which is enriched with ontology-specific features. One can also notice that the conceptual schema of a database, expressed in object form, is close to an ontology (a micro-ontology) of the application domain of the database. Therefore, most people dealing with health data have been dealing with ontologies, either explicitly or implicitly – most often implicitly. However, making explicit the notion of ontology has made it possible to formalize and unite various formalisms and practices. The current ontology standard in the web universe, namely OWL[1], might not be the final standard for ontologies, but it has initiated a movement towards the need for an agreement for such a standard.

Ontologies have their roots in Aristotle's categories, and particularly in Porphyry's tree-like representation (3rd century), which laid the foundations for modern ontologies. This tree-like structure is still present in ontologies and in most knowledge representation systems through the IS-A relationship. The attributes in object or frame-based systems and the roles in Description Logics provide the other relationships of a possibly corresponding ontology. However, the introduction of ontologies in the field of Computer Science by Gruber in the 90's was not motivated by philosophical considerations but by the need of a representation in first-order logic of knowledge-based systems in order to facilitate their interoperability (Gruber, 1991). Today's ontologies are still strongly linked to first-order logic, either through Description Logics, which constitute the main stream in the ontology domain, or through conceptual graphs, which also have a strong logic background. Ontologies have also become an unavoidable support to knowledge and data integration.

In order to provide a level of understanding of ontologies that enables the reader to comprehend their interest in data mining, we first present two examples to introduce the basic notions related to ontologies. We then make a short historical presentation of the notion of ontology, with its philosophical background and its introduction in the computer field in the 90's for knowledge sharing purposes. In the following section, we make a survey of classifications and ontologies in the medical and biological fields. We then address some issues related to ontologies: knowledge bases, terminology, information retrieval, and finally ontology building. We conclude by presenting a summary of recent and ongoing work on data mining with ontologies and mention some perspectives.

ONTOLOGY ESSENTIALS, ORIGIN AND DEFINITIONS

The basic notions necessary to approach ontologies are concepts, relations, vocabulary and definitions. We illustrate them through two examples taken from ongoing work involving ontology building and use.

Basic Concepts and Examples

A Concept-Based Terminology in the Field of Breast Cancer

The first example introduces the notions of concept and relationships, and illustrates the terminological aspects of ontologies. Some authors consider that an ontology does not contain any vocabulary, only universals describing "reality" (Smith, 2003). Such universals, anchored in "reality", are different from concepts, which are creations of the human mind. *Absent nipple* is an example of *concept* that is found in medical classifications. According to B. Smith, such a concept is not a universal, as an absent nipple does not exist in reality but is a creation of the human mind. Universals have to be named, but this name is conventional and the various terms used to designate an ontology component (usually called a concept) should be dealt with outside the ontology. Although we understand this view, which implies considering a *terminology* associated with - but not part of - the ontology, throughout this chapter we will adopt the common view of ontologies and consider the vocabulary associated with concepts as part of an ontology.

The problem addressed by the work presented below is that of the language used in medicine by different categories of users, namely health professionals and lay people. Most health professionals recognize that patients and other lay people are not familiar with medical terms. As these terms are used in health-related documents (texts, web sites) it makes it difficult for patients, and more generally for lay people, firstly to find these documents through queries, as their *natural* language is not the language used in the documents themselves, and secondly to understand them. Moreover, much of the health-related scientific literature is in English, which increases the problem of querying the web for some; this is also true for health professionals, who are not always familiar with the English language. One solution to this problem is to create an ontology of the considered domain (ideally the whole medical domain) and to associate with its concepts the terms in the relevant languages, e.g., professional-English, lay-English, professional-French, lay-French. This is the objective of the work undertaken by R. Messai for breast cancer in her PhD work (Messai et al., 2006). The ontology fragment presented in Figure 1 shows an example of a conceptual structure. *BREAST SURGERY*, *MASTECTOMY* and *LYMPH NODE REMOVAL* are concepts. The concept *MASTECTOMY* is linked to the concept *BREAST SURGERY* by the hierarchic relation *IS_A*. This means that the concept *MASTECTOMY* is more specific than the concept *BREAST SURGERY* (conversely, the concept *BREAST SURGERY* is more generic than the concept *MASTECTOMY*). Figure 1 shows three occurrences of pairs of concepts linked by the IS_A relationship:

BREAST RADIATION THERAPY IS_A BREAST CANCER TREATMENT
BREAST SURGERY IS_A BREAST CANCER TREATMENT
MASTECTOMY IS_A BREAST SURGERY

and three occurrences of non-IS_A relationships:

MASTECTOMY *Can_be_realized_with* LYMPH NODE REMOVAL
MASTECTOMY *Can_be_followed_by* BREAST RADIATION THERAPY
LYMPH NODE REMOVAL *Can_cause* LYMPHEDEMA OF ARM

The IS_A relationship provides the skeleton of the ontology (its taxonomic part), while other relationships provide information about the domain that can be exploited through logical reasoning, for example for information retrieval or question-answering purposes.

Although the concept names are in english, the concepts themselves are independent from the language, as is the ontology[2]. The name chosen to designate the concept in a given situation among several possible terms is somewhat arbitrary (for a presentation in french, french names would be chosen). Moreover, several terms can be used in the same language to designate a concept, e.G., mastectomy, mammectomy and breast removal, for the concept MASTECTOMY. These terms can be considered as synonyms and any of them could be used to designate the concept MASTECTOMY. However, it is common usage to choose a preferred term among these synonyms, in order to facilitate the communication between the different users of the ontology. In the context of the current project a preferred term has been chosen for each category of users considered: professional-English, lay-English, professional-French and lay-French. Examples of terms associated with the concepts of Figure 1 are given below (the preferred term is underlined).

Lymphedema of arm:

Lymphedema of arm, *arm lymphedema, edema of arm*	(professional-English)
Arm swelling	(lay-English)
Lymphœdème du bras, *œdème lymphatique du bras*	(professional-French)
Gros bras, *gonflement du bras*	(lay-French)

One important objective of this ontology is to support multilingual Information Retrieval. It is established that patients' query formulation leads to poor results since most health-related information is available in English and uses a specialized medical terminology. It is likely that they will search for "heart attack" rather than "myocardial infarction", "rash" rather than "exanthema" or "hair loss" rather than "alopecia" (McCray et al., 2003). Therefore, breast cancer terminology for lay people should contain terms specific to the patients' language, such as *"breast pain"* for *"mastodynia"* and *"breast removal"* for *"mastectomy"*, but also medical terms such as *"pyrexia"*, which they can encounter.

Through an ontology with a rich terminology covering English and French, professional and lay languages in the domain of breast cancer, lay people will be able to access and understand health-related data and knowledge in the breast cancer field, while using their own words and language. In order that access to web-based medical content be independent from the language and the scientific skill of the user, an ontology associated with a multilingual terminology will be used to index and query documents. Such an Information Retrieval system can also be used by health professionals, as their language

Figure 1. An example of a conceptual structure in the breast cancer field

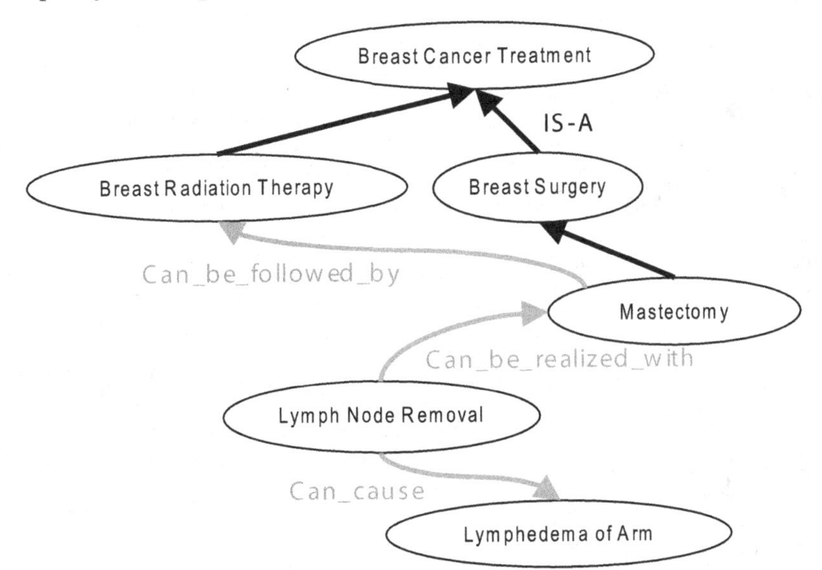

has also been employed in the indexing process, through the concept-based indexing approach that is applied (see §4.3).

The second example is taken from a former national French project on the mining of brain data (Bonnevay et al., 2003). This project aimed at discovering relationships between brain regions and cognitive functions through the results of cognitive tests performed on patients with brain injuries. To achieve this goal, knowledge about both the anatomical and functional aspects of the brain has been formalised through an anatomical ontology, a functional ontology and an ontology of cognitive tests. The knowledge about the brain domain (a.k.a. anatomo-functional ontology) is expressed through semantic relationships between the concepts of the three ontologies. Generally speaking, a given cognitive function (e.g., *memory, language*) is evaluated by a set of cognitive tests or subtests (e.g., *verbal agility test, picture naming test*). A particular area or region of the brain participates in the execution of a given cognitive function. For example, the *temporal lobe* is involved in *memory*. Figure 2 presents an example taken from the ontology built in this project. It illustrates two basic notions of ontologies: concepts and relationships. It also shows the use of a particular relation, namely *Part_Of*, which play with the *IS-A* relationships a key role in biomedical ontologies such as the Digital Anatomist Foundational Model of Anatomy (FMA) and the Gene (GO) ontology (§3.1). The *Part_Of* relation links an entity and its components, and is intended to be transitive.

This ontology has been used to support the discovery of relationships between the cognitive function and the anatomical regions of the brain in the French national project BC3 (Brain and Health Knowledge Base) (Bonnevay et al., 2003).

Basic Notions

The two previous examples have illustrated the notions of *concepts*, *relations* and *terminology*, which can be considered as the main constituents of an ontology. The IS_A relationship, which is central to ontologies, provides the taxonomic skeleton of the ontology.

Figure 2. An example of a conceptual structure in the brain field

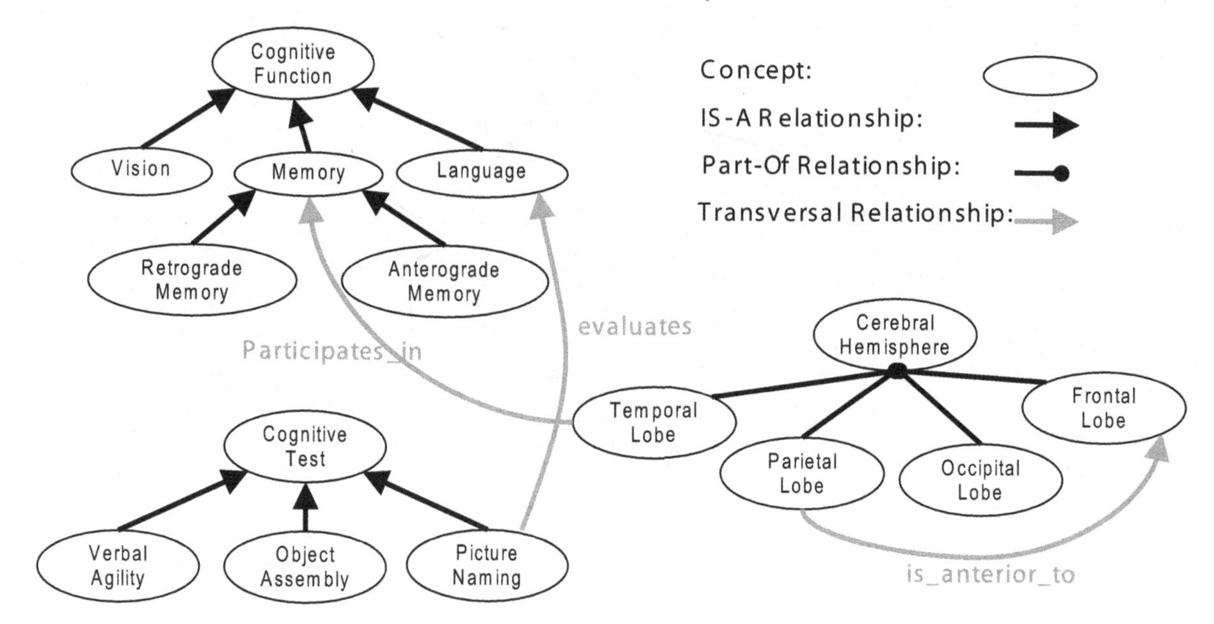

In the above examples, definitions were not associated with concepts. As an ontology aims at establishing a consensus within a community on a (general or specific) domain, it is necessary, during ontological engineering, i.e., the design and the building of the ontology, to provide definitions in natural language. Such definitions are often sufficient to reveal dissentions in the understanding of concepts, which often have different meanings in different groups, thus leading the group to look for a consensus.

Associating formal definitions with concepts and relationships requires the use of a formal language. First-order logic is well suited for that purpose, and was indeed used in the first formal work on ontologies, in the KIF/Ontolingua environments (Gruber, 1993). Today, Description Logics (DL), a meaningful subset of First-Order Logic, is the formalism most widely used to support formal ontological work. OWL, the current recommendation of W3C for ontology description, is based on Description Logics. The first and most well known formal work in medicine using DLs is the GALEN system (Rector et al., 1993). It uses a specific DL, namely GRAIL, whose author, I. Horrocks, is one of the designers of the OWL language.

Origins and Definitions

Aristotle's categories may be considered as the first tentative to build an ontology of what exists. It consisted in identifying and naming ten categories[3] into which any existing thing or being can be classified. These categories may seem awkward to us today but it was indeed an original and remarkable work at the time. They were provided as a flat list, but five centuries later, Porphyry (234?-305?) organized them into a tree structure and provided basic principles to differentiate child and parent nodes, as well as nodes at the same level (Figure 3).

These principles consist in identifying sets of characteristics that distinguish two close nodes. This principle is known as the differentia principle and it is the basis of contemporary approaches to ontology construction (Roche, 2003) (Troncy et al., 2002).

Figure 3. Porphyry tree[4]

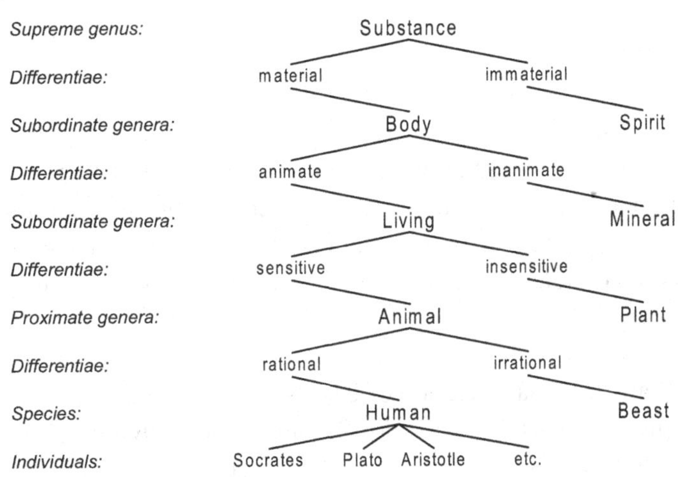

The Latin work *ontologia* first appeared in a text in 1613. The word "ontology" itself (in English) first appeared in a text in 1721 in *An Universal Etymological English Dictionary* by Nathaniel Bailey: *An Account of Being in the Abstract.* It first appeared in a title of a book in 1733 (Notes on the history of ontology http://www.formalontology.it/history.htm). It referred to the philosophical usage of the term. Barry Smith, a philosopher who is now working on ontologies in the biomedical field, gives the following definition: "Ontology as a branch of philosophy is the science of what is, of the kinds and structures of the objects, properties and relations in every area of reality … In simple terms it seeks the classification of entities. Each scientific field will of course have its own preferred ontology, defined by the field's vocabulary and by the canonical formulations of its theories" (Smith, 2003).

The contemporary use of the word "ontology" in computer science and particularly in the semantic web area originates in the work of the Knowledge Systems Laboratory at Stanford in the late 80's to provide a clear and logically defined meaning of knowledge bases, and as a consequence provide a methodology to ensure their sharing and reuse (Gruber, 1991). This resulted in the KIF (Knowledge Interchange Language) language and the Ontolingua language and project (Gruber, 1993).

The first definition referred to in Computer Science comes from the above group: " an ontology defines the basic terms and relations comprising the vocabulary of a topic area as well as the rules for combining terms and relations to define extensions to the vocabulary " (Neches et al., 1991). The most generally referred to definition of an ontology is that given by Grüber: *"an ontology is an explicit specification of a conceptualization"* (Gruber, 1993).

It should be emphasized that there is currently no definition of an ontology that is agreed upon by the computer science community. A fairly complete list of the many other definitions provided since the early 90's, can be found in (Corcho et al., 2003), as well as a survey of methodologies, tools and languages for building ontologies. The question of what is a good or sound ontology remains the subject of an intense debate. Reference authors in this domain are B Smith (http://ontology.buffalo.edu/smith), N Guarino (Guarino et al., 1995) (http://www.loa-cnr.it/guarino.html). In France the work on ontology is centered on terminology (Baneyx et al., 2005), (Roche, 2005).

ONTOLOGIES IN MEDICINE

Medical Classifications

Since Linne's classification of species in 1735, there has been an explosion of the number of classifications in the biomedical field, which poses the problem of reusing data based on different classification systems. With the proliferation of computer tools, this problem has become particularly acute in data mining, where the size of the data set plays an important role; hence, the need to group sets of data from different origins, which is impossible if these data sets use different coding systems. Among the best known and most used we can cite[5]:

- **ICD** (International Statistical Classification of Diseases and Related Health Problems), has been developed by The United Nations World Health Organization (WHO) in Geneva, in collaboration with 10 international centres. It is regularly revised to reflect advances in medicine. The main focus of this classification is *"to promote international comparability in the collection, classification, processing, and presentation of mortality statistics"*[6].
- **SNOMED CT** (Systematized NOmenclature of MEDicine – Clinical Terms) is a clinical terminology. It results from a merging between SNOMED-RT (Reference Terminology) developed by the College of American Pathologists (CAP) and the England and Wales National Health Service's Clinical Terms (a UK-based terminology for primary care previously known as the Read Codes). It was designed to give a common framework to capture and code information about a patient's history, illness and treatment. A new international organisation, the Health Terminology Standards Development Organisation (IHTSDO, also known as SNOMED SDO) acquired the ownership of SNOMED CT on 26 April 2007 and will be responsible for future maintenance and development.
- **MeSH** (Medical Subject Headings) is a medical Thesaurus used to index, catalogue and retrieve the world's medical literature, by PubMed, the NLM's interface to the MEDLINE database. There are 24,767 descriptors in the 2008 edition of the MeSH thesaurus. In addition to these headings, there are more than 172,000 headings called Supplementary Concept Records (formerly Supplementary Chemical Records) within a separate thesaurus. There are also over 97,000 entry terms that assist in finding the most appropriate MeSH Heading; for example, Vitamin C is an entry term to Ascorbic Acid[7].
- **The FMA** (Foundational Model of Anatomy) is a reference ontology in the field of anatomy. Its main focus is to represent anatomical entities, ranging from biological macromolecules to cells, tissues, organs, organ systems, and major body parts, including the entire body (Rosse, 2003). The different parts of the human body and their relationships are described in such a way that they are understandable to humans and can also be browsed, processed and interpreted by machines. The FMA currently contains around 75,000 anatomical items (concepts) and 120,000 terms.
- **GO**, the Gene Ontology, aims "to describe gene and gene product attributes in any organism". It can be broadly split into two parts. The first is the ontology itself (actually three ontologies), each representing a key concept in Molecular Biology: the molecular function of gene products; their role in multi-step biological processes; and their localization to cellular components. The ontologies are continuously updated, and the new version is made available on a monthly basis. The second part is annotation, the characterization of gene products using terms from the ontology.

The members of the GO Consortium submit their data and it is publicly available through the GO website[8].

While most classifications in the biomedical field were designed to answer specific needs, FMA and GO offer a more declarative view of the domain they cover, respectively anatomy and genetics. As a consequence, they are more open to a wide variety of applications.

UMLS[9]

To try to solve the problem of the explosion of biomedical classifications, the National Library of Medicine launched in 1986 the ambitious UMLS program. UMLS stands for Unified Medical Language System and aims at providing a unique entry point for any biomedical item that can be referred to in scientific medical and biological texts or studies. To do so, a so-called meta-thesaurus has been built – and is constantly evolving – in order to cover the whole medical and biological domain. An entry in the meta-thesaurus is a concept with a unique *CUI* (Concept Unique Identifier). The number of concepts in the meta-thesaurus is constantly growing and the 2006 AA release contains 1 276 301 concepts. This size makes it very difficult to manage and it is almost impossible to guarantee the consistency of this set of concepts. The concepts of the meta-thesaurus are linked through the IS_A relationship, which is the main relation, and through other relations such as *Associated_with* and *Occurs_in*. The 2006 version contains 57 different relations. Each UMLS concept is linked to the *same* concept in other classifications. UMLS considers currently 149 classifications. Therefore, it becomes possible, through UMLS, to use data from sources using different classifications, provided that each reference to a data item in a classification is transformed into its corresponding UMLS concept and the UMLS *cui* is used in the global study.

The UMLS program is still active. However, consistency issues are becoming more and more difficult to manage, due to the constantly growing size of the metathesaurus and the poor ontological quality of the UMLS structure. Currently, the OBO initiative appears to be one of the most promising enterprises in the domain of health-related ontologies.

OBO (Open Biology Ontologies)

Data need to be integrated for a better and easier access. One way to achieve data integration is to use ontologies or other terminological resources to annotate data. The absence of a solid theoretical background in the building and the formalization of ontologies have led to a proliferation of ontologies, which itself creates obstacles to integration.

In 2001, Ashburner and Lewis initiated a strategy in order to address the question of: *"how best to represent the proteins, organisms, diseases or drug interactions that are of primary interest in biomedical research"* (Smith et al., 2007) by creating OBO (Open Biology Ontologies), an organization that aims at gathering developers of life-science ontologies. OBO has established the key-principles of sound ontology building and sharing. According to these principles, ontologies must be open and available without any constraint or restriction; they must be scalable and receptive to modification as a result of community debate; they must be orthogonal to other ontologies to facilitate the combination of different ontologies through additional relationships and modular development; they must share the same syntax to facilitate shared software implementation; and they must employ a unique identifier space to enable backward compatibility with legacy annotations as the ontologies evolve.

OBO now holds over 60 ontologies, including the GO and the FMA. It is supported by the NIH Roadmap National Center for Biomedical Ontology (NCBO) through its BioPortal. A group of OBO ontologies developers have initiated the OBO Foundry, a collaborative experiment based on the voluntary acceptance by its participants of an evolving set of principles (available at http://obofoundry.org) that extend those of the original OBO by requiring in addition that ontologies must be developed in a collaborative effort, must use common relations that are unambiguously defined, have to provide procedures for user feedback and for identifying successive versions and have a clearly bounded subject-matter.

RELATED ISSUES

Ontologies and Knowledge Bases

The development of ontologies in Computer Science is anchored in that of Knowledge Bases. In Ross Quillian's PhD thesis (1966 - unpublished), the central theme was "What sort of representational format can permit the *meanings* of words to be stored, so that humanlike use of these meanings is possible? " (Ringland et al., 1987). This sounds today almost as an objective of the Semantic Web, and ontologies appear as an answer to this question. Quillian's answer was Semantic Networks, which made an intensive use of the IS_A relationship, now at the heart of ontologies. However, there was not a clear distinction between concept and instance nodes, and the IS_A relationship could hold between concepts (MALE IS_A HUMAN) as well as between an instance and a concept (John IS_A HUMAN). This made automatic reasoning complex, and Minsky's frames made a clear distinction between classes and instances (Minsky, 1975). The main reasoning process with frame-based systems was *instance classification*. A frame (class) is characterized by attributes (named *slots*) and by range constraints over these attributes. An instance is classified into a given frame (class), if and only if its own attribute values satisfy the range constraints of the same attribute in this frame. For example, the instance *John* with attribute *Age=40* is classified into the class ADULT as it satisfies the constraint Age>18 associated with this class.

In the same decade, the 70's, rule-based systems were developed independently. Their main function was also *instance classification* although this term was not explicitly used. Instead, their role was described as the process of deriving *conclusions* from initial values called *facts*. The experts who designed the Mycin rules, for example, clearly had in mind an underlying taxonomy, which can be guessed at through the rules (Buchanan et al., 1984). Considering the initial *facts* as the attribute values of an instance, the reasoning process supported by the Mycin set of rules can be understood as the classification of this instance in this implicit taxonomy. This was made explicit in the Centaur system, which was a re-writing of the former rule-based system Puff, replacing some rules by the corresponding taxonomy of classes, while other rules were used to calculate the value of an attribute from other attributes (Aikins, 1983).

Frame systems were much criticized because a hierarchy of frames could contradict the set inclusion property inherent to the IS_A relationship. For example, a class OSTRICH could be defined as a subclass of the class BIRD, with the class BIRD defined with the property *flies=true* and an exception *flies=false* attached to the class OSTRICH. This made sound reasoning with frames impossible and the KL-ONE language was designed to overcome this drawback (Brachman et al., 1985). Although the KL-ONE system was never fully implemented because of the complexity of the logic operations involved, it laid the foundations for Description Logics (initially called Terminological Logics). Description Logics are themselves the most widely used support today to represent formal ontologies, in particular through OWL (Ontology Web Language), which is the standard proposed by the W3C (World Wide Web Consortium) for ontology representation.

The two most important reasoning operations (also called inference) supported by Description Logics are *concept classification* and *instance classification.* Concept classification is the process of identifying the inclusion property between two concepts through their logical definition. For example, given the following two definitions:

ADULT ≡ PERSON and Age>18
SENIOR ≡ PERSON and Age>65

Concept classification will establish that SENIOR IS_A ADULT, which can also be read as SENIOR ➔ ADULT, SENIOR *implies* ADULT, ADULT *subsumes* SENIOR, or SENIOR *is subsumed by* ADULT. *Concept classification* is the discovery of the IS_A relationship (also called *subsumption*) between two concepts from their sole definition.

Instance classification can be seen as a particular case of concept classification and was dealt with in this way in the first DL systems. Given the instance defined by *John≡PERSON and Age=40*, considering it as a concept (the concept *JOHN* with the single instance *John*) would establish that *JOHN is subsumed by* ADULT. This is instance classification (the classification of the instance *John* into the class ADULT).

However, implementing instance classification through the concept classification process was too expensive, as concept classification is a complex operation, while instance classification can be implemented in a simpler and more efficient manner. Current DL systems distinguish the two operations, as does RACER, one of the most widely used reasoners associated with the implementation of the OWL language in the Protégé environment.

Consistency checking of a set of concepts in a DL is also a side effect of concept classification. If a concept is subsumed by no other concept, either it is a concept at the top of a hierarchy, or its definition is inconsistent (he cannot have a parent concept, due to an inconsistent definition).

Within the Noesis project (www.noesis-eu.org) we have implemented a subset of the MeSH thesaurus in OWL. Although the MeSH thesaurus cannot claim an ontology status, implementing it in OWL and applying the concept classification scheme made possible the discovery of a cycle in the taxonomy of concepts in the first version of the 2007 MeSH. This cycle has been removed in the following version.

One can see the advantages of a formal definition of an ontology, for example through a DL formalism. Non-explicit IS_A relationships between concepts can be discovered automatically, and the whole set of concepts can be checked for consistency. However, implementing an ontology in a formal language can be a difficult task, especially for large ontologies. This was done in the Galen project (Rector et al., 1993) for a subset of the medical field, using the GRAIL DL. The OWL language now offers the possibility of choosing three degrees of complexity in the description of an ontology, by proposing three sublanguages:

- **OWL lite**, which is syntactically simple and adapted to the description of simple hierarchies with simple constraints.

- **OWL DL**, based on Description Logics, which enables automated reasoning and checking for inconsistencies.
- **OWL Full**, which is highly expressive but which cannot guarantee decidability.

Ontology and Terminology

Terminologies focus on *words* and their relationships; where the main relationships are hyperonymy and its inverse, hyponymy. Ontologies focus on *concepts* and their relationships. Concepts are mainly organized through the *subsumption* (or IS_A) relationship, which corresponds to the hyperonymy/hyponymy relationships in terminologies and in thesauri. It organizes concepts by abstracting common characteristics, leading to a hierarchy of concepts corresponding to a taxonomic organization of objects (Roche, 2005). Moreover, ontologies offer the possibility to create new relationships, thus increasing their expressive power.

Ontologies and terminologies are used for the main purpose of providing a shared conceptualization of a specific part of the world to a community of users, aiming to facilitate knowledge communication. Gamper provides four criteria to distinguish the two notions (Gamper et al., 1999):

- **The formal framework of their definition:** The science of Terminology uses the plain text in the natural language to define the meaning of terms. The correct interpretation of the intended meaning depends on the user. Ontologies explicitly specify the conceptual knowledge by the use of a formal language with a clear semantic, which avoids ambiguous interpretation of terms;
- **Computational support:** The available tools differ for the two disciplines: most currently used terminologies provide little or no semantics for both an explicit representation of knowledge and for data maintenance. While for ontologies, through the use of formal representation language, e.g., Description Logics (Nardi and Brachman, 2003), it is possible to check their consistency, and to infer new knowledge.
- **Users:** terminologies are human user-oriented (translators and domain experts are their primary users). Ontologies are mainly developed for knowledge sharing between agents (human and machines);
- **Natural language usage:** The terminology focuses on knowledge transfer as a linguistic activity, i.e., natural language exploration in order to identify all terms used by people to talk about underlying concepts, whereas ontologies are intended mainly for computational use and can often ignore the importance of naming concepts with "understandable" terms (e.g., UMLS CUI)

In France, the ontology work is much anchored in terminology (Rousselo et al., 2002) (Roche, 2005).

Ontologies and Information Retrieval

Traditional information retrieval systems mostly rely on keyword-based search. They only take into account the co-occurrence of words to represent the documents and the query. However, a relevant document does not always contain the same words as the query. One of the promising solutions to this problem is the use of an external semantic resource in the information retrieval process. Such systems are characterized by the notion of a conceptual space in which documents and queries are represented, in opposition to the word space found in traditional models (Baeza-Yates et al., 99). Since the end of the nineties, ontologies offer this conceptual space upon which these systems depend to retrieve a part of the semantics of both documents and queries.

The identification of concepts in a document (concept mapping) is not an easy task. Moreover, one of the limitations of this approach is that the quality of the search depends on the coverage of the ontology. In order to support concept-based Information Retrieval, an ontology should contain all the terms that can be found in the documents searched for, and also the terms and the expressions used in the queries by people searching these documents.

Using the ontology of breast cancer presented in §2.1.1 to index documents and to interpret queries, any of the terms associated with the concept LYMPHEDEMA OF ARM would be equivalent in a user query. For instance, asking for *lymphedema of arm, arm lymphedema, edema of arm, arm edema, arm swelling, lymphœdème du bras, œdème lymphatique du bras, gros bras, gonflement du bras* would result in the same set of documents.

In the Noesis project, where objectives included concept-based Information Retrieval and annotation, a significant effort was made for the enrichment of the vocabulary of the concept-based terminology[10] that was used, in order to ensure a good coverage of texts to be indexed by this terminology (Simonet et al., 2006).

Ontology Design

Ontology building is not an easy task and one of the major bottlenecks in developing bio-ontologies is the lack of a unified methodology. Different methodologies have been proposed for different scenarios, but there is no agreed-upon standard methodology for building ontologies, contrary to the database domain, for example, with the Entity-Relationship Model. The building process usually involves domain experts to reflect current knowledge about the concerned domain.

Projects about ontology building started in the early 90's. In 1995, Ushold and King proposed a method to build an ontology from scratch (Ushold et al., 1995), which comprises four steps: identify the purpose, build the ontology by the identification of the key concepts and relationships in the domain of interest, evaluate it, and document it.

Literature scanning for deciding on the basic concepts and relationships to insert in the ontology may be useful to help building an ontology. However, since building an ontology from a huge amount of literature data is a difficult and time-consuming task, a number of tools such as TextToOnto (Maedche, 2004) and its successor Text2Onto (Cimiano, 2005), TERMINAE (Biebow et al., 1999), the ASIUM system (Faure, 1998), Ontologos (Roche, 2003) OntoLearn (Velardi, 2005) or OntoLT (Buitelaar, 2003) have been developed in order to support the user in constructing ontologies from a given set of (textual) data. The common element to these frameworks is the use of natural language processing for providing features to be used to learn ontological structures. For instance, OntoLT is an ontology learning plug-in for the Protégé ontology editor which basically makes use of the internal structure of noun phrases to derive ontological knowledge from texts. The OntoLearn framework (Velardi et al., 2005) mainly focuses on the problem of word sense disambiguation, i.e., finding the correct sense of a word with respect to a general ontology or lexical database. TextToOnto and Text2Onto are frameworks implementing a variety of algorithms for diverse ontology learning subtasks: relevance measures for term extraction, algorithms for taxonomy construction as well as techniques for learning relations between concepts. Text2Onto also takes into account the fact that the document collection can change and thus avoids starting the whole learning process from scratch every time a change occurs (Cimiano, 2005). TERMINAE is a tool that integrates the design and editing steps. It brings together both Natural Language Processing (NLP) Tools and Knowledge Engineering tools. NLP tools support the extraction of all the occurrences of the different terms, and the definition of the different meanings, called notions, of each term. Knowledge engineering tools associate concepts with terms and insert them into the ontology.

Ontology Representation

Several languages, based on the XML syntax, have been developed for the use of ontologies within the Semantic Web infrastructure. The most representative are RDF/RDFS, the W3C recommendation for metadata representation, OIL, DAML+OIL and now OWL which is the W3C recommendation for ontology representation.

SKOS is an area of work developing specifications and standards to support the use of knowledge organization systems (KOS) such as thesauri, classification schemes, subject heading systems and taxonomies within the framework of the Semantic Web. SKOS provides a standard way to represent knowledge organization systems using RDF, which allows it to be passed between computer applications in an interoperable way. The SKOS specifications are currently published as W3C Working Drafts but they will soon become a W3C recommendation. In the Noesis project, the OWL representation of the MeSH thesaurus also used SKOS elements that were necessary to represent multilingual aspects of the associated vocabulary (e.g., choose a preferred term for each language), which could not be easily achieved in pure OWL.

The Protégé environment is the most used ontology editor. However, its poor user-friendliness has led the OBO group to design their own ontology editor and format, better suited for use by non-IT people.

Although they are currently less in fashion than Description Logics, Conceptual Graphs offer a graphical representation formalism to implement ontologies (Sowa: Building, sharing and merging ontologies, http://www.jfsowa.com/ontology/ontoshar.htm).

DATA MINING AND ONTOLOGIES

The interaction between data mining and ontologies can be considered in two ways:

1. The use of ontologies in data mining processes, either to include domain knowledge in the input information or to represent the results.
2. The use of data mining techniques to build ontologies.

In both cases, it is mainly text mining that is concerned. Text mining aims to extract useful knowledge from textual data or documents (Chen, 2001) (Hearst, 1999). In the biomedical domain, this process is very useful since the huge and rapidly increasing volume of scientific literature makes finding relevant information increasingly difficult. For example, the identification of relationships among different biological entities, e.g., genes, proteins, diseases, drugs and chemicals, etc, is an important concern for biological researchers. While such information can be extracted from different types of biological data (e.g., gene and protein sequences, protein structures), a significant source of such knowledge is the biological textual research literature which is increasingly being made available as large-scale public-domain electronic databases (e.g., the Medline database). Automated extraction of such relationships (e.g., gene A *inhibits* protein B) from textual data can significantly enhance biological research productivity in several ways: by keeping researchers up-to-date with the state-of-the-art in their research domain, by helping them visualize biological pathways, and by generating likely new hypotheses concerning novel interactions, some of which may be good candidates for further biological research and validation (Palakal et al., 2005).

Examples of text mining applications include document classification, document clustering, concept extraction, information extraction and summarization. Using an ontology for document clustering has several advantages: it is possible to cluster documents written in several languages since concepts are *language-independent* and the use of concepts helps reduce the size of data, which, in turn, reduces processing time (Pham et al., 2007). Ontologies also offer a natural support to the extraction of semantic relations between entities. For example, the Genescene system utilizes an ontology-based approach to relation extraction by integrating the Gene Ontology, the Human Genome Nomenclature, and the UMLS (Leroy and Chen, 2005).

Ontologies offer a natural support to data mining in that they provide semantically sound classes to collect and organize data. One important principle behind the use of ontologies to represent the input data in data mining processes is that, by increasing the conceptual level of input data, one can also expect to obtain results at a higher conceptual level. This has been demonstrated in several papers. (Hotho et al., 2003) have shown that using ontologies as filters in term selection, prior to the application of the K-means clustering algorithm, increases the tightness and relative isolation of document clusters as a measure of improvement. Other examples can be found in a new book on data mining with ontologies that presents recent and ongoing research and industrial work in this domain (Nigro et al., 2007).

Text mining is also used in the construction and enrichment of ontologies (Mothe et al., 2007). The statistical analysis of texts of a domain may help exhibit clusters of terms that are candidate concepts for this domain (Karoui et al., 2006), and the discovery of relationships between such clusters of terms can evoke possible relationships between concepts. Although much work is done on the automation of ontology construction (Cimiano et al., 2005), the use of knowledge discovery in texts may help the ontology designer to identify concepts and structure them through IS_A and other relationships, in a semi-automatic way. Ontologos and Terminae are examples of such systems that use linguistic techniques to support the building of ontologies (Roche, 2003) (Biebow et al., 1999).

CONCLUSION

In this chapter, we have provided an overview of ontologies with the objective of helping people involved in Data Mining in the biological field to apprehend the possible contribution of ontologies to their discipline. We did not answer explicitly the question "What is an ontology" and this question is still open to debate. An ontology of ontologies would be needed to organize the various points of view on this question. The same problem arises concerning the term Knowledge Base, and the two notions are strongly related. We have shed some light on some aspects of ontologies that seem important to us. Some of these aspects would justify further developments and we have tried to provide references to major publications in the relevant fields.

Integration aspects are of vital importance in data mining as data from various sources can be used in the input data set. The principle of using an ontology to unify input data from different sources via the concepts of this ontology now appears obvious. However, its implementation with real and heterogeneous databases is not so simple and constitutes the matter of active research and technical work (Lenzerini, 2002). Database integration requires establishing mappings between the schemas of the constituent databases or between these schemas and a global schema built for that purpose and which reflects the conceptual structure of the ontology. Such mappings can be represented as SQL views but recent approaches use Description Logics to implement an ontology-based representation of them (Dejing et al., 2006). We can also note that integrating database schemas is a problem similar to that of integrating different ontologies on the same domain; this problem is known as ontology alignment (Euzenat et al., 2004).

Data mining aims at extracting knowledge from data, thus creating *a posteriori* knowledge, whereas ontologies provide *a priori* knowledge that can be used in the data mining process, as well at its start by providing semantically sound classes to collect and organize data, as at its end to represent the results. One key of the success of ontologies in many domains, including the biomedical field, is that they provide semantics of domain knowledge in a human as well as in a computer-readable form. Data mining techniques can also be used to help building ontologies from texts. Note that some concept-based terminology, e.g., wordnet, which is sometimes (improperly) considered as an ontology, could be used to process the input data by replacing words by low-level concepts of this ontology in the texts to be analyzed. This ontology represents *a priori* knowledge, while the ontology obtained through text mining constitutes *a posteriori* knowledge, and one expects the resulting ontology to provide a description of the domain at a higher conceptual level than the initial one.

We conclude by quoting the editors of a recent book, Data Mining with Ontologies (Nigro et al., 2007) where they recall that: "One of the most important and challenging problems in data mining is the definition of the prior knowledge: this can be originated from the process or the domain. This contextual information may help select the appropriate information, features or techniques, decrease the space of hypothesis, represent the output in a most comprehensible way and improve the whole process. Therefore we need a conceptual model to help represent this knowledge … As a result, ontological foundation is a precondition for efficient automated usage of knowledge discovery information".

REFERENCES

Aikins, J. S. (1983). Prototypal Knowledge in Expert Systems. *Artificial Intelligence, 20*(2),163-210.

Baeza-Yates, R. A., & Ribeiro-Neto, B. A. (1999). *Modern Information Retrieval.* ACM Press / Addison-Wesley.

Baneyx, A., Malaisé, V., Charlet, J., Zweigenbaum, P., & Bachimont, B. Synergie entre analyse distributionnelle et patrons lexico-syntaxiques pour la construction d'ontologies différentielles. *In Actes Conférence TIA-2005* (pp. 31-42). Rouen.

Biebow, B., & Szulman, S. (1999). Terminae: A linguistic-based tool for the building of a domain ontology. *In proceedings of the 11th European Workshop, Knowledge Acquisition, Modeling and Management (EKAW' 99)* (pp. 49-66). Dagstuhl Castle, Germany.

Bonnevay, S., & Lamure, M. (2003). Bases de connaissances anatomo-fonctionnelles : application au cerveau et au cœur. *Santé et Systémique*, *7*(3), 47-75, Hermès.

Brachman, R. J., & Schmolze, J. G. (1985). An overview of the KL-ONE knowledge representation system. *Cognitive Science 9*(2), 171-216.

Buchanan, B. G., & Shortliffe, E. H. (Eds.). (1984). *Rule-Based Expert Systems: The MYCIN Experiments of the Stanford Heuristic Programming Project.* Reading, MA: Addison-Wesley

Buitelaar, P., Olejnik, D., & Sintek., M. (2003). OntoLT: A protégé plug-in for ontology extraction from text. *In Proceedings of the International Semantic Web Conference (ISWC).*

Chen, H. (2001). *Knowledge Management Systems: A Text Mining Perspective.* Tucson, AZ: The University of Arizona.

Cimiano, P., & Vorlker, J. (2005). Text2Onto – A Framework for Ontology Learning and Data-driven Change Discovery. In Andres Montoyo, Rafael Munoz, Elisabeth Metais (Ed.), *the 10th International Conference on Applications of Natural Language to Information Systems (NLDB), Lecture Notes in Computer Science. Springer: 3513.* (pp. 227-238). Alicante, Spain.

Corcho, O., Lopez, M. F., & Perez, A. G. (2003). Methodologies, tools and languages for building ontologies. Where is their meeting point? *Data & Knowledge Engineering, 46*(1), 41-64.

Dejing, D., & Paea, L. (2006). Ontology-based Integration for Relational Databases. *In Proceedings of the 2006 ACM symposium on Applied computing* (pp. 461-466). Dijon, France.

Euzenat, J., Barrasa, J., Bouquet, P., Bo, J.D., et al. (2004). State of the Art on Ontology Alignment. *Knowledge Web, Statistical Research Division, Room 3000-4, Bureau of the Census, Washington, DC, 20233-9100 USA,* deliverable 2.2.3.

Faure, D., & Nedellec, C. (1998). A corpus-based conceptual clustering method for verb frames and ontology. *In Proceedings of the LREC Workshop on Adapting lexical and corpus resources to sublanguages and applications.*

Gamper, J., Nejdl, W., & Wolpers, M. (1999). Combining ontologies and terminologies in information systems. *In Proc. 5th International Congress on Terminology and knowledge Engineering.* Innsbruck, Austria.

Gruber, T. R. (1991). The Role of Common Ontology in Achieving Sharable, Reusable Knowledge Base. In J. Allen, Fikes and E. Sandewall, Eds. *Principles of knowledge representations and reasoning,* Cambridge, MA, Morgan Kaufmann.

Gruber, T. R. (1993). A translation approach to portable ontology specification. *Knowledge Acquisition,* 5(2), Special issue: Current issues in knowledge modeling, 199-220.

Guarino, N., Carrara, M., & Giaretta, P. (1995). Ontologies and knowledge bases: towards a terminological clarification. In N. Mars (Ed.), *Towards Very Large Knowledge Bases, Knowledge Building and Knowledge Sharing* (pp. 25-32). IOS Press, Amsterdam.

Hearst, M. A. (1999). Untangling Text Data Mining. In Proceedings of ACL'99: *the 37th Annual Meeting of the Association for Computational Linguistics* (pp. 20-26). Maryland.

Hotho, A., Staab, S., & Stumme, G. (2003). Ontologies improve text document clustering. *In Proceedings of the 3rd IEEE conference on Data Mining* (pp. 541-544). Melbourne, FL.

Karoui, L., Aufaure, M.A., & Bennacer, N. (2006). Context-based Hierarchical Clustering for the Ontology Learning. *The 2006 IEEE/WIC/ACM International Conference on Web Intelligence (WI-06) jointly with the 2006 IEEE/WIC/ACM International Conference on Data Mining (ICDM-06)* (pp. 420-427). Hong-Kong.

Maedche, A., & Staab, S. (2004). Ontology learning. In S. Staab and R. Studer (Ed.), *Handbook on Ontologies* (pp. 173-189). Springer.

McCray, A. T., & Tse, T. (2003). Understanding search failures in consumer health information systems. *Proc AMIA Symp* (pp. 430-434).

Messai, R., Zeng, Q., Mousseau, M., & Simonet, M. (2006). Building a Bilingual French-English Patient-Oriented Terminology for Breast Cancer. *In proceedings of MedNet 2006, Internet and Medicine.* Toronto, Canada.

Minsky, M. (1975). A Framework for Representing Knowledge. In The Psychology of Computer Vision (Ed.), *P.H. Winston, McGraw-Hill* (pp. 211-277). New York.

Mothe, J., & Hernandez, N. (2007). TtoO: Mining thesaurus and texts to build and update a domain ontology. In H. O. Nigro, S. G. Císaro, and D.Xodo. Idea Group Inc (Ed.), *Data Mining with Ontologies: Implementations, Findings, and Frameworks.*

Nardi, D., & Brachman, R. J. (2003). An introduction to description logics. In F. Baader, D. Calvanese, D.L. McGuinness, D. Nardi, P.F. Patel-Schneider (Ed.), *the Description Logic Handbook* (pp. 5-44). Cambridge University Press.

Neches, R., Fikes, R.E., Finin, T., Gruber, T.R., Senator, T., & Swartout, T. (1991). Enabling technology for knowledge sharing. *AI Magazine 12*(3), 36-56.

Nigro, H. O., Gonzalez Cisaro, S. E., & Xodo, D. H. (Ed.). (2007). *Data Mining with ontologies – Implementations, findings and frameworks.* Information Science Reference, IGI Gobal.

Palakal, M., Mukhopadhyay, S., & Stephens, M. (2005). Identification of Biological Relationships from Text Documents. *Book Series: Integrated Series In Information Systems. Book: Medical Informatics, 8*, 449-489.

Pham, M.H., Bernhard, D., Diallo, G., Messai, R., & Simonet, M. (2007). SOM-based Clustering of Multilingual Documents Using an Ontology. In H. O. Nigro, S. G. Císaro, and D.Xodo. Idea Group Inc (Ed.), *Data Mining with Ontologies: Implementations, Findings, and Frameworks.*

Rector, A. L., & Nowlan, W. A. (1993). The GALEN Project. *Computer Methods and Programs in Biomedicine, 45,* 75-78.

Ringland, G. A., & Duce, D. A. (1987). *Approaches in Knowledge Representation: An Introduction.* John Wiley& Sons.

Roche, C. (2003). *The Differentia Principle: a Cornerstone for Ontology.* Knowledge Management and Philosophy Workshop in WM 2003 Conference, Luzern.

Roche, C. (2005). Terminologie et ontologie. *LAROUSSE – Revue, 157,* 1-11.

Rosse, C., & Mejino, J. L. V. (2003). Reference ontology for bioinformatics: the Foundational Model of Anatomy. *J Biomed Inform, 36*(6), 478-500.

Simonet, M., Patriarche, R., Bernhard, D., Diallo, G., Ferriol, S., & Palmer, P. (2006). Multilingual Ontology Enrichment for Semantic Annotation and Retrieval of Medical Information. *MEDNET'2006,* Toronto - Canada.

Smith, B. (2003). Ontology. Chapter in L. Floridi (ed.), *Blackwell Guide to the Philosophy of Computing and Information* (pp. 155-166). Oxford, Blackwell.

Smith, B., Ashburner, M., Rosse, C., Bard, J., Bug, W., Ceusters, W., Goldberg, L. J., Eilbeck, K., Ireland, A., Mungall, C. J., Leontis, N., Rocca-Serra, P., Ruttenberg, A., Sansone, S., Scheuermann, R. H., Shah, N., Whetzel, P. L., & Lewis, S. (2007). The OBO Foundry: coordinated evolution of ontologies to support biomedical data integration. *Nat Biotech,* 25(11), 1251-1255.

Troncy, R., & Isaac, A. (2002). DOE: une mise en œuvre d'une méthode de structuration différentielle pour les ontologies. *In Actes 13e journées francophones sur Ingénierie des Connaissances (IC)* (pp. 63-74).

Uschold, M., & Jasper, R. (1999). A Framework for Understanding and Classifying Ontology Applications. *In: Proc.IJCAI99 Workshop on Ontologies and Problem-Solving Methods.* Stockholm.

Uschold, M., & King, M. (1995). *Towards a methodology for building ontologies.* Workshop on Basic Ontological Issues in Knowledge Sharing, held in conduction with IJCAI-95.

Velardi, P., Navigli, R., Cuchiarelli, A., & Neri, F. (2005). Evaluation of Ontolearn, a methodology for automatic population of domain ontologies. In P. Buitelaar, P. Cimiano, and B. Magnini (Eds), *Ontology Learning from Text: Methods, Applications and Evaluation.* IOS Press.

KEY TERMS

Data Mining: Data mining, also referred to as knowledge discovery in databases (KDD), is a process of finding new, interesting, previously unknown, potentially useful, and ultimately understandable patterns from very large volumes of data (Nigro et al., 2007)

Information Retrieval: Information Retrieval (IR) is concerned with the indexing and retrieval of information in documents. Although any kind of document can be indexed and searched for, IR has been first and mainly applied to texts. Active research is currently devoted to content-based indexing of other types of documents such as images, videos and audio content. Automatic indexing of texts relies on a thesaurus. Contemporary IR tends to use ontologies associated with multilingual terminologies in order to make the search less language-dependent (e.g., English documents can be returned for queries posed in French, provided they refer to the same concept).

Knowledge Base: The term "Knowledge Base" was first used in the seventies to designate a set of expert rules to be processed by an "inference engine" along with the " facts " that represent the current situation that the (expert) system is to identify though the chaining of expert rules. In modern systems, starting with frame-based systems, this operation is known as *instance classification.* The most recent KB systems, based upon Description Logics, also consider *concept classification,* which consists in ordering concepts through the subsumption (inclusion) relation.

Medical Classification: Medical classifications provide the terminology of the medical domain (or a part of it). There are more than 100 medical classifications currently in use, most of them being specific of a subdomain (e.g., brain) or oriented towards a specific usage (e.g., MeSH for bibliographical indexing).

Ontology: An ontology is a structured description of a domain under the form of concepts and relations between these concepts. The IS-A relationship provides a taxonomic skeleton while other relations reflect the semantics of the domain. Definitions (either formal or informal) can be associated with concepts, as well as terminological variants, possibly in different languages. Usual definitions are : "An ontology is a specification of conceptualization" (Gruber) and " An ontology describes the concepts and relationships that can exist and formalizes the terminology in a domain " (Gruninger & Lee)

Terminology: Terminology deals with terms definition and usage, in general or in a specific context (e.g., medical terminology). According to authors, the definition of terminology vary from the study of terms to the actual sets of terms of a domain, possibly structured, which brings terminological work near to ontological work. This closeness is illustrated by the neologism "ontoterminology" which has been proposed by C. Roche at the TOTh conference in 2007.

ENDNOTES

1. The Ontology Web Language : http://www.w3.org/2004/OWL/
2. This is not strictly true, as there are concepts that exist only in some culture and in a given language. However, in the scientific domain such an approximation is usually considered as valid.
3. Aristotle's categories: substance, quantity, quality, relation, place, time, position, state, action and affection.
4. http://faculty.washington.edu/smcohen/433/PorphyryTree.html accessed on April 14th, 2008
5. http://www.openclinical.org/medicalterminologiesLst.html
6. Colorado Department of Public Health and Environment. New International Classification of Diseases (ICD-10): the history and impact. Brief. Mar 2001; no.41.
7. http://www.nlm.nih.gov/pubs/factsheets/mesh.html
8. http://en.wikipedia.org/wiki/Gene_Ontology
9. The Unified Medical Language System. http://umlsks.nlm.nih.gov
10. In the course of the NOESIS project it was improperly called an ontology. Although it was represented in OWL, its structure was strictly that of the MeSH thesaurus.

Chapter III
Cost-Sensitive Learning in Medicine

Alberto Freitas
University of Porto, Portugal; CINTESIS, Portugal

Pavel Brazdil
LIAAD - INESC Porto L.A., Portugal;
University of Porto, Portugal

Altamiro Costa-Pereira
University of Porto, Portugal; CINTESIS, Portugal

ABSTRACT

This chapter introduces cost-sensitive learning and its importance in medicine. Health managers and clinicians often need models that try to minimize several types of costs associated with healthcare, including attribute costs (e.g. the cost of a specific diagnostic test) and misclassification costs (e.g. the cost of a false negative test). In fact, as in other professional areas, both diagnostic tests and its associated misclassification errors can have significant financial or human costs, including the use of unnecessary resource and patient safety issues. This chapter presents some concepts related to cost-sensitive learning and cost-sensitive classification and its application to medicine. Different types of costs are also present, with an emphasis on diagnostic tests and misclassification costs. In addition, an overview of research in the area of cost-sensitive learning is given, including current methodological approaches. Finally, current methods for the cost-sensitive evaluation of classifiers are discussed.

INTRODUCTION

Data mining and machine learning methods are important tools in the process of knowledge discovery and, in medicine, knowledge is crucial for biomedical research, decision making support and health management.

Classification methods, an important subject in data mining, can be used to generate models that describe classes or predict future data trends. Their generic aim is to build models that allow predicting the value of one categorical variable from the known values of other categorical or continuous variables. In its generic concept, classification is a common and pragmatic tool in clinical medicine. In fact, it is the basis for deciding for a diagnosis and, therefore, for the choice of a therapeutic strategy. In addition, classification can play an important role in evidence-based medicine as it can be used as an instrument for assessing and comparing results (Bellazzi and Zupan, 2008).

The majority of existing classification methods was designed to minimize the number of errors, but there are many reasons for considering costs in medicine. Diagnostic tests, such as other health interventions, are not free and budgets are limited. In fact, real-world applications often require classifiers that minimize the total cost, including misclassifications costs (each error has an associated cost) and diagnostic test (attribute) costs.

In medicine a *false negative* prediction, for instance failing to detect a disease, can have fatal consequences, while a *false positive* prediction although mostly being less serious (e.g. giving a drug to a patient that does not have a certain disease) can also induce serious safety consequences (e.g. being operated for a non-existing cancer). Each diagnostic test has also a financial cost and this may help us to decide whether to use it or not. It is thus necessary to know both misclassification and tests costs.

Misclassification and test costs are the most important costs, but there are also other types of costs. Cost-sensitive learning is the area of machine learning that deals with costs in inductive learning.

In this chapter we give an overview of different types of costs associated with data used in medical decision making, present some strategies that can be used to obtain cost-sensitive classifiers and discuss current cost-sensitive approaches in more detail. We also present some techniques to visualize and compare the performance of classifiers over the full range of possible class distributions and misclassification costs. Finally, we conclude and point out some future trends.

COST-SENSITIVE CLASSIFICATION

Classification is one of the main tasks in knowledge discovery and data mining (Mitchell, 1997). It has been object of study in areas as machine learning, statistics and neural networks. There are many approaches for classification, including decision trees, Bayesian classifiers, neural classifiers, discriminant analysis, support vector machines, and rule induction, among many others.

The goal of classification is to correctly assign examples to one of a finite number of classes. In classification problems the performance of classifiers is usually measured using an *error rate*. The error rate is the proportion of errors detected in all instances and is an indicator of the global classifier performance. A large number of classification algorithms assume that the errors have the same cost and, because of that, are normally designed to minimize the number of errors (the zero-one loss). In these cases, the error rate is equivalent to assigning the same cost to all classification errors. For instance, in the case of a binary classification, false positives and false negatives would have equal cost. Nevertheless, in many situations, each type error may have a different associated cost.

In fact, in the majority of daily situations, decisions have distinct costs, and a bad decision may have serious consequences. It is therefore important to take into account the different costs associated to decisions, i.e., classification costs.

In this context, we may designate *cost-sensitive classification* when costs are ignored during the learning phase of a classifier and are only used when predicting new cases. In the other hand, we may call *cost-sensitive learning* when costs are considered during the learning phase and ignored, or not, when predicting new cases. In general, the cost-sensitive learning is a better option, with better results, as it considers costs during the process of generation of a new classifier. Cost-sensitive learning is the sub-area of Machine Learning concerned with situations of non-uniformity in costs.

When speaking about cost-sensitive classification or cost-sensitive learning we normally consider it as the problem of minimizing total costs associated to decisions.

This area is of special importance in medicine. For instance, when a specific disease is not timely detected (because the result of the test was negative), it can have possible negative consequences. In a diagnostic test there is normally a higher cost for false negatives compared to false positives, that is, the cost is higher when the disease is present and the result of the test indicates the opposite. To avoid this type of situations, more sensitive tests are normally used as, for instance, in medical screening programmes. These tests are normally also more costly.

In other situations, to confirm a particular diagnosis or when a false positive result may have negative consequences to the patient (for instance, in a test for the detection of HIV – human immunodeficiency virus), diagnostic tests with high specificity should be used. In this case, the costs associated to decisions are much different when compared with the previous case.

For a decision-making model, and in addition to misclassification costs, it is important to consider also other costs, as those related to a specific medical test.

Some types of classifiers can be easily modified to incorporate costs. In the process of building a decision tree for instance, the information gain (or the gain ratio, or alternatively the Gini index) is traditionally used to determine which attribute to choose in each node of the tree. If our aim is to minimize costs it makes sense that the strategies for building the tree minimize both misclassification and test (attribute) costs. If attribute costs are not considered, then the most expensive attributes could be present in top nodes of the tree, in equality of circumstances with other less expensive ones. This could consequently lead to higher total costs as tests associated with top nodes of the tree have a higher probability of being requested than those at leaf nodes.

Let us suppose, for instance, that the class to predict is whether a patient has (or has not) a brain tumour. When the medical doctor receives a new patient with a headache he probably will not immediately request a CT scan (computerized axial tomography scan). Despite the high discriminative power of this diagnostic test, the doctor has also in mind the cost of the test and normally, first, he will start by asking questions to the patient and requesting other simpler and more economic tests (Núñez, 1991).

In medicine, a diagnostic test can be related to an attribute in machine learning: the medical test can be obtained at a cost (the cost of the attribute) and a wrong diagnosis has a cost (misclassification cost). Both types of costs (for diagnostic tests and for errors in the diagnosis) should be considered when building a medical classification model.

The minimization of costs is definitely an important issue, as medical interventions are not free and health budgets are limited (Eccles and Mason, 2001). In the next sections we discuss this issue in more detail.

Types of Costs

There are many possible types of costs that may occur in medical classification problems. Next, we will briefly present some of the main types including misclassification and test costs.

Turney (2000) provides a general overview of the many possible types of costs associated with classification problems. According to Turney, the majority of the machine learning literature ignores all types of costs. Only a few have investigated the costs of misclassification errors, and a small minority studied others types of costs.

In the same work Turney presents a taxonomy for many types of costs that may be involved in learning problems (e.g., in the induction of decision trees). The proposed taxonomy helps in the organization of the cost-sensitive learning literature. The costs are categorized as cost of misclassification errors, cost of tests, cost of classifying cases (by an expert), cost of intervention, cost of unwanted achievements, cost of computation, cost of cases, cost of human-computer interaction, and cost of instability:

- **Cost of misclassification errors:** In many classification problems the cost of errors is not equal for different classes. So, minimizing the costs of misclassified examples is more important than minimizing the number of misclassified examples.
- **Cost of diagnostic tests:** Many medical tests have an associated cost. Usually, tests (attributes) should only be measured if they cost less than misclassification costs.
- **Cost of classifying cases:** Before or during learning, the cost of asking an expert to classify examples with unknown class. In some situations unclassified examples are abundant but labelling (determining the correct class) is expensive. This type of learning problems is called *active learning.*
- **Cost of intervention:** Cost needed to modify a specific process that might change the cost of the attribute (this is not the cost of the attribute).
- **Cost of unwanted achievements:** Cost associated with incorrect predictions (misclassification errors) that result from changes in a specific process.
- **Cost of computation:** In certain circumstances the cost of computation should be considered. Different types of computational complexity can represent different type of costs to be considered.
- **Cost of cases:** Cost associated with the acquisition of examples for learning. Sometimes the acquisition of new cases is very expensive (one of the reasons for the use of the learning curve).
- **Cost of human-computer interaction:** Human cost associated with the utilization of the learning software, including data preparation, attribute selection, definition of parameters, output analysis, and model evaluation.
- **Cost of instability:** In learned models, instability can be seen as a cost and stability as a benefit (a repeated experiment should produce similar results).

In the previous enumeration, the cost of misclassification errors and the cost of tests are the ones that are most commonly used and probably are the most important. These costs can be measured in different units, such as monetary units, temporal units (minutes, hours, days), or units related to the quality of life of a patient (health-related quality of life).

Misclassification Costs

For a problem with n classes there is normally an associated cost matrix, where the element in line A and column B represents the cost of classifying a case from class A as a case from class B. Usually the cost is zero when $A = B$ (any cost matrix can be transformed to an equivalent matrix with zeros along the main diagonal). Typically, misclassification costs are constant, that is, the cost is the same for any instance classified in class A but belonging to class B. The traditional error rate measure occurs when the cost is 0 for $A = B$ and 1 for all other situations.

In some cases, the cost of misclassification errors could be conditional, that is, it could be dependent on specific features or dependent on a particular moment in time. In a bank, the cost associated with the non-detection of fraudulent transactions is clearly associated with the amount involved in each case, because the bank is responsible for the loss of money due to fraud (Elkan, 2001). The same situation occurs in the telecommunications fraud domain (Hollmén et al., 2000). In medicine, the cost of prescribing a specific drug to an allergic patient may be different than prescribing that drug to a non allergic patient. A wrong diagnosis may have different consequences (costs) for each patient as, for instance, for elder patients or for those with particular comorbidities.

The cost of misclassification can be associated with the particular moment it occurs. A medical device (incorporating sensor(s)) can issue an alarm when a problem occurs and, in this situation, the cost is dependent simultaneously on the correctness of the classification and on the time the alarm is issued, that is, the alarm will only be useful if there is time for an adequate action. Misclassification costs can also be dependent on the classification of other cases. In the previous example, if an alarm is correctly and consecutively issued for the same problem, then the benefit of the first alarm should be greater than the benefit of the others (Fawcett and Provost, 1999).

Costs of Diagnostic Tests

In medicine the majority of diagnostic tests has an associated cost (e.g., an *echography* or a *blood test*). These costs can be highly distinct for different tests (attributes). For instance, considering monetary costs, a *single photon emission computed tomography* (SPECT) scan can cost around 110 Euros, while a *positron emission tomography* (PET) scan can cost thirteen times more.

The costs of tests may be constant for all patients or may change according to specific patient features. A *bronchodilatation test*, for instance, has a higher cost for children less than 6 years, which means that the feature *age* has influence on the cost of the test.

Medical tests can also be very distinct when considering their influence on the *quality of life*. A range of tests are completely harmless for patients (e.g., *obstetric echography*), others can be dangerous and put patient life at risk (e.g., *cardiac catheterism*), and some can be (only) uncomfortable (e.g., *digestive endoscopy*).

There is also the possibility that tests with common characteristics be requested in conjunction. Some tests can be cheaper (and faster) when ordered together (in a group) than when ordered individually and sequentially (e.g., *renal*, *digestive* and *gynecological echographies*). Some tests can also have common costs that can be priced only once. *Blood tests*, for instance, share a common cost of collecting the blood sample, that is, blood is collected only once when the first test is ordered and there is no need to collect it again for associated blood tests (supposing the amount of blood is enough). Besides the financial reduction there is also a non-financial reduction in the cost of inconvenience for the patient. Blood tests ordered in group can also imply other kinds of savings: a financial reduction related to a lower group cost, and a time reduction (results may be available sooner).

A number of tests may depend of the results of other tests. As referred before, the test *age*, for instance, may influence the cost of the *bronchodilatation test*. Some tests can have an increased price as result of secondary effects. Other tests can have patient-specific, time-dependent or emergency-dependent costs. So, it is important that a cost-sensitive learning strategy considers and combines these types of costs.

In general, if misclassification costs are known, tests should only be requested if their costs are not superior to the costs of classification errors. Therefore, any test with a cost greater than the cost of misclassification errors is not worthwhile to be carried out. On the other hand, if the cost for a set of tests is less than the cost of misclassification errors, it is rational to order all possibly relevant tests. These aspects should similarly be considered in a strategy for cost-sensitive learning.

A Simple Example

Let us consider a simple example. Suppose we want to predict a cardiac disease using attributes *ECG*, *Cholesterol* and *Exercise test* and let us also suppose that these attributes have constant costs of $30, $15 and $60 respectively. Figures 1 and 2 show possible decision trees generated with and without using the costs of attributes in the learning phase. When costs are not considered, attributes that are equally informative, but have higher costs, have equal chances to be selected for the top nodes of the decision tree (root of the tree), as in Figure 1. On the other hand, when costs are considered in the learning phase, attributes with higher costs will be penalised and would normally not appear in top nodes of the tree. Note that the top node of the tree will always be used (and priced) when predicting a new case. In this example, for the model of Figure 1, the cost to predict a new case will be at least of $75 ($60+$15) while, for the cost-sensitive model (Figure 2), the minimum cost will be $45.

Obtaining Cost-Sensitive Classification by Manipulating Data

It is possible to manipulate training data or manipulate the outputs of the learned model in order to obtain cost-sensitive classifiers. This type of algorithm is known as meta-classifier (Domingos, 1999).

Figure 1. A simple decision tree for predicting cardiac disease generated without considering attribute costs in the learning phase

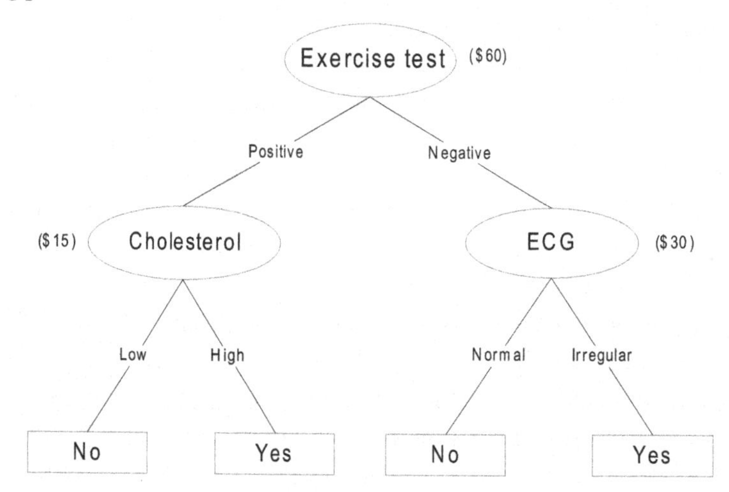

In cost-sensitive learning, a meta-classifier converts a cost-insensitive algorithm into a cost-sensitive one. A meta-classifier pre-processes the training data or post-processes the output of a base classifier. They can be applied to (almost) any type of classifier and provide classifications modified to minimize misclassification error costs. This method is also known as *cost-sensitive meta-learning*.

One common approach is to change the class distribution in order to minimize, in a specific way (by increasing specificity or sensitivity), the costs of new instances. These changes aim to give each class a distribution proportional to its importance (its cost). This process may be done by *stratification/rebalancing*, with the use of *undersampling* or *oversampling* in the implementation (Japkowicz and Stephen, 2002). In a medical classification problem, to increase or to reduce the number of positive cases of a specific disease is an example of this type of manipulation.

For a given instance, many classification algorithms produce a probability estimate for each class or can be modified to output class probabilities. In decision trees, the class distribution of examples in a leaf can be used to estimate the probability of each class for a particular instance. With the probabilities of each class it is then possible to modify the result of the classification, giving a weight to each class, i.e., adjusting to costs of misclassification errors (costs of false negatives and false positives, in the case of a binary classification).

Generically, meta-classifiers can be divided into those that use sampling to modify the learning data and those that do not. The *costing* technique (Zadrozny et al., 2003) is an example of a meta-classifier that uses sampling to produce a cost-sensitive classification from a cost-insensitive classifier. The other approach, without using sampling, can further be divided in three categories, specifically *re-labeling*, by exploiting the minimal expected cost (Michie et al., 1994); *weighting* (Ting, 2002); and *threshold adjusting* (Elkan, 2001). Re-labeling can be applied to training data, as in *MetaCost* (Domingos, 1999), or to test data, as in *CostSensitiveClassifier* (Witten and Frank, 2005).

Meta-classifiers work over built classifiers, and so they can only consider misclassification error costs and do not influence the process of deciding which attribute to use in each node of the tree.

MetaCost (Domingos, 1999) is an algorithm that manipulates the training data for making an arbitrary classifier sensitive to costs, with the classifier included within a cost-minimizing procedure. The

Figure 2. A similar decision tree generated considering attribute costs in the learning phase

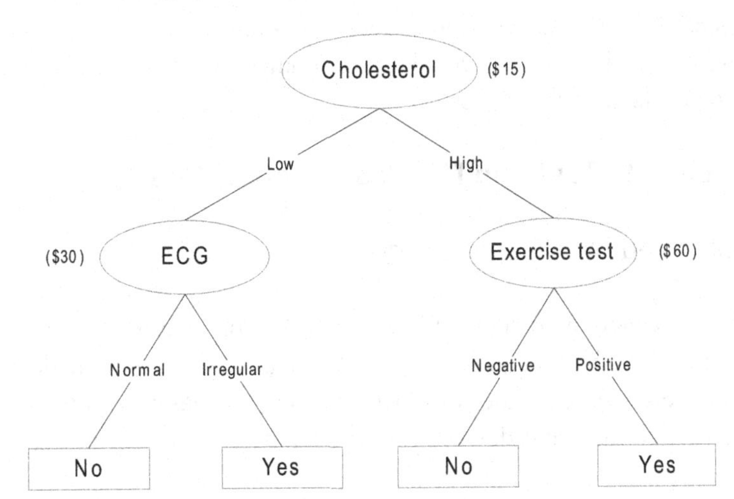

procedure is based on re-labeling training examples with their estimated minimal-cost classes, and using the modified training set to produce a final model.

In CostSensitiveClassifier (Witten and Frank, 2005) two methods can be used to make a classifier sensible to misclassification costs. One of the approaches is to reweight the training instances according to the total cost of each class (*weighting*). The other approach is to adjust the model to predict the class with minimum expected misclassification cost, as a substitute for predicting the most frequent class (*re-labeling*).

Obtaining Cost-Sensitive Classification by Modifying the Learning Algorithm

Another approach, other than manipulating the training data or manipulating the outputs, is to modify the learning algorithm. In this approach for cost-sensitive learning the training algorithm is internally modified to use information about costs when building the classifier.

The next section presents work in this area of cost-sensitive learning.

CURRENT COST-SENSITIVE APPROACHES

In inductive learning, the majority of the work is concerned with the error rate (or success rate). Yet, some work has been done considering *non-uniform misclassification costs*, that is, different costs for different types of errors, but without dealing with other costs, as attribute costs (Breiman et al., 1984; Domingos, 1999; Elkan, 2001).

This type of work can also be used to address the class imbalance problem (when, in a classification problem, there are many more instances of some classes than others, with ratios that exceeds 100:1) (Japkowicz and Stephen, 2002), as there is a relation between imbalanced classes and asymmetric costs (Drummond and Holte, 2000). The imbalanced class problem can be minimized by increasing the cost of misclassifying minority classes. On the other hand, one way to build an algorithm sensitive to costs is to imbalance the training set.

Other literature is paying attention to the cost of tests, without taking into account misclassification costs (Núñez, 1991; Melville et al., 2004).

There is also some work concerned with more than one type of costs. At this level, Turney (1995) was the first to consider both misclassification and test costs together.

Next, we give a brief overview of work considering simultaneously more than one type of cost: test costs, misclassification costs and other types of costs.

Different Approaches to Test and Misclassification Costs

Decision Tree Optimized by a Genetic Algorithm

The ICET system, implemented by Turney (1995), uses a genetic algorithm to build a decision tree to minimize the sum of misclassification and test costs. ICET is a hybrid genetic decision tree induction algorithm (it uses a two-tiered search strategy), sensitive to test and classification error costs, and capable of handling conditional test costs and delayed tests. ICET uses a two-tiered search strategy. Results showed that this system, although robust, is computationally expensive when compared with other algorithms, such as C4.5 (C4.5 is an algorithm developed by Ross Quinlan (1993) to generate decision trees). Turney considered that his approach for the cost-sensitive classification problem was, essentially, a reinforcement learning problem. Later, Lavrac et al. (1996) showed that in a pre-processing phase the elimination of irrelevant attributes can substantially improve the efficiency of learning. The cost-sensitive elimination of attributes increased the learning efficiency of the hybrid algorithm ICET.

Using Markov Decision Processes

Some authors formulated the problem of costs as a Markov decision process in which the transition model is learned from the training data (Zubek and Dietterich, 2002). They used an optimal search strategy (with a heuristic for the AO* algorithm (Nilsson, 1980)) which can be computationally very expensive. Previously, other authors also described the utilization of Markov decision processes, for instance for the induction of decision trees (Bonet and Geffner, 1998), but in the extension POMDP (Partially Observable Markov Decision Process) where partially observable states are allowed.

Considering Costs Related to Time

For a classification sensitive to costs related to time we can find the work of Arnt and Zilberstein (2004), in which they considered attribute (test) costs, misclassification costs and also a utility cost related to the time elapsed while measuring attributes. As in the work of Zubek and Dietterich (2002), they also modelled the problem as a Markov Decision Process and then used the search heuristic AO*. They tried to manage the trade-off between time and accuracy, and proposed an approach to attribute measurement and classification for a variety of time sensitive applications.

A Model that "Pays" for Attributes Using Active Learning with Naïve Bayes

The problem of learning optimal active classifiers was analyzed by Greiner et al. (2002) using a variant of the probably-approximately-correct (PAC) model. The proposed framework addressed learning and active classification together. The learner "pays" for any attributes it sees (learning costs) and has to predict the classification for each instance, with possible penalties. Lizotte et al. (2003) studied an active learning situation where the classifier (naïve Bayes), with a fixed budget, could "buy" data during training. Observing that each attribute of a training example has an associated cost, and the total cost during training must remain less than the fixed budget. They compared methods for sequentially deciding which attribute value to purchase next, considering budget limitations and knowledge about some parameters of the naïve Bayes model.

Cost-Sensitive Naïve Bayes Classifier

It is also possible to obtain cost sensitive naïve Bayes classifiers to minimize the sum of misclassification costs and test costs, as showed by Chai et al. (2004). For that, they included a test strategy to determine how unknown attributes are selected to be "purchased" (tested). In their framework they proposed sequential and batch test strategies.

Cost-Sensitive Decision Trees

Another approach to build and test decision trees sensitive for both types of costs was proposed by Ling et al. (2004). For attribute selection in tree generation (for the split), the algorithm chooses the attribute that minimizes the total cost, instead of minimal entropy (as in C4.5).

Generating Problem Specific Decision Trees and Hybrid Approaches

A lazy approach for learning cost-sensitive decision trees was proposed by Sheng et al. (2005a). Instead of building a single decision tree for all test examples, the proposed method builds a different tree for each new test example with a different set of unknown attributes. This lazy process considers costs only for attributes with unknown value (the test cost of known attributes is 0). In another paper, Sheng and Ling (2005b) propose a hybrid cost-sensitive decision tree to reduce the minimum total cost. The proposed model integrates cost-sensitive decision trees (to collect required tests) with cost-sensitive naïve Bayes. Zhang et al. (2005), studied missing data in cost-sensitive learning and argued that there is no need to impute values for missing data and the learning algorithms should only use known values, i.e., it is desirable to have missing values as they can be useful to reduce the total cost of tests and misclassifications. If a test is too expensive or too risky, compared with the expected reduction with misclassification costs, it is not rational to acquire it (it is preferable to skip it).

Later, Ling et al. (2006) updated their strategy to build decision trees sensitive to costs, with the inclusion of three medical test strategies, *sequential test, single batch* and *multiple batch*, to determine and order the attributes to carry out tests on.

Combining Several Types of Costs, Including a Penalization for Invasive or Delayed Tests

Recently, Freitas et al. (2007) presented an approach to combine several types of costs with relevance for health management. They defined algorithms for the induction of cost-sensitive decision trees, including misclassification costs, test costs, delayed costs and costs associated with risk. They used different strategies to test models, including group costs, common costs, and individual costs. The factor of "risk" was introduced to penalize invasive or delayed tests and to achieve patient-friendly and faster decision trees.

They adapted the decision tree splitting criteria to contemplate costs, that is, they defined a cost function based on a ratio between information gain and costs. When building a tree, for each node, the algorithm selects the attribute that maximizes the defined heuristic. Attributes without cost, as *age* and *gender*, are assigned the value 1. Attributes with higher costs lead to lower values of the heuristic and consequently have smaller chances to be selected.

In the implementation, they modified the C4.5 algorithm (Quinlan, 1993) to contemplate costs and, consequently, to generate cost-sensitive decision trees. Their framework also integrates a cost-sensitive meta-learner to consider the situations where misclassifications costs are different. Results showed that it outperforms the traditional, non cost-sensitive, C4.5 algorithm (Freitas, 2007).

In the next section we present methods for the cost-sensitive evaluation of classifiers.

EVALUATION OF CLASSIFIERS

Performance evaluation is a crucial stage in the development of classifiers. Some methods are useful for evaluating classifies in general, while others are useful also for cost-sensitive classification. In the following we review both the basic concepts and also some approaches for the cost-sensitive evaluation of classifiers.

Basic Concepts

In the area of medicine, we can find many examples using different measures for the evaluation of classifiers performance, as classification accuracy, sensitivity and specificity, and post-test probability (Lavrac, 1999). Nevertheless, there are also other methods to compare classifiers, with focus on problems with two classes. The misclassification error rate (1 minus classification accuracy), ROC (Receiver Operating Characteristics) graphs, and the Area Under ROC Curve (AUC) are on the most common.

Let us consider a classification problem with two classes. Given a classifier and an instance we have four possible results. If the instance belongs to the class positive and is classified as positive then the result is *true positive*, otherwise if the instance is classified as negative the result is *false negative*. On the other hand, if the instance belongs to the class negative and is classified as positive then the result is *false positive*, and if classified as negative the result is *true negative*.

Let us consider TP = True Positives, TN = True Negatives, FP = False Positives, and FN = False Negatives. In the confusion matrix, a two-by-two table (Table 1), values in the main diagonal (TP and TN) represent instances correctly classified, while the other cells represent instances incorrectly classified (FP and FN errors).

The confusion matrix is a useful tool to analyze how well a classifier is able to identify instances (tuples) from different classes. The confusion matrix in Table 1 has only two classes. For m classes, the confusion matrix grows to a $m * m$ matrix, with m correct classifications and $m^2 - m$ errors. The value $M_{i,j}$ in line i and column j in the confusion matrix represent the number of tuples from class i identified by the classifier as belonging to class j. A classifier with good accuracy (with few errors) should have the majority of tuples represented on the main diagonal of the confusion matrix (cells $M_{1,1}$ to $M_{m,m}$) and should have values near to zero in the other cells.

Table 1. Confusion matrix (contingency table)

		Real class		
		Positive	Negative	
Predicted class	Yes	True Positives (TP)	False Positives (FP)	**TP+FP**
	No	False Negatives (FN)	True Negatives (TN)	**FN+TN**
		TP+FN	**FP+TN**	

If we have a good classifier and a relation of order between classes (the dependent variable is ordinal), we may normally expect to find errors near the main diagonal. In this situation it is possible to define a cost for each error, which should increase as the distance to the main diagonal increases. The *Hadamard product of matrix* M with a *cost matrix* C ($m * m$) can be used to calculate the average cost (the expected misclassification cost). This measure of cost may be relevant in problems with more than two classes where it is important to distinguish between errors near the diagonal and errors far from the diagonal.

Considering the confusion matrix in Table 1, we may calculate some common metrics:

- $\textit{True Positive Rate (TP rate)} = \frac{\textit{Instances with positive class correctly classified}}{\textit{Total number of positive instances}} = \frac{TP}{TP+FN}$
- $\textit{False Positive Rate (FP rate)} = \frac{\textit{Instances with negative class incorrectly classified}}{\textit{Total number of negative instances}} = \frac{FP}{FP+TN}$
- $\textit{Precision} = \textit{Positive Predictive Value} = \frac{TP}{TP+FP}$
- $\textit{Negative Predictive Value} = \frac{TN}{FN+TN}$
- $\textit{Recall} = \textit{Sensitivity} = \textit{True Positive Rate}$
- $\textit{Specificity} = \frac{TN}{FP+TN} = 1 - \textit{False Positive Rate}$
- $\textit{Accuracy (proportion of correct predictions)} = \frac{TP+TN}{TP+TN+FN+FP} = 1 - \textit{error rate}$
- F-measure[1] $= \frac{2 \cdot precision \cdot recall}{precision + recall} = \frac{2}{1/precision + 1/recall}$

The overall precision and recall (for all the classes) can be obtained with measures *Micro-Average* and *Macro-Average* (Yang, 1999). Micro-Average gives the same importance to each instance (a benefit to most common classes), while Macro-Average gives equal importance to each class (rare or very frequent classes with equal importance). In Micro-Average, contingency tables for each class are grouped into one single table, where each cell (TP, FP, TN, FN) is the sum of corresponding cells in those local tables. In Macro-Average a contingency table is used for each class, local measures (precision and recall) are calculated and then global average values for precision and recall are calculated.

ROC Graphs

Receiver Operating Characteristic (ROC) graph is a useful technique to visualize and compare the performance of classifiers (Fawcett, 2004). ROC graphs are traditionally used in medical decision making (Swets et al., 2000), and recently they have been progressively adopted by the machine learning and data mining communities. In medicine, ROC graphs are very used in the evaluation of diagnostic tests. ROC graphs have some qualities that make them especially useful in domains with unequal distribution of classes and different costs for misclassification errors.

ROC graphs are represented in two dimensions, with True Positive Rate (TP rate) plotted on the Y axis and False Positive Rate (FP rate) on the X axis. This allows to visualize the relation between true positives and false negatives, i.e., the relation between sensitivity (recall) and 1 –specificity (FP rate = 1 – specificity).

In Figure 3 we can see a ROC graph with information from five classifiers, including three discrete classifiers. Considering only discrete classifiers, we can see in this example that classifier A is the one with higher TP rate and lower FP rate. Classifier C is the worst considering both criteria. The reference line, the diagonal $y=x$, represents the strategy of randomly guessing a class (by chance), that is, a good classifier should be far from this line, in the upper triangular region. A classifier in the lower triangular region performs worse than the random classifier.

The point (0, 1) represents perfect classification. The closer to this point, the best is the classifier, with higher TP rate and lower FP rate. Classifiers with low sensitivity and high specificity (low FP rate), the ones represented near the point (0, 0), are useful when the result is positive because it will normally be correct (FP rate is low); for these classifiers, negative results are not interesting, as they can be false negatives (sensitivity is low). On the other hand, classifiers with high sensitivity and low specificity (near the point (1, 0)), normally have good performance when classifying positive values, but with high FP rate (positive results may be false).

Discrete classifiers, such as decision trees, are designed to produce only one class decision, which corresponds only to a point in the ROC space. Probabilistic classifiers (such as naïve Bayes, some decision trees or neural networks) can be used with a threshold to produce several discrete classifiers. For each potential threshold the rate of true positives against the rate of false positives produces a point in the ROC space. All these different points are then used to define a curve in the ROC space, the so called

Figure 3. ROC graph for three discrete classifiers (A, B, C) and two probabilistic classifiers (Curves C1 and C2)

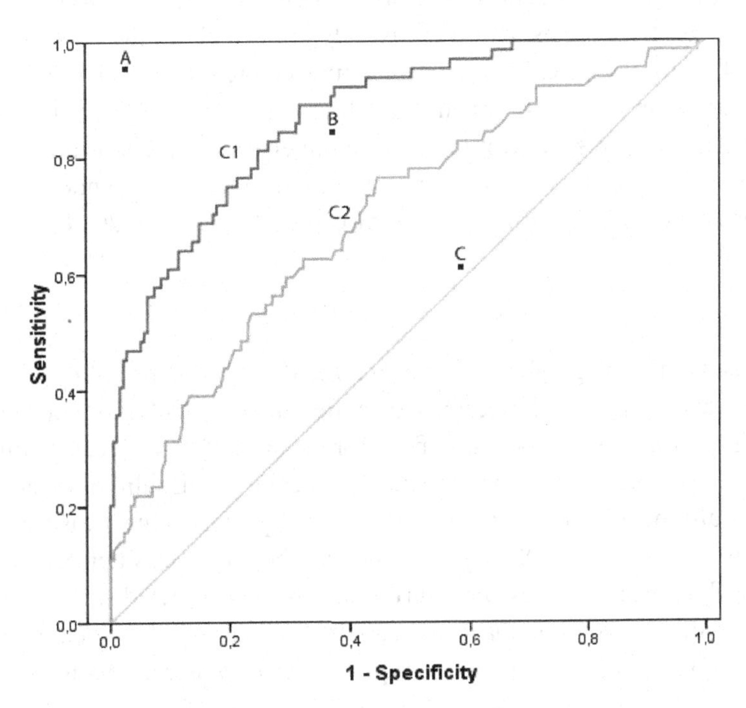

ROC curve. In Figure 3 we can see two ROC curves (Cl and C2) and we can notice that the model associated with curve Cl appears to perform better than the other.

The utilization of the single value Area Under the Curve (AUC) is usual when comparing several classifiers. This method (AUC) has important statistical properties, is equivalent to the Mann-Whitney-Wilcoxon (Hanley and McNeil, 1982) test, and is also closely related to the Gini index (Breiman et al., 1984). Generically, in a simple way, we may say that the larger the area (AUC), the best is the model.

Although the traditional use of the AUC is in two-class problems, it can be generalized to classification problems with more than two classes (Hand and Till, 2001). A method to deal with a *n* class problem is to produce *n* graphs, one for each class. In each instant, the class of reference has a positive value and the remaining set of classes has a negative value.

ROC curves are useful to compare and understand the relation between different classifiers, without considering class distribution or misclassification errors. For imprecise environments and in constant mutation (e.g., with variable misclassification costs), variants to this method can be used, as the ROCCH (ROC Convex Hull) proposed by Provost and Fawcett (2001).

Cost-Sensitive Evaluation of Classifiers

There are several approaches for the cost-sensitive evaluation of classifiers. Margineantu and Dietterich (2000) argue that it is important to use statistical methods (other than traditional) to compare cost-sensitive classifiers. In this sense, they proposed two statistical methods, one to construct a confidence interval for the expected cost of a single classifier, and another to construct a confidence interval for the expected cost difference of two classifiers. The basic idea behind these methods is to detach the problem of estimating probabilities for each cell in the confusion matrix from the problem of calculating the expected cost.

In order to facilitate comparing classifiers with costs, Adams and Hand (1999) proposed a method, the *LC index*, which results from the transformation of ROC curves. They argued that normally there is no precise information about costs, and there is only an idea about the relation between one error (FN) and the other (FP) (for instance, FN can cost ten times more than FP). The proposed method maps the ratio of error costs on an interval between 0 and 1, and transforms ROC curves into parallel lines, showing dominant classifiers in specific regions of the interval. LC index is a measure of confidence that indicates if a classifier is superior to another within an interval. LC index is only a measure of superiority, and does not express the differences between costs (Fawcett, 2004).

Cost Curves

Some of the limitations of ROC graphs can be overcome through the use of *cost curves* (Drummond and Holte, 2006). In fact, a single scalar performance measure (the AUC) cannot capture all aspects of the differences in the performance of two classifiers, for instance when the costs of misclassification are much different between classes. Cost curves are more powerful for visualizing cost-sensitive classifiers performance as they are specifically designed to the specific performance measure "expected cost". In cost curves, a line is associated to each classifier showing how the classifier performance varies with changes in class distribution and misclassification costs. Cost curves include the majority of ROC curves qualities and, additionally, they support the visualization of specific performance assessment that cannot be easily done with ROC curves. Among those types of performance assessment, cost curves permit the visualization of confidence intervals for a classifier performance and the statistical significance of the difference between the performances of two classifiers.

A simple classifier, or a confusion matrix, is represented by a point (FP, TP) in the ROC space. In the cost space this point is represented by a line joining the points (0, FP) and (1, FN). A set of points in ROC space is a set of lines in the cost space. While a ROC curve is defined by a set of connected ROC points, the cost curve is defined by the set of cost lines. Additional and detailed information about cost curves can be found in Witten and Frank (2005) or Drummond and Holte (2006).

CONCLUSION

In the area of health, costs are direct or indirectly present in the majority of situations. A variety of financial or human costs can be associated with a specific diagnostic test. The utilization of learning methods for the generation of diagnostic or prognostic models, that are sensitive to several types of costs, is an important step to transform the computer based process of knowledge acquisition into a more natural process, with tendency to be similar with mental processes used by medical doctors. On the other hand, these kinds of strategies can permit large financial savings and benefits in health-related quality of life costs.

It is important to notice that models can be adapted to the specificities (characteristics) of each patient. Costs may also be variable in different instants, and different medical tests may not be available in some periods. Strategies for cost-sensitive testing should consider these scenarios. Misclassification costs should also be naturally considered as, in many situations, false positives and false positives have different costs.

Because technologies are expensive and budgets are limited, it is rational to consider all the cost involved. A big challenge is to have better healthcare using less money.

FUTURE TRENDS

On the future, classification and learning methods will be focused on the integration of different costs in clinical decision support systems. Health-related quality of life (Guyatt et al., 1993) costs and other possible future costs related to diagnostic tests should be progressively considered when building and testing classification models in medicine. New strategies for urgent situations in obtaining test results, costs with staff and facilities, and other time-related costs, should also be considered.

REFERENCES

Adams, N. M., & Hand, D. J. (1999). Comparing classifiers when the misallocation costs are uncertain. *Pattern Recognition*, *32*(7), 1139-1147.

Arnt, A., & Zilberstein, S. (2004). Attribute measurement policies for time and cost sensitive Classification. In *Proceedings of the 4th IEEE International Conference on Data Mining* (ICDM'04), (pp. 323-326).

Bellazzi, R., & Zupan, B. (2008). Predictive data mining in clinical medicine: Current issues and guidelines. *International Journal of Medical Informatics, 77*(2), 81-97.

Bonet, B., & Geffner, H. (1998). Learning sorting and decision trees with POMDPs. In *Proceedings of the 15th International Conference on Machine Learning* (ICML), (pp. 73-81).

Breiman, L., Freidman, J. H., Olshen, R. A., & Stone, C. J. (1984). *Classification and regression trees*, Belmont, California: Wadsworth.

Chai, X., Deng, L., Yang, Q., & Ling, C. X. (2004). Test-cost sensitive naive Bayes classification. In *Proceedings of the 4th IEEE International Conference on Data Mining* (ICDM'2004).

Domingos, P. (1999). MetaCost: A general method for making classifiers cost-sensitive. In *Proceedings of the 5th ACM SIGKDD International Conference on Knowledge Discovery and Data Mining* (KDD-99), (pp. 155-164).

Drummond, C., & Holte, R. C. (2000). Exploiting the cost (in)sensitivity of decision tree splitting criteria. In *Proceedings of the 17th International Conference on Machine Learning* (ICML), (pp. 239-246).

Drummond, C., & Holte, R. C. (2006). Cost curves: An improved method for visualizing classifier performance. *Machine Learning, 65*, 95-130.

Eccles, M., & Mason, J. (2001). How to develop cost-conscious guidelines. *Health Technology Assessment, 5*(16), 1-69.

Elkan, C. (2001). The foundations of cost-sensitive learning. In *Proceedings of the 17th International Joint Conference on Artificial Intelligence* (IJCAI'01), (pp. 973-978).

Fawcett, T. (2004). *ROC graphs: Notes and practical considerations for researchers*. Technical report, HP Laboratories, Palo Alto.

Fawcett, T., & Provost, F. (1999). Activity monitoring: Noticing interesting changes in behavior. In *Proceedings of the 5th ACM SIGKDD International Conference on Knowledge Discovery and Data Mining* (KDD-99), (pp. 53-62).

Freitas, J. A., Costa-Pereira, A., & Brazdil, P. (2007). Cost-sensitive decision trees applied to medical data. In: I. Y. Song, J. Eder, & T. M. Nguyen (Eds.): *9th International Conference on Data Warehousing and Knowledge Discovery (DaWaK 2007), LNCS, 4654*, 303-312, Springer-Verlag Berlin Heidelberg.

Freitas, J. A. (2007). *Uso de Técnicas de Data Mining para Análise de Bases de Dados Hospitalares com Finalidades de Gestão*. Unpublished doctoral dissertation, University of Porto, Portugal.

Greiner, R., Grove, A. J., & Roth, D. (2002). Learning cost-sensitive active classifiers. *Artificial Intelligence, 139*(2), 137-174.

Guyatt, G. H., Feeny, D. H., & Patrick, D. L. (1993). Measuring health-related quality of life. *Annals of Internal Medicine, 118*(8), 622-629.

Hand, D. J., & Till, R. J. (2001). A simple generalisation of the area under the ROC curve for multiple class classification problems. *Machine Learning, 45*, 171-186.

Hanley, J. A., & McNeil, B. J. (1982). The meaning and use of the area under a receiver operating characteristic (ROC) curve. *Radiology, 143*(1), 29-36.

Hollmén, J., Skubacz, M., & Taniguchi, M. (2000). Input dependent misclassification costs for cost-sensitive classifiers. In *Proceedings of the 2nd International Conference on Data Mining*, (pp. 495-503).

Japkowicz, N., & Stephen, S. (2002). The class imbalance problem: A systematic study. *Intelligent Data Analysis, 6*(5), 429-449.

Lavrac, N., Gamberger, D., & Turney, P. (1996). Preprocessing by a cost-sensitive literal reduction algorithm: REDUCE. In *Proceedings of the Workshop Mathematical and Statistical Methods, at the International School for the Synthesis of Expert Knowledge* (ISSEK'96), (pp. 179-196).

Lavrac, N. (1999). Selected techniques for data mining in medicine. *Artificial Intelligence in Medicine, 16*, 3-23.

Ling, C. X., Sheng, V. S., & Yang, Q. (2006). Test strategies for cost-sensitive decision trees. *IEEE Transactions on Knowledge and Data Engineering, 18*(8), 1055-1067.

Ling, C. X., Yang, Q., Wang, J., & Zhang, S. (2004). Decision trees with minimal costs. In *Proceedings of the 21st International Conference on Machine Learning* (ICML).

Lizotte, D. J., Madani, O. & Greiner, R. (2003). Budgeted learning of naiveBayes classifiers. In *Proceedings of the 19th Conference in Uncertainty in Artificial Intelligence* (UAI'03), (pp. 378-385).

Margineantu, D. D., & Dietterich, T. G. (2000). Bootstrap methods for the cost-sensitive evaluation of classifiers. In *Proceedings of the 17th International Conference on Machine Learning* (ICML-2000), (pp. 583-590).

Melville, P., Saar-Tsechansky, M., Provost, F., & Mooney, R. (2004). Active feature-value acquisition for classifier induction. In *Proceedings of the 4th IEEE International Conference on Data Mining* (ICDM'04), (pp. 483-486).

Michie, D., Spiegelhalter, D. J., & Taylor, C. C. (1994) (eds). *Machine learning, neural and statistical classification*, Ellis Horwood Series in Artificial Intelligence, Prentice Hall.

Mitchell, T. M. (1997). *Machine Learning*, New York: McGraw-Hill.

Nilsson, N. (1980). *Principles of artificial intelligence*, Palo Alto: Tioga Publishing Co.

Núñez, M. (1991). The use of background knowledge in decision tree induction. *Machine Learning, 6*, 231-250.

Provost, F., & Fawcett, T. (2001). Robust classification for imprecise environments. *Machine Learning, 42*(3), 203-231.

Quinlan, J. R. (1993). *C4.5: Programs for machine learning*, Morgan Kaufmann Publishers.

Sheng, S., Ling, C. X., & Yang, Q. (2005a). Simple test strategies for cost-sensitive decision trees. In *Proceedings of the 16th European Conference on Machine Learning* (ECML), (pp. 365-376).

Sheng, S., & Ling, C. X. (2005b). Hybrid cost-sensitive decision tree. In *Proceedings of the 9th European Conference on Principles and Practice of Knowledge Discovery in Databases* (PKDD).

Swets, J. A., Dawes, R. M., & Monahan, J. (2000). Better decisions through science. *Scientific American, 283*(4), 82-87.

Ting, K. M. (2002). An Instance-Weighting Method to Induce Cost-Sensitive Trees. *IEEE Transactions on Knowledge and Data Engineering, 14*(3), 659-665.

Turney, P. (1995). Cost-sensitive classification: empirical evaluation of a hybrid genetic decision tree induction algorithm. *Journal of Artificial Intelligence Research, 2*, 369-409.

Turney, P. (2000). Types of cost in inductive concept learning. In *Proceedings of the Workshop on Cost-Sensitive Learning at the 17th International Conference on Machine Learning* (WCSL at ICML-2000), (pp. 15-21).

Witten, I. H., & Frank, E. (2005). *Data mining: Practical machine learning tools and techniques*, San Francisco: Morgan Kaufmann, 2nd Edition.

Yang, Y. (1999). An evaluation of statistical approaches to text categorization. *Information Retrieval, 1*(1-2), 69-90.

Zadrozny, B., Langford, J., & Abe, N. (2003). Cost-sensitive learning by cost-proportionate example weighting. In *Proceedings of the 3rd IEEE International Conference on Data Mining* (ICDM'03).

Zhang, S., Qin, Z., Ling, C. X., & Sheng, S. (2005). "Missing is useful": Missing values in cost-sensitive decision trees. *IEEE Transactions on Knowledge and Data Engineering. 17*(12), 1689-1693.

Zubek, V. B., & Dietterich, T. G. (2002). Pruning improves heuristic search for cost-sensitive learning. In *Proceedings of the 19th International Conference of Machine Learning* (ICML), (pp. 27-35).

KEY TERMS

Classification: Technique used to predict group membership for data instances (e.g., decision trees, neural networks).

Cost Curves: A graphical technique to visualize binary classifiers performance over the full range of possible class distributions and misclassification costs (a complement or an alternative to ROC curves).

Cost-Sensitive Learning: The sub-area of Machine Learning concerned with the questions of non-uniformity in costs.

Decision Tree: A predictive model; a mapping from observations about an instance to conclusions about its target class.

Error Rate: The rate of errors made by a predictive model (1 – accuracy).

False Negative: When an instance belongs to the class positive and is classified as negative (in a classification problems with two classes).

False Positive: When an instance belongs to the class negative and is classified as positive (in a classification problems with two classes).

Machine Learning: The study of computer algorithms that improve automatically through experience; a field of science and technology concerned with building machines that learn.

Model: A description that acceptably explains and predicts relevant data, and is normally much smaller than the data itself.

ROC: For a binary classifier, Receiver Operating Characteristic (ROC) is a graphical plot of the sensitivity vs. one minus specificity, for a range of different thresholds.

ENDNOTE

1 F-measure combines precision and recall (sensitivity) in a single number: F-measure is the weighted harmonic mean of precision and recall. Comparing with arithmetic mean, this measure (harmonic mean) only assumes high values when both measures (precision and recall) are high. In this situation, this measure is also known as F_1 since precision and recall have the same weight (a generic formula, not present here, allows weighting importance on precision over recall).

Chapter IV
Classification and Prediction with Neural Networks

Arnošt Veselý
Czech University of Life Sciences, Czech Republic

ABSTRACT

This chapter deals with applications of artificial neural networks in classification and regression problems. Based on theoretical analysis it demonstrates that in classification problems one should use cross-entropy error function rather than the usual sum-of-square error function. Using gradient descent method for finding the minimum of the cross entropy error function, leads to the well-known backpropagation of error scheme of gradient calculation if at the output layer of the neural network the neurons with logistic or softmax output functions are used. The author believes that understanding the underlying theory presented in this chapter will help researchers in medical informatics to choose more suitable network architectures for medical applications and that it helps them to carry out the network training more effectively.

INTRODUCTION

Medicine involves decision-making and classification or prediction is an important part of it. However, medical classification or prediction is usually a very complex and hard process at least from the following reasons:

- Much of the data that are relevant to classification or prediction, especially those received from laboratories, are complex or difficult to comprehend and can be interpreted only by experts.
- For reliable classification or prediction a large amount of data is frequently needed and some important anomalies in the data may be overlooked.

- When monitoring a patient, some for the patient dangerous events can be too rare and therefore it may be difficult to identify them in the continuous stream of data.

Thus computer-assisted support could be of significant help. With the increasing number of clinical databases it is likely that machine-learning applications will be necessary to detect rare conditions and unexpected outcomes. The needful methods and algorithms can be found first of all in the domain of mathematical statistics and artificial intelligence. From means of artificial intelligence rule based experts systems were primarily used. Today the most important applications utilize algorithms based on neural networks, fuzzy systems, neurofuzzy systems or evolution algorithms.

Classical statistical methods require certain assumptions about the distribution of data. Neural networks can constitute a good alternative when some of these assumptions cannot be verified. From this point of view neural networks constitute a special kind of nonparametric statistical methods. Therefore the most successful neural network architectures are implemented in standard statistical software packages, as there is for example STATISTICA. Thus the eligibility of neural network algorithms for the given decision making task can be easily tested on the sample data using one of these software packages.

From abstract mathematical point of view medical classification and prediction tasks fall into the scope of either classification or regression problems. A classification or pattern recognition can be viewed as a mapping from a set of input variables to an output variable representing the class label. In classification problems the task is to assign new inputs to labels of classes or categories. In a regression problem we suppose that there exists underlying continuous mapping $\mathbf{y} = f(\mathbf{x})$ and we estimate the unknown value of $\mathbf{y}$ using the known value of $\mathbf{x}$.

Typical case of classification problem in medicine is medical diagnostics. As input data the patient's anamnesis, subjective symptoms, observed symptoms and syndromes, measured values (e.g. blood pressure, body temperature etc.) and results of laboratory tests are taken. This data is coded by vector $\mathbf{x}$, the components of which are binary or real numbers. The patients are classified into categories $D_1, \ldots, D_m$ that correspond to their possible diagnoses $d_1, \ldots, d_m$.

Many successful applications of neural networks in medical diagnostics can be found in literature (Gant, 2001). The processing and interpretation of electrocardiograms (ECG) with neural networks was intensively studied, because evaluation of long term ECG recordings is a time consuming procedure and requires automated recognition of events that occur infrequently (Silipo, 1998). In radiology neural networks have been successfully applied to X-ray analysis in the domains of chest radiography (Chen, 2002) and (Coppini, 2003), mammography (Halkiotis, 2007) and computerized tomography (Lindahl, 1997), (Gletsos, 2003) and (Suzuki, 2005). Also classification of ultrasound images was successful (Yan Sun, 2005). Neural networks have been also successfully applied to diagnose epilepsy (Walczak, 2001) or to detect seizures from EEG patterns (Alkan, 2005).

Also prediction of the patient's state can be stated as classification problem. On the basis of examined data represented with vector $\mathbf{x}$ patients are categorized into several categories $P_1, \ldots, P_m$ that correspond to different future states. For example five categories with the following meaning can be considered: P_1 can mean death, P_2 deterioration of the patient's state, P_3 steady state, P_4 improvement of the patient's state and P_5 recovery.

Neural networks were applied with good results for prognosis of the hepatectomized patients with hepatocellular carcinoma (Hamamoto, 1995). Also neural network predictions for patients with colorectal cancer (Bottaci, 1997) or with bladder cancer (Wei, 2003) were successful.

The typical set up of a regression problem in medical decision-making is the following:

- It is necessary to estimate value of some physiological quantity that cannot be measured directly or a measurement of which would yield unacceptable risk or discomfort for the patient.
- The future value of some physiological quantity is to be estimated on the base of its known past values, i.e. for example the value $\mathbf{x}(t+1)$ is to be estimated knowing $\mathbf{x}(t-n)$, . . . , $\mathbf{x}(t-1)$, $\mathbf{x}(t)$.

Neural networks were applied with good results for prognosis of the time course prediction of blood glucose metabolism of a diabetic patient (Prank, 1998) and (Tresp, 1999), for prediction of lengths of patient stay on a post-coronary care unit (Mobley, 1995) or for modeling survival after treatment of intraocular melanoma (Taktak, 2004). Also an efficient decision support tool for allocating hospital bed resources and determining required acuity of care was based on neural networks (Walczak, 2003).

In classification problems multilayer feedforward architectures trained with backpropagation of error algorithm appeared to be the most successful. The good alternative to multilayer feedforward networks is Kohonen Self-Organizing Map (SOM) used together with one of the algorithms for Learning Vector Quantization (LVQ). Sometimes the categories of patients are not given a priori and the objective is to create the specified or unspecified number of categories automatically using similarities inherent in patient vectors $\mathbf{x}$. This task is known as cluster analysis and is traditionally pursued in mathematical statistics. Neural networks provide additional algorithms with new useful properties. For this task the most suitable neural network is Kohonen Self-Organizing Map. In the scope of regression problems instead of multilayer feedforward neural networks the so-called Radial Basis Function (RBF) networks have been also often applied.

In this chapter we focus on the mainstream solution of classification or regression problems consisting in utilizing feedforward multilayer neural networks. After introducing feedforward multilayer networks and the gradient decent search method generally used for their adaptation to real decision tasks, we analyze properties of adapted networks if the sum-of-square error function estimated on the training set has been minimized. The analysis shows that this adaptation strategy is for both classification or regression problems sound, if the size of training set goes to infinity. The more elaborate analysis using maximum likelihood approach, which is more proper for the real training sets, gives for regression problems the same result. However, for classification problems, the maximum likelihood approach leads to the conclusion that the more accurate estimates of probabilities of class membership can be acquired if instead of sum-of-square error function the cross-entropy error function is used. However, if the cross-entropy error function is used for an usual network architecture with liner neurons at the output layer, the standard backpropagation algorithm for weight updates ought to be recalculated. The other possibility is to change the output functions of the neurons at the output layer. If the output layer consists of one neuron only, the logistic output function should be used and if the output layer consists of more than one output neuron, the softmax functions should be used. Using those output functions, the weight updates can be calculated according to the standard backpropagation scheme.

In the paragraph that follows after the theoretical part of the chapter, the process of data preparation is at first discussed. Further usual difficulties encountered during training neural networks, as trapping in a local minimum or overfitting, are described and general hints for their overcoming are given. Eventually, concise overall guidelines for design and training of a neural network in a real application are presented and neural network solutions of two medical classification problems are described.

The general theory of neural networks can be found for example in monographs (Haykin, 1999) or (Mitchell, 1997). The principles, which maximum likelihood method of optimal network weights establishment is based on, are clearly explained in (Bishop, 1996).

MODEL OF A NEURON

For building up neural networks simple models of physiological neurons are used. These models we will call neurons. A neuron is a simple information-processing unit. It takes a vector of real-valued inputs, calculates a linear combination of these inputs, adds a constant value called bias and then on the resulting sum applies an output (activation) function. More precisely, given inputs $x_1, \ldots x_n$, the output y is computed according to the formula:

$$y = \varphi\left(\sum_{i=1}^{n} w_i x_i + b\right) \tag{1}$$

where each w_i is a real-valued constant called weight that determines the contribution of input x_i to the neuron output y, b is the bias and $\varphi(\cdot)$ is the output function. The computation of the neuron is illustrated in Figure 1.

To simplify notation we imagine an additional constant input x_0=1 with weight w_0=b, allowing us to write:

$$\sum_{i=1}^{n} w_i x_i + b = \sum_{i=0}^{n} w_i x_i \text{ and } y = \varphi\left(\sum_{i=0}^{n} w_i x_i\right) \tag{2}$$

or in vector form:

$$y = \varphi(\mathbf{w} \cdot \mathbf{x}) \tag{3}$$

where $\mathbf{w} = (w_0, \ldots, w_n)$, $\mathbf{x} = (x_0, \ldots, x_n)$ and operation $\cdot$ is scalar product.

Figure 1. Formal model of a physiological neuron

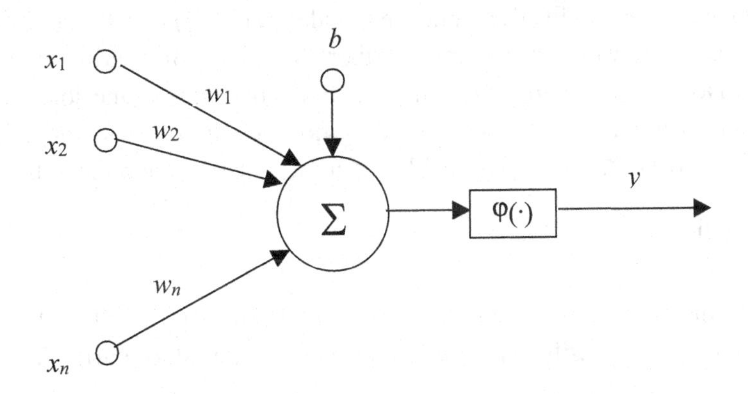

If one of the functions $\sigma(x)$ or $\mathrm{sgn}(x)$ is taken in the role of output function, we will get the neuron model firstly proposed by McCulloch and Pitts (1943), which is usually called Threshold Logic Unit (TLU). The functions $\sigma(x)$ and $\mathrm{sgn}(x)$ are defined:

$$\sigma(x) = \begin{cases} 1 & \text{if } y > 0 \\ 0 & \text{otherwise} \end{cases} \tag{4}$$

and:

$$\mathrm{sgn}(x) = \begin{cases} 1 & \text{if } y > 0 \\ -1 & \text{otherwise} \end{cases} \tag{5}$$

This type of neuron model was also the basic computing unit of the perceptron devised by Rossenblatt in fifties and therefore is sometimes called simple perceptron. In the following we will use instead of the term simple perceptron the shorter term perceptron.

Usually we assume that components of input vectors $\mathbf{x}$ are real numbers and therefore $\mathbf{x} \in \boldsymbol{R}^n$, where $\boldsymbol{R}$ is the set of real numbers. An input vector is called pattern and n-dimensional space $\boldsymbol{R}^n$ is called pattern space. A surface that separates the patterns into different classes is called a decision surface. Patterns belonging to the one class all lie on the one side of the decision surface, and patterns belonging to the other class lie on the other side of the decision surface. In the case of perceptron the decision surface is a hyperplane defined in the pattern space by scalar product:

$$\mathbf{w} \cdot \mathbf{x} = 0 \tag{6}$$

A perceptron categorizes a set of input patterns into two classes according to whether $\mathbf{w} \cdot \mathbf{x} < 0$ or $\mathbf{w} \cdot \mathbf{x} > 0$. Of course some classes cannot be separated by any hyperplane. Those that can be separated are called linearly separable sets of patterns.

If the inputs are binary, that is if the input vectors $\mathbf{x} \in \{0, 1\}^n$, then perceptron with the output function $\sigma(\cdot)$ represents a boolean function. It would be interesting to know the computational power of perceptron, i.e. can a perceptron represent all possible boolean functions? The answer is that a perceptron can represent only a small subset of boolean functions, which are called to be linearly separable. Linearly separable are those boolean functions, values of which can be separated by a hyperplane. For example from two-argument boolean functions are linearly separable boolean multiplication (AND) and boolean addition (OR) or their negations NAND and NOR. Linearly non-separable two-argument boolean functions are only two: equivalence (EQV) and non-equivalence (XOR) (see Figure 2).

In multilayer neural networks considered further the nonlinear continuous computing units are needed. Perceptron as computing unit is nonlinear but not continuous. One solution is the sigmoid unit or sigmoid neuron $y = f(\mathbf{w} \cdot \mathbf{x})$, where $f(\cdot)$ is so called sigmoid function. The sigmoid function is defined as a bounded, strictly increasing and differentiable function. The most popular is the sigmoid function:

$$f(x) = \frac{1}{1 + e^{-kx}}, \quad k > 0 \tag{7}$$

which forms a continuous approximation of the threshold function $\sigma(x)$. This function has the useful property that its derivative is easily expressed in terms of its output, in particular:

Figure 2. The AND function (a) is linearly separable, but the EQV function (b) is not

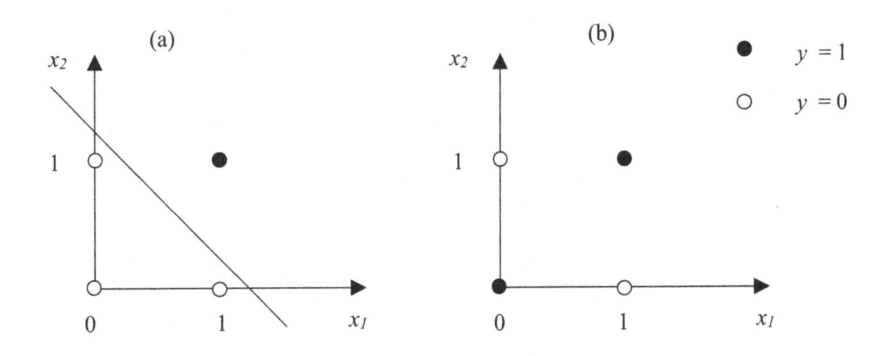

$$\frac{df(x)}{dx} = kf(x)(1 - f(x)) \quad (8)$$

A sigmoid function with $k = 1$ is called logistic function.

Sometimes neurons $y = \mathbf{w} \cdot \mathbf{x}$, i.e. neurons without output function are used. These neurons, called linear neurons, represent linear functions.

MULTILAYER FEEDFORWARD NETWORKS

Multilayer feedforward networks, also often called multilayer perceptrons, form an important class of neural networks. The network consists of a set of sensory units (receptors) that constitute the input layer, one or more hidden layers of computation nodes and an output layer that consists also of computation nodes. Computing units in hidden layers are threshold or sigmoid neurons. In the output layer usually linear neurons are used. Only neurons of the neighbor layers are connected and the input signal propagates through the network only in the forward direction (see Figure 3). The strength of the connection going from i-th neuron of the certain layer to the j-th neuron of the next layer is denoted w_{ji}. When we use the term L-layer network, we refer to a network with L layers of computing units. Thus we shall call a network with one hidden layer a two-layer network, a network with two hidden layers a three-layer network and so on. A layer network with n inputs and m outputs represents m functions with n arguments. These functions can be easily expressed explicitly. For example a two-layer network with n receptors, one output and m hidden units represents function:

$$y = \varphi\left(\sum_{j=0}^{m} W_j \, \psi\left(\sum_{i=0}^{n} w_{ji} x_i\right)\right) \quad (9)$$

Here W_j is the weight of connection between j-th neuron at the hidden layer and the output neuron and w_{ji} is the weight of the connection between the i-th input neuron and the j-th neuron at the hidden layer. All neurons in the hidden layer have the same output function $\psi(\cdot)$ and the output neuron has the output function $\varphi(\cdot)$.

Figure 3. Two-layer feedforward neural network

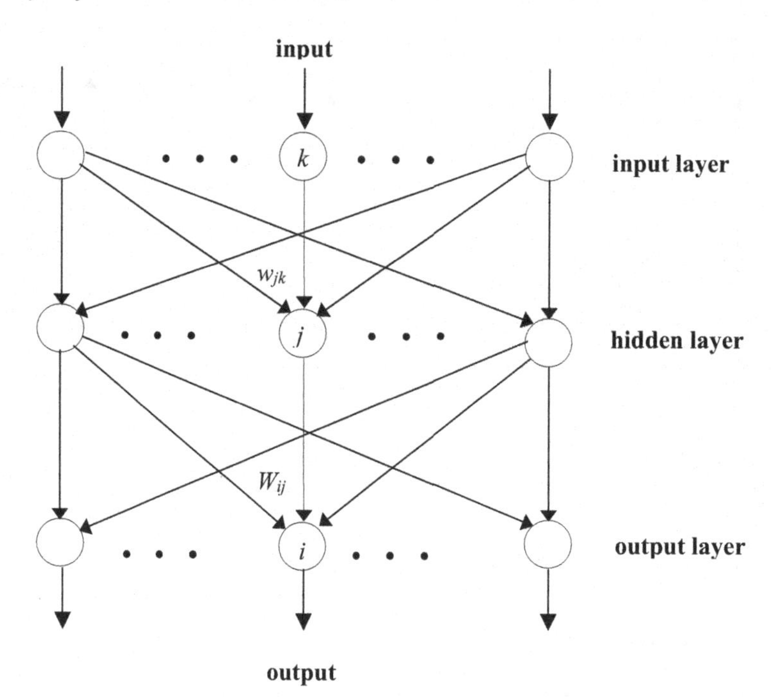

Consider the network with binary inputs, one output neuron and one or more hidden layers. Assume that all computing layers consist of neurons with threshold output function $\sigma(\cdot)$ defined by (4). Since the network output is also 0 or 1, the network computes a boolean function. We can easily show that a two-layer network can generate any boolean function, provided the number of hidden units is sufficiently large.

If the inputs are continuous, then three-layer network can classify two arbitrary disjunctive categories with arbitrary precision, see e.g. Bishop (1996).

In regression problems continuous functions are approximated. It was proved that an arbitrary bounded continuous function can be approximated to arbitrary accuracy with two-layer feedforward network with sigmoid neurons at the hidden layer and with linear neuron at the output layer (Cybenko, 1989; Hornik,1989). The number of hidden neurons required depends on the function to be approximated.

Moreover the following was proved. Any function can be approximated to arbitrary accuracy by a three-layer network (Cybenko, 1988). The output layer uses linear neuron and the two hidden layers consist of sigmoid neurons. The number of required neurons in hidden layers is not known in general and depends on the approximated function.

If a function $\varphi(x_1, \ldots, x_n) \in (0, 1)$ is continuous and bounded, it can be approximated with arbitrarily accuracy by means of a two-layer network with sigmoid neurons in the hidden as well as in the output layer. The prove of this assertion is based on the fact that sigmoid function $f(.)$ is increasing and therefore uniquely invertible. Thus the function $f^{-1}(\varphi(x_1, \ldots, x_n))$ is also continuous and bounded and therefore can be approximated to arbitrary accuracy with a two-layer network with linear output neuron according to Cybenko(1989) and Hornik (1989).

BACKPROPAGATION OF ERROR ALGORITHM

Multilayer feedforward networks can be used for solving different classification or regression problems. The behavior of a neural network is determined by the set of its weights. Therefore the crucial problem is how to determine the weights in a given problem to get the neural network with desired behavior.

The neural network approach involves parameter learning from examples. The neural networks are able of learning from its environment and improve their performance through learning. Neural network learning or training means to have an adaptive procedure in which the weights of the network are incrementally modified so as to improve a prespecified performance criterion. Such a procedure is called a learning rule (learning algorithm) and the adaptation may take place in supervised or in an unsupervised way. In supervised learning the set of training examples consists of known input-output pattern pairs. The learning process consists in updating the weights so that an error function dependent on the network output and the known target value is reduced. In the unsupervised learning the network also learns the association between input and output, but no feedback indicating whether the association is correct or not is not provided.

The performance criterion is often based on the sum-of-square error function $E(\mathbf{w})$ evaluated on the training set. Suppose that the multilayer network should learn s n-argument functions:

$$f_\alpha(x_1, \ldots, x_n) = f_\alpha(\mathbf{x}), \quad \alpha = 1, \ldots, s \tag{10}$$

and that the training set T consists of N samples:

$$T = \{(\mathbf{x}^i, \mathbf{t}^i), i = 1, \ldots, N\}, \ \mathbf{x}^i = (x_1^i, \ldots, x_n^i), \ \mathbf{t}^i = (t_1^i, \ldots, t_s^i). \tag{11}$$

Then:

$$E(\mathbf{w}) = \frac{1}{2}\sum_{i=1}^{N}\sum_{\alpha=1}^{s}(y_\alpha^i(\mathbf{x}^i, \mathbf{w}) - t_\alpha^i)^2 \tag{12}$$

where $\mathbf{w}$ is vector of the neural network weights and y_α^i is the output of the α-th output neuron if the sample vector $\mathbf{x}^i$ is on its input. If the network represents functions that are on the learning set identical to functions $f_\alpha(\mathbf{x})$, then $E(\mathbf{w}) = 0$. Therefore the problem of neural network approximation of functions $f_\alpha(\mathbf{x})$ on the training set $\boldsymbol{T}$ transforms into the problem of finding out such weight vector $\mathbf{w}^*$ for which $E(\mathbf{w}^*)$ reaches the minimum.

In the following we will simplify the notation of summing over the training set and instead of (12) we will write:

$$E(\mathbf{w}) = \frac{1}{2}\sum_{\mathbf{x}}\sum_{\alpha=1}^{s}(y_\alpha(\mathbf{x}, \mathbf{w}) - t_\alpha)^2 \tag{13}$$

Algorithm for searching minimum of $E(\mathbf{w})$ can be based on the gradient descent search. Gradient descent search starts with an arbitrary initial weight vector, which is then repeatedly modified in many steps. At each step the weight vector is altered in the direction of the steepest descent along the error surface. The process continues until a satisfactory small error $E(\mathbf{w})$ is reached.

Algorithm of gradient descent search:

1. At the beginning the weights are set equal to small random values.
2. At the n-th step the value of gradient $\text{grad}E(\mathbf{w}^{n-1})$ is estimated. For estimation one or more elements of learning set are used. Then the weight vector $\mathbf{w}^{n-1}$ is modified according to:

$$\mathbf{w}^n = \mathbf{w}^{n-1} - \varepsilon\, \text{grad}E(\mathbf{w}^{n-1}) + \mu\, \Delta\mathbf{w}^{n-1} \tag{14}$$

where $\varepsilon > 0$ determines the rate of weight vector change, $\Delta\mathbf{w}^{n-1} = \mathbf{w}^{n-1} - \mathbf{w}^{n-2}$ is the weight vector change in the previous n–1-th step of the algorithm and $0 \leq \mu \leq 1$ is a constant called the momentum. □

The use of momentum in the algorithm represents a minor modification of the classical gradient descent algorithm, yet it may improve the learning behavior of the algorithm. It has the effect of gradually increasing the step size of the search in regions where the gradient is unchanging and thus to accelerate the learning process. It also helps to prevent the learning process from terminating in some shallow local minimum of the error surface.

Gradient method guarantees convergence of weight vector to the vector $\mathbf{w}^*$ for which $E(\mathbf{w})$ reaches its local minimum. In the following we shall show how the gradient of error function can be determined in a multilayer network with one hidden layer. The equations for more hidden layers can be obtained in a similar way.

We assume that the network has n input neurons (so called receptors) denoted r_k with output values x_k (i.e. output values of receptors equal to their inputs values), m hidden neurons denoted n_j with output values o_j and s output neurons denoted N_i with output values y_i (see Figure 4). Neurons at hidden layer are sigmoid neurons with the output function $f(\cdot)$ and neurons at the output layer are linear neurons. The weights between neurons at hidden and input layer are denoted w_{jk} and the weights between hidden and output layer W_{ij}. The network represents s functions:

Figure 4. Feedforward network with one hidden layer

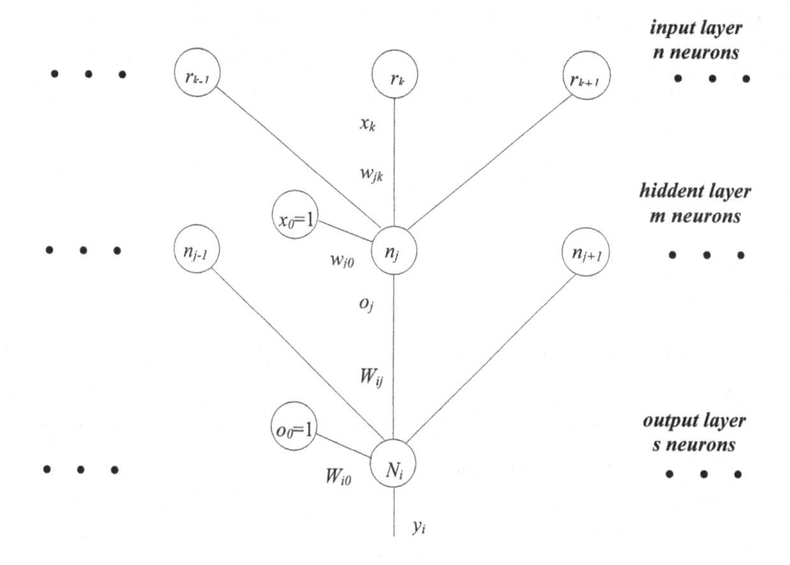

$$y_\alpha = \sum_{p=0}^{m} W_{\alpha p} f(\sum_{q=0}^{n} w_{pq} x_q), \quad \alpha = 1,\ldots,s \tag{15}$$

The gradient of the error function (13) is:

$$\text{grad } E(W_{ij}, w_{kl}) = \left(\frac{\partial E}{\partial W_{10}}, \frac{\partial E}{\partial W_{11}}, \ldots, \frac{\partial E}{\partial W_{sm}}, \ldots, \frac{\partial E}{\partial w_{10}}, \frac{\partial E}{\partial w_{11}}, \ldots, \frac{\partial E}{\partial w_{mn}} \right) \tag{16}$$

The partial derivatives of the error function E can be established as follows:

$$\frac{\partial E}{\partial W_{ij}} = \sum_{\mathbf{x}} \sum_{\alpha=1}^{s} (y_\alpha - t_\alpha) \frac{\partial y_\alpha}{\partial W_{ij}} = \sum_{\mathbf{x}} \sum_{\alpha=1}^{s} (y_\alpha - t_\alpha) \frac{\partial}{\partial W_{ij}} (\sum_{p=0}^{m} W_{\varphi} o_p) = \sum_{\mathbf{x}} (y_i - t_i) o_j = \sum_{\mathbf{x}} \Delta_i o_j \tag{17}$$

where:

$$\Delta_i = y_i - t_i \text{ and } o_j = f(\sum_{q=0}^{n} w_{jq} x_q) \tag{18}$$

When building up (17) we took into consideration that all derivatives:

$$\frac{\partial W_{\alpha p}}{\partial W_{ij}}, \quad \alpha = 1,\ldots,s, \quad p = 1,\ldots m$$

equal 0 except the derivative $\frac{\partial W_{ij}}{\partial W_{ij}}$ which equals 1.

In a similar way we are getting:

$$\frac{\partial E}{\partial w_{jk}} = \sum_{\mathbf{x}} \sum_{\alpha=1}^{s} (y_\alpha - t_\alpha) \frac{\partial y_\alpha}{\partial w_{jk}} = \sum_{\mathbf{x}} \sum_{\alpha=1}^{s} \Delta_\alpha \frac{\partial}{\partial w_{jk}} (\sum_{p=0}^{m} W_{\alpha p} o_p) = \sum_{\mathbf{x}} \sum_{\alpha=1}^{s} \Delta_\alpha \sum_{p=0}^{m} W_{\alpha p} \frac{\partial}{\partial w_{jk}} f(\sum_{q=0}^{n} w_{pq} x_q)$$

$$= \sum_{\mathbf{x}} \sum_{\alpha=1}^{s} \Delta_\alpha \sum_{p=0}^{m} W_{\alpha p} f'(\sum_{q=0}^{n} w_{jq} x_q) \frac{\partial}{\partial w_{jk}} (\sum_{q=0}^{n} w_{pq} x_q) = \sum_{\mathbf{x}} \sum_{\alpha=1}^{s} \Delta_\alpha W_{\alpha j} f'(\sum_{q=0}^{n} w_{jq} x_q) x_k = \sum_{\mathbf{x}} \delta_j x_k \tag{19}$$

where:

$$\delta_j = \sum_{\alpha=1}^{s} \Delta_\alpha W_{\alpha j} f'(\sum_{q=0}^{n} w_{jq} x_q) \tag{20}$$

Again all derivatives $\frac{\partial w_{pq}}{\partial w_{jk}}$ in (19) equal 0 except the derivative $\frac{\partial w_{jk}}{\partial w_{jk}}$ that equals 1.

Thus to gain the estimate of grad $E(W_{ij}, w_{kl})$, the values:

$$\Delta_i o_j \text{ and } \delta_j x_k \text{ , where } i = 1,\ldots\alpha;\ j = 1,\ldots,m;\ k = 1,\ldots,n \tag{21}$$

are to be evaluated for all training samples. This evaluation can be carried out according to the equations (18) and (20).

The calculation of δ_i can be described more clearly as so called backpropagation of error.

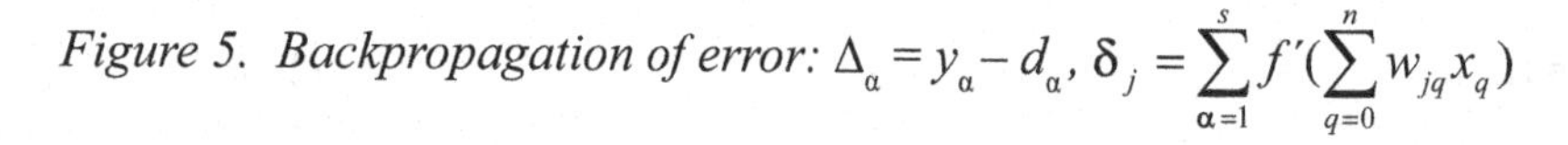

Figure 5. Backpropagation of error: $\Delta_\alpha = y_\alpha - d_\alpha$, $\delta_j = \sum_{\alpha=1}^{s} f'(\sum_{q=0}^{n} w_{jq} x_q)$

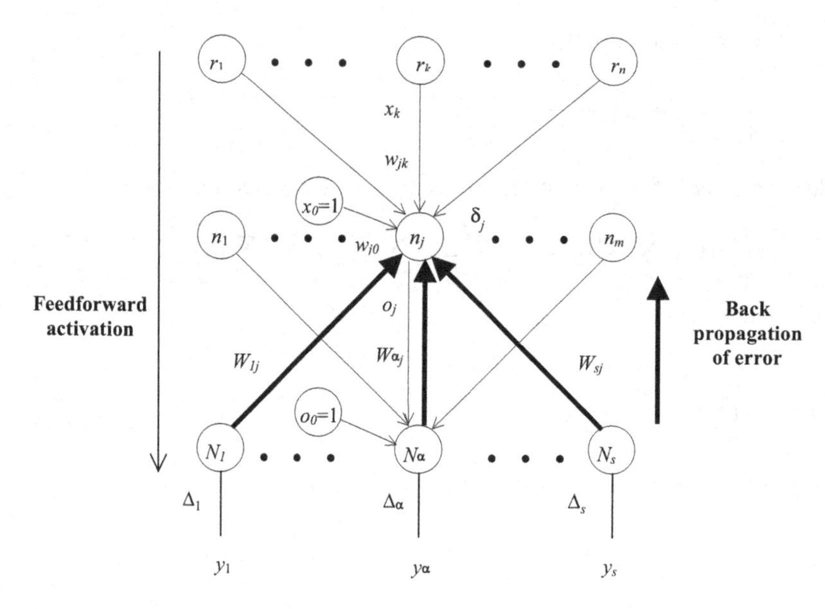

Backpropagation of error:

1. The input **x** is propagated forward to the network output **y**.
2. The output errors $\Delta_\alpha = y_\alpha - d_\alpha$, $\alpha = 1, \ldots, s$ are evaluated.
3. The output errors Δ_α are propagated back to the hidden layer (see Figure 5). This propagation results in associating new errors δ_i to all neurons at the hidden layer:

$$\delta_j = \sum_{\alpha=1}^{s} \Delta_\alpha W_{\alpha j} f'(\sum_{q=0}^{n} w_{jq} x_q),\ \Delta_\alpha = y_\alpha - d_\alpha\ ,\ j = 1, \ldots, m \qquad (22)\ \square$$

The equations (16)-(21) form the theoretical basis for use of so called batch gradient descent method. The batch gradient descent method uses the training rule that updates weights after all samples from training set are presented and their individual weight updates summed. But very often a modification of this method, called incremental gradient descent method, is used. This method uses incremental training rule that updates weights incrementally after each training sample is presented and its individual weight update calculated. So incremental gradient descent method iterates over training examples and can be considered to be a reasonable approximation of the original gradient descent method. Both these gradient descent methods are commonly used in practice.

So far we considered neural network training as a problem of finding the minimum of the pre-defined error function, which is highly nonlinear function of the network weights. Numerical mathematics provides different optimization methods for finding the minimum. The basic one is the above used gradient descent search method. Gradient descent search method uses linear approximation of error function and its convergence might be sometimes very slow. In such case numerical mathematics offers more efficient methods based on the second order approximation of error surface. These methods use for calculation of weight updates Hessian matrix, which consists of second order derivatives of error function. Therefore to compute weight updates is more time-consuming. However, the quicker convergence might outweigh this drawback. Conjugate-gradient method, quasi-Newton method or Levenberg-Marquardt method are mostly used second order optimization methods.

Generally it is not possible to say that the second order methods are better. Often better results are obtained with the standard gradient descent method after a long period of training. However using one of the second order methods we may acquire efficient networks architectures faster. Therefore the second order methods are mainly used at the beginning so that to gain quicker insight into behavior of different network architectures in the considered decision task.

NEURAL NETWORKS IN REGRESSION AND CLASSIFICATION PROBLEMS

The goal of the network training is not to memorize the training data but rather to model the underlying generator of the data so that the best possible predictions for the output can be made when the trained network is presented with a new, in the training set not contained, input vector. The underlying generator, from which training samples are independently drawn, is completely described if the probability density $p(\mathbf{x}, \mathbf{t})$ in the joint input-target space is known.

Assume that a neural network represents functions $y_\alpha(\mathbf{x}, \mathbf{w})$, $\alpha = 1, \ldots, s$ and that the training samples constitute the training set $T = \{(\mathbf{x}^i, \mathbf{t}^i), i = 1, \ldots, N\}$. Consider the average value $e_N(\mathbf{w})$ of the sum-of-square error $E(\mathbf{w})$:

$$e_N(\mathbf{w}) = \frac{1}{2N}\sum_{n=1}^{N}\sum_{\alpha=1}^{s}(y_\alpha(\mathbf{x}^i, \mathbf{w}) - t_\alpha^i)^2 \tag{23}$$

If the size N of the training set goes to infinity, the quantity $e_N(\mathbf{w})$ converges to the expectation value $\langle e_N(\mathbf{w})\rangle$, for which holds:

$$\langle e(\mathbf{w})\rangle = \lim_{N\to\infty} e_N(\mathbf{w}) = \frac{1}{2}\sum_{\alpha=1}^{s}\iint(y_\alpha(\mathbf{x}, \mathbf{w}) - t_\alpha)^2\, p(\mathbf{x}, t_\alpha)dt_\alpha d\mathbf{x} \tag{24}$$

The conditional expectations $\langle t_\alpha \mid \mathbf{x}\rangle$ and $\langle t_\alpha^2 \mid \mathbf{x}\rangle$ of the variables t_α and t_α^2 are:

$$\langle t_\alpha \mid \mathbf{x}\rangle = \int t_\alpha p(t_\alpha \mid \mathbf{x})dt_\alpha \tag{25}$$

and $$\langle t_\alpha^2 \mid \mathbf{x}\rangle = \int t_\alpha^2 p(t_\alpha \mid \mathbf{x})dt_\alpha \tag{26}$$

Using the well known identity $p(\mathbf{x}, t) = p(t \mid \mathbf{x})p(\mathbf{x})$ gives:

$$\langle e(\mathbf{w})\rangle = \frac{1}{2}\sum_{\alpha=1}^{s}\int_{t_\alpha}\int_{\mathbf{x}}(y_\alpha(\mathbf{x}, \mathbf{w}) - t_\alpha)^2\, p(t_\alpha \mid \mathbf{x})p(\mathbf{x})dt_\alpha d\mathbf{x} = \frac{1}{2}\sum_{\alpha=1}^{s}\int_{\mathbf{x}} I_\alpha(\mathbf{x})p(\mathbf{x})d\mathbf{x} \tag{27}$$

where:

$$I_\alpha(\mathbf{x}) = \int_{t_\alpha}(y_\alpha(\mathbf{x}, \mathbf{w}) - t_\alpha)^2\, p(t_\alpha|\mathbf{x})dt_\alpha \tag{28}$$

$I_\alpha(\mathbf{x})$ can be rewritten equivalently as:

$$I_\alpha(\mathbf{x}) = \int_{t_\alpha}\{(y_\alpha(\mathbf{x}, \mathbf{w}) - \langle t_\alpha \mid \mathbf{x}\rangle) + (\langle t_\alpha \mid \mathbf{x}\rangle - t_\alpha)\}^2\, p(t_\alpha \mid \mathbf{x})dt_\alpha \tag{29}$$

In the following equations we shall use another well-known identity of probability theory, namely:

$$\int_{t_\alpha} p(t_\alpha \mid \mathbf{x}) dt_\alpha = 1 \tag{30}$$

We are getting:

$$\int_{t_\alpha} (y_\alpha - \langle t_\alpha \mid \mathbf{x} \rangle)^2 p(t_\alpha \mid \mathbf{x}) dt_\alpha = (y_\alpha - \langle t_\alpha \mid \mathbf{x} \rangle)^2 \int_{t_\alpha} p(t_\alpha \mid \mathbf{x}) dt_\alpha = (y_\alpha - \langle t_\alpha \mid \mathbf{x} \rangle)^2 \tag{31}$$

$$\int_{t_\alpha} (y_\alpha - \langle t_\alpha \mid \mathbf{x} \rangle)(\langle t_\alpha \mid \mathbf{x} \rangle - t_\alpha) p(t_\alpha \mid \mathbf{x}) dt_\alpha = (y_\alpha - \langle t_\alpha \mid \mathbf{x} \rangle) \int_{t_\alpha} (\langle t_\alpha \mid \mathbf{x} \rangle - t_\alpha) p(t_\alpha \mid \mathbf{x}) dt_\alpha = \tag{32}$$

$$= (y_\alpha - \langle t_\alpha \mid \mathbf{x} \rangle)(\langle t_\alpha \mid \mathbf{x} \rangle \int_{t_\alpha} p(t_\alpha \mid \mathbf{x}) dt_\alpha - \int_{t_\alpha} t_\alpha p(t_\alpha \mid \mathbf{x}) dt_\alpha) = (y_\alpha - \langle t_\alpha \mid \mathbf{x} \rangle(\langle t_\alpha \mid \mathbf{x} \rangle - \langle t_\alpha \mid \mathbf{x} \rangle) = 0$$

and:

$$\int_{t_\alpha} (\langle t_\alpha \mid \mathbf{x} \rangle - t_\alpha)^2 p(t_\alpha \mid \mathbf{x}) dt_\alpha = \langle t_\alpha \mid \mathbf{x} \rangle^2 \int_{t_\alpha} p(t_\alpha \mid \mathbf{x}) dt_\alpha - 2\langle t_\alpha \mid \mathbf{x} \rangle \int_{t_\alpha} t_\alpha p(t_\alpha \mid \mathbf{x}) dt_\alpha + \int_{t_\alpha} t_\alpha^{\ 2} p(t_\alpha \mid \mathbf{x}) dt_\alpha \tag{33}$$

$$= \langle t_\alpha \mid \mathbf{x} \rangle^2 - 2\langle t_\alpha \mid \mathbf{x} \rangle^2 + \langle t_\alpha^2 \mid \mathbf{x} \rangle = \langle t_\alpha^2 \mid \mathbf{x} \rangle - \langle t_\alpha \mid \mathbf{x} \rangle^2$$

Putting (29) together with (31)-(33) gives:

$$I_\alpha(\mathbf{x}) = (y_\alpha(\mathbf{x}, \mathbf{w}) - \langle t_\alpha \mid \mathbf{x} \rangle)^2 + (\langle t_\alpha^2 \mid \mathbf{x} \rangle^2 - \langle t_\alpha \mid \mathbf{x} \rangle^2 \tag{34}$$

and due to (27):

$$\langle e(\mathbf{w}) \rangle = \frac{1}{2} \sum_{\alpha=1}^{s} \int_{\mathbf{x}} (y_\alpha(\mathbf{x}, \mathbf{w}) - \langle t_\alpha \mid \mathbf{x} \rangle)^2 p(\mathbf{x}) d\mathbf{x} + \frac{1}{2} \sum_{\alpha=1}^{s} \int_{\mathbf{x}} (\langle t_\alpha^2 \mid \mathbf{x} \rangle - \langle t_\alpha \mid \mathbf{x} \rangle^2) p(\mathbf{x}) d\mathbf{x} \tag{35}$$

The second term on the right hand side of the equation (35) is the variance of the distribution of t_α averaged over **x**. It represents the intrinsic variability of the learning data and can be regarded as noise. Because it is independent of weight vector **w**, the expectation value $\langle e(\mathbf{w}) \rangle$ is minimized by a vector $\mathbf{w}_{min}$ for which:

$$y_\alpha(\mathbf{x}, \mathbf{w}_{min}) = \langle t_\alpha \mid \mathbf{x} \rangle \tag{36}$$

Thus minimization of $\langle e(\mathbf{w}) \rangle$ provides a network that represents the conditional expectation of the target data $\langle t_\alpha \mid \mathbf{x} \rangle$. According to this important result the minimization of the sum-of-square error leads to the approximation of conditional expectation values of the target data.

If we can assume that the underlying probability density $p(\mathbf{x}, \mathbf{t})$ has a specific parametric form, then for search of the optimal network weights a method known in statistics as maximum likelihood method can be used. Maximum likelihood method seeks to find the optimum values for the parameters by maximizing likelihood function derived from the training data set. Because the samples are drawn independently from the same distribution, the likelihood $\Lambda(T)$ of the training set T is:

$$\Lambda(T) = \prod_{x} p(\mathbf{x}, \mathbf{t}) = \prod_{x} p(\mathbf{t} \mid \mathbf{x}) p(\mathbf{x}) \tag{37}$$

where the product is taken over all elements of the training set T. If we assume that the conditional distributions $p(t_\alpha \mid \mathbf{x})$ of the target variables t_α are independent, we can write:

$$p(\mathbf{t} \mid \mathbf{x}) = \prod_{\alpha=1}^{s} p(t_\alpha \mid \mathbf{x}), \ \alpha = 1, \dots, s \tag{38}$$

and $$\Lambda(T) = \prod_{x} p(\mathbf{x}, \mathbf{t}) = \prod_{x} \prod_{\alpha=1}^{s} p(t_\alpha \mid \mathbf{x}) p(\mathbf{x}) \tag{39}$$

REGRESSION PROBLEMS

At first consider a regression problem. Here a network is to represent values of continuous functions with added noise. More precisely it is reasonable to assume that target variables t_α are independent and given by deterministic functions $h_\alpha(\mathbf{x})$ with added Gaussian noise ε with zero mean and standard deviation σ which does not depend on $\mathbf{x}$ and α:

$$t_\alpha = h_\alpha(\mathbf{x}) + \varepsilon \tag{40}$$

$$p(t_\alpha \mid \mathbf{x}) = \frac{1}{(2\pi\sigma^2)^{\frac{1}{2}}} \exp\left(-\frac{(h_\alpha(\mathbf{x}) - t_\alpha)^2}{2\sigma^2} \right) \tag{41}$$

The functions $h_\alpha(\mathbf{x})$ are to be approximated with neural network outputs $y_\alpha(\mathbf{x}, \mathbf{w})$.

According to the (36) the gradient descent algorithm minimizing sum-of-square error leads to a network weights $\mathbf{w}^*$ that approximate conditional expectation values of target variables t_α:

$$y_\alpha(\mathbf{x}, \mathbf{w}^*) \cong \langle t_\alpha \mid \mathbf{x} \rangle = h_\alpha(\mathbf{x}) \tag{42}$$

Let us now analyze the considered regression problem using maximum likelihood method. If the network output $y_\alpha(\mathbf{x}, \mathbf{w})$ represents the functions $h_\alpha(\mathbf{x})$, then the likelihood function $\Lambda(T)$ of the training set T is:

$$\Lambda(T) = \prod_{\mathbf{x}} \prod_{\alpha=1}^{s} p(t_\alpha \mid \mathbf{x}) p(\mathbf{x}) = \prod_{x} \prod_{\alpha=1}^{s} \frac{1}{(2\pi\sigma^2)^{\frac{1}{2}}} \exp\left(-\frac{(y_\alpha(\mathbf{x}, \mathbf{w}) - t_\alpha)^2}{2\sigma^2} \right) p(\mathbf{x}) \tag{43}$$

To maximize $\Lambda(T)$ means to minimize $-\log \Lambda(T)$. We are getting

$$-\log \Lambda(T) = -\sum_{\mathbf{x}} \sum_{\alpha=1}^{s} \log(p(t_\alpha \mid \mathbf{x}) p(\mathbf{x})) = -\sum_{\mathbf{x}} \sum_{\alpha=1}^{s} \log p(t_\alpha \mid \mathbf{x}) - \sum_{\mathbf{x}} \sum_{\alpha=1}^{s} \log p(\mathbf{x}) \tag{44}$$

Because the last sum in (44) does not depend on the network weights, to minimize (44) means to minimize the expression:

$$-\sum_{\mathbf{x}} \sum_{\alpha=1}^{s} \log p(t_\alpha \mid \mathbf{x}) = \frac{Ns}{2\sigma^2} \log(2\pi\sigma^2) + \frac{1}{2\sigma^2} \sum_{\mathbf{x}} \sum_{\alpha=1}^{s} (y_\alpha(\mathbf{x}, \mathbf{w}) - t_\alpha)^2 \tag{45}$$

The first component of the sum on the right side of the equation (45) is constant and does not depend on network weights. Therefore (45) is minimized by a network that minimizes the second expression on the right side of (45). However, minimization of this second expression is equivalent to minimization of the sum-of-square error (13). Thus also according to the maximum likelihood method getting the best approximation of the target functions corresponds to searching for weights that minimize the sum-of-square error.

CLASSIFICATION PROBLEMS

In a classification problem vectors $\mathbf{x}$ are assumed to be members of finite number of classes or categories C_α, $\alpha = 1, \ldots, s$. There are various ways how the class membership can be coded. For more than two classes or for two classes that are not mutually exclusive a so-called 1-of-s coding scheme using a vector $\mathbf{t}$ of length s is mostly used. According to this scheme the element t_α of $\mathbf{t}$ takes the value 1 if the input vector $\mathbf{x}$ belongs to the class C_α and takes the value 0 otherwise. The obvious advantage of this classification scheme is that the conditional expectation values of variables t_α equal to the conditional probabilities of classes:

$$p(C_\alpha \mid \mathbf{x}) = \langle t_\alpha \mid \mathbf{x} \rangle \ , \alpha = 1, \ldots, s \tag{46}$$

For two mutually exclusive classes a more simple way of coding can be adopted. Instead of vector $\mathbf{t}$ a single scalar target variable t is used, the value of which is 1 if the vector $\mathbf{x}$ belongs to the class C_1 and 0 if it belongs to the class C_2. Clearly:

$$p(C_1 \mid \mathbf{x}) = \langle t \mid \mathbf{x} \rangle \text{ and } p(C_2 \mid \mathbf{x}) = 1 - \langle t \mid \mathbf{x} \rangle \tag{47}$$

The goal of network training is to obtain a network, the outputs of which approximate the conditional probabilities of classes as accurately as possible. One possibility that we have immediately at hand is to utilize the result (36) and to minimize the sum-of-square error using backpropagation algorithm. However we may try to get more accurate approximation by means of maximum likelihood method that should be, as parametric method, on limited data sets more efficient.

Two Mutually Excluded Classes

To start with, we consider the problems involving two mutually excluded classes. We assume to have a training set $T = \{(\mathbf{x}^i, t^i), i = 1, \ldots, N\}$ and a neural network with one output y. The value of y should represent the posterior probability $p(C_1|\mathbf{x})$. If this is true, then the probability of observing $t = 1$ for $\mathbf{x}$ falling into C_1 is y and the probability of observing $t = 0$ for $\mathbf{x}$ falling into C_2 is $1 - y$. We may combine both these cases into expression:

$$p(t \mid \mathbf{x}) = y^t (1 - y)^{1-t} \tag{48}$$

The likelihood $\Lambda(T)$ of the training data set T is then:

$$\Lambda(T) = \prod_{\mathbf{x}} p(t \mid \mathbf{x}) p(\mathbf{x}) = \prod_{\mathbf{x}} y^t (1-y)^{1-t} p(\mathbf{x}) \tag{49}$$

It is again more convenient instead of maximizing the likelihood function to minimize its negative logarithm:

$$-\log \Lambda(T) = -\sum_{\mathbf{x}} (t \log y + (1-t)\log(1-y)) - \sum_{\mathbf{x}} \log p(\mathbf{x}) \tag{50}$$

Because the last sum in (50) does not depend on the network, the minimization of $-\log\Lambda(T)$ leads to minimization of the so called cross-entropy error function:

$$E^* = -\sum_{\mathbf{x}} (t \log y + (1-t)\log(1-y)) \tag{51}$$

This result differs from the result we have obtained before and is considered to be more appropriate for applications. Therefore in classification tasks the gradient descent algorithm minimizing the cross-entropy error function, instead of minimizing the sum-of-square error function, is commonly used.

To be able to use the cross-entropy error function in the gradient descent algorithm, we must recalculate the expressions (17)-(20). For networks with only one linear output, neuron equations (17)-(20) take the form:

$$\frac{\partial E}{\partial W_j} = \frac{\partial}{W_j}\left(\frac{1}{2}\sum_{\mathbf{x}}(y-t)^2\right) = \sum_{\mathbf{x}}(y-t)\frac{\partial y}{\partial W_j} = \sum_{\mathbf{x}} \Delta o_j\,,\ \Delta = (y-t),\ o_j = f\left(\sum_{q=0}^{n} w_{jq}x_q\right) \tag{52}$$

and

$$\frac{\partial E}{\partial w_{jk}} = \frac{\partial}{w_{jk}}\left(\frac{1}{2}\sum_{\mathbf{x}}(y-t)^2\right) = \sum_{\mathbf{x}}(y-t)\frac{\partial y}{\partial w_{jk}} = \sum_{\mathbf{x}} \delta_j x_k\,,\quad \delta_j = \Delta W_j f'\left(\sum_{q=0}^{n} w_{jq}x_q\right) \tag{53}$$

If we use instead of the sum-of-square error function E the cross-entropy error function E^*, we are getting:

$$\frac{\partial E^*}{\partial W_j} = -\frac{\partial}{\partial W_j}\left(\sum_{\mathbf{x}} t\log y + (1-t)\log(1-y)\right) = \sum_{x}\left(\frac{t}{y}\frac{\partial y}{\partial W_j} + (1-t)\frac{-1}{(1-y)}\frac{\partial y}{\partial W_j}\right) =$$

$$= \sum_{\mathbf{x}} \frac{y-t}{y(1-y)}\frac{\partial y}{\partial W_j} = \sum_{\mathbf{x}} \Delta^* o_j \tag{54}$$

where:

$$\Delta^* = \frac{y-t}{y(1-y)}\ ,\ o_j = f\left(\sum_{q=0}^{n} w_{jq}x_q\right) \tag{55}$$

and:

$$\frac{\partial E^*}{\partial w_{jk}} = -\frac{\partial}{\partial w_{jk}}\left(\sum_{\mathbf{x}} t\log y + (1-t)\log(1-y)\right) = \sum_{\mathbf{x}} \frac{y-t}{y(1-y)}\frac{\partial y}{\partial w_{jk}} = \sum_{\mathbf{x}} \delta_j^* x_k \tag{56}$$

where:

$$\delta_j^* = \Delta^* W_j f'\left(\sum_{q=0}^{n} w_{jq}x_q\right) \tag{57}$$

The equations (54)-(57) show that the calculation of the gradient falls under the same scheme of backpropagation of error as before, if instead of error Δ the error Δ^* is used.

In a non-trivial classification problem the network should approximate probabilities, which take values from interval (0, 1). For this task also a network with sigmoid output neuron can be used. If the output sigmoid function of the output neuron is logistic function, i.e. sigmoid function given in (7) with $k = 1$, the following expressions for gradient components of cross-entropy error function E^* can be easily obtained:

$$\frac{\partial E^*}{\partial W_j} = \sum_{\mathbf{x}} y(1-y)\frac{y-t}{y(1-y)}\frac{\partial y}{\partial W_j} = \sum_{\mathbf{x}} \Delta o_j \tag{59}$$

$$\frac{\partial E^*}{\partial w_{jk}} = \sum_{\mathbf{x}} y(1-y)\frac{y-t}{y(1-y)}\frac{\partial y}{\partial w_{jk}} = \sum_{\mathbf{x}} \delta_j x_k \tag{60}$$

where Δ and δ_j are the same as those in (52) and (53). In the derivation of (59) and (60) the property of sigmoid function derivative, given in (8), was used.

Thus for the network architecture with logistic output neuron the gradient of cross-entropy function can be calculated using the same scheme (22), that was used in calculating the gradient of sum-of-square error function for the network with linear output neuron.

Multiple Independent Classes

In some applications vectors might be categorized into s ($s > 2$) classes that are not mutually exclusive and we wish to use a network with s outputs that will determine particular probabilities of class membership.

Suppose that the classes are mutually independent. If the network output y_α represents the probability $p(C_\alpha \mid \mathbf{x})$, then the posterior probability of target value $\mathbf{t}$ of the input vector $\mathbf{x}$ is:

$$p(\mathbf{t}|\mathbf{x}) = \prod_{\alpha=1}^{s} p(t_\alpha|\mathbf{x}) = \prod_{\alpha=1}^{s} y_\alpha^{t_\alpha}(1-y_\alpha)^{1-t_\alpha} \tag{61}$$

Therefore the likelihood of the training data set T is:

$$\Lambda(T) = \prod_{x}\prod_{\alpha=1}^{s} y_\alpha^{t_\alpha}(1-y_\alpha)^{1-t_\alpha} p(\mathbf{x}) \tag{62}$$

Minimization of $-\log \Lambda(T)$ leads to minimization of cross-entropy function:

$$E^* = -\sum_{\mathbf{x}}\sum_{\alpha=1}^{s}(t_\alpha \log y_\alpha + (1-t_\alpha)\log(1-y_\alpha)) \tag{63}$$

Under assumption that at output layer linear neurons are used, we will get the following expressions for calculating the gradient components of E^*:

$$\frac{\partial E^*}{\partial W_{ij}} = \sum_{\mathbf{x}}\sum_{\alpha=1}^{s}\frac{(y_\alpha - t_\alpha)}{y_\alpha(1-y_\alpha)}\frac{\partial y_\alpha}{\partial W_{ij}} \tag{64}$$

$$\frac{\partial E^*}{\partial w_{jk}} = \sum_{\mathbf{x}}\sum_{\alpha=1}^{s}\frac{(y_\alpha - t_\alpha)}{y_\alpha(1-y_\alpha)}\frac{\partial y_\alpha}{\partial w_{jk}} \tag{65}$$

Comparing (64) with (17) and (65) with (19) we see that the gradient components can be calculated according to the same classical backpropagation scheme (17)-(20) if we substitute the error Δ_α with error Δ^*_α, where:

$$\Delta^*_\alpha = \frac{y_\alpha - t_\alpha}{y_\alpha(1-y)} \tag{66}$$

Suppose now that we will use a network with logistic neurons at its output layer. Then we will get:

$$\frac{\partial E^*}{\partial W_{ij}} = \sum_{\mathbf{x}}\sum_{\alpha=1}^{s} y_\alpha(1-y_\alpha)\frac{(y_\alpha - t_\alpha)}{y_\alpha(1-y_\alpha)}\frac{\partial y_\alpha}{\partial W_{ij}} = \sum_{\mathbf{x}}\sum_{\alpha=1}^{s}(y_\alpha - t_\alpha)\frac{\partial y_\alpha}{\partial W_{ij}} \tag{67}$$

$$\frac{\partial E^*}{\partial w_{jk}} = \sum_{\mathbf{x}}\sum_{\alpha=1}^{s} y_\alpha(1-y_\alpha)\frac{(y_\alpha - t_\alpha)}{y_\alpha(1-y_\alpha)}\frac{\partial y_\alpha}{\partial w_{jk}} = \sum_{\mathbf{x}}\sum_{\alpha=1}^{s}(y_\alpha - t_\alpha)\frac{\partial y_\alpha}{\partial w_{jk}} \tag{68}$$

We see that for this network architecture the gradient of cross-entropy function can be computed according to the classical backpropagation scheme (22).

Multiple Excluded Classes

Consider now the classification problem involving more than two mutually excluded classes:

$$C_1, \ldots, C_s, s > 2$$

coded according to the 1-of-s coding scheme, where each classified input is a member of one and only one class $C_1, \ldots, C_s$.

Assume that the classification network has at its output layer s neurons with so called softmax output functions

$$y_i = \theta_i(a_1,\ldots,a_s) = \frac{\exp(a_i)}{\sum_{j=1}^{s}\exp(a_j)}, \quad i = 1, \ldots, s \tag{69}$$

Here the real variables $a_1, \ldots, a_s$ are excitation inputs into the output neurons (see Figure 6):

$$a_i = \sum_{j=0}^{m} W_{ij} o_j \tag{70}$$

and $o_j, j = 1, \ldots, m$ are outputs of neurons at hidden layer

$$o_j = \sum_{k=0}^{n} f(w_{jk} x_k) \tag{71}$$

Obviously the network with softmax output neurons represents continuous mapping from the n-dimensional Euclidian input space into the space $(0, 1)^s$. The partial mappings y_i are continuous functions with values in the interval (0, 1). Their sum for all network inputs equals 1. Thus this network is well suited for here considered classification problem.

We shall show that using the maximum likelihood method for establishing the optimal network weights leads to the standard backpropagation scheme (22).

Figure 6. Neural network with softmax output neurons

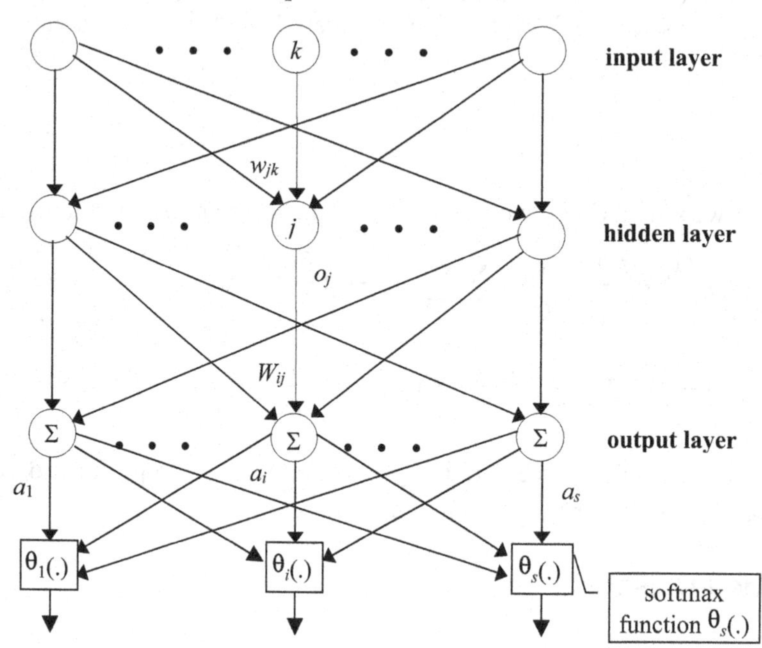

In the following we will need derivatives of softmax functions that can be easily calculated:

$$\frac{\partial y_l}{\partial a_k} = \delta_{lk} y_l - y_l y_k, \quad l, k = 1, \ldots, s \tag{72}$$

where δ_{lk} equals one if $l = k$ and equals zero otherwise.

If values y_l represent class membership posterior probabilities $p(C_l \mid \mathbf{x})$, then the probability of target vector **t** can be written as:

$$p(\mathbf{t}|\mathbf{x}) = \prod_{l=1}^{s} y_l^{t_l} \quad l = 1, \ldots, s \tag{73}$$

The likelihood of the training set is then:

$$\Lambda(T) = \prod_{\mathbf{x}} \prod_{l=1}^{s} y_l^{t_l} p(\mathbf{x}) \tag{74}$$

Instead of maximization of (74) we can minimize:

$$-\log \Lambda(T) = -\sum_{\mathbf{x}} \sum_{l=1}^{s} \log y_l^{t_l} - \sum_{\mathbf{x}} \sum_{l=1}^{s} \log p(\mathbf{x}) \tag{75}$$

Because the last double sum in (75) is constant, the expression (75) is minimized if cross-entropy function E is minimized:

$$E = -\sum_{\mathbf{x}} \sum_{l=1}^{s} \log y_l^{t_l} = -\sum_{\mathbf{x}} \sum_{l=1}^{s} t_l \log y_l \tag{76}$$

For the gradient of the error function E we are getting:

$$\frac{\partial E}{\partial W_{ij}} = -\frac{\partial}{\partial W_{ij}} \sum_{\mathbf{x}} \sum_{l=1}^{s} t_l \log y_l = -\sum_{\mathbf{x}} \sum_{l=1}^{s} \frac{t_l}{y_l} \frac{\partial y_l}{\partial W_{ij}} = -\sum_{\mathbf{x}} \sum_{l=1}^{s} \frac{t_l}{y_l} \sum_{\alpha=1}^{s} \frac{\partial y_l}{\partial a_\alpha} \frac{\partial a_\alpha}{\partial W_{ij}} \quad (77)$$

The substitution (72) into (78) provides:

$$\frac{\partial E}{\partial W_{ij}} = -\sum_{\mathbf{x}} \sum_{l=1}^{s} \sum_{\alpha=1}^{s} \frac{t_l}{y_l} (\delta_{l\alpha} y_l - y_l y_\alpha) \frac{\partial a_\alpha}{\partial W_{ij}} = \sum_{\mathbf{x}} \sum_{\alpha=1}^{s} \sum_{l=1}^{s} (t_l y_\alpha - t_l \delta_{l\alpha}) \frac{\partial a_\alpha}{\partial W_{ij}} =$$

$$= \sum_{\mathbf{x}} \sum_{\alpha=1}^{s} \left(\sum_{l=1}^{s} (t_l y_\alpha) - \sum_{l=1}^{s} t_l \delta_{l\alpha} \right) \frac{\partial a_\alpha}{\partial W_{ij}} = \sum_{\mathbf{x}} \sum_{\alpha=1}^{s} \left(y_\alpha \sum_{l=1}^{s} t_l - t_\alpha \right) \frac{\partial a_\alpha}{\partial W_{ij}} \quad (78)$$

As the sum of t_l over l must equal to one, we have:

$$\frac{\partial E}{\partial W_{ij}} = \sum_{\mathbf{x}} \sum_{\alpha=1}^{s} (y_\alpha - t_\alpha) \frac{\partial a_\alpha}{\partial W_{ij}} = \sum_{\mathbf{x}} \Delta_i o_j \quad (79)$$

where Δ_i and o_j are given by (18).

Similarly we are getting:

$$\frac{\partial E}{\partial w_{jk}} = \sum_{\mathbf{x}} \sum_{\alpha=1}^{s} (y_\alpha - t_\alpha) \frac{\partial a_\alpha}{\partial w_{jk}} = \sum_{\mathbf{x}} \delta_j x_k \quad (80)$$

where δ_j is given according to (18) and (20).

Thus in the case of mutually excluded classes the maximum likelihood method leads to minimization of the cross-entropy error function E given by (76). If a network with softmax output neurons is used, then, quite surprisingly, the gradient components of this error function can be calculated according to the standard backpropagation of error scheme (22).

TRAINING NEURAL NETWORKS

Preparing Data

Before training the neural network the data are often transformed into some new representation. It is not necessary, since neural networks can perform any arbitrary mapping between input and output variables. Nevertheless in many applications such pre-processing leads to the better performance of the final trained network.

The simplest pre-processing consists in normalization of input data. In regression problems also output data are usually normalized. Normalization of a variable x is a linear transformation:

$$x' = \frac{x - \bar{x}}{\sigma} \quad (81)$$

where $\bar{x}$ is the mean and σ the standard deviation of x. Obviously the new variable x' has zero mean and unit standard deviation.

Another possibility how to pre-process the input data is to map it onto interval $\langle 0, 1 \rangle$ using linear transformation:

$$x' = \frac{x - x_{\min}}{x_{\min} - x_{\max}} \qquad (82)$$

In medicine we often deal with categorical data. A categorical variable takes values from an unordered set of values. For example variable eye color might have values blue, green or brown. For this data the coding scheme 1-of-*s*, introduced in paragraph 5, can be used. This coding scheme is more appropriate than to use a code that imposes some artificial ordering on the data as for example the code that assigns to blue, green and brown the values 0.0, 0.5 and 1.0.

More sophisticated pre-processing may involve reduction of the dimensionality of the input data and is commonly called feature extraction. There are many methods we may choose from. For regression problems very often the well-known statistical method PCA (Principal Component Analysis) is used. The goal of the PCA method is to extract m normalized orthogonal vectors in the input space that account for as much of the data variance as possible. Then by projecting n-dimensional input vectors into m orthogonal directions, the dimensionality reduction with minimal loss of information is achieved.

In classification problems with discrete input variables methods based on results of information theory are used. Here the information content of input variables is calculated and input variables with the greatest information content are then chosen.

Also neural networks provide methods for dimensionality reduction. For example consider a feed-forward network with one hidden layer that is trained to repeat the input vectors on its output (so called auto-associative network). If the number m of neurons at the hidden layer is less than the number n of neurons at the input and the output layers and if the training has been successful, then the weights between the input and the hidden layer determine the linear transformation from n-dimensional input space into a reduced m-dimensional feature space.

In many applications it happens that some of the input values are missing for some input vectors from the data set. This deficiency must be settled before training. The simplest solution is to discard the vectors with missing values from the data set. This is possible only if the quantity of data available is sufficiently large. Also if the mechanism, responsible for omission of data values depends on data itself, this approach cannot be adopted, because we might modify the underlying data distribution. Various heuristic methods have been proposed for situations in which the discarding of incomplete data patterns cannot be used. The simplest one is to fill the missing value of the variable with its mean value. A more elaborate approach is to express the variable that has missing values in terms of other variables and then to fill the missing values according to the regression function.

Local Minima and Overfitting

There are two main troubles with network training: trapping in a local minimum and overfitting. Backpropagation algorithm implements a gradient descent search through the weight space reducing the value of defined error function. Because the error surface may contain many different local minima, the algorithm can be trapped in one of these. As a result the backpropagation algorithm is only guaranteed to converge toward some local minimum of the error function and not necessarily to its global minimum.

The second trouble is phenomenon known as data overfitting. The network should correctly map inputs to corresponding target values not only for previously used training data but also for new inputs. If we train a network with many hidden neurons, the error will be decreasing and the network will adapt very well to the training data. But usually such network will fail to map well new, previously unseen input data, i.e. it will have poor generalization ability.

The essence of the overfitting trouble can be easily explained on a simple example of regression. Assume that the training data are generated from distribution given by deterministic function $h(x)$ with added Gaussian noise (see Figure 7). For sufficiently large training data set the output of the network would be according to (42) $y(x) \cong h(x)$. However, if the training data set contains only few samples and if a network with good generalization ability is taken (i.e. a network with many hidden neurons), then, if not trapped in a local minimum, the network after sufficiently long training period might closely approximate the partly linear function $\varphi(x)$. Though the network will fit training data very well, this solution is not what we had in mind. Surely we would prefer, for example, the straight line solution $\psi(x)$.

Since the goal of network training is to find the network with the best performance on new data, it is necessary to evaluate the error function using data which is independent of that used for training. This independent data form so called validation set. Using different network architectures and varying learning parameters of backpropagation algorithm we get many network configurations, performance of which is then compared by evaluating the error function using this validation set. The network having the smallest error with respect to the validation set is then selected. Because this procedure itself can lead to a selection of a network with small error only on this validation set, the performance of the selected network should be confirmed by measuring its performance on a third independent data set called test set.

In many applications the amount of data available for training, validating and testing is limited. To find a good network we wish use as much of the available data as possible for training. However if the validation and test data sets are small, the accuracy of the network performance estimates is poor. Therefore sometimes so called cross-validation is used. In the S-fold cross-validation the available data is partitioned into S groups. Then $S - 1$ groups are chosen and used for training a set of neural networks. The performance of the trained networks is evaluated on the remaining group considered as a validation set. This procedure is repeated for all possible S choices of the validation set (see Figure 8). As ultimate

Figure 7. Overfitting training data

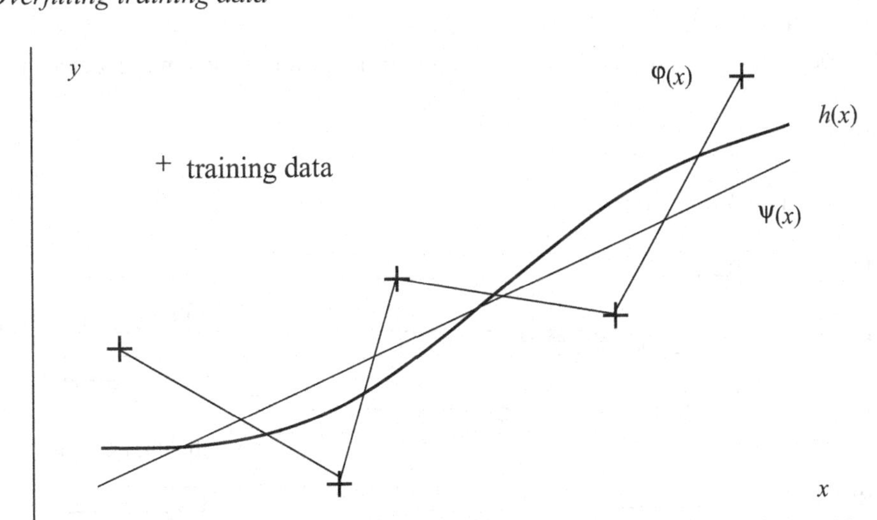

performance estimates of trained networks the averages over all S choices of validation set are taken and the network with the best average is chosen as the best solution.

To escape trapping in local minima a technique called regularization is commonly used. The technique of regularization prefers smooth network mappings by adding a penalty Ω to the error function:

$$E'(\mathbf{w}) = E(\mathbf{w}) + \delta\Omega \tag{83}$$

The weight decay is the regularization technique mostly used. If descent search algorithm starts with small weights, the output function of the network represents in weight space roughly linear surface. The reason is that neuron output functions are sigmoid functions, which are near zero approximately linear. Thus to keep weights small means to have smoother error surface which helps the algorithm to escape local minima. To achieve this goal we might add to the error function $E(\mathbf{w})$ an expression penalizing big weight vectors:

$$E'(\mathbf{w}) = E(\mathbf{w}) + \frac{1}{2}\delta|\mathbf{w}|^2 = E(\mathbf{w}) + \frac{1}{2}\delta\sum_j w_j^2 \quad , \delta > 0 \tag{84}$$

and search for minimum of the function $E'(\mathbf{w})$ instead of $E(\mathbf{w})$.

Gradient of error function $E'(\mathbf{w})$ is then:

$$\text{grad } E'(\mathbf{w}) = \text{grad } E(\mathbf{w}) + \delta\,\mathbf{w} \tag{85}$$

Thus in the descent search algorithm the expression for weight vector modification after n−1-th step of the algorithm will change into:

$$\mathbf{w}^n = \mathbf{w}^{n-1} - \varepsilon\ \text{grad}E(\mathbf{w}^{n-1}) - \gamma\,\mathbf{w}^{n-1} + \mu\,\Delta\,\mathbf{w}^{n-1}, \quad \gamma = \varepsilon\delta \tag{86}$$

The most powerful and the mostly used technique of avoiding overfitting is so called early stopping. The network is iteratively trained on samples taken from training set. During the training the error measured on the training set is typically decreasing. However the error measured with respect to the independent validation set usually shows decrease only at first and then it starts to increase. The reason is that the network learned to fit particularities of the training examples that are not inherent in the underlying distribution. Training can therefore be stopped at the point of the smallest error measured on

Figure 8. S-fold cross-validation (S = 4)

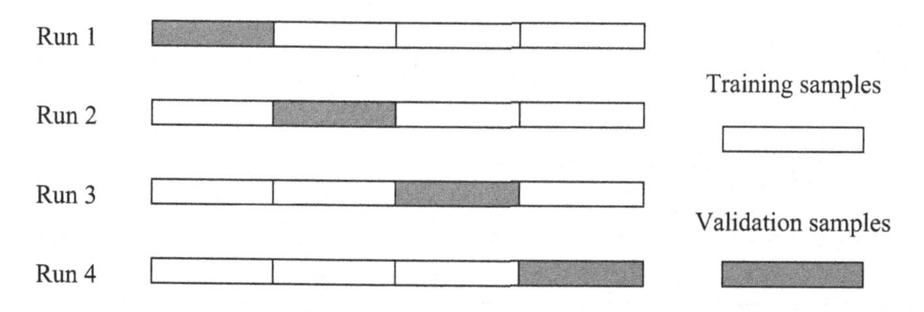

the validation set, because this gives the network with the best expected generalization performance. Of course if we did not used the S-fold cross-validation, the performance of the network must be confirmed on the independent test set.

NEURAL NETWORK APPLICATION GUIDELINES

It is difficult to give an overall general guidelines for building up a suitable neural network solution of a regression or a classification task. However, at least general recommendations may be provided.

At the beginning the data must be attentively scrutinized and input vectors with missing component values must be either discarded or missing values must be substituted with their probable values. For this purpose some standard statistical method can be used.

For non-categorical data the simplest substitution utilizes the main value of the missing component, computed over the whole data set. After getting rid of missing values the data should be normalized according to (81) or (82).

For categorical data we may estimate probabilities of particular values and substitute missing values according to this probability distribution estimate.

If we suspect data to be very redundant we ought to consider its transformation into a feature space with reduced dimension.

The data should be randomly separated into training, validation and test sets. Of course, greater training set leads to the better trained networks. On the other hand, smaller validation and testing sets mean that gained results will be less reliable. Therefore some compromise must be adopted. If we have too little data at our disposal, we should think of the use of cross-validation technique.

The choice of the proper network architecture is the most troublesome task. The numbers of neurons at the input layer and at the output layer are given by the task to be solved. However, the choice of the proper number of hidden layers and the choice of the proper numbers of neurons at each of them is a difficult problem that cannot be resolved beforehand. Usually we start with a network with one hidden layer and change the number of its neurons. More neurons means better approximation ability, however, as we saw before, networks with great approximation ability are susceptible to the overfitting. If we anticipate, due to the supposed complexity of the given data, that a network with greater approximation ability will be needed, we may try also network architectures with two hidden layers.

The output functions of neurons at the hidden layers are always sigmoid functions (7). However, to choose correctly the output functions of neurons at the output layer is the trickiest point concerning network architecture. A good choice can be made if the theoretical results, explained in the preceding paragraphs, are taken into account. These results offer more variants. Here we mention only those commonly used:

a. In regression problems the sum-of-square error function (13), calculated over the training set, should be minimized. The neurons at the output layer should be linear and gradient components used for weight updates should be computed according to the classical backpropagation scheme (22).
b. If we tackle the most usual classification problem, i.e. the problem with two mutually excluded classes, network with only one output neuron can be used. In this case the so call cross-entropy error function (51) should be minimized. To accomplish the minimization easily we can use at the

output layer of the network the logistic neuron (i.e. the neuron with sigmoid output function (7), where k=1). The gradient components used for weight updates then are to be calculated according to the classical backpropagation scheme (22). The other possibility is to use 1-of-2 class coding scheme. Then the corresponding neural network will have 2 output neurons and the error function to be minimized will be the cross-entropy error function (76). Using output neurons with softmax output functions will facilitate computation of weight updates as they can be calculated according to the classical backpropagation scheme (22).

c. For classification problems with s (s>2) classes the so called 1-of-s coding scheme is the best choice.
   - If the classes are mutually excluded (i.e. each classified input falls into one and only one class), then the cross-entropy error function (76) should be minimized. The usual practice is to use the network with softmax functions at the output layer. Strictly speaking this architecture does not fall under the paradigm of layer network, as the output function of each output neuron depends not only on the excitation input into the same output neuron, but also on the excitation inputs into all other output neurons (see Figure 6). However, using this architecture leads to the standard calculation of weight updates, i.e. the calculation of gradient components of the error function (76) leads to the usual backpropagation scheme (22).
   - If the classes are not mutually excluded, then there exist two possibilities:
     - We may decompose the s-class problem into s independent 2-class problems and create s independent networks, letting each of them to discriminate between two mutually excluded classes C_i and $\neg C_i$.
     - The second possibility is to assume mutual independence of classes. Then we will use one network with s neurons at the output layer and the error function to be minimized will be the cross-entropy function (63). If we use in the output layer neurons with logistic output function, then the gradient components necessary for weight updates are to be calculated according to the classical backpropagation scheme (22).

After establishing the network architecture we may start the network training:

a. We choose values for training parameters. These values are to be preferably taken from intervals that proved to be good in similar experiments referred to in literature. For the rate of weight change ε it is usually interval $\langle 0.001, 0.1\rangle$, for momentum μ interval $\langle 0.1, 0.9\rangle$ and for weight decay γ interval $\langle 0.0001, 0.001\rangle$.

b. We assign small random real values to initial weights and start training. One efficient way how to stop training is to follow the training process on line and stop it if the network error, computed on the validation set starts to increase. Programs that carry out the training process usually calculate both training and validation errors after each training epoch and cache the weights with the smallest validation error. The training process should be repeated tens times, each time for new randomly initialized weights and those weights, which have proved to be the most successful when tested on the validation set should be taken as the best one.

c. The values of training parameters should be systematically changed and the step b) should be repeated.

After behavior of the current network architecture has been systematically examined, experiments with new network architectures should be carried out.

At the end of the training the network with the least validation error should be chosen as the optimal solution of the given classification or regression problem. Eventually its performance should be tested on the independent test data set.

APPLICATION 1: ISCHEMIC HEART DISEASE

Ischemic heart disease is characterized by reduced blood supply to the heart muscle (myocardium), usually due to atherosclerosis of the coronary arteries. Myocardial perfusion imaging is a form of functional cardiac imaging commonly used for the diagnostics of ischemic heart disease. Imaging is usually done by means of the Single Photon Emission Computed Tomography (SPECT).

SPECT is a nuclear tomographic imaging technique using gamma rays. To conduct the scan a small amount of radioisotope is injected into the blood circulation of the examined patient. The radioisotope emits positrons that after traveling up to few millimeters annihilates with electrons producing pair of photons moving in the opposite directions. Photon pairs are detected with gamma camera and multiple 2-D images (projections) from multiple angles are aquired. From these projections the 3-dimentional structure of the scanned area can be then established applying a tomographic reconstruction algorithm. On the scan, the areas where the radioisotope has been absorbed will show up differently than the areas that have not absorb it due to decreased blood flow to the area.

The underlying principle of the myocardial perfusion imaging is that under stress conditions diseased myocardium receives less blood flow than normal myocardium. SPECT imaging is performed under stress (during physical exercise) and at rest. Diagnosis is made by comparing stress images to images obtained at rest.

In the application 1 we pursue a diagnostic problem to discriminate between healthy individuals (normal) and individuals with ischemic heart disease (abnormal) after myocardial perfusion SPECT scan. The pictures obtained by SPECT scan were divided into 22 regions of interest. Each region of interest was described by integer value from interval $\langle 0, 100 \rangle$. As each patient was scanned under stress and at rest, the vector describing a patient consists of 44 components or features. The patient vector database contained 267 patient vectors (212 normal and 55 abnormal) without any missing values.

Utilized data comes from machine learning data repository of University of California in Irvine that serves as a benchmark for testing machine learning algorithms, including neural networks (UCI Machine Learning, 2007). Neural networks training was carried out using neural network module of commercial statistical software package STATISTICA, version 7.1.

The patient vectors were normalized and randomly parted into three sets. The training set consisted of 135 patients (109 normal, 26 abnormal), the validation set consisted of 66 patients (56 normal, 10 abnormal) and the test set consisted of 66 patients (47 normal, 19 abnormal). According to the paragraph Neural network application guidelines the network architectures with one hidden layer, 44 input neurons and one output neuron with logistic output function was used. In the role of the error function to be minimized the cross-entropy function was taken.

The results of training are given in Table 1. For all architectures (i.e. for each chosen number of hidden neurons) the values of weight change rate ε and that of the momentum μ were varied. The training

Table 1. Classification of cardiac patients into normal or abnormal classes

neurons in hidden layer	ε	μ	N	E_{valid}	P_{train}	P_{valid}	P_{test}
20	.001	.2	800	.5153	.8518	.6970	.7576
	.005	.2	200	.5420	.7259	.6970	.6364
	.001	.3	600	.5762	.7481	.7121	.6667
	.005	.3	300	.5328	.7852	.7727	.7878
30	.001	.2	400	.5173	.8444	.8030	.7424
	.005	.2	150	.5050	.7556	.6364	.6970
	.001	.3	400	.5291	.7630	.7273	.7121
	.005	.3	300	.5328	.7630	.6818	.6818
40	**.001**	**.2**	**340**	**.4416**	**.8667**	**.8789**	**.7273**
	.005	.2	200	.5181	.8370	.6818	.7121
	.001	.3	800	.4601	.9037	.8636	.7576
	.005	.3	200	.5244	.8296	.7121	.7272

for each particular combination of ε and μ values was carried out approximately twenty times, each time with different, randomly generated, initial values. During a particular training run the estimate of the error function on the validation set E_{valid} and the estimate of the error function on the training set E_{train} were calculated at the end of every training epoch. The courses of the error estimates E_{train}, E_{valid} were observed on-line and when the overfitting (i.e. the increase of the error estimate E_{valid}) turned out to be obvious, the training process was stopped. During each training run the program stored the most successful weights and these weights constituted the resulting configuration of the run. The number N in Table 1 provides the total number of epochs used for training. As performance measure the ratio of correctly classified vectors to the number of all classified vectors was taken. The performance was tested on all three sets and thus three performance measures P_{train}, P_{valid} and P_{test} were obtained.

After training the network with the least validation error E_{valid} was chosen and its performance was tested. From Table 1 we see that the most successful was the network with validation error $E_{valid} = 0.4416$, performance of which estimated on the test set was $P_{test} = 0.73$. The confidence interval of P_{test} for the 95 % confidence level can be calculated as follows (see for example Mitchell (1997)):

$$P_{test} \pm 1.96\sqrt{\frac{P_{test}(1-P_{test})}{N_{test}}} = 0.73 \pm 0.11 \qquad (87)$$

where $N_{test} = 66$ is the size of the test data set.

APPLICATION 2: BREAST CANCER

Mammography is the most effective method for breast cancer screening available. However, to discriminate between benign and malignant mammographic data is a hard task. Therefore several computer-aided diagnosis systems have been proposed. These systems help physicians in their decision to perform a breast biopsy immediately or to perform short term follow up examination instead.

The Breast Imaging Reporting and Data System (BI-RADS), developed by the American College of Radiology, provides a standardized classification for mammographic studies. According to BI-RADS mammographic data can be classified into 7 assessment categories: incomplete = 0, negative = 1, benign finding = 2, probably benign finding = 3, suspicious abnormality = 4, highly suspicious of malignancy = 5, biopsy-proven malignancy = 6. All categories reflect the radiologist's level of suspicion for malignancy, and these assessment categories have been shown to be correlated with the likelihood of malignancy.

In application 2 we explored the possibility to use neural networks as decision support system that would help physicians to discriminate between benign and malignant mammography findings. We used the data set that originated from UCI Machine Learning Repository (UCI Machine Learning Repository, 2008) and that was collected at University of Erlangen-Nuremberg between 2003 and 2006 (Elter, 2007). It contained 961 screened patients with mass lesions. Each patient was described with six parameters: BI-RADS assessment category (1-5), age (in years), three BI-RADS attributes characterizing mass lesion (mass shape, mass margin, mass density) and severity (benign=0, malignant=1).

BI-RADS attributes were the following:

Mass shape: Round = 1, oval = 2, lobular = 3, irregular = 4
Mass margin: Circumscribed = 1, microlobulated = 2, obscured = 3, ill-defined = 4, speculated = 5
Mass density: High = 1, iso = 2, low = 3, fat-containing = 4

The BI-RADS assessment was assigned to each patient in double-review process by physicians. As BI-RADS assessment was a subjective parameter we did not include it into the classification model. Thus vectors describing patients included patient's age and three BI-RADS attributes. The BI-RADS attributes were categorical and therefore they were coded using 1-of-*s* coding scheme. Thus 4 input neurons were necessary to code the mass shape, 5 input neurons to code mass margin and 4 neurons to code mass density.

The data set contained missing values. As the data set was sufficiently large, we simply discarded all input vectors with missing values. The resulting data set consisted of 427 benign and 402 malignant individuals. For modeling we used the neural network module of STATISTICA 2008. The data set was randomly separated into training set (60% of cases), validation set (20% of cases) and test set (20% of cases).

According to the Neural network application guidelines recommendation the coding scheme of classes 1-of-2 was chosen. The network had 14 input neurons, 1 hidden layer and 2 output neurons with softmax output functions. The minimized error function was cross-entropy function (76).

According to Neural network application guidelines we systematically changed the network architecture (number of neurons in hidden layer). For each particular architecture we varied values of the weight change rate ε and that of the momentum μ and we calculated the performance measures on training set P_{train}, validation set P_{valid} and test set P_{test}. Then the network configuration with the highest value P_{valid} was chosen as the resulting network. From Table 2 we see that it was the network with $P_{valid} = .8242$. Eventually the confidence interval of P_{test} for the 95 % confidence level was calculated with the result $P_{test} = .81 \pm .06$.

Table 2. Discrimination between benign and malignant mammographic data

neurons in hidden layer	ε	μ	*N*	P_{train}	P_{valid}	P_{test}
5	.1	.3	600	.8336	.8060	.8181
	.05	.3	600	8136	8060	8000
	.01	.3	1200	.8256	.8121	.8181
10	.1	.3	1200	.8356	.8121	.8121
	.1	.3	600	.8336	.8121	.8121
	.05	.3	600	.8336	.8060	.8181
	.01	.3	600	.8336	.8121	.8181
15	**.1**	**.3**	**1200**	**8316**	**.8242**	**.8121**
	.1	.2	1200	.8476	.8121	.7939
	.1	.4	1200	.8376	.8060	.8121
	.1	.3	600	.8376	.8060	.8121
	.05	.3	600	.8316	.8000	.8181
	.01	.3	1200	.8316	.8060	.8181
	.01	.3	600	.8196	.8121	.8121
20	.1	.3	600	.8216	.7939	.8181
	0.05	.3	600	.8396	.8000	.8181
	.01	.3	1200	.8336	.8060	.8181

CONCLUSION

Classification and prediction are important parts of today medical decision-making. Since the amount and the complexity of patient's data that must be considered when crucial decisions are taken is all the time increasing, the significance of automatic algorithms emerges. Although they cannot substitute decisions of a medical doctor yet they may support them. In last decade many algorithms that proved to be well suited to medical decision support appeared also in the field of neural networks. The most important of them showed to be those based on feedforward layer networks.

To develop a successful neural network application is far from simple and straightforward process. The knowledge of basics of neural network theory is necessary for the correct choice of network architecture as well as some experience in training for choosing proper parameter values.

In the first part of this chapter those parts of neural network theory that are crucial for network architecture design have been presented. Although theoretical analysis cannot determine the architecture unequivocally, it still may give helpful suggestions that enable to exclude improper variants and make the search for proper network architecture more efficient.

The network training is often cumbersome process requiring a lot of computing. Though the underlining troubles as trapping in a local minimum or overfitting are intuitively well understood, no theory permitting to avoid them exists. Thus the training requires rather engineering experience than theoretical analysis. Therefore in the last part of this chapter we have given at least general hints for network training in the form of neural network application guidelines and demonstrated its use on two medical classification problems taken from the field of cardiology and radiology.

ACKNOWLEDGMENT

This work has been supported by the Ministry of Education of the Czech Republic (program MSM 6046070904).

REFERENCES

Alkan, A., Koklukaya, E., & Subasi, A. (2005). Automatic seizure detection in EEG using logistic regression and artificial neural network. *Journal of Neuroscience Methods, 148*, 167–176.

Bishop, CH. M. (1996). *Neural Networks for Pattern Recognition*. Oxford, Oxford University Press.

Bottaci, L., & Drew, P. J. (1997). Artificial Neural Networks Applied to Outcome Prediction for Colorectal Cancer Patients in Separate Institutions. *Lancet, 350*(16), 469-473.

Chen, D., Chang, R., Kuo, W., Chen, M., & Huang, Y. (2002). Diagnosis of breast tumors with sonographic texture analysis using wavelet transform and neural networks. *Ultrasound in Medicine & Biology, 28*(10), 1301-1310.

Coppini, G., Diciotti, S., Falchini, M., Villari, N., & Valli, G. (2003). Neural networks for computer-aided diagnosis: detection of lung nodules in chest radiograms. *IEEE Transactions on Information Technology in Biomedicine, 7*(4), 344-357.

Cybenko, G. (1988). *Continuous valued neural networks with two hidden layers are sufficient* (Technical Report). Department of Computer Science, Medford, Tufts University.

Cybenko, G. (1989). Approximation by superpositions of a sigmoidal function. *Mathematics of Control, Signals and Systems, 2*, 303-314.

Elter, M., Schulz-Wendtland, & Wittenberg, T. (2007). The prediction of breast cancer biopsy outcomes using two CAD approaches that both emphasize an intelligible decision process. *Medical Physics, 34*(11), 4164-4172.

Gant, V., Rodway, S., & Wyatt, J. (2001). Artificial neural networks: Practical considerations for clinical applications. In V. Gant, R. Dybowski (Eds.), *Clinical applications of artificial neural networks* (pp. 329-356). Cambridge, Cambridge University Press.

Gletsos, M., Mougiakakou, S. G., Matsopoulos, G. K., Nikita, K. S., Nikita, A. S., & Kelekis, D. (2003). A computer-aided diagnostic system to characterize CT focal liver lesions: Design and optimization of a neural network classifier. *IEEE Transaction on Information Technology in Biomedicine, 7*(3), 153-162.

Halkiotis, S., Botsis, T., & Rangoussi, M. (2007). Automatic detection of clustered microcalcifications in digital mammograms using mathematical morphology and neural networks. *Signal Processing, 87*(3), 1559-1568.

Hamamoto, I., Okada, S., Hashimoto, T., Wakabayashi, H., Maeba, T., & Maeta, H. (1995). Predictions of the early prognosis of the hepatectomized patient with hepatocellular carcinoma with a neural network. *Comput Biol Med, 25*(1), 49-59.

Hornik, M., Stinchcombe, M., & White, H. (1989). Multilayer feedforward networks are universal approximators. *Neural Networks*, 2, 359-366.

Haykin. S. (1999). *Neural Networks*. London: Prentice Hall.

Lindahl, D., Palmer, J., Ohlsson, M., Peterson, C., Lundin, A., & Edenbrand, L. (1997). Automated interpretation of myocardial SPECT perfusion images using artificial neural networks. *J Nucl Med, 38*, 1870-1875.

McCulloch, W. S., & Pitts, W. (1943). A logical calculus of the ideas immanent in neurons activity. *Bulletin of Mathematical Biophysics*, 5, 115-133.

Mitchell, T. M. (1997). *Machine Learning*. Boston, McGraw-Hill.

Mobley, B., Leasure, R., & Davidson, L. (1995). Artificial neural network predictions of lengths of stay on a post-coronary care unit. *Heart Lung, 24*(3), 251-256.

Prank, K., Jurgens, C., Muhlen, A., & Brabant, G. (1998). Predictive Neural Networks for Learning the Time Course of Blood Glucose levels from the Complex Interaction of Counterregulatory Hormones. *Neural Computation, 10*(4), 941-954.

Silipo, R., & Marchesi, C. (1998). Artificial Neural Networks for automatic ECG analysis. *IEEE Transactions on Signal Processing, 46*(5), 1417-1425.

Suzuki, K., Feng Li, Sone, S., & Doi, K. (2005). Computer-aided diagnostic scheme for distinction between benign and malignant nodules in thoracic low-dose CT by use of massive training artificial neural network. *IEEE Transactions on Medical Imaging, 24*(9), 1138 – 1150.

Taktak, A. F. G., Fisher, A. C., & Damato, B. (2004). Modelling survival after treatment of intraocular melanoma using artificial neural networks and Bayes theorem. *Physics in Medicine and Biology, 49*(1), 87-98.

Tresp, V., Briegel, T., & Moody, J. (1999). Neural-network models for the blood glucose metabolism of adiabetic. *IEEE Transactions on Neural Networks, 10*(5), 1204-1213.

UCI Machine Learning Repository, University of California, Irvine. Retrieved November 15, 2007, from http://mlearn.ics.uci.edu/ MLRepository.html.

Yan Sun, Jianming Lu, & Yahagi, T. (2005). Ultrasonographic classification of cirrhosis based on pyramid neural network. *Canadian Conference on Electrical and Computer Engineering*, 1678-1681.

Walczak, S., & Nowack, W.J. (2001). An artificial neural network to diagnosing epilepsy using lateralized burst of theta EEGs. *Journal of Medical Systems, 25*(1), 9–20.

Walczak, S., Pofahl, W. E., & Scorpio, R. J. (2003). A decision support tool for allocating hospital bed resources and determining required acuity of care. *Decision Support Systems, 34*(4), 445-456.

Wei Ji, Naguib, R. N. G., Macall, J., Petrovic, D., Gaura, E., & Ghoneim, M. (2003). Prognostic prediction of bilharziasis-related bladder cancer by neuro-fuzzy classifier. *Information Technology Applications in Biomedicine*, 181-183.

KEY TERMS

Artificial Neuron (neuron): An abstraction of a biological neuron and the basic unit of an artificial neural network.

Backpropagation of Error Algorithm: A common method of teaching artificial neural networks how to perform a given task based on gradient descent search.

Cross-Entropy Error Function: A function used for solving classification tasks that is minimized during neural network training.

Gradient Descent Search: An optimization method for finding a local minimum of a function. One takes steps proportional to the negative of the gradient of the function at the current point.

Multilayer Feedforward Neural Network: An artificial neural network that consists of an input layer, an output layer and one or more hidden layers of neurons. Each neuron in one layer connects with a certain weight to every other neuron in the following layer.

Neural Network Training (learning): It means to carry out an adaptive procedure, in which the weights of the network are incrementally modified so as to improve a prespecified performance criterion.

Overfitting: A neural network correctly maps only inputs previously used for training and fails to map correctly new, previously unseen inputs.

Softmax Function: A neural activation function used in layered neural networks for neurons at output layer.

Sum-of-Square Error Function: A function used for solving classification and mainly regression tasks that is minimized during neural network training.

Chapter V
Preprocessing Perceptrons and Multivariate Decision Limits

Patrik Eklund
Umeå University, Sweden

Lena Kallin Westin
Umeå University, Sweden

ABSTRACT

Classification networks, consisting of preprocessing layers combined with well-known classification networks, are well suited for medical data analysis. Additionally, by adjusting network complexity to corresponding complexity of data, the parameters in the preprocessing network can, in comparison with networks of higher complexity, be more precisely understood and also effectively utilised as decision limits. Further, a multivariate approach to preprocessing is shown in many cases to increase correctness rates in classification tasks. Handling network complexity in this way thus leads to efficient parameter estimations as well as useful parameter interpretations.

INTRODUCTION

Decision limits, in the sense of discrimination values used for interpretative purposes (Solberg, 1987), are arrived at through traditional bio-statistical approaches to medical data analysis (see e.g. (Armitage & Berry, 1994)). In discrimination (or classification), such as typically used in differential diagnosis, involving several attributes, this analysis should not be performed on univariate level. Attributes cannot be analysed one by one, since synthesization of these decision limits must then be considered separately. Such a discriminator is then like a hybrid, with isolated univariate analysis composed with a classification network, where network parameters are trained independently from the level of univariate decision limits. This would provide a separation of univariate decision limits and discrimination, which is unfavourable for correctness rates. Furthermore, efforts to increase correctness rates are typically based on increase of network complexities, leading to other complications such as overtraining and difficulties to interpret network parameters. An analytical presentation of the usefulness to correlate data complexity with network complexity is outside the scope of this chapter. We refer e.g. to (Duda et. al., 2001) for further reading.

In this chapter, we propose to use preprocessing perceptrons which include a preprocessing layer allowing establishing optimal multivariate decision limits. Classification networks coupled with preprocessing can be kept small, and, indeed, with a network complexity in correlation with data complexity. The classification network coupled with preprocessing can be ordinary logistic regression, i.e., a perceptron using neural network terminology. Several other classification networks can be used but it has been shown (Eklund, 1994) difficult to establish significantly higher correctness rates with classifiers of higher complexities.

Hybrid networks, used either in classification or closed-loop problems, are often used in order to increase network complexity to cope with higher data complexity. Typical examples include moving from character to voice recognition or applications of intelligent control. The hybrid described in this chapter is intended to enhance decision limit related preprocessing within the classifier itself. Careful preprocessing with parameter estimations, also for the preprocessing layer, enables the use of classifier networks with low complexities. We support our claims by using some typical case studies in binary classification. Examples are drawn from chromosomal anomalies, endocrinology and virology.

This chapter is organised as follows; First, a description of the proposed preprocessing perceptron is given, including the mathematical formulas behind it. In the next section, three case studies, where the preprocessing perceptron has been used, are described together with the methods used and the results. The results are compared with the results of a multilayer perceptron run on the same data. Next, univariate versus multivariate decision limits are discussed and the final section in this chapter contains a conclusion of the chapter.

THE PREPROCESSING PERCEPTRON

A linear regression is given by the weighted sum:

$$y = \gamma + \sum_{i=1}^{n} w_i x_i$$

where x_i are inputs and w_i and γ are parameters of the linear function. A logistic regression performs a sigmoidal activation of the weighted sum, i.e.:

$$y = \frac{1}{1 + e^{\left(-\gamma + \sum_{i=1}^{n} w_i x_i\right)}}$$

Note that a logistic regression function is precisely a (single-layer) perceptron in the terminology of neural networks (Duda et. al., 2001). The preprocessing perceptron consists similarly of a weighted sum but includes preprocessing functions for each input variable. Suitable preprocessing functions are sigmoids (sigmoidal functions):

$$g[\alpha, \beta](x) = \frac{1}{1 + e^{-\beta(x-\alpha)}},\ \beta \neq 0 \tag{1}$$

where α is the parameter representing the position of the inflexion point, i.e., the soft cut-off or decision limit, and β corresponds[1] to the slope value at the inflexion point. Often the sigmoid is also used as an activation function in neural networks. In this case, α is usually set 0 and β is set to 1, i.e.:

$$\sigma(x) = \frac{1}{1+e^{-x}} \quad (2)$$

More formally, a preprocessing perceptron, including methods for parameter estimation, can be described as follows. For an input pattern $\overline{x}_p = (x_1,\ldots,x_n)$, and an output pattern $\overline{y}_p = (y_1,\ldots,y_n)$, a parameterised input/output-function is written as:

$$\overline{y}_p = f\left[\overline{s}\right]\left(\overline{x}_p\right)$$

where $\overline{s} = (s_1,\ldots,s_k)$ represents the parameters of the function. Gradient descent is, in these contexts, one of the most widely used techniques for parameter estimation. Given a pattern $\overline{x}_p$, a single parameter s_j is updated according to:

$$s_j^{new} = s_j^{previous} \oplus_j \Delta_p s_j \quad (3)$$

and:

$$\Delta_p s_j = -\eta \frac{\partial E_p}{\partial s_j}$$

where $\oplus_j$ is the corresponding addition in the range of s_j, η the learning rate, and E_p is a function measuring the error of the output with respect to some target (expected) values $\overline{t}_p = (t_1,\ldots,t_m)$. In the neural network literature, s_j is the weights in the network and $\oplus_j$ is the ordinary addition. Equation (3) is the well-known *delta rule.*

If s_j is allowed to range over the whole real line, then $\oplus_j$ is the ordinary addition. If s_j ranges in an (open) interval $]a,b[$ then addition in the interval can be done with the help of a invertible function $h :]a,b[\rightarrow \Re$, i.e.:

$$s_j^{new} = h^{-1}\left(\Delta_p s_j + h\left(s_j^{previous}\right)\right)$$

The mapping h can be given in many ways. We have utilised the half circle h_c, given by:

$$h_c(x) = \sqrt{R^2 - (x - x_0)^2}$$

where:

$$x_0 = \frac{a+b}{2}$$

and:

$$R = \frac{b-a}{2}$$

to provide the mapping h, according to:

$$h(x) = x_0 + \frac{R}{\sqrt{R^2 - (x - x_0)^2}}$$

The application of the function h for the half-circle function is shown in Figure 1. We have a value x in the interval $]a,b[$ and want to transform it to the real interval. This is done by calculating $h(x)$ or, geometrically, by finding the point where the normal to the point $h_c(x)$ is crossing the real line (which has been transformed to $y=R$).

If s_j ranges in $]a,\infty[$, addition can similarly obtained by using e.g.:

$$h(x) = \begin{cases} \ln(x-a) & \text{if } x > a \\ -\infty & \text{otherwise} \end{cases}$$

and

$$h^{-1}(x) = a + e^x$$

In practice, it is recommended to use normalised settings, i.e., to work within the intervals $]0,1[$ and $]0,\infty[$. Alternative functions, h, can be given, but they are expected to have little, if any, effect on the classification performance (Eklund, 1994; Eklund & Forsström, 1995). Note also how these mappings h^{-1} are candidates for use as activation functions in neural networks (Eklund, 1994; Eklund et. al., 1991).

Typically, E_p is given by the square sum:

$$E_p\left[\bar{s}\right] = \frac{1}{2}\sum_{i=1}^{m}(t_i - y_i)^2$$

and thus the selected parameter estimation technique solves the minimal least squares problem. Often the errors are calculated for a set of patterns and there is a possible utility of epoch sizes in training sequences. This is applied in ordinary manner.

Now let σ be a differentiable activation function and y_p a single-layer perceptron:

Figure 1. This provides an illumination of corresponding calculations of using the half-circle to define addition in the interval]a,b[

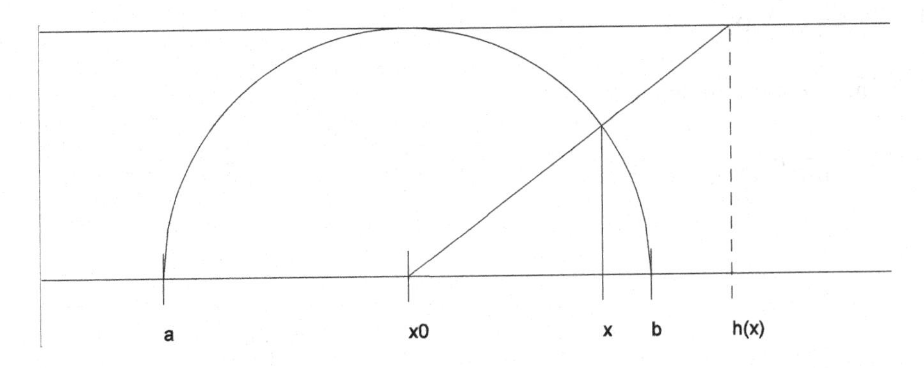

$$\bar{y}_p = f[\bar{w}](\bar{x}_p) = \sigma\left(\sum_{i=1}^{n} w_i x_i\right)$$

if σ is a sigmoid, i.e., as in Equation (2), we obtain:

$$\Delta_p w_i = -\eta \frac{\partial E_p}{\partial w_i} = \eta (t_i - y_i)\sigma'(z_i) x_i$$

where $z_i = \sum_{i=1}^{n} w_i x_i$ and the derivative of σ is given by:

$$\sigma'(z_i) = \sigma(z_i)(1 - \sigma(z_i)) \qquad (4)$$

Given the notation above, the preprocessing perceptron can now be defined as:

$$\begin{aligned} \bar{y}_p &= f[\bar{s}](\bar{x}_p) = f[w_1,\ldots,w_n,\alpha_1,\ldots,\alpha_n,\beta_1,\ldots,\beta_n](x_1,\ldots,x_n) \\ &= \sigma\left(\sum_{i=1}^{n} w_i g[\alpha_i,\beta_i](x_i)\right) \end{aligned}$$

where $g[\alpha_i, \beta_i]$ is given by Equation (1). With $\sigma'(z_i)$ defined as in Equation (4) and $g'(x_i)$ defined in the same manner:

$$g'(x_i) = g[\alpha_i,\beta_i](x_i)(1 - g[\alpha_i,\beta_i](x_i))$$

the corresponding learning rules are based on:

$$\begin{aligned} \Delta_p w_i &= -\eta_{weights} \frac{\partial E_p}{\partial w_i} = -\eta_{weights} (t_p - y_p)\sigma'(\sum_{i=1}^{n} w_i g[\alpha_i,\beta_i](x_i)) g[\alpha_i,\beta_i](x_i) \\ \Delta_p \alpha_i &= -\eta_{cutoffs} \frac{\partial E_p}{\partial \alpha_i} = +\eta_{cutoffs} (t_p - y_p)\sigma'(\sum_{i=1}^{n} w_i g[\alpha_i,\beta_i](x_i)) w_i g'[\alpha_i,\beta_i](x_i)\beta_i \\ \Delta_p \beta_i &= -\eta_{slopes} \frac{\partial E_p}{\partial \beta_i} = -\eta_{slopes} (t_p - y_p)\sigma'(\sum_{i=1}^{n} w_i g[\alpha_i,\beta_i](x_i)) g'[\alpha_i,\beta_i](x_i)(x_i - \alpha_i) \end{aligned}$$

respectively, and we update w, α and β values according to:

$$\begin{aligned} w_i^{new} &= w_i^{previous} + \Delta_p w_i, \\ \alpha_i^{new} &= \alpha_i^{previous} \oplus_{]0,1[} \Delta_p \alpha_i, \\ \beta_i^{new} &= \beta_i^{previous} \oplus_{]0,\infty[} \Delta_p \beta_i \end{aligned}$$

As a rule of thumb, we recommend to use:

$$\eta_{weights} = \frac{1}{10}\eta_{alphas} = \frac{1}{100}\eta_{betas}$$

with:

$$\eta_{betas} = 1$$

or less. It can also be useful to regularise training in the sense that parameter classes are trained separately. In this case it is suitable to start with the weight values, with cut-off values, i.e. (univariate) decision limits, initialised to the centre of respective data intervals. Weights can be retrained each time cut-offs have gone through a training sequences. Outliers must be handled in the data set. If used at all, they should be truncated; otherwise the data distribution becomes skewed. Further, cut-off values should not approach the data interval boundaries, since the utility of the cut-off value as a decision limit becomes less credible. Similar recommendations can be given for slope values even if slopes values tend to have less impact on discriminant capacity. Moreover, where cut-off are seen as decision limits, the interpretation and use of slope values in decisions is less obvious even if slope value tuning provides a further decrease of error values in training procedures.

CASE STUDIES

We will demonstrate the use of the preprocessing perceptron in three typical case studies. For a more detailed description of the case studies see (Eklund & Forsström, 1995; Kallin et. al., 1998). Some of the data sets used in this chapter have been narrowed down to provide illumination rather than best classification rates.

Data Sets

The first case study, Scandinavian mild form of **Nephropathia Epidemica (NE),** is a virus-infection caused by the Puumala virus. It has a sudden onset with fever, headache, backpain and gastrointestinal symptoms, but sometimes worse symptoms such as internal hemorrhaging and it can even lead to death. However, the majority of infected individuals is asymptomatic or develops only mild symptoms, and the disease does not spread from human to human.

The data is collected from three different hospitals and the inputs are CRP (C-reactive protein), ESR (erythrocyte sedimentation rate), creatinine (μ mol/l) thrombocytes and myopia (as a binary value). Output is the possible presence of the virus (Puumala virus (Lahdevirta, 1971)) established in a virological test. The data set consists of 280 cases where 140 have the diagnosis and 140 have not. The data set contains missing data which in this case is set to 0.5 after normalisation.

The second case study is **Down's syndrome (DS)**, also known as 21-trisomy. Down's syndrome is due to an extra copy in chromosome #21. The frequency of DS is 1/770 in live born babies. The incidence in conception is greater, but more than 60% are spontaneously aborted in the first trimester of pregnancy. The case study is again a multicentre study (Spencer et. al., 1992) and the inputs are mother's age (years), alpha-foetoprotein (AFP, measured in MoM, the specific multiple of the median of this marker in each week of pregnancy) and free β-subunit of human chorion gonadotropin β-hCG measured in MoM). The output is the possible chromosomal anomali observed after birth. The data set consists of 873 cases where 450 have the diagnosis and 423 have not. There is no missing data in this data set.

In the third case study, **Pima-Indians-Diabetes (D)**, the data were originally collected by the National Institute of Diabetes and Digestive and Kidney Diseases. It was found in the UCI Repository of machine learning databases (Asuncion & Newman, 2007). The eight inputs are number of times pregnant, plasma glucose concentration a 2 hours in an oral glucose tolerance test, diastolic blood pressure

Table 1. Sizes of data sets used for respective case studies

Data characteristics	NE	DS	D (D1/D2)
Total number of cases	280	873	768
Number of negatives	140	450	500
Number of positives	140	423	268
Negatives/Positives in training set	69/71	300/282	375/201
Negatives/Positives in test set	71/69	150/141	125/67
Missing data	Yes	No	Yes

(mm Hg), triceps skin fold thickness (mm), 2-Hour serum insulin (μU/ml), body mass index (kg/m^2), diabetes pedigree function, and age (years). Output is the possible diagnose of diabetes.

The set consists of 768 cases where 268 have the diagnosis diabetes and 500 have the diagnose non-diabetes. In the text, accompanying the data set, it is claimed that there is no missing data in the set. However, if the set is examined more closely, zeros will be found in six out of eight columns that are clearly markers of missing data. For example there are zeros in the column "body mass index" and in the column "triceps skin fold thickness". There are also a substantial amount of zeros in the column representing "number of times pregnant". In that column, it is impossible to decide if the zeros are missing data or not. As will be explained in the subsection below, we will handle the missing data in two different ways resulting in two data sets Dl and D2.

In Table 1, a summary of the information about the cases, e.g. the size of the different training sets, are shown.

Method

In all case studies, we have transformed the values to the unit interval with the use of maximum and minimum values from the training set. When applying the normalisation to the test set, values outside the boundaries are truncated to fit into the unit interval.

Classification results are obtained for the preprocessing perceptron (PPP) and the multi-layer perceptron (MLP), respectively. All computations were done in the MATLAB environment using the neural network toolbox for the MLPs and implementations of the preprocessing perceptrons according to recommendations in the previous section. All MLPs were trained using the gradient descent method. There are several other methods available in MATLAB but we chose this since gradient descent is also applied for learning parameters in the preprocessing perceptron.

It is well known that any function can be learned with an arbitrary accuracy by a three-layer network and that every bounded continuous function can be learned with a small error by a two-layer network (Hornik et. al., 1989). However it is more difficult to decide how many nodes there should be in each layer of the network to obtain a high accuracy for a given data set. Several suggestions has been given as to choose the number of hidden nodes N in an MLP. In (Sartori & Antsaklis, 1991), it is said that for a training set with p inputs, a MLP with p-1 hidden nodes can perfectly learn the training set. In our case studies this corresponds to 140 (NE), 582 (DS), and 576 (D) hidden nodes, respectively. Usually this number can be reduced. Another suggestion is found in (Kasabov, 1996), namely $N \geq (p-1)/(N_{in}+2)$, where p in this suggestion also denotes the number of training examples and N_{in} is the number of inputs of the network. In our case studies it would correspond to 140/7 = 20 (NE), 582/5 ≈ 117 (DS), and 576/10 ≈ 58 (D) weights, which corresponds to approximately 3, 16, and 8 hidden nodes respectively. Further, in (Duda et. al., 2001), it is recommended that the number of hidden nodes should be chosen so that the total number of weights in the net is approximately $p/10$. In our case studies we then obtain 14, 58, and 58 hidden nodes. As can be seen, there are differences among such recommendations. However, the most important goal is to have a number large enough to avoid underfitting, i.e. the function cannot be learned, without introducing overfitting, i.e. the model does not provide an ability to generalise.

In order to find the best network structure for each of the case studies, the data sets were divided into training and test data in five random ways. These data sets were then used to train different network structures and the resulting mean accuracy of the test sets, applied on a specific net structure, were used to select the network structure. Networks were trained with 1, 2, 3, ..., 10, 20, 50, 100, and 200 nodes in order to get an overview of the magnitude of the nodes needed. The same sets were also used for training networks with two layers containing all possible combinations of the numbers of nodes above. It was soon clear, that a network with more than 10 nodes leads to overfitting. Network structures that were finally chosen are shown in Table 2.

The preprocessing perceptron has, in all three cases, used sigmoids as preprocessing functions.

Results

The total accuracy, i.e., total number of correctly classified patients, has been compared at three different points; when the sensitivities are 95%, the specificities are 95%, and when the optimal efficiency is reached. Significance levels are computed using Minitab's test for two proportions.

Table 3 illuminates these comparison points. If both target (previously made diagnosis) and test are positive, it is called a *true positive* (TP). The probability of a TP to occur is estimated by counting the true positives in the test set and divide by the size of the test set. If the target is positive and the test is negative it is called a *false negative* (FN). *False positive* (FP) and *true negative* (TN) are defined similarly.

Table 2. Multi-layer perceptron architectures used in respective case studies

Network characteristics	**NE**	**DS**	**D**
Number of hidden layers	1	2	1
Number of nodes in each layer	5	3/6	8

Table 3. Relations between the measurement probabilities of the outcome, prevalence, and level of a test defined in the text

	Test result		
Target	Positive	Negative	
Positive	TP	FN	P
Negative	FP	TN	P'
	Q	Q'	1

Sensitivity, SE, is the probability of having a positive test among the cases that have a positive target:

$$SE = TP/(TP + FN) = TP/P$$

Specificity, SP, is the probability of having a negative test among the cases that have a negative target:

$$SP = TN/(FP + TN) = TN/P'$$

Since sensitivity and specificity both are related to the level Q of the test, their ideal value of 100% might not be achievable. Two quality measurements are derived in (Kraemer, 1992) and their values lies in the interval [0,1]:

$$\kappa(1,0) = (SE - Q)/Q'$$
$$\kappa(0,0) = (SP - Q')/Q$$

Furthermore, these quality measurements are weighted together and efficiency are considered in a third measurement, the optimal efficiency (Kraemer, 1992):

$$\kappa(0.5,0) = \frac{PQ'\kappa(1,0) + P'Q\kappa(0,0)}{PQ' + P'Q}$$

As we can see in Table 4, the accuracies are similar for the two methods. In fact, there is significant difference between the methods in only two cases. The first case is comparing accuracies for D2 when sensitivity is forced to be 95%. Remember that D2 is the case where missing data was set to 0.5 after normalisation. That seems to be favourable for the preprocessing perceptron with an accuracy at 70.8% compared to the accuracy for the MLP at 59.4% (p=0.018). The second case is for NE when specificity is forced to be 95% with the accuracy for PPP at 85% and for the MLP at 67.9% (p = 0.001). It seems that the results from the multilayer perceptron and the preprocessing perception are comparable using this type of medical data.

Accuracies in these results are not very high. This is due to the nature of the data sets, and we wanted indeed to select data sets that have shown to be somewhat more difficult when used in classification

Table 4. Accuracies are presented for the case studies when sensitivity is 95%, specificity is 95% and optimal efficiency is reached, respectively

	SE		DS		D1		D2	
Accuracies	MLP	PPP	MLP	PPP	MLP	PPP	MLP	PPP
Sens = 95%	68.6	76.4	74.6	69.8	62.0	62.0	59.4	70.8
Spec = 95%	67.9	85.0	75.3	71.5	75.0	77.1	72.9	77.6
Optimal eff.	82.1	85.0	82.1	82.5	78.1	79.2	78.7	77.6

tasks. For DS, these are accuracies you reach, which is known from previous studies, e.g. (Kallin et. al., 1998). Of course, if combined with other facts, such as information delivered e.g. by ultrasound observations on the foetus, accuracies are even higher. Similarly, the original data set for NE contains 28 variables, from which we selected five for the purpose of this chapter. Using all 28 variables we can expect to have accuracies of up to 89% (Eklund, 1994).

UNIVARIATE VS MULTIVARIATE DECISION LIMITS?

Decision limits are usually treated in a univariate manner. Threshold values are computed to reach specific specificity and/or sensitivity levels based on patient material and clinical requirements. In multivariate classification it seems natural to preprocess individual variables according to traditional methods for establishing decision limits. In (Ellenius et. al., 1997), preprocessing perceptrons were used with α's and β's as fixed values in the preprocessing perceptron. Thus only weights were trained. The obvious question is whether decision limit fixing in this way provides optimal classification as compared to training all parameters.

In order to provide a comparison, we use the following setup for network models. In the first model, denoted by PPP95, each α is set to the value needed to reach a 95% sensitivity on univariate levels, i.e. fixing the cut-offs, for learning data, in a way that each univariate classification provides a 95% sensitivity on learning data. Networks are then trained according to recommendations provided in a previous section.

Table 5 shows how training of all parameters improves classification rates. In three cases, the performance is significantly lower for the fixed net. This is when the sensitivity is set to be 95% (recall that this is what the α's were manually set to handle). In the NE case the p-value is 0.001 and in the Down case the p-value is 0.001. The third case is when the specificity is set to 95% in the NE case (p=0.003).

Tables 6 and 7 present preprocessing perceptron parameters after training, exemplified in the NE and DS case studies. Cut-offs are normalised within the unit interval. In particular we see how the trained α values differ from the corresponding ones fixed with respect to univariate 95% sensitivity levels. The interpretations of α's in the PPP95 model are clear, i.e. they are arrived at using the criteria of a 95% sensitivity in univariate view. However, α's in the PPP model cannot be viewed *in casu*, and are indeed to be utilised as decision limits altogether in a multivariate sense. Interpretations of β's are, as remarked earlier, less clear. Intuitively, such a slope value, converging to be rather steep, means that the value of the corresponding α value is very sensitive to being shifted. Even rather small manual ad hoc adjust-

Table 5. Accuracies are again presented for the case studies when sensitivity is 95%, specificity is 95% and optimal efficiency is reached, respectively

	NE		DS	
Accuracies	PPP	PPP95	PPP	PPP95
Sens = 95%	76.4	57.9	69.8	60.1
Spec = 95%	85.0	70.7	71.5	69.1
Optimal eff.	82.6	82.1	82.5	79.4

ments of the α value would change preprocessing of data and thereby classification performance of the network as a whole. It is also clear that the α values do not respect a 95% based decision limit even if the overall classification rate is designed so as to provide a multivariate sensitivity level of 95%. This clearly indicates that one has to be cautious concerning individual decision limits when working in a multivariate setting. The preprocessing perceptron is thus one solution for such an analysis.

CONCLUSION

The broad acceptance of neural network techniques stem from their powerful classification capacities and from their general superiority over regression techniques. Regression techniques do not possess universal approximation capacities and is thus generally speaking prone to providing worse discriminant performance e.g. as compared with multilayer perceptron type neural networks. On the other hand, overtraining of neural networks is always at risk. Typical difficulties arise when we adapt models to data collected at a certain time and from a certain location. When trying to use the adapted model at subsequent time periods and/or different locations, measurement cultures may have changed, or are different, and thus data selections used in a testing environment are different to those used in a learning phase. In such transferability situations robustness of models is difficult to reach, and neural network superiority over regression techniques is less obvious.

In this chapter, we have explained these phenomena by providing the preprocessing perceptron method that has a classification capacity comparable to those of multilayer networks, yet providing network simplicity and interpretability comparable to regression techniques.

The preprocessing perceptron, providing a network complexity between perceptron networks and multilayer networks, is shown to be well suited for medical data analysis and also robust from learning point of view in that classification performance is not sensitive to parameter initialisations or stopping

Table 6. Weight values together with α (normalised) and β values within the NE case study, i.e. including five weights and together with five α and five β values, respectively

NE	PPP	PPP95
w	0.54 0.28 1.54 1.97 1.30	0.52 0.50 1.30 -0.22 1.06
α	0.45 0.47 0.47 0.32 0.55	0.66 0.67 0.10 0.91 0
β	1.42 1.39 1.87 2.42 1.86	1.30 1.30 1.30 1.30 1.30

Table 7. Weight values together with α (normalised) and β values within the DS case study, i.e. including three weights, three α, and three β values, respectively

DS	PPP	PPP95
w	3.39 2.14 5.83	0.28 2.62 6.11
α	0.80 0.28 0.19	0.15 0.08 0.06
β	15.3 -12.5 11.9	15 -15 15

conditions for learning. Overtraining is rare and the classification is comparable to those given by networks with higher complexity.

REFERENCES

Armitage, P., & Berry, G. (1994). *Statistical Methods in Medical Research*, Oxford: Blackwell Science.

Asuncion, A., & Newman, D. J. (2007). *UCI Machine Learning Repository* [http://www.ics.uci.edu/~mlearn/MLRepository.html]. Irvine, CA: University of California, Department of Information and Computer Science.

Duda, R. O., Hart, P. E., & Stork, D. G (2001). *Pattern Classification*, New York: John Wiley & Sons.

Eklund, P. (1994). Network size versus preprocessing, In R.R. Yager and L.A. Zadeh (Ed.), *Fuzzy Sets, Neural Networks and Soft Computing*, (pp 250-264). New York: Van Nostrand Reinhold.

Eklund, P., & Forsström, J. (1995). Computational intelligence for laboratory information systems, *Scandinavian Journal of Clinical and Laboratory Investigation*, *55(Suppl. 222)*, 75-82.

Eklund, P., Riissanen, T., & Virtanen, H. (1991). On the fuzzy logic nature of neural Nets. In *Neural Networks \& their Applications: Proceedings of Neuro-Nimes '91* (pp293-300), Nimes, France, November 4-8.

Ellenius, J., Groth, T., Lindahl, B., & Wallentin, A. (1997). Early Assessment of Patients with Suspected Acute Myocardial Infarction by Biochemical Monitoring and Neural Network Analysis. *Clinical Chemistry*, *43*, 1919-1925.

Hornik, K., Stinchcombe, M., & White, H. (1989). Multilayer feedforward networks are universal approximators. *Neural Networks (2)*, 359-366.

Kallin, L. , Räty, R., Selén, G., & Spencer, K. (1998). A Comparison of Numerical Risk Computational Techniques in Screening for Down's Syndrome. In P. Gallinari and F. Fogelman Soulie, (Eds.), *Industrial Applications of Neural Networks* (pp.425-432). Singapore: World Scientific.

Kasabov, N. (1996), *Neural Networks, Fuzzy Systems and Knowledge Engineering.* USA:MIT Press.

Kraemer, H. C. (1992), *Evaluating Medical Tests.* Newbury Park, CA: Sage Publications.

Lähdevirta, J. (1971). Nephropathia epidemica in Finland: A clinical, histological and epidemiological study. *Annals of clinical research, 3(Suppl 8)*, 1-154.

Sartori, M. A., & Antsaklis, P. J. (1991). A Simple Method to Derive Bounds on the Size and to Train Multilayer Neural Networks. *IEEE Transactions on Neural Networks,* 4*(2),* 467-471.

Solberg, H. E. (1987). Approved recommendation (1986) of the theory of reference values, Part I. The Concept of reference values. *Journal of Clinical Chemistry & Clinical Biochemistry*, *25*, 337-342.

Spencer, K., Coombes, E. J., Mallard, A. S., & Ward A. M. (1992). Free beta human choriogonadotropin in Down's syndrome screening: a multicentre study of its role compared with other biochemical markers. *Annals of clinical biochemistry, 29(Suppl 216),* 506-518.

KEY TERMS

Preprocessing Perceptron: A single-layer perceptron with non-linear preprocessing function for each input.

Sensitivity (SE): The probability of having a positive test among the cases that have a positive target.

Specificity (SE): The probability of having a negative test among the cases that have a negative target.

ENDNOTE

[1] If s is the slope value, the actual relation between slope and β values is $\beta = 4s$.

Section II
General Applications

Chapter VI
Image Registration for Biomedical Information Integration

Xiu Ying Wang
BMIT Research Group, The University of Sydney, Australia

Dagan Feng
BMIT Research Group, The University of Sydney, Australia;
Hong Kong Polytechnic University, Hong Kong

ABSTRACT

The rapid advance and innovation in medical imaging techniques offer significant improvement in healthcare services, as well as provide new challenges in medical knowledge discovery from multi-imaging modalities and management. In this chapter, biomedical image registration and fusion, which is an effective mechanism to assist medical knowledge discovery by integrating and simultaneously representing relevant information from diverse imaging resources, is introduced. This chapter covers fundamental knowledge and major methodologies of biomedical image registration, and major applications of image registration in biomedicine. Further, discussions on research perspectives are presented to inspire novel registration ideas for general clinical practice to improve the quality and efficiency of healthcare.

INTRODUCTION

With the reduction of cost in imaging data acquisition, biomedical images captured from anatomical imaging modalities, such as Magnetic Resonance (MR) imaging, Computed Tomography (CT) and X-ray, or from functional imaging modalities, such as Positron Emission Tomography (PET) and Single Photon Emission Computed Tomography (SPECT), are widely used in modern clinical practice. However, these ever-increasing huge amounts of datasets unavoidably cause information repositories to overload and pose substantial challenges in effective and efficient medical knowledge management, imaging data retrieval, and patient management.

Biomedical image registration is an effective mechanism for integrating the complementary and valuable information from diverse image datasets. By searching the optimal correspondence among the multiple datasets, biomedical image registration enables a more complete insight and full utilization of heterogeneous imaging resources (Wang and Feng, 2005) to facilitate knowledge discovery and management of patients with a variety of diseases.

Biomedical image registration has important applications in medical database management, for instance, patient record management, medical image retrieval and compression. Image registration is essential in constructing statistical atlases and templates to extract common patterns of morphological or functional changes across a large specific population (Wang and Feng, 2005). Therefore, registration and fusion of diverse imaging resources is important component for clinical image data warehouse and clinical data mining.

Due to its research significance and crucial role in clinical applications, biomedical image registration has been extensively studied during last three decades (Brown, 1992; Maintz et al., 1998; Fitzpatrick et al. 2000). The existing registration methodologies can be catalogued into different categories according to criteria such as image dimensionality, registration feature space, image modality, and subjects involved (Brown, 1992). Different Region-of-Interests (ROIs) and various application requirements and scenarios are key reasons for continuously introducing new registration algorithms. In addition to a large number of software-based registration algorithms, more advanced imaging devices such as combined PET/CT and SPECT/CT scanners provide hardware-based solutions for the registration and fusion by performing the functional and anatomical imaging in the one imaging session with the one device. However, it remains challenging to generate clinically applicable registration with improved performance and accelerated computation for biomedical datasets with larger imaging ranges, higher resolutions, and more dimensionalities.

CONCEPTS AND FUNDAMENTALS OF BIOMEDICAL IMAGE REGISTRATION

Definition

Image registration is to compare or combine multiple imaging datasets captured from different devices, imaging sessions, or viewpoints for the purpose of change detection or information integration. The major task of registration is to search for an appropriate transformation to spatially relate and simultaneously represent the images in a common coordinate system for further analysis and visualization. Image registration can be mathematically expressed as (Brown, 1992):

$$I_R(X_R) = g(I_S(T(X_S))) \qquad (1)$$

where I_R and I_S are the reference (fixed) image and study (moving) image respectively; $T:(X_S) \rightarrow (X_R)$ is the transformation which sets up spatial correspondence between the images so that the study image X_S can be mapped to and represented in the coordinate system of reference image X_R; $g:(I_s) \rightarrow (I_R)$ is one-dimensional intensity calibration transformation.

Framework

As illustrated in Figure 1, in registration framework, the study dataset is firstly compared to the reference dataset according to a pre-defined similarity measure. If the convergence has not been achieved yet, the optimization algorithm estimates a new set of transformation parameters to calculate a better spatial match between the images. The study image is interpolated and transformed with the updated transformation parameters, and then compared with the reference image again. This procedure is iterated until the optimum transformation parameters are found, which are then used to register and fuse the study image to the reference image.

Major Components of Registration

Input Datasets

The characteristics of input datasets, including modality, quality and dimensionality, determine the choice of similarity measure, transformation, interpolation and optimization strategy, and eventually affect the performance, accuracy, and application of the registration.

The input images for registration may originate from identical or different imaging modality, and accordingly, registration can be classified as monomodal registration (such as CT-CT registration, PET-PET registration, MRI-MRI registration) or multimodal registration (such as CT-MRI registration, CT-PET registration, and MRI-PET registration). Monomodal registration is required to detect changes over time due to disease progression or treatment. Multimodal registration is used to correlate and integrate the complementary information to provide a more complete insight into the available data. Comparatively, multimodal registration proves to be more challenging than monomodal, due to the heterogeneity of data sources, differing qualities (including spatial resolution and gray-level resolution) of the images, and insufficient correspondence.

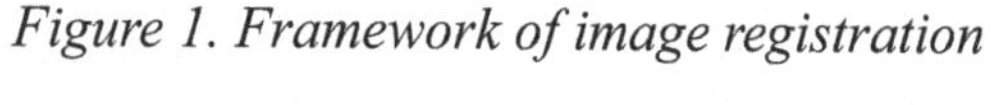

Figure 1. Framework of image registration

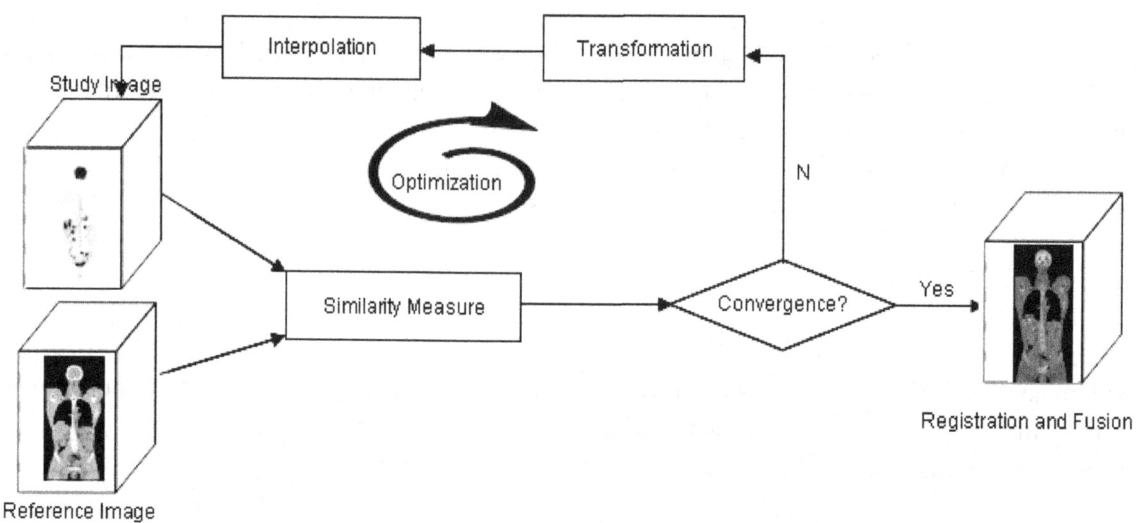

Registration algorithms for the input datasets with different dimensionalities are used for other applications and requirements. For instance, two-dimensional image registration is applied to construct image mosaics to provide a whole view of a sequence of partially overlapped images, and is used to generate atlases or templates for a specific group of subjects. Although three-dimensional image registration is required for most clinical applications, it is challenging to produce an automatic technique with high computational efficiency for routine clinical usages. Multidimensional registration is demanded to align a series of three-dimensional images acquired from different sessions for applications such as tumor growth monitoring, cancer staging and treatment assessment (Fitzpatrick et al, 2000).

Registration Transformations

The major task of registration is to find a transformation to align and correlate the input datasets with differences and deformations, introduced during imaging procedures. These discrepancies occur in the form of variations in the quality, content, and information within the images, therefore posing a significant obstacle and challenge in the area of image registration. In addition, motions, either voluntary or involuntary, require special attention and effort during the registration procedure (Wang et al., 2007; Fitzpatrick et al., 2000).

- **Rigid-body Transformations** include rigid and affine transformations, and are mainly used to correct simple differences or to provide initial estimates for more complex registration procedures. Rigid transformation is used to cope with differences due to positional changes (such as translations and rotations) in the imaging procedure and is often adopted for the registration of brain images, due to the rigid nature of the skull structure. In addition, affine transformation can be used to deal with scaling deformations. However, these transformations are usually limited outside of the brain.
- **Deformable Transformations** are used to align the images with more complex deformations and changes. For instance, motions and changes of organs such as lung, heart, liver, bowel, need to be corrected by more comprehensive non-linear transformations. The significant variance between subjects and changes due to disease progression and treatment intervention require nonlinear transformations with more degrees of freedom. In deformable registration, a deformation field which is composed of deformation vectors, needs to be computed. One displacement vector is decided for each individual image element (pixel for 2D or voxel for 3D). Compared to rigid-body transformations, the complexity of deformable transformations will slow down the registration speed, and efficient deformable registration remains a challenging research area.

Interpolation Algorithms

Interpolation is an essential component in registration, and is required whenever the image needs to be transformed or there are resolution differences between the datasets to be registered. After the transformation, if the points are mapped to non-grid positions, interpolation is performed to approximate the values for these transformed points. For the multimodal image registration, the sample space of the lower-resolution image is often interpolated (up-sampled) to the sample space of the higher-resolution image. In the interpolation procedure, the more neighbouring points are used for the calculation, the better accuracy can be achieved, and the slower the computation. To balance interpolation accuracy and computational complexity, bilinear interpolation technique which calculates the interpolated value based on four points, and trilinear interpolation, are often used in registration (Lehmann et al., 1999).

Optimization Algorithms

Registration can be defined as an iterative optimization procedure (Equation 2) for searching the optimal transformation to minimize a cost function for two given datasets:

$$T_{optimal} = \underset{(T)}{\arg\min}\, f(T(X_S), X_R) \tag{2}$$

where T is the registration transformation; f is the cost function to be minimized.

- **Gradient-based optimization methods** are often used in registration, in which the gradient vector at each point is calculated to determine the search direction so that the value of the cost function can be decreased locally. For instance, Quasi-Newton methods such as Broyden-Fletcher-Goldfarb-Shanno (BFGS), has been investigated and applied in medical image registration (Unser, Aldroubi, 1993; Mattes et al., 2003).
- **Powell optimization** (Powell, 1964) is another frequently adopted searching strategy in registration. Powell method performs a succession of one-dimensional searches to find the best solution for each transformation parameter, and then the single-variable optimizations are used to determine the new search direction. This procedure is iterative until no better solution or further improvement over the current solution can be found. Because of no derivatives required for choosing the searching directions, computational cost is reduced in this algorithm.
- **Downhill Simplex optimization** (Press et al., 1992) does not require derivatives either. However, compared with Powell algorithm, Downhill Simplex is not so efficient due to more evaluations involved. For a given n-dimensional problem domain, the Simplex method searches the optimum solution downhill through a complex n-dimensional topology through operations of reflection, expansion, contraction, and multiple contractions. Because it is more robust in finding the optimal solution, Simplex optimization has been widely used in medical registration.
- **Multi-resolution optimization schemes** have been utilized to avoid being trapped into a local optimum and to reduce computational times of the registration (Thévenaz ,Unser, 2000; Borgefors, 1988; Bajcsy, Kovacic, 1989; Unser, Aldroubi, 1993). In multi-resolution registration, the datasets to be registered are firstly composed into multiple resolution levels, and then the registration procedure is carried out from low resolution scales to high resolution scales. The initial registration on the global information in the low resolution provides a good estimation for registration in higher resolution scales and contributes to improved registration performance and more efficient computation (Wang et al, 2007).

Spline based multi-resolution registration has been systematically investigated by Thévenaz (Thévenaz, Unser, 2000) , and Unser (Unser, Aldroubi, 1993). In these Spline-based registration, the images are filtered by B-spline or cubic spline first and then down-sampled to construct multi-resolution pyramids. Multi-resolution B-spline method provides a faster and more accurate registration result for multimodal images when using mutual information as a similarity measure.

BIOMEDICAL IMAGE REGISTRATION METHODOLOGIES AND TECHNIQUES

Registration methods seek to optimize values of a cost function or similarity measure which define how well two image sets are registered. The similarity measures can be based on the distances between certain homogeneous features and differences of gray values in the two image sets to be registered (Wang et al, 2007). Accordingly, biomedical image registration can be classified as feature-based or intensity-based methods (Brown, 1992).

Feature-Based Registration

In feature-based registration, the transformation required to spatially match the features such as landmark points (Maintz, et al, 1996), lines (Subsol, et al, 1998) or surfaces (Borgefors, 1988), can be determined efficiently. However, in this category of registration, a preprocessing step is usually necessary to extract the features manually or semi-automatically, which makes the registration, operator- intensive and dependent (Wang et al, 2007).

Landmark-Based Registration

Landmark-based registration includes identifying homologous points which should represent the same features in different images as the first step, and then the transformation can be estimated based on these corresponding landmarks to register the images. The landmark points can be artificial markers attached to the subject which can be detected easily or anatomical feature points.

- **Extrinsic landmarks (fiducial markers)**, such as skin markers, can be noninvasive. However, skin markers cannot provide reliable landmarks for registration due to elasticity of human skin. The invasive landmarks such as stereotactic frames are able to provide robust basis for registration, and can be used in Image Guided Surgery (IGS) where registration efficiency and accuracy are the most important factors. Since they are easily and automatically detectable in multiple images to be registered, extrinsic landmarks can be used in both monomodal and multimodal image registration.
- **Intrinsic landmarks** can be anatomically or geometrically (such as corner points, intersection points or local extrema) salient points in the images. Since landmarks are required to be unique and evenly distributed over the image, and to carry substantial information, automatic landmark selection is challenging task. Intensive user interaction is often required to manually identify the feature points for registration (Wang et al, 2007). Iterative closest point (ICP) algorithm (Besl, MaKey 1992) is one of most successful landmark-based registration methods. Because no prior knowledge on correspondence between the features is required, ICP eases the registration procedure greatly.

Line-Based Registration and Surface-Based Registration

- **Line-based registration** utilizes line features such as edges and boundaries extracted from images to determine the transformation. "Snakes" or active contours (Kass et al, 1988) provide effective contour extraction techniques and have been widely applied in image segmentation and shape modelling, boundary detection and extraction, motion tracking and analysis, and deformable registration (Wang and Feng 2005). Active contours are energy-minimizing splines, which can detect the closest contour of an object. The shape deformation of an active contour is driven by both internal forces, image forces and external forces. To handle the difficulties of concavity and sensitivity during initialization, classic snakes, balloon model (Cohen and Cohen 1993) and gradient vector flow (GVF) (Xu and Prince 1998) were proposed.

- **Surface-based registration** uses the distinct surfaces as a registration basis to search the transformation. The "Head-and-Hat" algorithm (Chen, et al, 1987) is a well-known surface fitting technique for registration. In this method, two equivalent surfaces are identified in the images to be registered. The surface extracted from the higher-resolution images, is represented as a stack of discs, and is referred to as "head", and the surface extracted from the lower-resolution image volume, is referred to as "hat", which is represented as a list of unconnected 3D points. The registration is determined by iteratively transforming the hat surface with respect to the head surface, until the closest fit of the hat onto the head is found. Because the segmentation task is comparatively easy, and the computational cost is relatively low, this method remains popular. More details of surface-based registration algorithms can be found in the review by Audette et al, 2000.

Intensity-Based Registration

Intensity-based registration can directly utilize the image intensity information without segmentation or intensive user interaction required, and thereby can achieve fully automatic registration. In intensity-based registration, a similarity measure is defined on the basis of raw image content and is used as a criterion for optimal registration. Several well-established intensity-based similarity measures have been used in the biomedical image registration domain.

Similarity measures based on intensity differences including sum of squared differences (SSD) (Equ. 3) and sum of absolute differences (SAD) (Equ.4) (Brown, 1992), are the simplest similarity criteria which exhibit minimum value for perfect registration. As these methods are too sensitive to the intensity changes and significant intensity differences may lead to false registration, SAD and SSD are limited in application and as such, are mainly used to register monomodal images (Wang et al, 2007):

$$SSD = \sum_{i}^{N} (I_R(i) - T(I_S(i)))^2 \quad (3)$$

$$SAD = \frac{1}{N} \sum_{i}^{N} |I_R(i) - T(I_S(i))| \quad (4)$$

where $I_R(i)$ is the intensity value at position i of reference image R and $I_S(i)$ is the corresponding intensity value in study image S; T is geometric transformation.

Correlation techniques were proposed for multimodal image registration (Van den Elsen, et al, 1995) on the basis of assumption of linear dependence between the image intensities. However, as this assumption is easily violated by the complexity of images from multiple imaging devices, correlation measures are not always able to find optimal solution for multimodal image registration.

Mutual information (MI) was simultaneously and independently introduced by two research groups of Collignon et al (1995) and Viola and Wells (1995) to measure the statistical dependence of two images.

Because of no assumption on the feature of this dependence and no limitation on the image content, MI is widely accepted as multimodal registration criterion (Pluim et al., 2003).

For two intensity sets $R = \{r\}$ and $S = \{s\}$, mutual information is defined as:

$$I(R,S) = \sum_{r,s} p_{RS}(r,s) \log \frac{p_{RS}(r,s)}{p_R(r) \cdot p_S(s)} \tag{5}$$

where $p_R(r,s)$ is the joint distribution of the intensity pair (r,s); $p_R(r)$ and $p_S(s)$ are the marginal distributions of r and s.

Mutual information can be calculated by entropy:

$$\begin{aligned} I(R,S) &= H(R) + H(S) - H(R,S) \\ &= H(R) - H(R \mid S) \\ &= H(S) - H(S \mid R) \end{aligned} \tag{6}$$

$H(S|R)$ is the conditional entropy which is the amount of uncertainty left in S when R is known, and is defined as:

$$H(S \mid R) = \sum_{r \in R} \sum_{s \in S} p_{RS}(r,s) \log p_{S|R}(s \mid r) \tag{7}$$

If R and S are completely independent, $p_{RS}(r,s) = p_R(r) \cdot p_S(s)$ and $I(R,S) = 0$ reaches its minimum; if R and S are identical, $I(R,S) = H(R) = H(S)$ arrives at its maximum. Registration can be achieved by searching the transformation parameters which maximize the mutual information. In implementation, the joint entropy and marginal entropies can be estimated by normalizing the joint and marginal histograms of the overlapped sections of the images. Although maximization of MI is a powerful registration measure, it cannot always generate accurate result. For instance, the changing overlap between the images may lead to false registration with maximum MI (Studholme, et al., 1999).

Case Study: Inter-subject Registration of Thorax CT Image Volumes Based on Image Intensity

The increase in diagnostic information is critical for early detection and treatment of disease and provides better patient management. In the context of a patient with non-small cell lung cancer (NSCLC), registered data may mean the difference between surgery aimed at cure and a palliative approach by the ability to better stage the patient. Further, registration of studies from healthy lung and the lung with tumor or lesion is critical to better tumor detection.

In the example (Figure 2), the registration between healthy lung and the lung with tumor is performed based on image intensity, and normalized MI is used as similarity measure. Figure 2 shows that affine registration is not able to align the common structures from different subjects correctly and therefore deformable registration by using spline (Mattes, et al 2003) is carried out to further improve the registration accuracy.

Hardware Registration

Although continued progress in image registration algorithms (software-based registration) has been achieved, the software-based registration might be labor intensive, computationally expensive, and with

Figure 2. Registration for thoracic CT volumes from different subjects

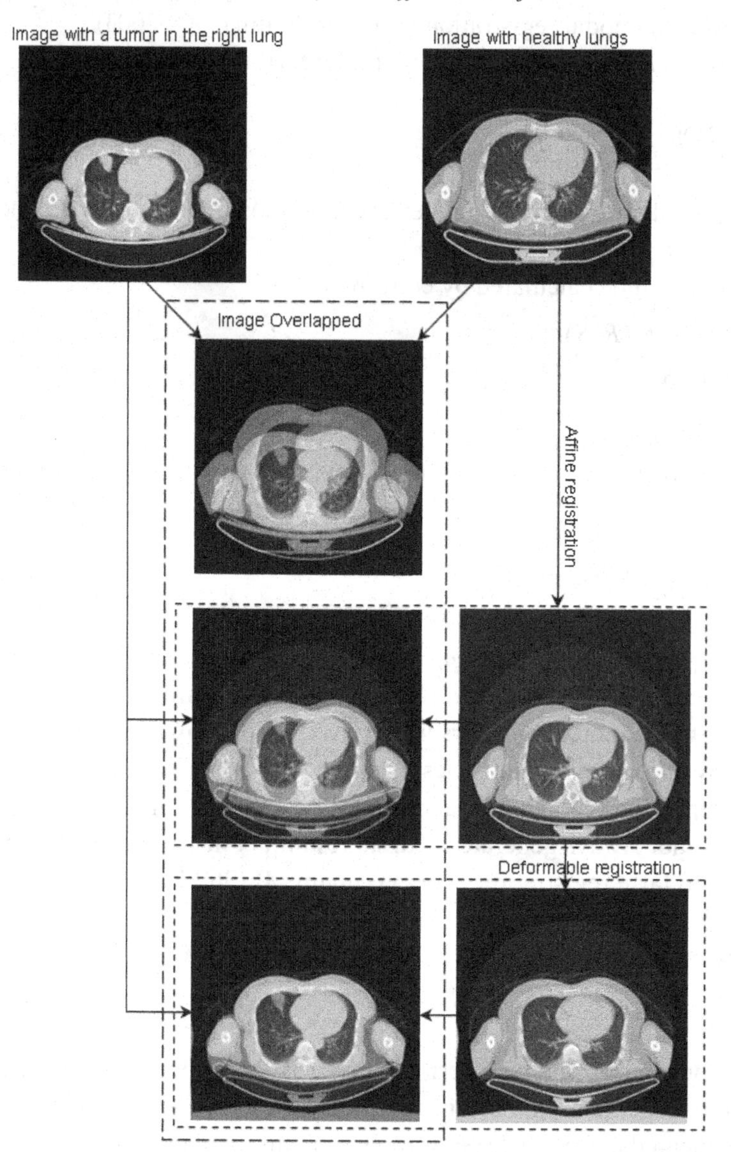

limited accuracy, and thus is impractical to be applied routinely (Townsend, et al, 2003). Hardware registration, in which the functional imaging device, such as PET is combined with an anatomical imaging device such as CT in the one instrument, largely overcomes the current limitations of software-based techniques. The functional and anatomical imaging are performed in the one imaging session on the same imaging table, which minimizes the differences in patient positioning and locations of internal organs between the scans. The mechanical design and calibration procedures ensure that the CT and PET data are inherently accurately registered if the patient does not move. However, patient motion can be encountered between the CT and PET. This not only results in incorrect anatomical localization, but also artifacts from the attenuation correction based on the misaligned CT data (Wang et al, 2007).

Misalignment between the PET and CT data can also be due to involuntary motion, such as respiratory or cardiac motion. Therefore, although the combined PET/CT scanners are becoming more and more popular, there is a clear requirement for software-registration to remove the motions and displacements from the images captured by the combined imaging scanners.

APPLICATIONS OF BIOMEDICAL IMAGE REGISTRATION

Biomedical image registration is able to integrate relevant and heterogeneous information contained in multiple and multimodal image sets, and is important for clinical database management. For instance, registration is essential to mining the large medical imaging databases for constructing statistical atlas of specific disease to reveal the functional and morphological characteristics and changes of the disease, and to facilitate a more suitable patient care. The dynamic atlas in turn is used as a pattern template for automated segmentation and classification of the disease. Image registration is also critical for medical image retrieval of a specific type of disease in a large clinical image database, and in such a scenario, the functional or anatomical atlas provides prior knowledge and is used as a template for early-stage disease detection and identification (Toga, Thompson, 2001).

Registration has a broad range of clinical applications to improve the quality and safety of healthcare. Early detection of tumors or disease offers the valuable opportunity for early intervention to delay or halt the progression of the disease, and eventually to reduce its morbidity and mortality. Biomedical image registration plays an important role in detection of a variety of diseases at an early stage, by combining and fully utilizing complementary information from multimodal images. For instance, dementias are the major causes of disability in the elderly population, while Alzheimer's disease (AD) is the most common cause of dementia (Nestor, et al, 2004).. Registration of longitudinal anatomical MR studies (Scahill, et al, 2003) allows the identification of probable AD (Nestor, et al, 2004) at an early stage to assist an early, effective treatment. Breast cancer is one of major cause of cancer-related death. Registration of pre- and post-contrast of a MR sequence can effectively distinguish different types of malignant and normal tissues (Rueckert, et al, 1998) to offer a better opportunity to cure the patient with the disease (Wang et al, 2007).

Biomedical image registration plays an indispensable role in the management of different diseases. For instance, heart disease is the main cause of death in developed counties (American Heart Association 2006) and cardiac image registration provides a non-invasive method to assist in the diagnosis of heart diseases. For instance, registration of MR and X-ray images is a crucial step in the image guided cardiovascular intervention, as well as in therapy and treatment planning (Rhode, et al, 2005). Multimodal image registration such as CT-MR, CT-PET allows a more accurate definition of the tumor volume during the treatment planning phase (Scarfone et al 2004). These datasets can also be used later to assess responses to therapy and in the evaluation of a suspected tumor recurrence (Wang et al, 2007).

FUTURE TRENDS

Image registration is an enabling technique for fully utilizing heterogeneous image information. However, the medical arena remains a challenging area due to differences in image acquisition, anatomical and functional changes caused by disease progression and treatment, variances and differences across subjects, and complex deformations and motions of internal organs. It is particularly challenging to seamlessly integrate diverse and complementary image information in an efficient, acceptable and applicable manner for clinical routine. Future research in biomedical image registration would need to continuously focus on improving accuracy, efficiency, and usability of registration.

Deformable techniques are in high demand for registering images of internal organs such as liver, lung, and cardiac. However, due to complexity of the registration transformation, this category of registration will continuously hold research attention.

Insufficient registration efficiency is a major barrier to clinical applications, and is especially prevalent in the case of whole-body images from advanced imaging devices such as the combined PET/CT scanners. For instance, whole-body volume data may consist of more than 400 slices for each modality from the combined PET/CT machine. It is a computationally expensive task for registering these large data volumes. With rapid advance in medical imaging techniques, greater innovation will be achieved, for instance, it is expected that a combined MRI/PET will be made available in near future, which will help to improve the quality of healthcare significantly, but also pose a new set of challenges for efficiently registering the datasets with higher resolution, higher dimensionality, and wider range of scanning areas. Multi-scale registration has the potential to find a more accurate solution with greater efficiency.

Graphics Processing Units (GPUs) may provide a high performance hardware platform for real-time and accurate registration and fusion for clinical use. With its superior memory bandwidth, massive parallelism, improvement in the programmability, and stream architecture, GPUs are becoming the most powerful computation hardware and are attracting more and more research attention. The improvement in floating point format provides sufficient computational accuracy for applications in medical areas. However, effective use of GPUs in image registration is not a simple issue (Strzodka, et al 2004). Knowledge about its underlying hardware, design, limitations, evolution, as well as its special programming model is required to map the proposed medical image registration to the GPU pipeline and fully utilize its attractive features. Medical image registration, particularly for high-dimensional data, which fully utilizes the outstanding features of graphics hardware to facilitate fast and cost-saving real-time clinical applications, is new and yet to be fully explored.

CONCLUSION

Registration of medical images from multiple imaging devices and at multiple imaging times is able to integrate and to facilitate a full utilization of the useful image information, and is essential to clinical diagnosis, treatment planning, monitoring and assessment. Image registration is also important in making the medical images more ready and more useful to improve the quality of healthcare service, and is applicable in a wide array of areas including medical database management, medical image retrieval, telemedicine and e-health.

Biomedical image registration has been extensively investigated, and a large number of software-based algorithms have been proposed alongside the developed hardware-based solutions (for instance, the combined PET/CT scanners). Among the comprehensive software-based registration, the feature-based techniques are more computationally efficient, but require a preprocessing step to extract the features to be used in registration, which make this category of registration user-intensive and user-dependent. The intensity-based scheme provides an automatic solution to registration. However, this type of registration is computationally costly. Particularly, image registration is a data-driven and case-orientated research area. It is challenging to select the most suitable and usable technique for specific requirement and datasets from various imaging scanners. For instance, although maximization of MI has been recognized as one of the most powerful registration methods, it cannot always generate accurate solution. A more general registration is more desirable. The combined imaging devices such as PET/CT provide an expensive hardware-based solution. However, even this expensive registration method is not able to always provide the accurate registration, and software-based solution is required to fix the mis-registration caused by patient motions between the imaging sessions. The rapid advance in imaging techniques raises more challenges in registration area to generate more accurate and efficient algorithms in a clinically acceptable time frame.

ACKNOWLEDGMENT

This work is supported by the ARC and UGC grants.

REFERENCES

American Heart Association (2006). *Heart and stroke statistical update.* Http://www.american heart.org

Audette, M., Ferrie, F., & Peters, T. (2000). An algorithm overview of surface registration techniques for medical imaging. *Medical Image Analysis*, 4(4), 201-217.

Bajcsy, R., & Kovacic, S. (1989). Multiresolution elastic matching. *Comp Vision Graphics Image Processing, 46*, 1–21, April 1989

Besl, P. J., & MaKey, N. D. (1992). A method for registration of 3-D shapes. *IEEE Trans. PAMI*, 14(2), 239-256.

Borgefors, G. (1988). Hierarchical Chamfer Matching: A Parametric Edge Matching Algorithm. *IEEE Transactions on Pattern Analysis and Machine Intelligence, 10*, 849-865.

Brown, L. G. (1992). A survey of image registration techniques. *ACM Computing Surveys, 24*(4), 325-376.

Chen, C., Pellizari, C. A., Chen, G. T. Y., Cooper, M. D., & Levin, D. N. (1987). Image analysis of PET data with the aid of CT and MR images. *Information processing in medical imaging*, 601-611.

Cohen, I., & Cohen, I. (1993, November). Finite-element methods for active contour models and balloons for 2-D and 3-D images. *IEEE Pattern Anal. Machine Intelligence*, 15, 1131-1147.

Collignon, A., Maes, F., Delaere, D., Vandermeulen, D., Suetens, P., & Marchal, G. (1995). Automated multimodality image registration based on information theory. In *Proc. 14th International Conference of Information Processing in Medical Imaging 1995,* vol.3, (Bizais, Y., Barillot, C. and Di Paola, R. eds.), Ile Berder, France, pp. 263–274, June 1995.

Fitzpatrick, J.M., Hill, D.L.G. & Maurer, C.R. (2000). *Handbook of medical imaging*, (pp. 375-435). Bellingham, WA: SPIE Press.

Kass, M., Witkin, A., & Terzopoulos, D. (1988). Snakes: active contour models. *International Journal of Computer Vision*, pp.321-331.

Lehmann, T. M., Gönner, C., & Spitzer, K. (1999). Survey: Interpolation methods in medical image processing. *IEEE Transactions on Medical Imaging, 18*(11), 1049-1075.

Maintz, J. B. A., van den Elsen, P. A. & Viergever, M. A. (1996). Evaluation of ridge seeking operators for multimodality medical image registration. *IEEE Trans. PAMI, 18*(4), 353-365.

Maintz, J. B. A. & Viergever, M. A. (1998). A Survey of Medical Image Registration. *Medical Image Analysis, 2*(1), 1-36.

Mattes, D., Haynor, D. R., Vesselle, H., Lewellen, T. K., & Eubank, W. (2003) PET-CT image registration in the chest using free-form deformations. *IEEE Transactions on Medical Imaging*, 23(1), 120-128.

Nestor, P. J., Scheltens, P., & Hodges, J. R. (2004, July). Advances in the early detection of Alzheimer's disease. *Nature Reviews Neuroscience, 5*(Supplement), S34-S41.

Pluim, J. P., Maintz, J. B. A., & Viergever, M. A. (2003, August) Mutual-information-based registration of medical images: a survey. *IEEE Transactions on Medical Imaging*, 22(8), 986-1004.

Powell, M. J. D. (1964). An efficient method for finding the minimum of a function of several variables without calculating derivatives. *Comput. J., 7*, 155-163.

Press, W. H., Teukolsky, S. A., Vetterling, W. T., & Flannery, B. P. (1992). *Numerical Recipes in C.* Cambridge Univ. Press, Cambridge, U.K.

Rhode, K. S., Sermesant, M., Brogan, D., Hegde, S., Hipwell, J., Lambiase, P., Rosenthsal, E., bucknall, C., Qureshi, S. A., Gill, J.S., Razavi, R., & Hill, D. L.G. (2005, November). A system for real-time XMR guided cardiovascular intervention. *IEEE Transactions on Medical Imaging,* 24(11), 1428-1440.

Rueckert, D., Hayes, C., Studholme, C., Summers, P., Leach, M., & Hawkes, D. J. (1998). Non-rigid registration of breast MR images using mutual information. *MICCAI'98 lecture notes in computer science*, Cambridge, pp.1144-1152.

Scahill, R. I. Frost, C., Jenkins, R., Whitwell, J. L., Rossor, M. N., & Fox, N.C. (2003, July). A longitudinal study of brain volume changes in normal aging using serial registered magnetic resonance imaging. *Archives of Neurology*, 60(7), 989-994.

Scarfone, C., Lavely, W. C., Cmelak, A. J., Delbeke, D., Martin, W. H., Billheimer, D., & Hallahan, D. E. (2004). Prospective feasibility trial of radiotherapy target definition for head and neck cancer using 3-dimensional PET and CT imaging. *Journal of Nuclear Medicine*, 45(4), 543-552, Apr 2004.

Subsol, G., Thirion, J. P., & Ayache, N. (1998). A scheme for automatically building three dimensional morphometric anatomical atlases: application to a skull atlas. *Medical Image Analysis*, 2(1), 37-60.

Strzodka, R., Droske, M., & Rumpf, M. (2004) Image registration by a regularized gradient flow - a streaming implementation in DX9 graphics hardware. *Computing, 73*(4), 373–389.

Studholme, C., Hill, D. L. G., & Hawkes, D. J. (1999) An overlap invariant entropy measure of 3D medical image alignment. *Pattern Recognition, 32*, 71–86.

Thévenaz, P., & Unser, M. (2000). Optimization of mutual information for multiresolution registration. *IEEE Transaction on Image Processing*, 9(12), 2083-2099.

Toga, A. W., & Thompson P. M. (2001, september) The role of image registration in brain mapping. *Image and Vision Computing Journal*, 19, 3–24.

Townsend, D. W., Beyer, T., & Blodgett, T. M. (2003). PET/CT Scanners: A Hardware Approach to Image Fusion. *Semin Nucl Med* XXXIII(3), 193-204.

Unser, M., & Aldroubi, A. (1993, November). A multiresolution image registration procedure using spline pyramids. Proc. of SPIE 2034, 160-170, Wavelet Applications in Signal and Image Processing, ed. Laine, A. F.

Van den Elsen, P. A., Maintz, J. B. A., Pol, E. -J. D., & Viergever, M. A. (1995, June). Automatic registration of CT and MR brain images using correlation of geometrical features. *IEEE Transactions on Medical Imaging, 14*(2), 384 – 396.

Viola, P. A., & Wells, W. M. (1995, June) Alignment by maximization of mutual information. In *Proc. 5th International Conference of Computer Vision*, Cambridge, MA, 16-23.

Wang, X., S. Eberl, Fulham, M., Som, S., & Feng, D. (2007) Data Registration and Fusion, Chapter 8 in D. Feng (Ed.) *Biomedical Information Technology*, pp.187-210, Elsevier Publishing

Wang, X., & Feng, D. (2005). Active Contour Based Efficient Registration for Biomedical Brain Images. *Journal of Cerebral Blood Flow & Metabolism, 25*(Suppl), S623.

Wang, X., & Feng, D. (2005). Biomedical Image Registration for Diagnostic Decision Making and Treatment Monitoring. Chapter 9 in R. K. Bali (Ed.) *Clinical Knowledge Management: Opportunities and Challenges*, pp.159-181, Idea Group Publishing

Xu, C., & Prince, J. L. (1998, March). Snakes, shapes, and gradient vector flow. *IEEE Trans. Image Processing, 7*, 359-369.

KEY TERMS

Image Registration: The process to search for an appropriate transformation to spatially align the images in a common coordinate system.

Intra-Subject Registration: Registration for the images from same subject/person.

Inter-Subject Registration: Registration for the images from different subjects/persons.

Monomodal Images: Refers to images acquired from same imaging techniques.

Multimodal Images: Refers to images acquired from different imaging.

Chapter VII
ECG Processing

Lenka Lhotská
Czech Technical University in Prague, Czech Republic

Václav Chudáček
Czech Technical University in Prague, Czech Republic

Michal Huptych
Czech Technical University in Prague, Czech Republic

ABSTRACT

This chapter describes methods for preprocessing, analysis, feature extraction, visualization, and classification of electrocardiogram (ECG) signals. First we introduce preprocessing methods, mainly based on the discrete wavelet transform. Then classification methods such as fuzzy rule based decision trees and neural networks are presented. Two examples - visualization and feature extraction from Body Surface Potential Mapping (BSPM) signals and classification of Holter ECGs – illustrate how these methods are used. Visualization is presented in the form of BSPM maps created from multi-channel measurements on the patient's thorax. Classification involves distinguishing between Holter recordings from premature ventricular complexes and normal ECG beats. Classification results are discussed. Finally the future research opportunities are proposed.

INTRODUCTION

Electrocardiogram (ECG) analyses have been used as a diagnostic tool for decades. Computer technology has led to the introduction of ECG analysis tools that aim to support decision making by medical doctors. This chapter will introduce the reader to ECG processing as an example of a data-mining application. Basic methods of preprocessing, analysis, feature extraction, visualization, and classification will be described. First, clinical features of ECGs are presented. These features are the basic characteristics used in temporal analysis of ECGs. Then four types of ECG signal measurement are briefly described.

The next section focuses on preprocessing, analysis, and feature extraction. Since the measured ECG signal contains noise, the first step is denoising. Then we introduce the wavelet transform as a method for detecting the characteristic points of ECG. Feature extraction is a necessary step before classification can be performed. The quality of the classification depends strongly on the quality of the features. We present an overview of techniques for extracting ECG diagnostic and morphological features. Feature extraction from BSPM is shown as an example. The final step in ECG processing is classification. In the section on classification, several supervised and unsupervised methods are described. Classification of Holter ECGs is presented as an example, and we discuss the results achieved using the algorithms presented here. The chapter concludes with a look at future trends and problems to be addressed.

THE PHYSIOLOGICAL BASIS OF ECGS AND ECG MEASUREMENT

ECG signals

An electrocardiogram (ECG) is a recording of the electrical activity of the heart in dependence on time. The mechanical activity of the heart is linked with its electrical activity. An ECG is therefore an important diagnostic tool for assessing heart function.

ECG signals, measurements of which will be described here, can provide a great deal of information on the normal and pathological physiology of heart activity. An ECG as an electrical manifestation of a human activity is composed of heartbeats that repeat periodically. Several waves and interwave sections can be recognized in each heartbeat. The shape and length of these waves and interwave sections characterize cardiovascular diseases, arrhythmia, ischemia and other heart diseases. Basic waves in ECG are denoted by P, Q, R, S, T, and U - see Figure 1. The denotation (and length) of the intervals and segments is derived from these. The time axis uses the order of milliseconds, while the potential axis uses the order of mV.

Figure 1. ECG temporal analysis – parameters of a heartbeat

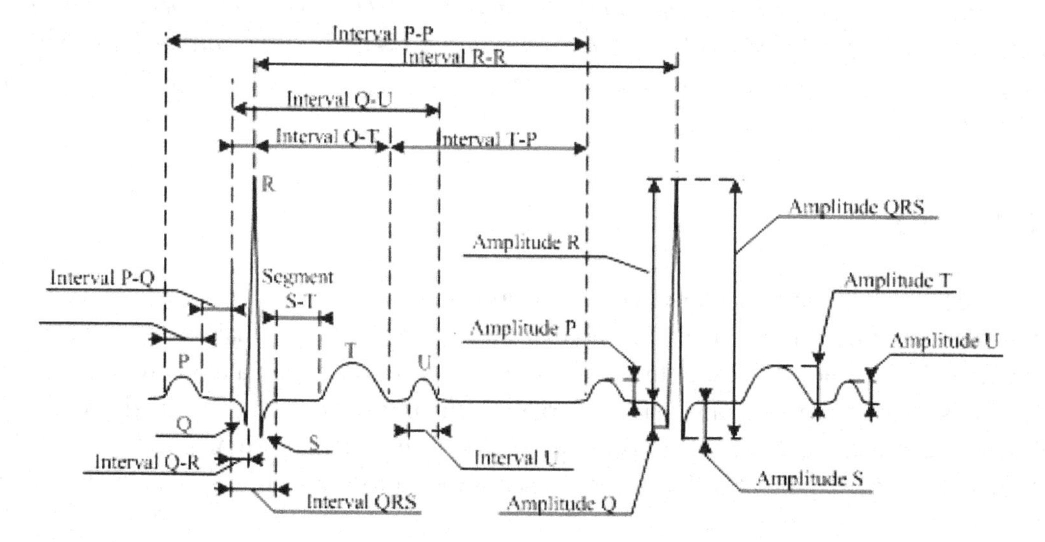

The P wave emerges when there is atrial depolarization. The P-Q interval is measured between the beginning of the P wave and the beginning of the Q wave. If the Q wave is missing, the interval is measured between the beginning of the P wave and beginning of the R wave, and is denoted as the P-R interval. The interval represents the time needed for atrial depolarization (P wave) and the time for conducting the electrical potential from the atria to the ventricle through the atrio-ventricular node. The length of the interval depends on the heartbeat frequency.

The Q wave represents depolarization of the interventricular septum. The depth of the Q-wave depends on the lead system that is used – in the standard 12-lead ECG system the Q wave may be deep, and in a VR lead it may even be dominating. The Q wave is usually very low, and may disappear when there is intensive inhalation (depending on the heart position).

The R wave is any positive wave of the QRS complex. It represents depolarization of the anterior, posterior and lateral walls of the ventricles, thus representing the beginning of the ventricular systole. In the case of a QRS complex split, an additional R wave (usually denoted R') may appear. This is often a symptom of pathology. Lower amplitude of the R wave, for example, appears both in the case of vast myocardial processes (e.g. myocardial infarction), or diseases such as emphysema.

The S wave representing the final phase of heart depolarization is a negative wave ending with a J-point and continuing to the ST segment.

The ST segment is the time interval from the end of the QRS complex to the beginning of the T wave. This corresponds to the time when depolarization of the ventricles finishes and their slow repolarization starts. The ST segment is normally isoelectric.

The T wave represents rapid repolarization of the ventricles. Both the orientation and the amplitude of the T wave are evaluated. The T wave is usually oriented to the same side as the main wave of the QRS complex. The amplitude of the T wave is in a certain relation with the amplitude of the R wave (the standard is 1/8 to 2/3 of the amplitude of the R wave).

The QT interval is measured from the beginning of the QRS complex - Q wave to the end of the T wave. The length of this interval depends on the heartbeat frequency and other factors, such as drugs used by the patient. All new drugs must be tested against the QT interval to show that there are no interferences between the drug and heart function.

ECG Signal Pathology

An ECG of a healthy heart is regular and may vary slightly in frequency, amplitude and length of the individual parts of the P-QRS-T complex. For example, the normal length of the P-R interval is 0.12 – 0.2 sec; with certain disorders, the interval can be shorter (abnormalities in conduction from atrium to ventricle) or longer (e.g. 0.36 sec for a 1st degree heart block).

An ECG is of great importance for diagnosing arrhythmias – it cannot be replaced by any other examination. Some arrhythmias are not perceived by the patient, and some arrhythmias are frequent among patients monitored at coronary units after an acute heart attack. However arrhythmias often cause complaints that are temporary, so that the patient may feel in good order when examined by the doctor. Detection of arrhythmias, especially from long-term ECG records, is therefore a significant task. Figure 2 illustrates four examples of normal ECGs and ECGs with various types of arrhythmia.

Cardiac arrhythmias are usually caused by one or a combination of the following abnormalities in the rhythmicity-conduction system of the heart: abnormal rhythmicity of the pacemaker; shift of the

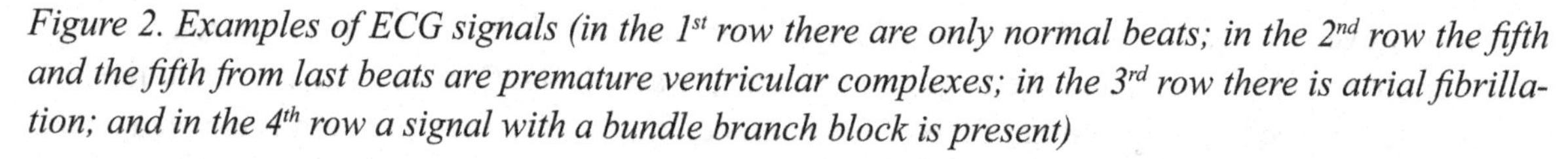

Figure 2. Examples of ECG signals (in the 1st row there are only normal beats; in the 2nd row the fifth and the fifth from last beats are premature ventricular complexes; in the 3rd row there is atrial fibrillation; and in the 4th row a signal with a bundle branch block is present)

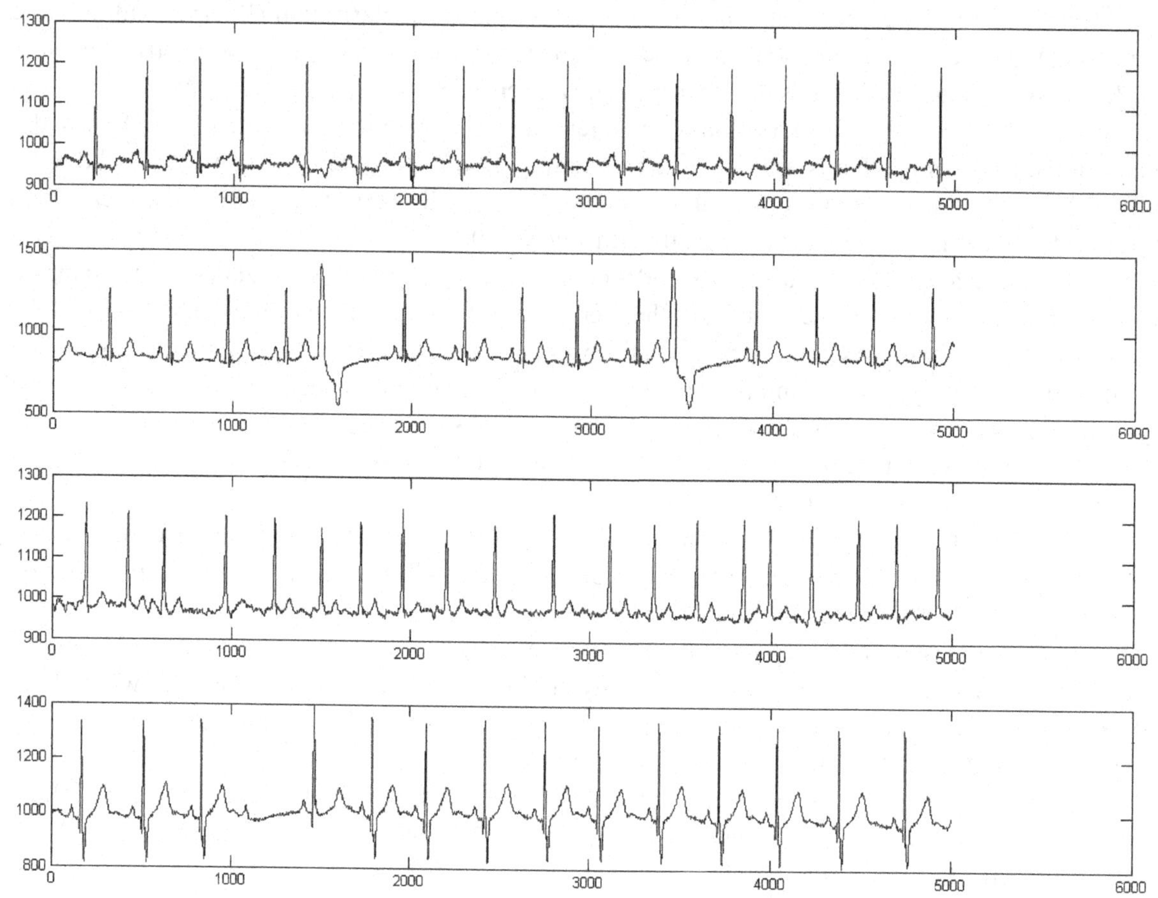

pacemaker from the sinus node to other parts of the heart; blocks at various points in the transmission through the heart; spontaneous generation of abnormal impulses in almost any part of the heart.

For example, bradycardia is a slow and persistent sinus rhythm, tachycardia is a fast and persistent sinus rhythm, extrasystola means the occurrence of sporadic early contractions; if activation of the atria or ventricles is chaotic, then fibrillation occurs. We have mentioned only a few examples of pathological changes of ECGs as an illustration of the complexity of ECG signal analysis.

Descriptions of physiological ECGs and pathological changes in ECGs can be found in numerous publications, e.g. in (Khan, 2003).

ECG Temporal Analysis

In medical practice, ECG analysis is performed for temporal analysis almost to the exclusion of other methods. Other methods, such as frequency analysis of QRS or ST complexes, are mostly limited to experimental environments. When interpreting an ECG, physicians first locate the P waves, QRS complexes, T complexes and U waves. Then they interpret the shapes (morphology) of these waves and complexes; in addition they calculate the heights and the interval of each wave, such as the RR interval, PP interval, PR interval, QT interval, and ST segment. From the technical point of view, the assumption for ECG analysis is the existence of perfect ECG signals (i.e. signals with sufficient dynamics and a minimum of artifacts). It follows from the physicians' approach that three related problems are usually distinguished and must be considered when designing a system for ECG analysis and classification:

- Recognition of several primary characteristic ECG elements. In a selected ECG segment (usually one or several heart beats), these elements, i.e., waves, points and complexes, are identified.
- Graphoelement quantification. The curvature of the arcs, and the length of the waves and complexes are calculated (or visually evaluated); their amplitudes are measured, etc. Measurement of individual cardiac intervals is also important. In the simplest case, a certain number of characteristic points and intervals are determined on a single ECG period (see Figure 1). The characteristic points are selected in such a way that the co-ordinates can be determined in order to calculate all important graphoelements of the corresponding ECG segment.
  Undesirable effects such as breathing waves (which have period T equal to 3 - 5 s) and slow waves must be sufficiently removed for successful separation of significant diagnostic ECG features. For automatic analysis, it is necessary to define the amplitudes of the individual graphoelements with a maximum error of ±5 per cent. An error of 10 per cent is usually acceptable for time intervals. When analyzing the QRS complex and P and T waves, the corresponding areas above and below the isoline are calculated (see Figure 1) and the velocity of the potential change in the QRS complex is determined.
- Classification into certain diagnostic classes is performed on the basis of appropriately defined features.

There exist classification systems that are able to localize pathological changes in ECG records, detect the QRS complex, the ST segment (Jager, 1994), find the RR interval (Azuaje, 1998), the appearance of individual waves (Jeras, 2001), and many other values. Based on this data, and supported by such a classification system, the doctor can determine the diagnosis.

From the point of view of ECG signal classification, four types of ECG signal measurement can be described:

- **Ambulatory "classical" 12-lead ECG:** This is a measurement where the patient lies in a relatively steady state, the electrode placements are very strictly defined, consisting of 3 Einthoven leads, 3 augmented leads and 6 unipolar Goldberger leads. The purpose of ambulatory 12-lead ECG is to assess the morphological quality of the heart muscle. Signs of acute myocardial infarction or signs of old infarction are usually sought; other structural damage can also be diagnosed on the basis of the measurement. The measurement takes about 10 seconds of recording, during which approximately 5-10 beats are acquired. For further work with the ECG, the averaged beat is computed as a representative of the most common beats in the recording - all beats with unusual timing such as premature ventricular contractions are skipped, and the rest are used for creating the averaged representative. The beat averaging approach allows us to measure out the characteristics of the heartbeat much more precisely than for example Holter ECG measurement.

- **Holter ECG:** Long-term ECG monitoring focuses on a search for deficiencies in heart rhythm (Holter, 1961). Holter measurement usually takes 24hours (and measurements up to 7 days are now available). During this extensive period of time the patient wears the device (and its electrodes) while performing his/her usual daily activities. The task of ECG signal processing and classification in particular is very different from ambulatory ECG evaluation. The computer program has to deal with more than 100 000 beats, with the morphology of the beats varying not only according to patient's physiognomy or pathology, but also due to normal circadian changes in heart function and the quality of the recording – the patient should live his/her unrestricted daily life. The main purpose of Holter ECG diagnostics is to make a clear distinction between various types of beats. Correct diagnostics of such clusters (subgroups) of the signal is only a secondary step. Many different methods have been proposed for solving the problem of discriminating between normal 'N' and premature ventricular 'V' beats. Some of these are based on beat-shape description parameters (de Chazal, 2004; Cuesta-Frau, 2003), while others use frequency-based features (Lagerholm, 2000). The software in Holter devices is intended to ease the burden imposed on doctors/nurses, who would otherwise need to process an incredible amount of data – comparable with the data in EEG sleep or coma monitoring. A more detailed description of the Holter ECG classification will be discussed below.
- **Telemedicine applications:** Applications in telemedicine usually record very simple (mostly just one-lead) ECGs, using cheap widely-available devices such as PDAs or mobile phones. These applications will spread in the future, especially in connection with the shift of focus toward home care and transferring more responsibility to individuals for their own health. Since telemedical applications have certain limitations, they require a special approach to classification. The very low resolution of the ECG signal means that the position of the QRS complex is often the only feature that can be extracted. Various methods dealing with heart rate variability (HRV) analysis have been proposed for diagnosing atrial fibrillation (Malik, 1995).
- **Body Surface Potential Mapping:** Body surface potential mapping is a method first described in 1963 (Taccardi, 1963). The aim of the method was to improve the resolution of the ECG to such an extent that it could substitute invasive catheter measurement when searching for an infarction lesion or an arrhythmogenetic part of the heart muscle, thus providing better diagnostic values (Kornreich, 1997). BSPM systems may use up to several hundreds of electrodes, which can also lead to some drawbacks, e.g. more complicated measurement and electrode positioning. Advances in imaging techniques, such as PET and SONO, and also the very steep decrease in complications in the use of invasive catheter operations, have edged BSPM methods to the very border between clinical medicine and research (Lux, 1982). BSPM has been used in recent times when searching for inverse problem solutions and also in physiological experiments on the human heart during artificial blood occlusion in certain parts of the myocardium, for example during the PTCA (percutaneous transluminal coronary angioplasty) procedure. The most frequently used body surface maps are isopotential maps, which give the distribution of the potential at a specific moment, and isointegral maps, which provide the distribution of the sum of potentials over a specified time interval.

From the classification point of view, classification as in ambulatory ECG measurement is possible, or alternatively we can use a completely different approach based on map (image) comparison using features derived from the isopotential maps that are described in the section headed *Example of feature extraction from BSPM.*

There are other variants of ECG measurement devices, such as ergometry and ergospirometry, where the signal is preprocessed in the same way, but classification poses its own particular problems. In ergometry, the main focus is on assessing the ability of the heart muscle to function properly under a load. Due to space limitations, the reader is referred to books such as (Kjaer, 2003).

PREPROCESSING AND PROCESSING OF ECGs

This section introduces specific steps in ECG preprocessing and processing. There are three basic steps: preprocessing, analysis and feature extraction. We will discuss noise signals that corrupt the ECG signal and methods for removing them, mainly by means of filtering. ECG analysis is based on localizing the characteristic points in each beat of the record. Feature extraction from analyzed signal will now be described.

Preprocessing of ECGs

An ECG signal is corrupted by many different noise signals. The following list shows the most frequent types of noise and describes them briefly. This section is based on (Acharya, 2007; Clifford, 2006).

Power line noise (A/C interference) is made up of 50/60 Hz. baseline wandering, and ECG amplitude modulation is caused by respiration. The drift of the baseline with respiration appears in the ECG signal as an added sinusoidal component at the frequency of respiration. The frequency of this component is between 0.15 and 0.6 Hz. Muscle contractions (electromyographic, EMG) cause artifactual millivolt-level potentials to appear in the ECG recording. The frequency content of the EMG is from 0 Hz to 10.000 Hz. Motion artifacts are caused by movement or vibration in the subject. They change the skin-electrode interface and thereby also the impedance of the interface.

Electrode contact noise is caused by poor electrode contact between the subject and the electrode. This can happen if the subject moves during the recording, and the electrode disconnects from the skin surface. It can happen during Holter measurement. In the ECG this phenomenon manifests as a rapid step baseline transition which decays to the baseline value.

Non-adaptive and adaptive filters in ECG processing are introduced in (Thakor, 1991; Ferrara, 1981). These methods are usually used in preprocessing to filter power line noise, respiration frequency and muscle contraction. Baseline wandering correction using the wavelet transform is described in (Daqrouq, 2005). A further description of ECG noise and its removal can be found in (Acharya, 2007; Clifford, 2006).

Wavelet Transform

The basic signal transform from the time domain to the frequency domain is the Fourier transform (FT), which is defined as (Daubechies, 1992):

$$F(\omega) = \int_{-\infty}^{\infty} f(t)e^{-j\omega t}dt$$

The signal transformed by the Fourier transform is called the frequency spectrum. The spectrum shows the intensity of signal frequencies contained in the signal. The main problem is that we see only a summary of the frequency character of the signal.

The Short-Time Fourier Transform (STFT) allows us to observe both frequency and time. The STFT is defined as (Daubechies, 1992):

$$(T^{win} f)(t_0,\omega_0) = \int_{-\infty}^{\infty} f(t) g(t - t_0) e^{-j\omega_0 t} dt$$

The main problem is based on the Heisenberg uncertainty principle, namely it is not possible to identify exactly what frequency components occur in given times.

The Short-Time Fourier Transform divides the time-frequency space into equal parts. This means that the decomposition of the signal always has the best resolution in time or frequency, irrespective of the values. Thus, if a thin window is chosen we obtain good resolution in time, but poor resolution in frequency. By contrast, obviously, if a wide window is chosen we get good resolution in frequency but poor resolution in time. Though the Heisenberg uncertainty principle is valid irrespective of the transform, its effect can be restricted. The wavelet transform is also based on decomposition to set the scanning function. The basic and greatest difference is that the scanning functions - wavelets - are functions of both time and frequency. Thus they represent the time-frequency dependence of the transform.

Wavelet transform (WT) analysis began in the mid 1980s for analyzing interrogate seismic signals. Since the early 1990s, wavelet transform analysis has been utilized in science and engineering.

The continuous wavelet transform (CWT) is a time-frequency analysis method which differs from the short-time Fourier transform by allowing arbitrarily high localization in time of the high-frequency signal feature. The continuous wavelet transform of function f(t) with respect to this wavelet family is defined as (Daubechies, 1992; Mallat, 1992):

$$(T^{wav} f)(a,b) = \int f(x) \frac{1}{\sqrt{a}} \psi\left(\frac{x-b}{a}\right)$$

where a, b $\in$ R, a $\neq$ 0, and a is scaling and b is translation of mother wavelet ψ. Thus, if we define ψ a,b(t) as the translated and scaled ψ(t), then ψa,b(t) is given by:

$$\psi_{a,b}(t) = \frac{1}{\sqrt{a}} \psi\left(\frac{t-b}{a}\right)$$

The following conditions need to be satisfied for the function ψ(t) to behave as a wavelet (Daubechies, 1992) average value: $\int \psi(t)dt = 0$; energy signal; $\int |\psi(t)|^2 dt = 0$; admissibility of wavelet; $C_\psi = 2\pi \int |\hat{\psi}(\omega)|^2 / |\omega| d\omega < \infty$.

The continuous wavelet transform is also very useful for displaying the time-frequency distribution of a signal. Figure 3 shows the distribution of frequency a) before baseline correction, b) after baseline correction. The horizontal axis shows time, and the vertical axis shows frequency on the logarithmic scale (low frequency at the bottom). The Morlet wavelet (Daubechies, 1992) is used for decomposition into 60 levels.

Most computer implementations use the Discrete Wavelet Transform (DWT). In DWT, time t is not discretized, but variables a and b are discretized instead. The scaling parameter a is discretized as a = p^j, j $\in$ Z , p $\neq$ 0. The equation for the wavelet transform is given as (Daubechies, 1992):

Figure 3. CWT of an ECG signal before and after removal of low frequency and baseline wandering

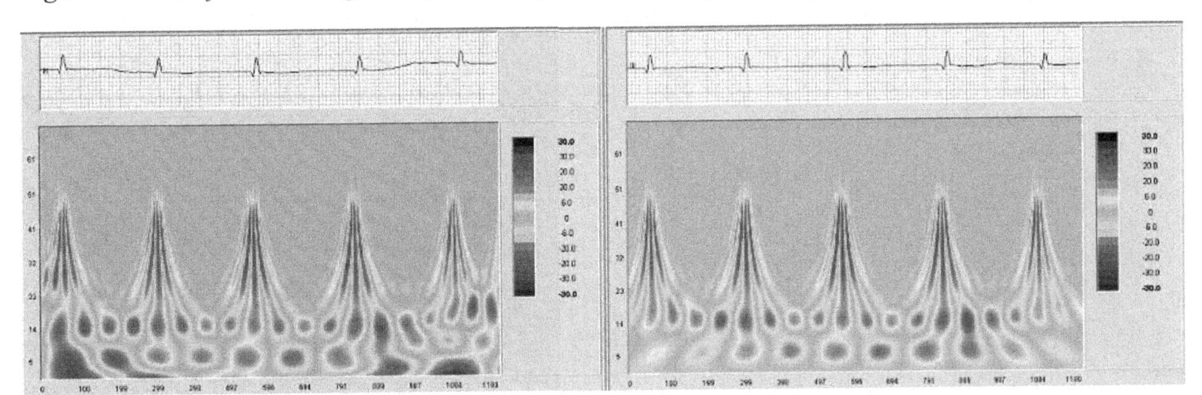

$$\psi_{j,b}(x) = \frac{1}{\sqrt{p^j}}\psi\left(\frac{x - nbp^j}{p^j}\right) = \frac{1}{\sqrt{p^j}}\psi\left(p^{-j}x - nb\right)$$

If $p = 2$ and $n = 2^{-j}$, the sampling of time-frequency space is called dyadic. Then the wavelet function has the following form:

$$\psi_{j,k}(x) = \frac{1}{\sqrt{2^j}}\psi\left(2^{-j}x - 2^{-j}b\right) = \frac{1}{\sqrt{2^j}}\psi\left(2^{-j}x - k\right) \quad \text{where } k = 2^{-j}b$$

Multi-Resolution Analysis (MRA) is the most important part of wavelet theory. The idea of MRA has been developed by Mallat and Meyer. In MRA, a function is decomposed into an approximation (representing slow variances in function) and a detail (representing rapid variances in function), level by level, by scaling and wavelet function (examples - see Figure 4). Both scaling and wavelet functions create a form for wavelet multi-resolution analysis.

Thus, let the signal f(t) be described by wavelet function $\varphi_k(t)$ and $\psi_{j,k}(t)$ by (Daubechies, 1992) as:

$$f(t) = \sum_{k=-\infty}^{\infty} c_k \varphi_k(t) + \sum_{j=0}^{\infty}\sum_{k=-\infty}^{\infty} d_{jk}\Psi_{jk}(t)$$

where $\varphi_k(t)$ is scaling function, $\psi_{jk}(t)$ is wavelet function, c_k is called approximation and d_{jk} is called signal detail.

In practice, filter banks (quadrature mirror filters - QMF) and Mallat's algorithm are often used for performing the discrete wavelet transform . The impulse response of a low pass filter corresponds with the scaling function. This means that the output signal from a low pass filter ($\bar{h}$,h) is an approximation. The impulse response of a high pass filter ($\bar{g}$,g) corresponds with the wavelet function. The output signal from a high pass filter is a detail. The relation between a coefficients and h,g coefficients is shown in (Daubechies, 1992).

For filters in a bank the following assumptions must be valid (Daubechies, 1992):

Figure 4. a) Example of four approximations, b) example of four details from an ECG signal

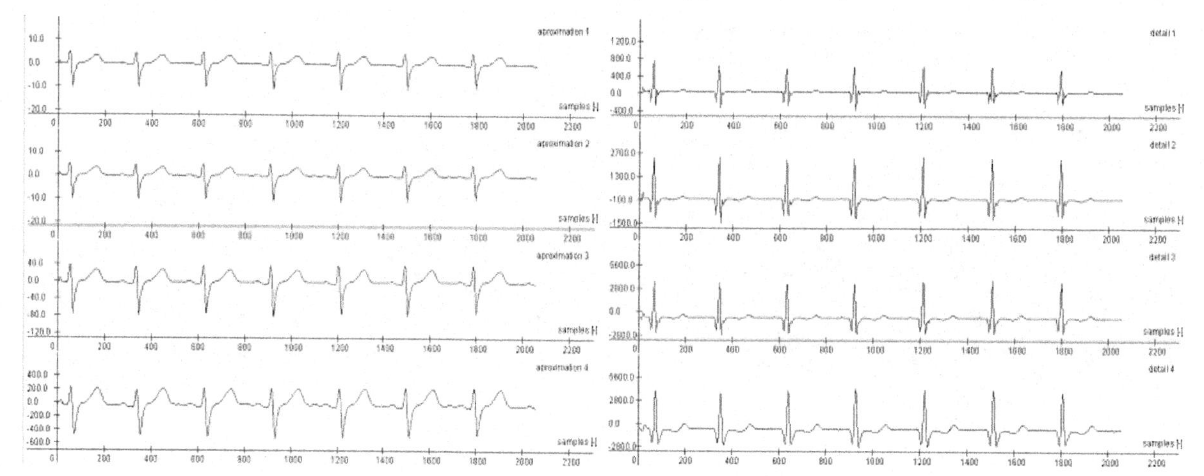

$$\tilde{a}^0(z)a^0(z)+\tilde{a}^1(z)a^1(-z)=0$$
$$a^1(z)=a^0(-z)$$
$$\tilde{a}^0(z)=a^0(z)$$
$$\tilde{a}^1(z)=-a^0(-z)$$

From this equation it results that we need only a^0 coefficients in order to calculate all bank filter coefficients. However we want to obtain the coefficients of the impulse response.

For the relation between a coefficients and h,g coefficients, it holds (Daubechies, 1992):

$$h(z^{-1})=a^0(z),\text{so}\quad h(z)=\tilde{a}^0(z)$$

Between low pass and high pass coefficients the relation holds:

$$g(L-1-n)=(-1)^n h(n),\ \text{resp.}$$
$$g(n)=(-1)^n h(-n+1)$$

From the equation we obtain the coefficients for reconstruction filters. For decomposition filters the previous equation is suitable:

$$\bar{h}(n)=\overline{h(-n)},\ \text{and}\ \bar{g}(n)=\overline{g(-n)}$$

Reconstruction filter g(n) is calculated as the complement of filter h(n), and decomposition filters $\bar{h}(n),\bar{g}(n)$ are defined as the time reverse sequence of h(n), g(n) filters.

Analysis and Feature Extraction

ECG analysis is a necessary step for ECG beat classification. The principle of the analysis is based on identifying important waves that represent individual functional steps of heart activity. The accuracy of the analysis is dependent on the quality of the signal. The better the signal-to-noise ratio, the higher the accuracy is.

Figure 5. Principle of detecting characteristic points on the 1st and 4th details from wavelet transform decomposition

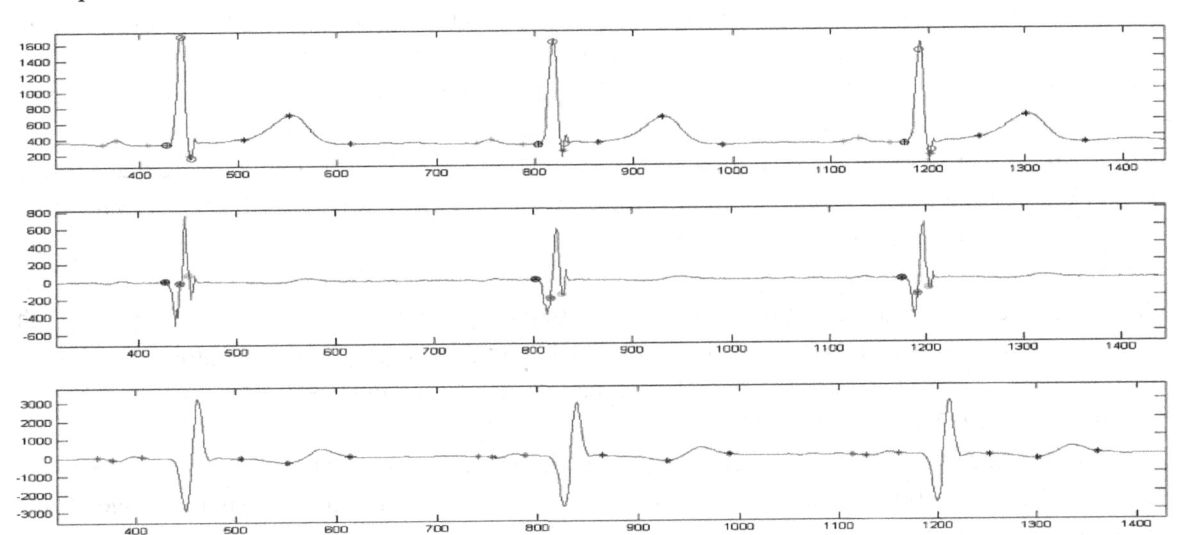

Most frequently, the first part of the heartbeat that is found is the R wave, because it is recognizable even in a very noisy signal. Thus, the R wave defines single beats of recorded signal. Before the R wave there is the Q wave, and after the R wave the S wave is localized. The Q wave, the R wave and the S wave form the QRS complex, which represents mainly the ventricular depolarization. Basic works about QRS analysis are (Li, 1995; Acharya, 2007;). The wavelet transform for the QRS complex detector is used in (Kadambe, 1999).

The P wave is usually located before the QRS complex. Finding the P wave is very dependent on the scale of the signal noise. One method for highlighting the P wave can be P wave averaging (Ferrara, 1981).

The last wave in the heartbeat is the T wave, which is located after the QRS complex. The T wave represents ventricular repolarization. The onset of the T wave is important with respect to analysis of the ST segment. Elevation or depression of the ST segment is an important factor in diagnosing myocardial infarction (Acharya, 2007; Clifford, 2006; Jager, 1994). The T wave offset is important for QT segment detection (Braga, 2004). T wave end analysis is shown in (Clifford, 2006). Locating the end of the T wave is a difficult task, because of noise.

Eleven characteristic points are defined in a single ECG period - maximum amplitude of the R wave, beginning and maximum amplitude of the Q wave, maximum amplitude and end of the S wave, and the beginning, maximum amplitude and end of the P and T waves (Li, 1995; Huptych, 2006).

The characteristic points are found on a decomposition signal by the discrete wavelet transform. This process is displayed in Figure 5. The transform has four levels and a quadratic spline as a wavelet. First, the R wave maximum is found as the zero crossing on all details. Then Q onset, Q peak, S peak, and S offset, based on the position of the R wave as the zero crossing, and the maxima in the defined time window on the 1st detail are localized. The final step is to locate the onsets, peaks and offsets of the P and T waves. These are detected similarly as the Q and S waves parameters, but on the 4th detail.

The next step in ECG processing is feature extraction. Extraction of basic features from a standard ECG is based on segmenting the signal into characteristics points. For example, important features of the heartbeat can be QRS width, QT interval length, Q wave amplitude, and T wave polarity. We can define the following features: P peak - maximum P wave amplitude; P wave interval – from P wave onset to P wave offset; PR interval – from P wave onset to R wave maximum amplitude; QRS complex interval - from Q wave onset to S wave offset; S interval - from S wave offset to S wave offset; ST interval - from S wave offset to T wave onset; T peak - maximum of T wave amplitude; R peak - maximum of R wave amplitude; T wave interval - from T wave onset to T wave offset; QT interval - from P wave onset to P wave offset.

Determining the heart rate is also based on the analysis described here. It is computed from the interval between the R waves of single beats, so it is usable on very noise data and/or in a system with limited computing possibilities (e.g. pacemakers). The heart rate is a very important parameter of heart function. There are many works on using HRV as the only heart function description parameter (Acharya, 2007; Clifford, 2006; Malik, 1995).

Advanced methods of feature extraction use a description of waves in terms of shape. Typical points chosen in (Christov, 2004; Malik, 1995) are similar to those given in Figure 1. An advantage of this approach is that it decreases the computational burden. Unfortunately these points depend very heavily

Figure 6. Two time-sampling methods for extracting ECG morphology features, as shown in (© 2004 IEEE. Used with permission.)

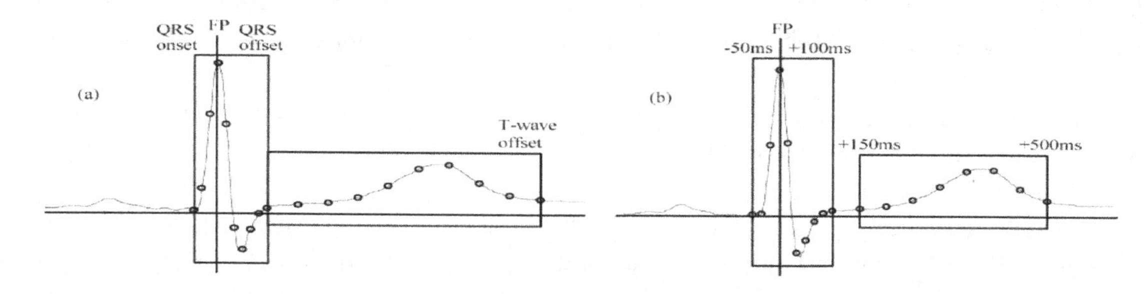

Figure 7. Some of the pattern recognition parameters obtained from ECG leads (left) and from a vectorcardiogram (VCG) (right), as shown in (©2006 Ivaylo Christov. Used with permission.)

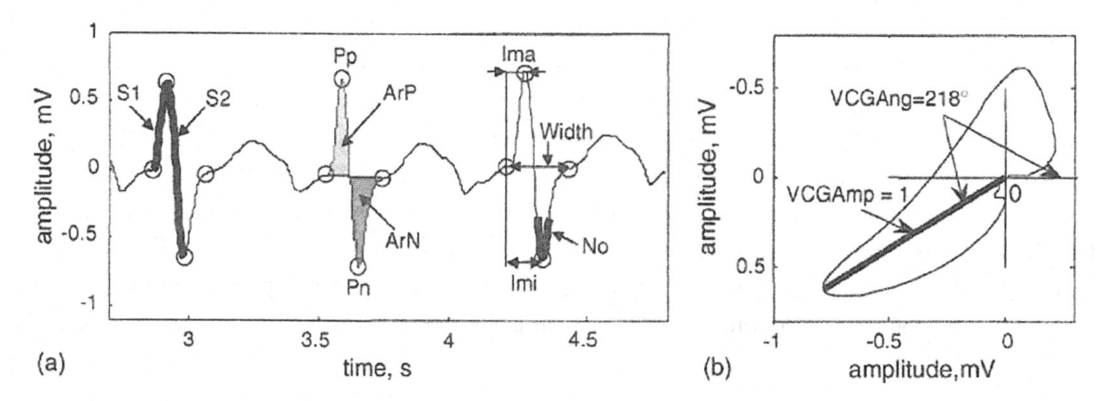

not only on the type of disease of the patient, measurement problems and sampling frequency, but also on correct analysis of the ECG signal. Further feature extraction methods use morphological description as an input for a pattern recognition technique (see Figures 6 and 7).

We have already described features identified from the original signal in the time domain. Another approach is to use a transform for feature extraction. Feature extraction using the wavelet transform can be divided into two cases. In the first case, the wavelet transform for ECG analysis is used (Li, 1995). The features are extracted by means of the methods described above. In the second case, the features are extracted from the transformed signal. Discrete wavelet transform (DWT) coefficients can be used for classifying ECG signals, e.g., as inputs of artificial neural networks (ANN). When using DWT to obtain a compact wavelet representation of the signal data, we must choose how many wavelet coefficients are needed to describe the signal adequately. One way to determine the significance of a particular coefficient is to look at its variance. When ordering the coefficients from lowest to highest resolution, we reach a point when adding components of higher resolution no longer makes a difference to the information content of the wavelet representation. The information required to distinguish between classes might be gained from a low number of wavelet coefficients.

A clustering set for Holter analysis is introduced in (Cuesta-Frau, 2003). The clustering set contains amplitude coefficients, trace segmentation, polygonal approximation and wavelet coefficients.

In BSPM, classification features are not commonly used. They are usually knitted together on an ad-hoc basis for the problem, based on the known electrophysiology of the expected disease. In rare cases, computers are used for classification. In our work we have used features such as maximum and minimum, as well as some others that can be found, for example, in (Casale, 1987). Feature extraction from BSPM of atrial fibrillation using a combination of continuous wavelet transform and entropy is proposed in (Gramatikov, 2000).

Example of Feature Extraction from Body Surface Potential Mapping

Mapping on one period of a signal, based on the lead signal, has turned out to be fundamental for the best display of immediate potential maps and integral maps. The mapped interval for generating maps is defined unambiguously for all electrodes. Thus, it allows better variability for creating maps in accordance with the user's choice from different periods. The features extracted from BSPM maps are divided into global features of BSPM maps, local features of BSPM maps, and global and local features belonging to different types of maps.

The global features of BSPM maps comprise the position of the global maximum and minimum of the integral map, the position of the local maxima and minima of the integral map, and the zero-line of the map (Chudacek, 2006).

The local features of BSPM maps include the distribution of positive, negative and neutral pixels in each of 40 leads from the anterior part of the thorax. Different types of maps are used, namely integral maps from QRS and QRST intervals and immediate potential maps for computing the maxima and minima of the map movement.

For further feature extraction the map is divided into 60 rectangles, as illustrated in Figure 8. Figure 9 shows rectangles in which the zero line was identified.

Figure 8. Dividing the QRS integral map into a square box according to the individual electrodes. The locations of the global and local maxima and minima are marked

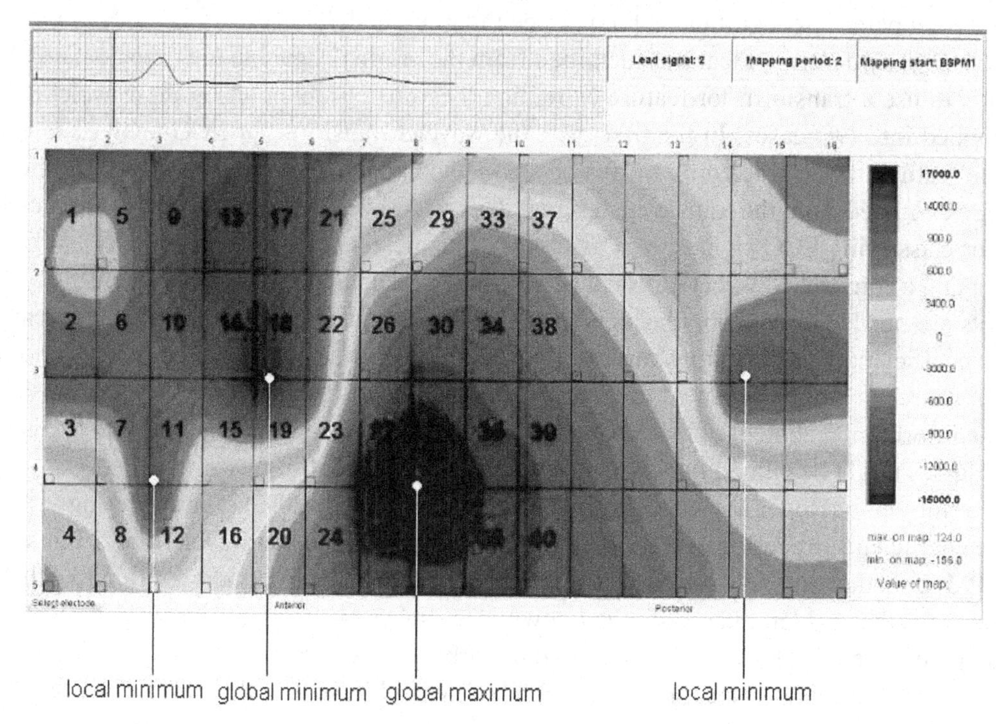

Figure 9. a) Extracting the zero line from a QRS integral map, b) description of one box by means of three numbers: positive, neutral and negative area)

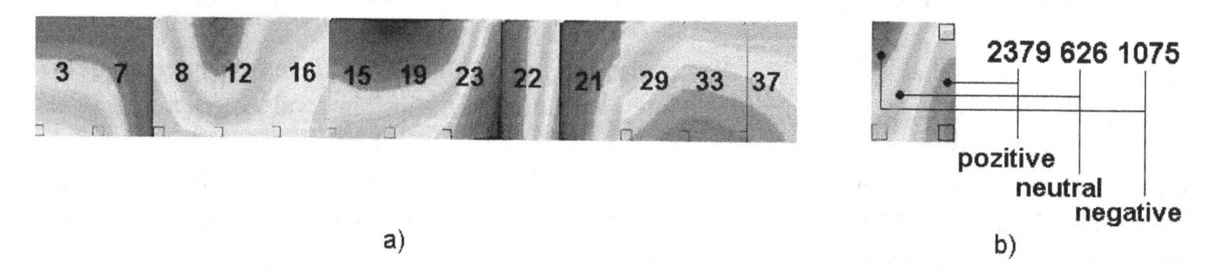

CLASSIFICATION

There are many approaches to ECG analysis and classification, including filtering algorithms, transforms, and machine learning methods. In some cases, combinations of two or more methods are used. The most frequently used (or cited) ECG classification methods include neural network classifications, expert systems (Gargasas, 1999), machine learning methods (Kukar, 1999), fuzzy systems (Kundu, 1998), wavelet transform (Li, 1995), and genetic algorithms (Poli, 1994). Bortolan et al. (1991) combine two pattern recognition techniques, namely cluster analysis and neural networks, in the problem of diagnostic classification of 12-lead electrocardiograms. Several neural networks were obtained either by varying the training set or by adjusting some components of the architecture of the networks.

Wavelet analysis, neural networks or digital filtering may provide good results in direct detection and classification of events. However, they do not express the relations between signals and process states, even if these exist. Attempts have therefore been made to discover such relations. In order to acquire knowledge for monitoring cardiac patients, formalisms such as expert rules (Bratko, 1989), attributed grammars (Kókai, 1997), fuzzy rules (Kundu, 1998), fuzzy sets (Bortolan, 2002), and inductive logic programming (Wang, 2001) have been used.

For classifying ECGs, a very wide selection of algorithms is available. We can divide these algorithms according to various attributes; a mixture of the most suitable attributes then has to be selected to tackle the problems described above.

- **Supervised vs. Unsupervised algorithms:** Supervised algorithms are those that classify beats into certain diagnostic groups, such as premature ventricular complex (PVC) in the case of the Holter ECG algorithm, and require training set in advance. All clustering methods such as k-means and the SOM approach are considered to be unsupervised algorithms (Cuesta-Frau, 2003). Rules and expert systems can also be considered, at least in this case, to be unsupervised learning methods, since they do not require training. Mixed approaches are sometimes used: clustering methods are used to generate a few representative beats on which more time-consuming operations can subsequently be performed.
- **Fast vs. Slow:** When dealing with large amounts of data, the speed of the algorithm and also memory demand can be of great importance. Simple, fast algorithms are therefore often used, e.g., methods such as decision trees and k-nn. More complex methods, such as the support vector machine (SVM) , and template matching, are not only slower but sometimes also much more vulnerable to overtraining, especially when an extensive training set is not available. In telemedicine applications, real-time measurement is very often performed and only interesting parts of the signal are stored for future more detailed evaluation on more powerful machines.
- **Accepted by clinicians vs. reluctantly accepted:** Medicine is a relatively conservative field, and explicit and transparent representation of the decision making process and the results supplied by a computer system are usually requires. "Black box" methods are not accepted without hesitation. Methods using, for example, rules or a decision table, i.e. more transparent representation, are considered more acceptable.
- **Using signal transform vs. temporal signal features:** Since clinicians perform only visual analysis manually, they work in the temporal domain and do not utilize information that may be acquired from different signal transforms. Many approaches utilizing transforms for feature extraction have been developed in the last two decades, for example the Karhunen-Loeve transform for myocardial infarction, Fourier transform features, features based on a wavelet transform (Addison, 2005), Empirical Mode Decomposition (Blanco-Velasco, 2006), the Hilbert transform (Nunes, 2005), and Hermite functions (Mugler, 2002). These approaches enable extraction of additional features to those acquired from temporal analysis, and thus enhance the information gain. However, they require rather extensive and representative training sets. In contrast, the temporal features used by clinicians allow a straight comparison of results reached by an algorithm and by a clinician. Most of the publications describing rule-based and expert-system approaches also deal with temporal features.

Figure 10. Example of a testing set (top left) and a cluster from RBDT- the white line represents the median of the clusters

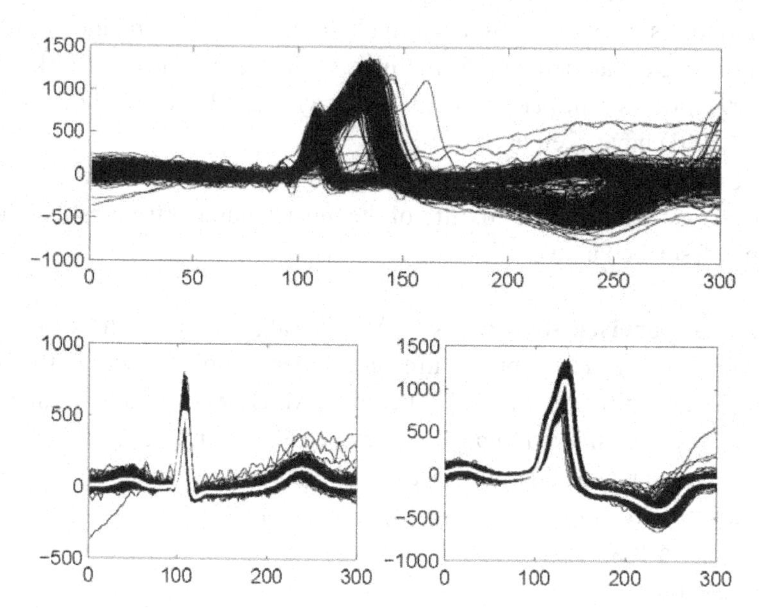

Rule-Based Decision Tree

The *Rule-Based Decision Tree* (RBDT) was first used for ECG beat clustering, and each cluster was represented by its median (see Figure 10). The rules included knowledge retrieved from the literature as well as from clinicians.

The clustering is performed by dividing the domain of each parameter into intervals. For each ECG beat we specify to which interval it belongs. The strength of this method lies in its ability to decrease the number of beats that must be considered before the final classification step – classification of the cluster median using a more detailed decision tree.

Rule-Based Decision Tree Clustering Based on Fuzzy Intervals

The RBDT that was described in the previous section has a drawback when dealing with borderline cases: two very similar ECG-beats can be classified differently only because their parameters are very close to the borderline of an interval, resulting in each of them being categorized in a different class. Generalization of the RBDT, replacing the crisp intervals by fuzzy intervals is presented, and more information can be found in (Zadeh, 1965).

When we describe the generalization of RBDT to fuzzy sets (fuzzy RBDT for short), the situation is similar to RBDT, the only difference being that the intervals are fuzzified – the fuzzy intervals overlap.

Thus for example an ECG-beat whose Q-wave amplitude value is near a border will partially belong to both intervals. Fuzzy RBDT is based on selecting groups of ECG-beats according to all reasonable combinations of values of the parameters, and finding medians of such groups. First we select a fuzzy set of ECG-beats and then a fuzzy membership degree is assigned to each of them. The fuzzy median of this selection is then computed.

GAME ANN

The *Group of Adaptive Models* (GAME) artificial neural network (ANN) is based on an inductive approach (Kordík, 2006). This means that both the parameters and the structure of the ANN are parts of a learning process (values for the parameters are selected and the ANN is constructed from certain basic blocks during the learning process). GAME is a feed-forward ANN, which extends the concept of the *Group Method of Data Handling* (GMDH) network. GMDH allows only one type of basic block – neurons can have one transfer function only, whereas in GAME ANN there are neurons with many different transfer functions. GAME ANN is built from scratch during the training phase. Each new layer is constructed in the following way: first a large number of new neurons are generated; the neurons differ in the transfer function and in the number of neurons in the previous layer that the new neuron is connected to. The next step is to find the optimal set of internal parameters and the best connections to neurons in the previous layer. To do this, GAME uses an advanced genetic algorithm. The population consists of neurons in every new layer and every neuron is coded to a genome. Genome coding contains information about neurons in the previous layer, which are connected to the neuron, the type of transfer function and some parameters of the transfer function. At the end of the genetic algorithm run, all neurons in a new layer are evaluated using a separate testing set, and the worst neurons are removed from the layer. The remaining neurons in the layer are "frozen" and the algorithm continues with the creation of a new layer. This is repeated until a neuron with the desired accuracy is found; this neuron is the output of the network.

Support Vector Machines

Support Vector Machines (SVMs) are learning systems that are trained using an algorithm based on optimization theory (Burges, 1998). The SVM solution finds a hyperplane in the feature space that keeps the empirical error small while maximizing the margin between the hyperplane and the instances closest to it. Each new pattern **x** is classified to one of the two categories (in the case of dichotomizing problems $y_i \in \{-1,1\}$) through:

$$f(\mathbf{x}) = sign\left(\sum_{i=1}^{n} y_i a_i K(\mathbf{x}, \mathbf{x}_i) + b\right)$$

where b is a threshold parameter. The coefficients a_i are found by solving a maximization quadratic programming problem which is "controlled" by a penalty factor C, and are assigned to each of the training patterns x_i. The kernel function K implicitly performs the mapping from the input space to the feature space. In our experimental procedure we have only employed the radial basis function kernels, where the width σ, which is common to all kernels, was specified a priori by the user.

Back Propagation Network

Back Propagation is probably the best-known supervised learning technique used for training artificial neural networks. It trains feed-forward networks with one or more hidden layer.

In the recall phase the sample is presented to the network and values are propagated from inputs to outputs of the network. During the training phase the training samples are presented to the network. The difference between desired and actual outputs is calculated formulating the error of the network. This error is propagated backwards from output neurons toward inputs. For each neuron, its contribution to the output error is calculated and the weights of its connections are adjusted accordingly. The weights are adjusted using the gradient deschen algorithm, which has the disadvantage of getting trapped in the local minimum. To overcome this, techniques like the addition of a momentum term, or the delta-bar-delta rule, are used.

SOM Network

The *Self Organizing Map* (SOM) is an unsupervised clustering algorithm. The network consists of neurons organized on a regular low-dimensional grid. Each neuron is represented by a d-dimensional weight vector, where d is equal to the dimension of the input vectors. Each neuron is connected to adjacent neurons by a neighborhood relation, which dictates the structure of the map.

The SOM is trained iteratively. In each training step, one sample is presented to the network. The distance between the sample and all the weight vectors of the SOM is calculated using the selected distance measure. The closest neuron is called the Best-Matching Unit (BMU). After finding the BMU, the weights in the SOM are updated so that the BMU is moved closer to the input vector in the input space. This is repeated until the stopping criterion (e.g., a number of learning steps) is reached. Then a template matching algorithm is used on the cluster median.

Template Matching

The *template matching* method is a sorting method which uses templates in order to distinguish to which group the sorted element belongs. In our case, the ECG-beats are sorted into two groups called N or V (i.e. "normal" or "premature ventricular" ECG-beats). Five templates are computed for each group. The computation is based on random selection of 21 ECG beats classified as N or V. For such a group, a median is computed which serves as the template. To sort an ECG beat into the N group or the V group we compare it with all the 10 templates (5 for the N group and 5 for the V group). The comparison is made with the help of correlation coefficients. The medians are compared with five different templates for each classification group, i.e., N and V. Correlation coefficients are computed and for the final decision on the median of cluster membership - majority voting for 2 of the first 3 coefficients is used. Finally all ECG beats in the particular cluster are classified as N or V, according to the result of the voting.

Example of Holter ECG Classification

The task of this classification example is to distinguish Premature Ventricular Complexes (V) from Normal beats (N) on a Holter ECG recording. The used features are: width of the QRS interval, presence of the P-wave, amplitudes of the Q, R, S and T waves, the QT interval, the RR interval, and the prematurity of the beat. The above-described methods are used, namely a decision tree using crisp and fuzzy rules, GAME, Support Vector Machine, Back-propagation Network, and the SOM clustering algorithm with template matching. Two approaches are selected for training the classifiers, namely the local approach, which uses randomly selected beats from the first five minutes of each MIT database recording (Goldberger, 2000), and the global approach, where all even recordings of the MIT database are used.

For testing the classifiers, the testing data is selected accordingly to the type of training. For the local approach, all beats over the first five minutes of each MIT database recording are used. For the global approach, all odd recordings from the MIT database are selected. The notions of sensitivity and specificity are used for comparing the results. These notions are described below.

Training and Testing Sets

Most academic studies have been carried out on free open access databases from the physionet (Goldberger, 2000). The ECG arrhythmia database is the most used. This database consists of just fifty 30-minute recordings, so the training and testing sets are very often compromised. A solution that complies with the European norm is presented in (de Chazal, 2004).

Results Comparison

Sensitivity and specificity are two statistical measures that are well established in medical applications. Computation of these two measures is based on *"true positive"*, *"true negative"*, *"false positive"*, and *"false negative"* elements (i.e., ECG-beats) of clusters.

- "True positives" . . . correctly classified as abnormal (group V in our example)
- "True negatives" . . . correctly classified as normal (group N in our example)
- "False positives" . . . normal, incorrectly classified as abnormal
- "False negatives" . . . abnormal, incorrectly classified as normal

General Definition of Sensitivity and Specificity

The cardinality C(S) of a finite set S is the number of elements that it contains. Let TN be a finite set of true negatives and let FP be a finite set of false positives. Specificity Sp is a real number from the interval [0, 1], defined as follows:

$$Sp(TN, FP) = \frac{C(TN)}{C(TN) + C(FP)}$$

Let TP be a finite set of true positives and let FN be a finite set of false negatives. Sensitivity Se is a real number from the interval [0, 1], defined as follows:

$$Se(TP, FN) = \frac{C(TP)}{C(TP) + C(FN)}$$

Sensitivity and specificity are defined as real numbers between 0 and 1. However, percentage values are easier to understand. The values are therefore usually multiplied by 100%.

A high sensitivity value means that most of the normal elements are classified correctly. A high specificity value means that most of the abnormal elements are classified correctly. Thus high values of both sensitivity and specificity mean that the classification method performs well.

Table 1. Results for all used methods

Method	Local training/testing Sensitivity [%]	Local training/testing Specificity [%]	Global training/testing Sensitivity [%]	Global training/testing Specificity [%]
RBDT	92.23	91.75	75.79	74.25
fuzzyRBDT	92.28	89.13	77.81	79.28
BP NN	90.17	85.20	76.86	77.06
GAME NN	48.79	95.13	42.57	83.68
RBF	87.94	85.35	72.28	77.06
SOM	94.32	65.28	77.00	35.21
SVM	91.20	91.01	73.80	81.93

Results

The results achieved using all the methods described above are shown in Table 1. They clearly illustrate the basic problems of Holter ECG classification. Although the global approach is very general, it is sensitive to the selection of the training set. If the training set is totally disconnected from the testing set, as in our case, the training set must be very large to cover all (or nearly all) possible shapes of beats to be classified. For the local approach, which can be used for example in telemedicine applications, many of the problems are solved by including the parts of the testing signals in the training set. This difference is due to the fact that the interpersonal variability of the ECG signal is much higher than the intrapersonal variability.

CONCLUSION

This chapter has tried to address the most important issues in ECG signal processing and to offer a brief description of the whole process, from signal denoising, though feature extraction to final classification. Clearly, we cannot expect to present all relevant methods and applications in a single chapter. Nevertheless, the key problems and solution principles have been discussed. We have presented the basic clinical features characterizing ECG in the temporal domain. Then the wavelet transform was briefly introduced as a tool for filtering and extracting additional features in time-frequency space. Finally, several supervised and unsupervised classification methods were used for classifying Holter ECGs, and the results were discussed.

Although there are many different approaches to signal preprocessing and feature extraction, future trends should include the development of more advanced preprocessing methods, which will be less sensitive to noise and artifacts. These methods will also offer more robust feature extraction. There is an open space, for example, for the development of advanced methods for detecting transient ST episodes and for more precise QT interval measurement. Another issue is a more appropriate morphological description that could be used for feature extraction. Advanced mathematical approaches, e.g., probabilistic modeling, information theory based learning, optimization methods for defining an optimum combination of learning parameters or extracted features deserve further investigation. Last but not least, hierarchical classification, hybrid classifiers, or integration of many classifiers may also improve the quality of ECG classification.

ACKNOWLEDGMENT

This work has been supported by the research program "Information Society" under grant No. 1ET201210527 "Knowledge-based support of diagnostics and prediction in cardiology".

REFERENCES

Acharya, U.R., Suri, J.S., Spaan, J., & Krishnan, S.M. (2007). *Advances in Cardiac Signal Processing.* Springer Berlin Heidelberg.

Addison, P.S. (2005). Wavelet transforms and the ECG: A review. *Physiological Measurement* 26 (pp. 155-199), Institute of Physics Publishing.

Azuaje, F. (1998). Knowledge discovery in electrocardiographic data based on neural clustering algorithms. In *Proceedings Medicon '98 of the International Federation for Medical & Biological Engineering.*

Barro, S., Ruiz, R., Cabello, D., & Mira, J. (1989). Algorithmic sequential decision-making in the frequency domain for life threatening ventricular arrhythmias and imitative artefacts: A diagnostic system. *Journal of Biomedical Engineering,* 11, 320–328.

Blanco-Velasco, M., Weng, B., & Barner, K. E. (2007). ECG signal denoising and baseline wander correction based on the empirical mode decomposition. *Computers in Biology and Medicine.*

Braga, F., Caiani, E. G., Locati, E., & Cerutti, S. (2004). Automated QT/RR Analysis Based on Selective Beat Averaging Applied to Electrocardiographic Holter 24 H. *Computers in Cardiology 31.* IEEE Computer Soc. Press.

Bortolan, G., & al. (1991). ECG classification with neural networks and cluster analysis. *Computers in Cardiology, 20, 177-180.* IEEE Computer Soc. Press.

Bortolan, G. & Pedrycz, W. (2002). An interactive framework for an analysis of ECG signals. *Artificial Intelligence in Medicine, 24* 109-132.

Bratko, I., Mozetic, I. & Lavrac, N. (1989). *Kardio: A study in deep and qualitative knowledge for expert systems.* MIT Press.

Burges, C. J. C: (1998). A Tutorial on Support Vector Machines for Pattern Recognition. *Data Mining and Knowledge Discovery,* 2, 121-167.

Casale, P. N., Devereux, R. B., Alonso, D., Campo, E., & Kligfield, P. (1987). Improved sex-specific criteria of left ventricular hypertrophy for clinical and computer interpretation of electrocardiograms: validation with autopsy findings. *Circulation, 75,* 565-572.

Christov, I., & Bortolan, G. (2004). Ranking of pattern recognition parameters for premature ventricular contractions classification by neural networks. *Physiogical Measurement* 25, 1281–1290) .

Christov, I., Herrero, G., Krasteva, V., Jekova, I., Grotchev, A., & Egiazarian, K. (2006). Comparative Study of Morphological and Time-Frequency ECG Descriptors for Heartbeat Classification. *Medical Engineering & Physics*, 28, 876 – 887. Elsevier.

Chudáček, V., Lhotská, L., & Huptych, M. (2006). Feature Selection in Body Surface Potential Mapping. In *IEEE ITAB International Special Topics Conference on Information Technology in Biomedicine,* Piscataway: IEEE.

Clifford, G. D., Azuaje, F., & McSharry, P. E. (2006). *Advanced Methods and Tools for ECG Data Analysis*. Artech House, Inc., Norwood, MA.

Cuesta-Frau, D., Perez-Cortes, J. C., & Andreu-Garcıa, G. (2003). Clustering of electrocardiograph signals in computer-aided Holter analysis. *Computer Methods and Programs in Biomedicine* 72,179-196.

Daubechies, I. (1992). Ten lectures on Wavelets. CBMS-NSF, *SIAM*, 61, Philadelphia, Pennsylvania, USA.

Daqrouq, K. (2005). ECG Baseline Wandering Reduction Using Discrete Wavelet Transform. *Asian Journal of Information Technology 4*, 989-995.

de Chazal, P., & Reilly, R. (2004). Automatic classification of heart beats using ECG morphology and heart beat interval features. *Journal of Electrocardiology,* 32, 58–66.

Ferrara, E., & Widrow, B. (1981). The time-sequenced adaptive filter. *IEEE Trans. 28*, 519-523.

Gargasas, L., Ruseckas, R. & Jurkoniene, R., (1999). An expert system for diagnosis of coronary heart disease (CHD) with analysis of multicardiosignals. *Medical & Biological Engineering Computing 37(Supplement 2*), 734-735.

Goldberger, A. L., Amaral, L., Glass, L., Hausdorf, J. M., Ivanov, P. C., Moody, G., Peng, C. K., & Stanley, H. E. (2000). PhysioBank, PhysioToolkit, and PhysioNet: Components of a New Research Resource for Complex Physiologic Signals. *Circulation*, 101(23), 215-220.

Gramatikov, B., Brinker, J., Yi-Chun, S., & Thakor, N. V. (2000) Wavelet Analysis and Time-Frequency Distribution of the Body Surface ECG Before and After Angioplasty. *Computer Methods and Programs in Biomedicine* (pp. 87-98). Elsevier Science Ireland Ltd.

Holter, N.J. (1961). New methods for heart studies. *Science 134,* 1214.

Huptych, M., Burša, M., & Lhotská, L. (2006). A Software Tool for ECG Signals Analysis and Body Surface Potential Mapping. In *IEEE ITAB International Special Topics Conference on Information Technology in Biomedicine*. Piscataway: IEEE.

Jager, F., Moody, G. B., Divjak, S., & Mark, R.G. (1994). Assessing the robustness of algorithms for detecting transient ischemic ST segment changes. *Computers in Cardiology* (pp. 229–232).

Jeras, M., Magjarević, R., & Paćelat, E. (2001). Real time P-wave detection in surface ECG. *Proceedings Medicon 2001 of the International Federation for Medical & Biological Engineering.*

Kadambe, S., Murray, R., & Boudreaux-Bartels, G. F. (1999). Wavelet transformed-based QRS complex detector. *IEEE Trans. Biomed. Eng.* 46, 838–848.

Khan, M. G. (2003). *Rapid ECG Interpretation.* Elsevier Inc. New York

Kjaer, M., Krogsgaard, M., & Magnusson, P., et al. (2003). *Textbook of sports medicine.* Oxford: Blackwell Publishing.

Kókai, G., Alexin, Z., & Gyimóthy, T., (1997). Application of inductive logic programming for learning ECG waveforms. *Proceedings of AIME97,* 1211,126-129.

Kordík, P. (2006). *Fully Automated Knowledge Extraction using Group of Adaptive Models Evolution.* Doctoral thesis, Czech Technical University in Prague.

Kornreich, F. (1997). Appropriate electrode placement in evaluating varied cardiac pathology. In Liebman J. (ed) *Electrocardiology '96. From the cell to the body surface.* Publ.World Scientific 1997.

Kukar, M. & al. (1999). Analysing and improving the diagnosis of ischaemic heart disease with machine learning. *Artificial Intelligence in Medicine,* 16, 25-50.

Kundu, M., Nasipuri, M. & Basu, D.K., (1998). A knowledge based approach to ECG interpretation using fuzzy logic. *IEEE Trans. System, Man and Cybernetics, 28,*237-243.

Lagerholm, M., & al. (2000). Clustering ECG complexes using Hermite functions and self-organizing maps. *IEEE Transaction on Biomedical Engineering, 47*(7), 838-848.

Li, C., Zheng, C., & Tai, C.(1995). Detection of ECG Characteristic Points Using Wavelet Transforms. *IEEE Transaction on Biomedical Engineering,* 42, 21-28.

Lux, R.L (1982): Electrocardiographic body surface potential mapping CRC. *Crit. Rev. Biomed. Eng.,* 8, 253 – 279.

Malik, M., & Camm, A. J. (1995). *Heart rate variability.* New York, 52-60, 533-539.

Mallat S. (1992). Characterization of Signals from Multi-scale Edges. *IEEE Trans. Pattern Anal. Machine Intelligen*ce, 14, 710-732.

Mugler, D. H., & Clary, S. (2000). Discrete Hermite Functions. *Proceedings of the Int'l Conf. on Scientific Computing and Mathematical Modeling, IMACS.*

Nunes, J.C., & Nait Ali, A. (2005). Hilbert Transform-Based ECG Modeling. *Biomedical Engineering, 39(3).* New York: Springer.

Poli, R., Cagnoni, S., & Valli, G., (1994). *A genetic algorithm approach to the design of optimum QRS detectors.* University of Florence Technical Report No. 940201, Florence, Italy.

Taccardi, B. (1963). Distribution of heart potentials on the thoracic surface of normal human subjects. *Circ. Res.,* 12, 341-52.

Thakor, N. V., & Yi-Sheng, Z. (1991). Application of Adaptive Filtering to ECG Analysis noise cancellation and arrhythmia detection. *IEEE Transaction on Biomedical Engineering,* 38,785-94.

Wang, F., Quinion, R., Carrault, G., & Cordier, M. O. (2001). Learning structural knowledge from the ECG. in: J. Crespo, V. Maojo, F. Martin, eds., *Medical Data Analysis - Second International Symposium,* LNCS 2199. *ISMDA 2001.* Springer Verlag.

Zadeh, L. A., (1965). *Fuzzy sets.* Inform. Control (pp. 338–353).

KEY TERMS

ECG: Recording of the electrical activity of the heart in dependence on time.

BSPM: An extension of conventional electrocardiography that provides a refined non-invasive characterisation of cardiac activity; the systems may use from 30 to 300 electrodes; increased spatial sampling on the body surface provides more in-depth information on the cardiac generated potentials.

Holter ECG: Long-term ECG monitoring focused on a search for deficiencies in heart rhythm (arrhythmias) or silent ischemia.

Heart Rate: Frequency of the cardiac cycle; usually calculated as the number of contractions (beats) of the heart in one minute and expressed as "beats per minute" (bpm).

Wavelet: A member of a family of functions generated by taking translations [eg.: w(t) → w(t 1)] and scaling [eg.: w(t) → w(2t)] of a function w(t), called the "mother" wavelet.

Rule - Principle: A basic generalization that is accepted as true and that can be used as a basis for reasoning or conduct.

Feature: A prominent aspect of the ECG signal.

Chapter VIII
EEG Data Mining Using PCA

Lenka Lhotská
Czech Technical University in Prague, Czech Republic

Vladimír Krajča
Faculty Hospital Na Bulovce, Czech Republic

Jitka Mohylová
Technical University Ostrava, Czech Republic

Svojmil Petránek
Faculty Hospital Na Bulovce, Czech Republic

Václav Gerla
Czech Technical University in Prague, Czech Republic

ABSTRACT

This chapter deals with the application of principal components analysis (PCA) to the field of data mining in electroencephalogram (EEG) processing. The principal components are estimated from the signal by eigen decomposition of the covariance estimate of the input. Alternatively, they can be estimated by a neural network (NN) configured for extracting the first principal components. Instead of performing computationally complex operations for eigenvector estimation, the neural network can be trained to produce ordered first principal components. Possible applications include separation of different signal components for feature extraction in the field of EEG signal processing, adaptive segmentation, epileptic spike detection, and long-term EEG monitoring evaluation of patients in a coma.

INTRODUCTION

Computer-assisted processing of long-term electroencephalogram (EEG) recordings has been gaining in importance. The aim is to simplify the work of a physician who needs to make a visual evaluation of EEG recordings many hours in length. At present, EEGs of patients may be recorded over a time span of tens of minutes up to 24 or 48 hours, depending on their purpose. Automatic systems cannot fully replace a physician, but aim to make his/her work more efficient. They identify segments of the signal where there are deviations from standard brain activity, and in this way they save some of the time that would be required for visual inspection of the whole recording.

This chapter deals with the issue of applying advanced methods to the analysis of EEG signals. It describes the design and implementation of a system that performs an automatic analysis of EEG signals.

First, EEG is briefly introduced. Then there is a description of the phases of EEG signal processing. The chapter focuses on the most important parts of this process, namely segmentation, application of principal component analysis (PCA) to feature extraction, and shape detection. The explanation is illustrated by examples of EEGs of comatose and epileptic patients. The chapter concludes with a look at future trends and problems to be addressed in EEG processing.

ELECTROENCEPHALOGRAM

An electroencephalogram (EEG) is a recording of spontaneous brain electrical activity by means of electrodes located on the scalp. The placing of the electrodes is constrained by natural physical limits, namely by the size of the electrodes, which limits the maximum number of electrodes that can be used. Another limitation is the mutual influence of electrodes located close to each other. Standardized placement of the basic number of electrodes is done in accordance with the scheme designed by Dr. Jasper (Jasper, 1958). This is nowadays known as the International 10-20 system.

In the frequency domain we can distinguish four basic frequency bands on an EEG signal, namely delta, theta, alpha, and beta activities.

The delta band corresponds to the slowest waves in the range of 0-4 Hz. Its appearance is always pathological in an adult in the waking state. The pathological significance increases with increasing amplitude and localization. The existence of a delta wave is normal for children up to three years of age, in deep sleep and hypnosis. During sleep the waves can be higher than 100 μV in amplitude.

The theta band corresponds to waves in the range of 4-8 Hz. Their existence is considered as pathological if their amplitude is at least twice as high as the alpha activity or higher than 30 μV if alpha activity is absent. The presence of a theta wave is normal if its amplitude is up to 15 μV and if the waves appear symmetrically. In healthy persons they appear in central, temporal and parietal parts. This activity is characteristic for certain periods of sleep.

The alpha band corresponds to waves in the range of 8-13 Hz. In the waking state in mental and physical rest the maximum appears in the occipital part of the brain. Its presence is highly influenced by open or closed eyes. The amplitude is in the range of 20-100 μV, most frequently around 50 μV.

The beta band corresponds to the fastest waves in the range of 13-20 Hz. The maximum of the activity is mostly localized in the frontal part, and it decreases in the backward direction. The rhythm is mostly symmetrical or nearly symmetrical in the central part. The amplitude is up to 30 μV. The activity is characteristic for concentration, logical reasoning and feelings of anger and anxiety.

An EEG contains a great deal of information about the state of a patient's health. It has the advantage of being non-invasive and applicable over a comparatively long time span (up to 24 hours, if necessary). This is an important feature in cases where we want to follow disorders that are not permanently present but appear incidentally (e.g., epileptic seizures) or under certain conditions (various sleep disorders) (Daube, 2002).

EEG of Epileptic Patients

The term epilepsy refers to a group of neurological disorders characterized by the recurrence of sudden reactions of brain function caused by abnormalities in its electrical activity, which is clinically manifested as epileptic seizures. Manifestations of epileptic seizures vary greatly, ranging from a brief lapse of attention to a prolonged loss of consciousness; this loss is accompanied by abnormal motor activity affecting the entire body or one or more extremities. The basic classification of epilepsy and epileptic seizures into partial and generalized seizures is widely accepted (Hornero, 1999). Among generalized epilepsy, grand mal and petit mal seizures are the most prevalent.

Coma

Coma is a state of brain function. It can be very roughly compared to sleep. However, an individual cannot awaken purposefully from a coma, using either an internal or an external stimulus. Comatose states may have a number of causes, from head injury in a serious accident, through cerebral vascular diseases, infectious diseases, brain tumours, metabolic disorders (failure of liver or kidney), hypoglycemia, to drug overdosing, degenerative diseases, and many more. A patient in coma does not manifest any notion of higher consciousness, does not communicate, and the functions of his/her inner organs are frequently supported by devices. Great efforts have been devoted to scaling comatose states into different levels according to seriousness, depth, and prediction of the probable development of the state of the patient. In practice, use has been made of relative terms, such as mild, moderate and severe coma. These terms cannot serve for more extended research, because there are no exact definitions. They are a source of misunderstandings. The first attempt to unify coma classification was the Glasgow classification of unconsciousness (Glasgow Coma Scale - GCS), described in 1974 (Teasdale, 1974). GCS has become widely used, and is a reliable scale for classifying coma depth. It is highly reproducible and fast, and it is a suitable tool for long-term monitoring of patient coma. In the decades that followed, more coma classification systems were developed, for example the Rancho Los Amigos Scale and the Reaction Level Scale RLS85 (Starmark, 1998), both classifying into 8 levels, the Innsbruck Coma Scale, the Japan Coma Scale, etc. Individual coma classification systems differ in numbers of levels, ways of examining, precision, etc.

PHASES OF EEG SIGNAL PROCESSING

EEG signal processing is a complex process consisting of several steps: data acquisition and storing, pre-processing, visualization, segmentation, extraction of descriptive features, and classification. We briefly describe each of these steps, and then we focus on segmentation, feature extraction and classification as the most important steps that are decisive for the success of the whole process.

- **Data acquisition:** An EEG signal is recorded digitally and saved in a defined format in files on a PC.
- **Pre-processing:** The aim of pre-processing is to remove noise and thus prepare the signal for further processing. The operations include removal of the DC part of the signal, signal filtering, and removal of certain artifacts (Smith, 1997).
- **Digital Filtering:** A digital filter is a computer program or algorithm that can remove unwanted frequency components from a signal. As in the case of analog filters, they may be classified as low-pass, high-pass, band-pass, or notch filters. The two commonly used types of digital filters are the finite impulse response (FIR) filter and the infinite impulse response (IIR) filter. The output of an FIR filter is a linear combination only of the input signal at the current time and at past times. The output of an IIR filter is a linear combination of both the input signal at the current time and at past times and the output signal at past time (Maccabee, 1992).
- **Segmentation:** If we use a signal divided into intervals of constant length for acquisition of informative attributes, non-stationariness of the signal may distort the estimation of the characteristics. Segments defined in this way may contain a mixture of waves of different frequencies and shapes. It depends strongly on the segment length. It is therefore preferable to divide the signal into segments of different interval lengths that are quasi-stationary (piece-wise stationary, depending on the length of the segment). There are several approaches to adaptive segmentation (Bodenstein, 1977; Krajca, 1991) that divide signals into quasi-stationary segments of variable length.
- **Principal Component Analysis** is a technique used to reduce multidimensional data sets to lower dimensions for analysis and to extract informative features. The principal components may be computed either using a covariance matrix (Murtagh, 1999) or using artificial neural networks (Sanger, 1989).
- **Extraction of descriptive features** is closely linked with segmentation and PCA (Cohen, 1986). In automatic signal analysis, extraction of informative features with the greatest possible discriminative ability is an important task. The feature vector consists of an ordered set of features. The values of the individual features may differ by several orders, and for this reason feature normalization is performed. The output of this step is a vector of normalized features for each segment.
- **Classification** involves assigning a class to unknown objects. A class is a group of objects with certain shared properties. In our case, the objects are segments described by vectors of normalized features, and the classes correspond to different groups of graphoelements representing, for example, normal and pathological states or different degrees of coma. The result of a classification is a signal divided into segments where each segment is assigned to a certain class. We used cluster analysis for classifying the segments (Jain, Dubes 1987, Krajca 1991).

SEGMENTATION

EEG signals are stochastic signals. Stochastic signals can be divided into two basic groups: stationary and non-stationary. Stationary stochastic signals do not change their statistical characteristics in time.

Non-stationary signals may have variable quantities in time, for example mean value, dispersion, or frequency spectrum. EEG signals are non-stationary, like most real signals. Therefore spectral analysis or other similar techniques cannot be directly applied to the signal. It is first necessary to divide the signal into stationary (or quasi-stationary) segments whose statistical parameters are constant. This is the main idea of signal segmentation. In principle, there are two basic approaches: constant segmentation and adaptive segmentation.

Constant segmentation divides a signal into segments of constant length. In general, this is the simplest type of segmentation. However, it has the disadvantage that the resulting segments are not necessarily stationary. Our modification suggests the use of individual segments that overlap. Using a small shift and suitable length of segments, we can achieve very good results for correct division directly into individual graphoelements.

Constant segmentation divides signal x[n], where n = 0, 1,..., N-1, into segments s_i[m], where m = 0, 1,..., N_i-1. The length of segment s_i[m] is then N_i. Let us assume that constant P is the value of a shift during segmentation and constant step M. If we allow M < P we achieve segment overlapping. For length of segments N_i and total number of segments S it holds:

$$\forall i : N_i = D,\ \mathrm{i} = 0, 1, ..., \mathrm{S} - 1, \mathrm{D} \in \mathbf{\mathit{N}}$$

Constant segmentation is based on dividing a signal into segments of length D with successive shift of the starting point in each step by the value M. For exact classification, it would be advantageous to acquire segments that contain a single graphoelement each. In this way we would achieve the most precise results in automatic detection of graphoelements. Therefore we have to set small values of step M and mean value D. A constant value of D is not optimal, and it is therefore impossible to achieve exact results. Moreover, an excessive number of segments are generated, resulting in increased demands on computation. Consequently, adaptive segmentation is preferred.

Adaptive segmentation is based on the principle of dividing the signal into quasi-stationary segments. These segments are relatively stationary and in general they have different length N_i for each segment in dependence on the presence of individual stationary parts in the signal. The method utilizes the principle of sliding two joint windows (Krajca, 1992), where the two windows have the same fixed length D. It is based on calculating the differences of the defined signal parameters of two windows. The following procedure enables us to indicate segment borders: Two joint windows slide along the signal. For each window the same signal characteristics are calculated. This measure corresponds to the difference of the signals in the two windows. If the measure of the difference exceeds the defined threshold, the point is marked as a segment border. The difference is frequently calculated from the spectra of the two windows, using the fast Fourier transform (FFT). The method is very slow because the difference is calculated using FFT for each window shift.

The method uses two characteristics for computing the measure of the difference of the two windows. The principle of the method is illustrated in Figure 1.

The two characteristics reflect certain properties of the signal in both the time and frequency domains. This method can be used for computing segment boundaries in all channels. However, this means that the segment boundaries computed in each channel independently from each other are positioned "asynchronously" at different places in different channels (see Figure 2).

Figure 1. Adaptive segmentation capable of independent processing of several channels

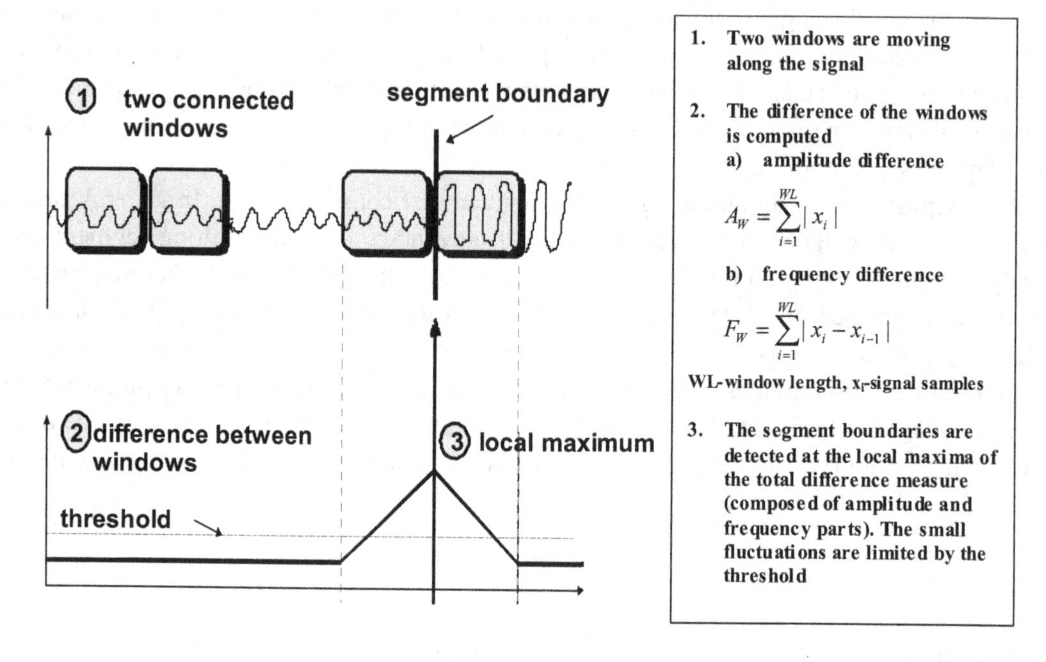

This approach may by useful for example for identifying epileptic spikes. However, crucial EEG indicators such as the "burst-suppression pattern" in deep coma occur simultaneously in several channels. Lehman (Lehman, 1987) and Wackerman et al. (Wackerman, 1993) used space-oriented (global) adaptive segmentation of multichannel EEG by segmenting a sequence of maps. Recently, Agarwal (Agarwal, 1998) used an averaged difference measure to segment multichannel EEG recordings.

PRINCIPAL COMPONENT ANALYSIS

Principal components analysis (PCA) (Jollife, 2002) is a technique used to reduce multidimensional data sets to lower dimensions for analysis. Depending on the field of application, it is also named the discrete Karhunen-Loève transform, the Hotelling transform, or proper orthogonal decomposition (POD).

PCA is mostly used as a tool in exploratory data analysis, for making predictive models, and more recently for feature extraction. It involves calculating the eigenvalue decomposition or singular value decomposition of a data set, usually after mean centering the data for each attribute. PCA can be used for dimensionality reduction in a data set by retaining those characteristics of the data set that contribute most to its variance, by keeping lower-order principal components and ignoring higher-order components. Such low-order components often contain the "most important" aspects of the data.

If the input data vector X is assumed to have dimension N, the purpose of PCA is to find those M (M<N) components of the elements of X which reduce the dimensionality of the input vector in a mean squared error sense. One approach to this problem is to project the data along orthogonal basis vectors through eigen decomposition of the covariance estimate of the input. For further details, refer to (Cohen, 1986; Dony, 1995).

Figure 2. Multichannel adaptive segmentation of an EEG signal. The numbers indicate the order of segments

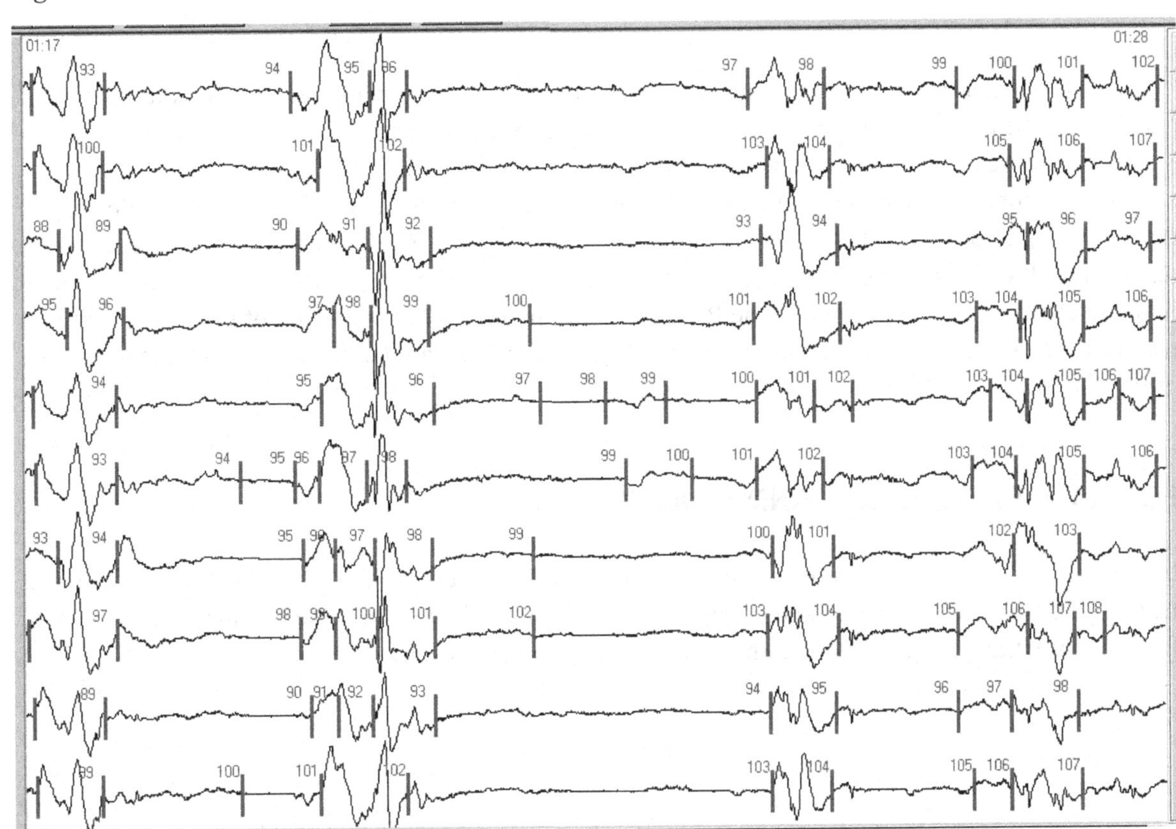

Self-Organized PCA

The alternative to the above-mentioned computationally complex procedure is to use self-organized principal components analysis. Self-organized (unsupervised) learning consists in repeated modification of the synaptic weights in response to activation until a final configuration develops. It is based on Hebb's postulate of learning: a synaptic weight w_i varies with time n, growing strong when presynaptic signal x_i and postsynaptic signal y coincide.

$$w_i(n+1)=w_i(n)+\eta\, y(n)x_i(n) \qquad (1)$$

where η is learning rate parameter. Oja was the first to show that the synaptic weight vector w(n) of a self-organized linear neuron operating under the modified Hebbian learning rule (which includes a stabilizing term) converges to a vector of unit Euclidean length, which lies in the maximal eigenvector direction of the correlation matrix of the input vector (Oja, 1982). Oja's rule was generalized from a single neuron to a single layer of linear neurons by Sanger. The weights of the net are computed by the Generalized Hebbian Algorithm (Sanger, 1989), which can compute the leading M principal components by a one-layer linear network. Sanger's rule for computing the weights:

$$w_{ji}(n+1)=w_{ji}(n)+\eta \{ y_j(n)x_i(n) - \sum_{k=0}^{j} w_{kj}(n)\, y_k(n)\} \tag{2}$$

Instead of performing computationally complex operations for eigenvector estimation, the neural network can be trained to produce the ordered first principal components.

The structure of a time delayed neural net for performing this task is shown in Figure 3.

The principal components are ordered with decreasing variance, and the output of the node reflects the increasing frequencies. The first trace explains the greatest variance of the input signal and therefore reflects the slowest frequencies of the EEG. With increasing number of PC, the frequency of the signal in the relevant trace also increases. The PCA provides "natural" decomposition of the signal based on raw data. The signal can be reconstructed again, by simply adding all the traces. The higher the number of PC, the lower the reconstruction error is (Krajca, 1996).

FEATURE EXTRACTION AND CLASSIFICATION

In the following section we present an application of adaptive segmentation and PCA to two types of EEG signals: EEGs of comatose and epileptic patients. A combination of these two methods is used for feature extraction. The extracted features are used for successive classification.

Figure 3. Structure of a neural net for PCA computing

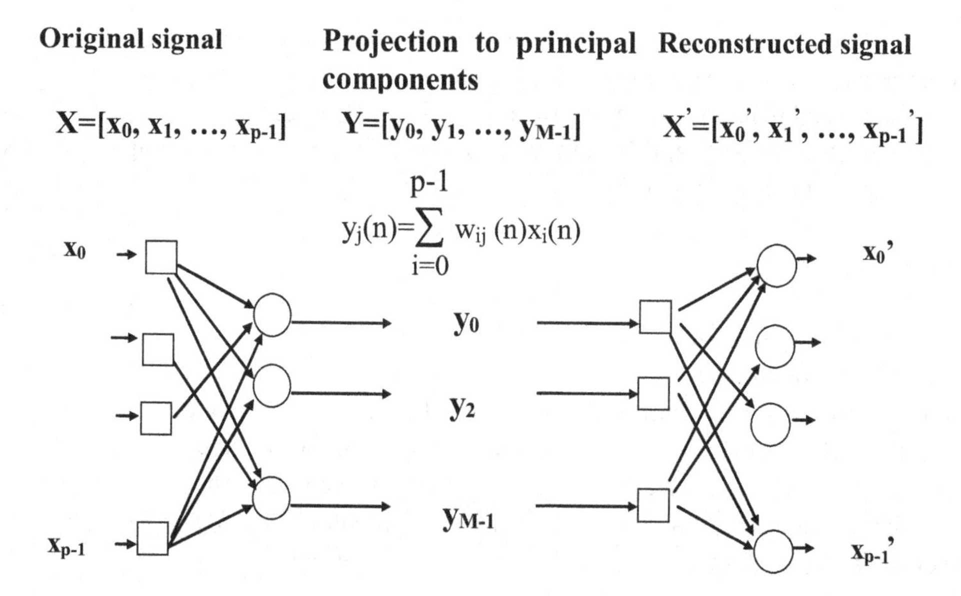

EEG of Comatose Patients

Feature Extraction from the EEG of Comatose Patients by Global Adaptive Segmentation

Long-term narcosis improves the outcome of treatment in acute brain disorders. EEG monitoring is employed to control the proper depth of narcosis in coma.

As a rule, evaluation of the EEG requires the assistance of a competent neurophysiologist. An automatic method would be more practical, but conventional spectrum analysis cannot be applied to a non-stationary EEG in coma. If the features are extracted from the segments with a fixed epoch length, the time structure of the signal may be lost.

The objective is to prepare a set of robust EEG indicators for automatic assessment of coma scales. There is a correlation between the EEG indicators and the clinical scores in comatose patients. One possible approach to pattern recognition is to apply a learning classifier. During the learning phase of the classifier tuning, the teacher provides the set of etalons (standards), extracted from the signal, and labels them visually according to the coma scale. Such epochs can serve as the prototypes of the appropriate class. Because of the non-stationary character of the EEG changes, the parametric signal description may not be correct, if the features are estimated from a fixed epoch length.

We use a strategy based on projecting a multichannel EEG on to the first principal component (Krajca, 1997). The signal, transformed in this way, is then used to summarize the activity from a multichannel EEG. Then adaptive segmentation is performed on the first principal component. The segment boundaries are projected backward to the original EEG traces.

An example of this algorithm is shown in Figure 4 (the first principal component is on the bottom line, and the ten original EEG traces are on the top).

The whole process of feature extraction and classification can be described by the following steps:

1. Using Principal Component Analysis (PCA), the relevant information from several EEG channels is concentrated in a single curve, corresponding to the first principal component (explaining most of the variance of the data). The PC is estimated by eigen decomposition of the covariance matrix of the data.
2. The first PC is processed by means of adaptive segmentation.
3. A set of features is calculated for each segment.
4. The features are used for classifying the individual segments.
5. The individual classes, or a sequence of individual classes, should correspond to the grades on the "coma scale", as used for the visual classification.

The EEG segments detected by adaptive segmentation are described by ten features (see Figure 5). The most important parameters for distinguishing the EEG activity between the two sleep states are amplitude variance, the power in the frequency bands: delta, theta, and alpha, mean frequency in the segment, and the first and second derivative of the signal (Krajča, 1991). The features describe the frequency characteristics and also the time characteristics of the EEG graphoelements.

In the formulas given below, N_s = number of samples in the segment; x_i = instantaneous sample value; $i = 1, 2, \ldots N_s$:

Figure 4. Global PCA based adaptive segmentation. The same signal is used as in Figure 2. The crucial indicators, such as the "EEG burst-suppression pattern", in deep coma occur simultaneously in several channels.The segment boundaries are projected from the first PC (bottom trace) computed from all channels to the original EEG traces

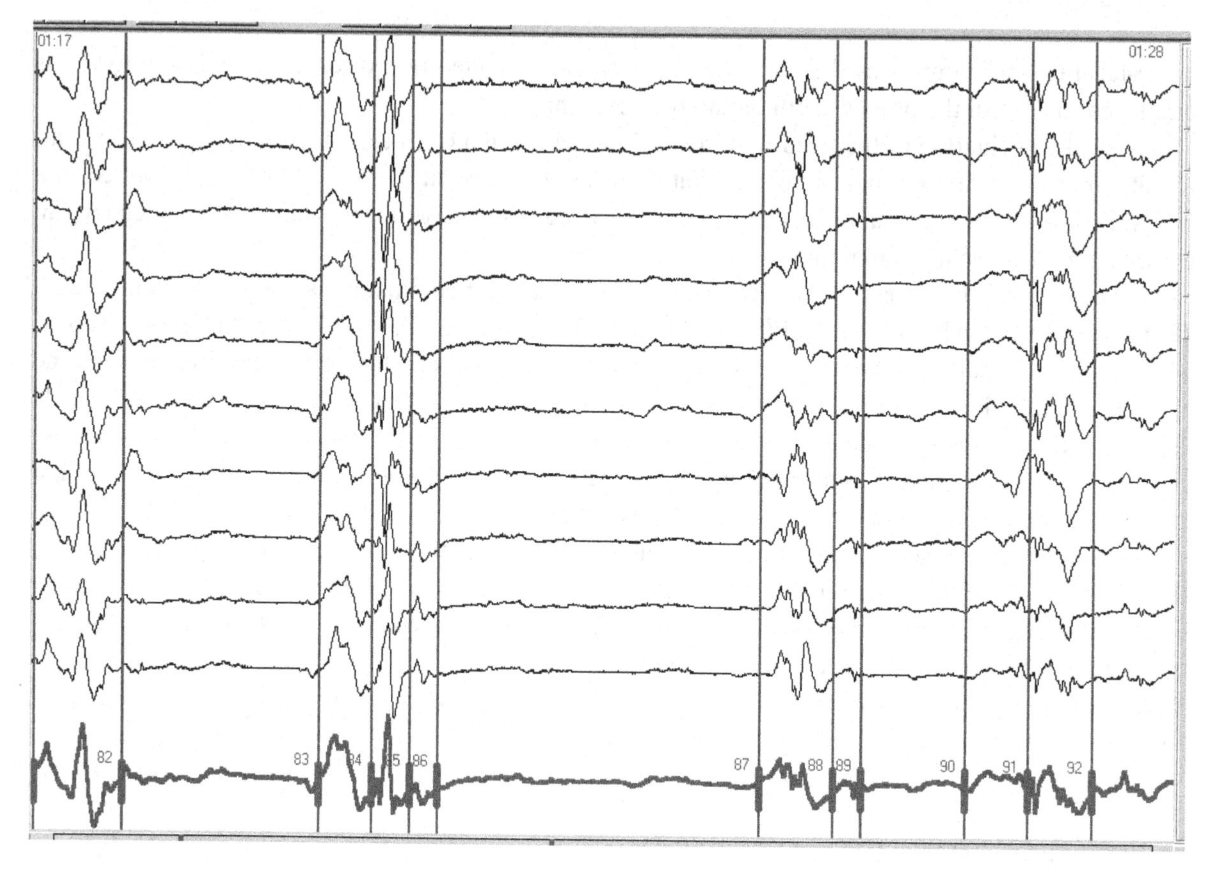

(1) Standard deviation of the sample values in the segment, calculated from:

$$AV = \sqrt{\frac{\sum_{i=1}^{N_S} x_i^2}{N_S} - \overline{A}_{DC}^2} \qquad \overline{A}_{DC} = \frac{\sum_{i=1}^{N_S} x_i}{N_S}$$

(2) Difference between the maximal positive and minimal negative values of the samples in the segment, calculated from:

$$Mm = x_{\max+} - x_{\min-}$$

$$x_{\max+} = \max_i \{x_i, x_i \geq 0, i = 1, \ldots.., N_S\}$$

$$x_{\min-} = \min_i \{x_i, x_i < 0, i = 1, \ldots.., N_S\}$$

Figure 5. Feature extraction from the segments. The left part of the picture shows the frequency spectrum from the 5 selected channels. The features are represented by the histogram on the left

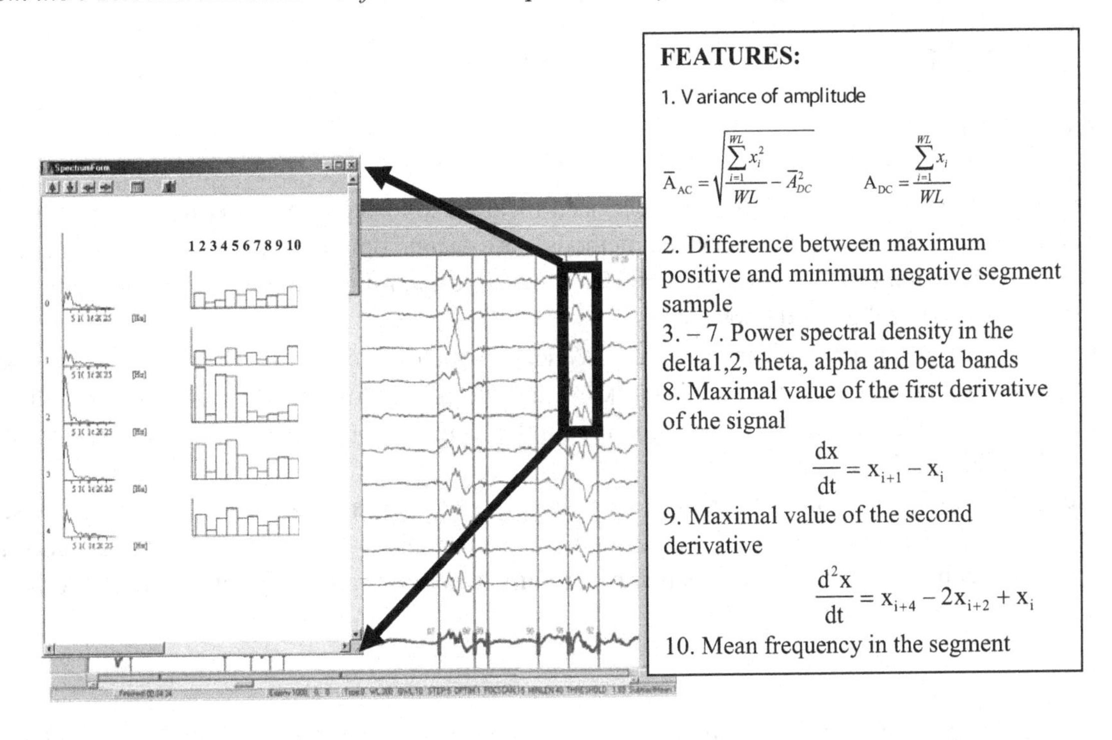

(3) Square root of power spectral density (PSD) in the 0,5 – 1,5 Hz band
(4) Square root of PSD in the 1,6 – 3 Hz band
(5) Square root of PSD in the 3,1 – 5 Hz band
(6) Square root of PSD in the 5,1 – 8 Hz band
(7) Square root of PSD in the 8,1 – 25 Hz band

The PSDs are calculated using the Fast Fourier Transform. The PSDs for the individual segments are calculated from the averages of the one-second epochs. If an epoch exceeds the boundary of a segment, it is not considered. If the segment is shorter than one second, it is considered to be an epoch.

(8) *D1* – maximum of the absolute values of the first derivative of the samples in the segment, determined by:

$$D1 = x_{i+1} - x_i$$

(9) *D2* – maximum of the absolute values of the second derivative of the samples in the segment, determined by:

$$D2 = x_{i+4} - 2x_{i+2} + x_i$$

(10) *MF* – average frequency of the EEG activity in the segment, calculated from:

$$MF = \frac{1}{N_S}\sum_{i=1}^{N_S}\left|x_i - x_{i-1}\right|$$

Classification

In classification, both supervised and unsupervised methods are used. Here, a k-means algorithm is selected as a representative of unsupervised methods. As a second option we use a k-NN classifier and a radial basis function (RBF) neural network for supervised learning. We describe a non-traditional way of using expert background knowledge.

In the case of unsupervised learning, the EEG segments characterized by the above features are classified into six classes by cluster analysis (k-means algorithm) (Anderberg, 1974). An example of classification is shown in Figure 6. The segments can be identified in the original EEG traces by different colors (Figure 7).

The k-NN classifier (Nearest Neighbour classifier) is a basic classification method in supervised learning. It is based on closest training examples in the feature space. A classified object is assigned to the class most common amongst its k nearest neighbours, where k is a small positive integer. A radial

Figure 6. Cluster analysis of the segments (the classes are ordered according to increasing amplitude)

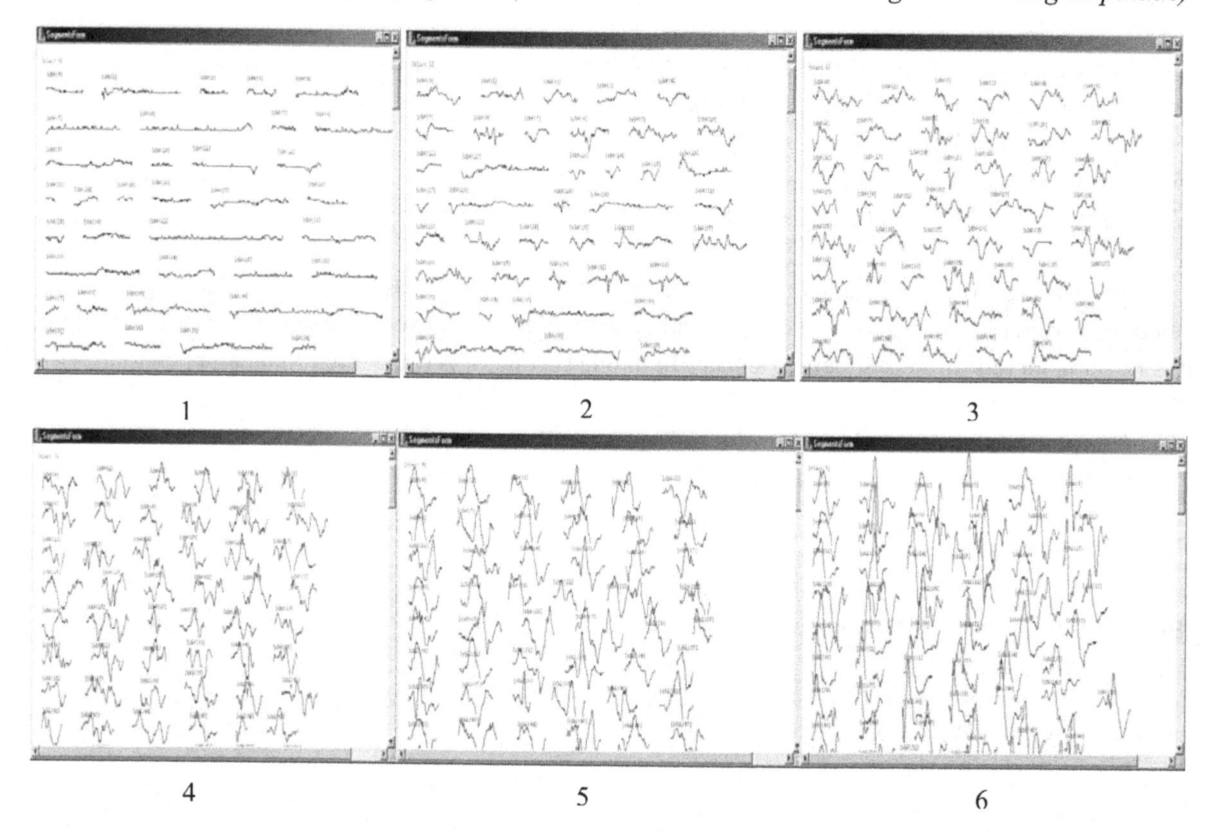

basis function is a function whose characteristic property is a monotonous decrease or increase from its central point. RBFs are used as activation functions of hidden neurons in Multi-Layer Perceptrons. Their advantage is that they do not suffer from getting stuck in local minima.

Now we describe an application of a k-NN classifier and an RBF neural network in comatose EEG classification. It is well known that the classification quality of a supervised learning method depends highly on the training set. Since comatose EEG is a relatively difficult type of data, the training set is developed in a non-traditional way using expert background knowledge (Rieger, 2004).

The basic steps can be described as follows:

1. We saved a total of 453 eight-second periods of 18-electrode EEG, where the classification into levels 1 thru 10 (provided by an experienced neurophysiologist) was known.
2. Since the training set that was created showed unacceptable cross-validation error, it was necessary to edit the training set to make it acceptable.
3. Segments unsuitable for further processing, e.g., those containing artifacts, were excluded from the training set. The number of segments decreased to 436.
4. The core of the training set was generated by cluster analysis - only those segments that agreed with the expert's original classification were included for classification by cluster analysis. Where

Figure 7. Automatic description of signal patterns – color identification of the segments according to their class membership (class 5 red, class 4 green, etc.). The numbers indicate the order of segment/class membership

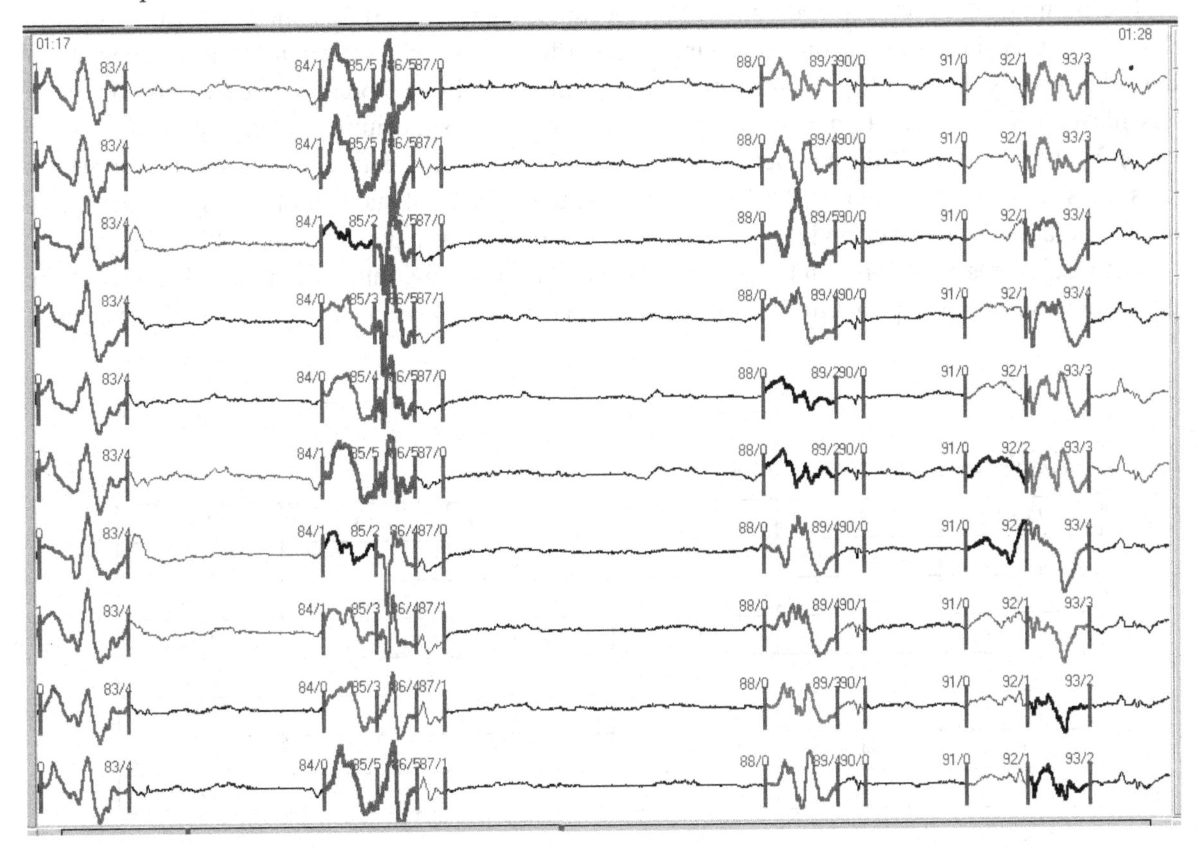

there was repeated clustering, a search was made for a metrics of the feature space that resulted in corresponding classification for the highest number of segments. The core of the training set generated in this way contains 184 segments.

5. Using classification by nearest neighbour and parallel visual control of the results, some of the segments excluded in the previous step were added to the training set. However, their classification was frequently changed by 1 to 2 levels. The resulting training set had 349 segments.
6. Using RBF implementation of a neural network (Haykin, 1999), the cross-validation error was computed. The data was randomly divided in a 1:1 ratio into training and testing sets. The RBF network was learned on the training set and the error was computed using the testing data. This procedure was repeated many times (in the order of hundreds) for different random distribution training/testing sets. The resulting error was computed as the average error of these distributions. Repeatedly incorrectly classified segments in the second phase of computation were excluded from the resulting training set.
7. The resulting training set created in the previous steps contains 319 segments classified into levels 1 thru 10 of coma. The average cross-validation error computed using the RBF neural network does not exceed a value of 3 percent.

The approach was tested on a real EEG recording for which the classification was known. A combination of non-adaptive and adaptive segmentation was used. The length of the segments for non-adaptive segmentation was set to 32 seconds (at a sampling rate of 256 Hz, 8192 samples correspond to 32 seconds, and this value was selected for successive computation of FFT). The intervals containing artefacts were determined by adaptive segmentation.

The training set developed according this procedure, containing 319 segments classified into 10 classes, was used for classifying the two-hour EEG recording. For the classification, the nearest neighbour algorithm was used. The whole classification lasted 2 minutes. Table 1 presents the success rate of the classification. The classified signal contained levels 1 thru 7. P1 is the number of segments assigned to a level by the expert, P2 is the number of successfully classified segments with no error, U1 represents the success rate as a percentage (P2/P1), P3 contains the number of successfully classified segments with a tolerance of one level, and U2 represents the success rate as a percentage (P3/P1).

The results presented here can be summarized as follows. Taking into account the character of the application, we cannot expect a 100% success rate. When an exact classification is required, we achieve

Table 1. Success rate of the classification

Level	P1	P2	U1	P3	U2
1	36	27	75%	33	92%
2	24	19	79%	21	88%
3	15	14	93%	15	100%
4	43	36	84%	40	93%
5	18	12	66%	15	83%
6	45	41	91%	42	93%
7	23	14	61%	20	87%

a success rate of approximately 80%. When we have a tolerance of one level of coma, the success rate increases to 90%. A more exact evaluation of the error has no practical sense because the expert himself considers that his classification is burdened by non-zero error.

EEG of Epileptic Patients

Application of Neural Networks Based Principal Component Analysis for Epileptic Spike Detection

If we are interested in long-term monitoring of multi-channel EEG recordings, one of the problems might be in detecting epileptic spikes. There are a large number of different spike detection algorithms. Some use the template matching (Salzberg, 1971), inverse autoregressive filtering (Lopes da Silva, 1975), signal decomposition into half-waves (Gotman, 1981), electrographic parameters (Ktonas, 1983), multichannel correlation and expert systems (Glover, 1986), median filtering (Nieminen, 1987), and many others. The multilayer perceptron was used in (Eberhart, 1989) for spike detection and classification.

In this example, we borrow an approach used in (Qian, 1988; Krajca, 1992). It consists in signal pre-processing (conditioning) by enhancing the frequency components that are common for epileptic graphoelements. The resulting signal is then squared and smoothed and compared with a threshold. Threshold crossing indicates the possible presence of a spike.

Figure 8. Signal decomposition into three PCs. The third principal component is used as the detection signal. It is squared, smoothed and compared with the threshold (bottom trace)

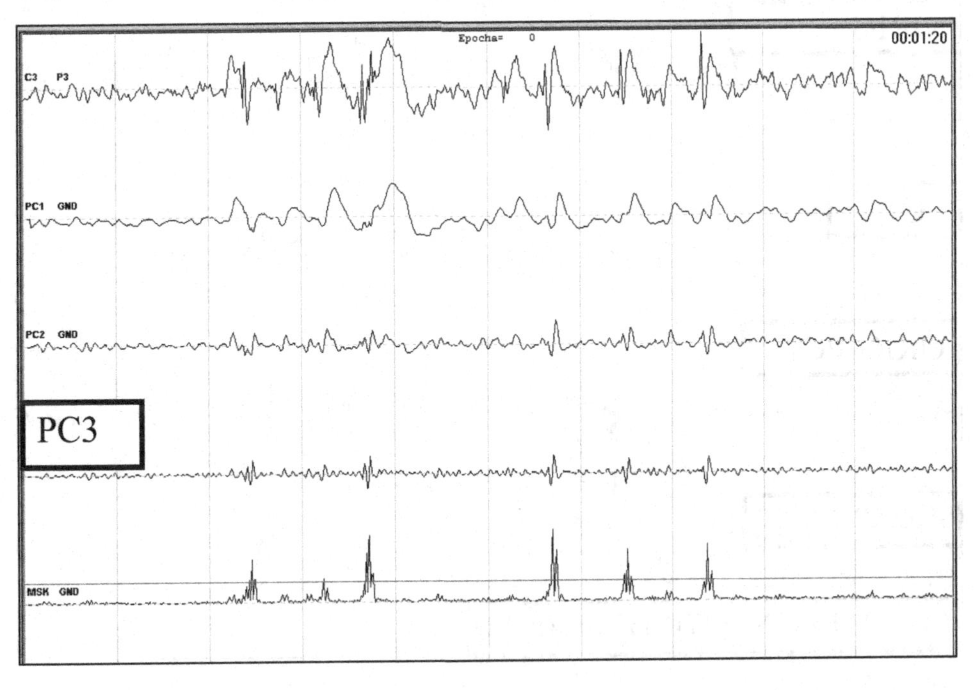

PCA Signal Decomposition and its Application to Spike Detection

Decomposition of a signal into time traces corresponding to the first three principal components is shown in Figure 8. The first trace is the original EEG, and the subsequent traces show the first three principal components. The last trace shows the detection curve.

The above-mentioned property of the PCA filter can be exploited for detecting epileptic spikes. There are basically two approaches to this task. The **first method** (designated PC3) uses the third PC, which reflects the sharp components of the signal (see Figure 8.) This signal is squared and smoothed and is used as the detection signal (lowest trace of the picture). The vertical lines represent the threshold for spike detection, set experimentally.

The **second method** (designated SUB) uses the first principal component (the second trace), which reflects only the slow frequency component (the PCA filter – the first PC acts as the low pass filter). This trace is subtracted from the original signal, resulting in the sharp component of the signal third trace. This detection curve is squared and smoothed and compared with the threshold again. The results are shown in Figure 9.

This method is applied to several recordings of the EEG of patients diagnosed with epilepsy. Application to an EEG with genuine spikes is shown in Figures. 8, 9.

All experiments are performed on a neural net with 10 inputs (window length), and the number of learning iterations is 25. The results show that this approach is very promising - the PCA3 method is not sensitive to the amplitude artefacts, and the influence of muscle artifacts can be suppressed by a simple FIR filter, which does not deteriorate the performance of the method on genuine epileptic spikes. One

Figure 9. Subtraction of the first PCA from the signal and smoothing of the result for detection of EEG epileptic spikes

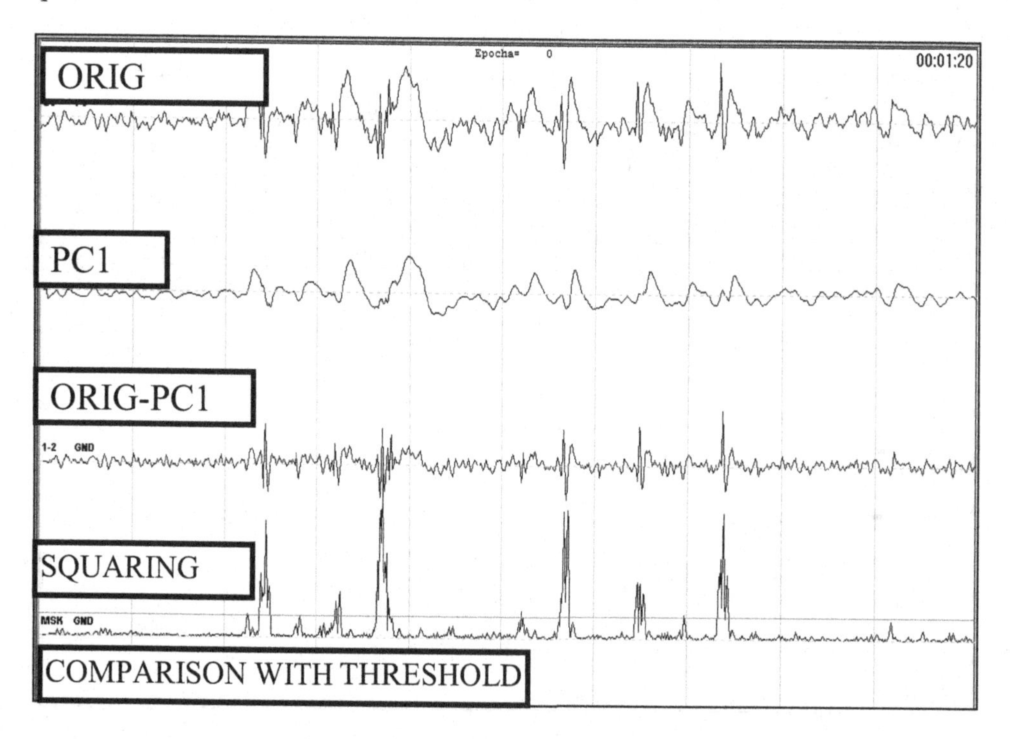

question to be solved in the future concerns the optimal number of taps, which influence the filtering properties of PCA net, and also the optimal threshold setting. PCA can be used in a single learning run after initial adaptation to the first part of the signal: after weight stabilising on the initial EEG page, the self-organised PCA can be applied without learning to the whole EEG of the same patient. This means very efficient computing, requiring only a small number of simple mathematical operations (multiplications and additions).

CONCLUSION

This chapter has tried to address some of the most important issues in EEG signal processing. By its nature, an EEG signal is the most complex signal that can be measured on the human body. It exhibits different characteristics according to the age of the person, mental activity, or state (normal, abnormal, sleep, wake, coma, etc.). It is therefore impossible to develop a single general method that would successfully classify all possible types of EEG signal. We have tried to point out key aspects of EEG processing and to show on the basis of two examples how to approach the task.

We have demonstrated the task of feature extraction and classification on two examples: EEGs signal containing epileptic graphoelements, and EEGs of comatose patients.

A combination of Principal Component Analysis and Global Adaptive Segmentation can provide a reliable description of the structure of an EEG, and can be used as the first step in automatic EEG processing during long-term narcosis. The results confirm that the individual segments can be detected and classified in a way that is compatible with the conventional "coma scale". For practical application, a further adjustment of the classification criteria is planned, using existing training material (100 EEGs of 5 min duration, obtained from 22 patients with brain contusion, intracranial hemorrhage or status epilepticus). Tests show that indicators of consciousness level, such as the burst-suppression pattern, could be correctly defined. It is anticipated that the use of global adaptive segmentation will be suitable for automatic feature extraction in coma and deep narcosis.

Neural network-based Principal Component Analysis allows rather fast and efficient computation of components. It is therefore suitable for processing long EEG records.

For the future there are still many open issues. The first of these is the development of new preprocessing methods that can detect artifacts easily and efficiently, and separate them from the useful signal. The second issue is better detection of typical graphoelements that have a specific morphological structure. More advanced optimization techniques also need to be developed that will define the optimal setup of learning parameters or optimal feature selection. Finally, it is desirable to develop new hierarchical, hybrid or multiple classifiers.

ACKNOWLEDGMENT

This work has been supported by the research program "Information Society" under grant No. 1ET101210512 "Intelligent methods for evaluation of long-term EEG recordings" and by IGA MZ CR grant No. 1A8600.

REFERENCES

Agarwal, R., Gotman, J., Flanagan, D., & Rosenblatt, B. (1998). Automatic EEG analysis during long-term monitoring in the ICU. *Electroenceph. clin. Neurophysiol*, 10744-58

Anderberg M.R. (1974). *Cluster Analysis for Applications*. Academic Press, New York

Bodenstein, G. & Praetorius, H.M. (1977). Feature extraction from the electroencephalogram by adaptive segmentation. In *Proc. IEEE*, 65, 642-652

Bradie, B. (1996). *Wavelet Packed-Based Compression of Single Lead ECG. IEEE Trans. Biomed. Eng.*, 43, 493-501.

Cohen, A. (1986). *Biomedical Signal Processing*. CRC Press, Boca Raton, Florida,USA.

Daube, J. R. (2002). *Clinical Neurophysiology Second Edition*. Mayo Foundation for Medical Education and Research, New York.

Dony, R. D. & Haykin, S. (1995). Neural Network Approaches to Image Compression. In *Proc. IEEE*, 83, 288-303.

Eberhart, R. C., Dobbins, R. W. & Webber,W. R. S.(1989). EEG Analysis using CaseNet. In *Proceedings of the IEEE-EMBS 11th Annual Conference*, Seattle, WA, 2046-2047.

Glover, J., Ktonas, P., Raghavan, N., Urnuela, J., Velamuri, S., & Reilly, E.(1986). A multichannel signal processor for the detection of epileptogenic sharp transients in the EEG. *IEEE Trans. Biomed. Eng.*, *33*(12), 1121-1128.

Gotman, J. (1981). Quantitative EEG-Principles and Problems. *Electroenceph. Clin. Neurophysiol.*, *52*, 626-639.

Haykin S. (1994). *Neural Networks. A Comprehensive Foundation*. Macmillan, New York.

Hornero, R., Espino, P., Alonso, A. & Lopez, M. (1999). Estimating Complexity from EEG Background Activity of Epileptic Patients. *IEEE Engineering in Medicine and Biology*, Nov./Dec. 1999, 73-79.

Jalaleddine, S. M. S. , Hutchens, Ch. G. , Strattan, R. D. & Coberly, W. A.(1990). ECG Data Compression Techniques - A Unified Approach. *IEEE Trans.Biomed.Eng.*, *37*, 329-343.

Jasper, H. H. (1958). Report of the Committee on Methods of Clinical Examination in Electroencephalography. *Electroenceph. Clin. Neurophysiol*, *10*, 370-1.

Jollife, I.T. (2002). *Principal Component Analysis*. Springer.

Krajča, V., Petránek, S., Patáková, I., & Värri A. (1991). Automatic identificaton of significant graphoelements in multichannel EEG recordings by adaptive segmentation and fuzzy clustering. *Int. J. Biomed. Comput.*, 28, 71-89.

Krajča, V., & Petránek, S. (1992). Automatic epileptic spike detection by median filtering and simple arithmetic sharp transient detector: a clinical evaluation. In *Proc. VI Mediterranean Conference on Medical and Biological Engineering*, 1, 209-212. Capri, Italy.

Krajča, V., Principe, J. C., Petránek, S., & Vyšata, O. (1996). Use of time-delayed self-organized principal components analysis for feature extraction from the EEG. *Third International Hans Berger Congress*, Jena, p. 50.

Krajča, V., Matoušek, M., Petránek, S., Grießbach, G., Ivanova, G., & Vršecká, M.(1997). Feature extraction from the EEG of comatose patients by global adaptive segmentation, *42. Internationales wissenschaftliches Kolloquium* TU Ilmenau, Band 2, pp.156-161.

Krajča, V., Principe, J.C. & Petránek S.. (1997). Dimensionality reduction and reconstruction of the EEG signal by self-organized principal components analysis. *First European Conference on Signal Analysis and Prediction*, Prague.

Ktonas, P. Y. (1983). Automated analysis of abnormal electroencephalograms, *CRC Crit. Rev. Bioeng.*, 9., 39-97.

Lehman, D., Ozaki, H., & Pal I. (1987). EEG alpha map series: brain micro states by space oriented adaptive segmentation. *Electroenceph. clin. Neurophysiol.*, *67*, 271-288

Lopes da Silva, F., Dijk, A., & Smits, H. (1975). Detection of nonstationarities in EEGs using the autoregressive model - An application to EEGs of epileptics. In *CEAN-Computerized EEG analysis*, G.Dolce, H.Kunkel Eds., Stuttgart, Germany, G. Fischer Verlag, pp.180-199.

Maccabee, P. J., & Hassan, N. F. (1992). Digital filtering: basic concepts and application to evoked potentials. *Muscle Nerve,* 15, 865-875.

Murtagh, F., Heck A. (1987). *Multivariate Data Analysis.* Kluwer Academic Publishers, Dordrecht

Murtagh, F. (1999) *Multivariate Data Analysis with Fortran, C and Java Code.* Queen's University Belfast and Astronomical Observatory Strasbourg.

Nave, G. & Cohen, A. (1990). *ECG Compression Using Long-Term Prediction.* IEEE Trans. Biomed. Eng., *40*, 877-885.

Nicoletti, D.W., & Onaral, B. (1991). The Application of Delta Modulation to EEG Waveforms for Database Reduction and Real-time Signal Processing. *Annals of Biomedical Engineering, 19*, 1-14.

Nieminen, A., & Neuvo, Y. (1987). EEG spike detection based on median type filters. In *Proc. of Int. Conf. on Digital Signal Processing*, Florence, Italy, 559-563.

Oja, E. (1982). A simplified neuron model as a principal component analyzer. *J.Math.Biol.*, *15*, 267-273.

Qian, J., Barlow, J. S., & Beddoes, M. P. (1988). A simplified arithmetic detector for EEG sharp transients - preliminary results. *IEEE Trans. Biomed. Eng.*, *35*(1), 11-17.

Rieger, J., Lhotská, L., Krajča, V., & Matoušek, M. (2004). Application of Quantitative Methods of Signal Processing to Automatic Classification of Long-Term EEG Records. In *Biological and Medical Data Analysis*. Springer Verlag, 2004, 333-343.

Salzberg, B. & Heath, R. (1971). The detection of surface EEG correlates of deep brain spiking in schizophrenic patients using matched digital filters. *Electroenceph.Clin.Neurophysiol.*, *38*, 550.

Sanger, T. D. (1989). Optimal unsupervised learning in a single-layer linear feedforward neural network. *Neural Networks,* 12, 459-473.

Siegwart, D. K., Tarassenko, L., Roberts, S. J., Stradling, J.R. & Parlett J. (1995). Sleep apnoea analysis from neural network post-processing. *Artificial Neural Networks*, 26-28 June 1995.Conference Publication No. 409, IEE pp. 427-437.

Smith, S. W. (1997). *Digital Signal Processing.* California Technical Publishing, San Diego, CA, USA.

Soong, A. C. K. & Koles, Z. (1995). Principal component localisation of the sources of the background EEG. *IEEE Trans. Biomed.Eng.*, 42, 59-67.

Starmark, J. E., Stalhammar, D., & Holmgren, E. (1998). The Reaction Level Scale (RLS85). Manual and Guidelines. *Acta Neurochirurgica, 91*(1), 12-20.

Teasdale, G., & Jennet, B. (1974). Assessment of coma and impaired consciousness. A practical scale. *The Lancet*, ii, 81-84.

Wackermann, J., Lehmann, D., Michel, C. M., & Strik, W. K. (1993). Adaptive Segmentation of Spontaneous EEG Map Series into Spatially Defined Microstates. *International Journal of Psychophysiology,* 14(3), 269-283.

KEY TERMS

Artifact: A signal in the EEG that is of non-cerebral origin; it contaminates the EEG signal; it may have either a biological or a technical origin.

EEG: A recording of the electrical activity of the brain in dependence on time.

Filtering: A process for removing unwanted frequency components from the signal.

Graphoelement: A pattern in an EEG signal having a characteristic waveform, e.g. a spike, a sharp wave, alpha rhythmic activity, K-complex.

Nonstationary Signal: A signal having variable quantities in time, e.g., mean value, dispersion, or frequency spectrum.

Principal Component Analysis: A statistical technique for finding patterns in data of high dimension.

Segmentation: A process for dividing a non-stationary signal into (quasi-)stationary segments; there are two basic approaches: constant segmentation and adaptive segmentation.

Chapter IX
Generating and Verifying Risk Prediction Models Using Data Mining

Darryl N. Davis
University of Hull, UK

Thuy T.T. Nguyen
University of Hull, UK

ABSTRACT

Risk prediction models are of great interest to clinicians. They offer an explicit and repeatable means to aide the selection, from a general medical population, those patients that require a referral to medical consultants and specialists. In many medical domains, including cardiovascular medicine, no gold standard exists for selecting referral patients. Where evidential selection is required using patient data, heuristics backed up by poorly adapted more general risk prediction models are pressed into action, with less than perfect results. In this study, existing clinical risk prediction models are examined and matched to the patient data to which they may be applied using classification and data mining techniques, such as neural nets. Novel risk prediction models are derived using unsupervised cluster analysis algorithms. All existing and derived models are verified as to their usefulness in medical decision support on the basis of their effectiveness on patient data from two UK sites.

INTRODUCTION

Risk prediction models are of great interest to clinicians. They offer the means to aide the selection of those patients that need referral, to medical consultants and specialists, from a general medical population. In many medical domains, including cardiovascular medicine, no gold standard exists for selecting referral patients. Existing practice relies on clinical heuristics backed up by poorly adapted generic risk prediction models. In this study existing clinical risk prediction models are examined and matched to the patient data to which they may be applied using classification and data mining techniques, such as neural nets. The evidence from earlier research suggests that there are benefits to be gained in the utilization of neural nets for medical diagnosis (Janet, 1997; Lisboa, 2002).

In this chapter, the cardiovascular domain is used as an exemplar. The problems associated with identifying high risk patients, (i.e. patients at risk of a stroke, cardiac arrest or similar life threatening event), are symptomatic of other clinical domains where no gold standard exists for such purposes. In routine clinical practice, where domain specific clinical experts are unavailable to all patients, the patient's clinical record is used to identify which patient's are most likely to benefit from referral to a consulting clinician. The clinical record typically, although not always, contains generic patient data (for example age, gender etc.), a patient history of events related to the disease (for example, past strokes, cardiovascular related medical operations), and a profile of measurements, and observations from medical examinations, that characterize the nature of the patient's cardiovascular system. The general practitioner may use a risk prediction model, together with observations from medical examinations, as an aid in determining whether to refer the patient to a consultant. Currently, any such risk prediction model will be based on a general clinical risk prediction system, such as APACHE (Rowan et al., 1994) or POSSUM (Copeland, 2002; Yii & Ng, 2002), which generate a score for patients. Clinicians expert in the disease may well use further risk prediction models, based on their own research and expertise. Such risk prediction models are described in more detail in the second section. The strengths and flaws of the available models for the current clinical domain are explored in the third section, where they are used in conjunction with supervised neural nets. It should be noted, that although this chapter predominantly reports on the use of supervised neural nets and unsupervised clustering in predicting risk in patients, a wide range of other techniques, including decision trees, logistic regression, Bayesian classifiers (Bishop, 2006; Witten & Eibe, 2005) have been tried. The results from applying these other techniques are not given, but typically are similar to or worse than the results presented here. The fourth and fifth sections present an alternative to the coercion of outcome labels, arising from current risk prediction models, with the use of unsupervised clustering techniques. The results from these sections are discussed in the sixth section. The problems associated with making available to clinicians, risk prediction models that arise from the application of data mining techniques, are discussed in that and the concluding section.

RISK PREDICTION MODELS

In this section, two forms of risk prediction model, as used in routine clinical practice, are introduced. The first, POSSUM, typifies the application of generic models to specific medical disciplines. The second set reflect the clinical heuristics regularly used in medicine. The data used throughout this case study is from two UK clinical sites. The attributes are a mixture of real number, integer, Boolean and categorical values. The data records typically contain many default and missing values. For both sites there is typically too high a data value space (i.e. the space of all possible values for all attributes in the raw data) for the data volume (i.e. the number of records) to perform naïve data mining, and some form of data preprocessing is required before using any classifier if meaningful results are to be obtained.

Furthermore, as can be seen in the tabulated results, the data once labeled is class-imbalanced; with low risk patients heavily out numbering high risk patients.

The main characteristics of the cardiovascular data from Clinical Site One (98 attributes and 499 patient records) are:

- Many redundant attributes such as date or time attributes with mostly null values, or explanatory attributes. These attributes bear little relevance to the risk prediction models and experiments. For example, the attribute labelled as "*THEATRE_SESSION_DATE*" shows the date of a patient's operation. This is ignored in these experiments, and so this feature can be removed. Other examples are "empty features", containing mostly null values. For example, the attribute labelled as "*LOWEST_BP*" is an attribute representing the lowest blood pressure of the patients during an operation. All of its values are null except for four patient entries. Such attributes are best removed.
- Data has 7018 out of 42914 cells (16%) with missing values after removing the type of redundant attributes described above; leaving 86 "meaningful" attributes.
- Noisy and inconsistent data such as abbreviations in categorical attributes and outlier values in some numerical attributes; these are replaced with "meaningful" values.
- Data includes the scored values (*PS* and *OSS* explained below) for the POSSUM and PPOSSUM risk prediction systems.

The data from Clinical Site Two includes 431 patient records with 57 attributes. The nature and structure of the data has similar characteristics to the first site, with many redundant and noisy attributes, missing values, etc., as follows:

- The redundant attributes have the same characteristics as above. For example, the attribute "*ADMISSION_DATE*" shows the patient's date of operation - it can be removed. Two attributes labelled as "*Surgeon name1*" and "*Surgeon name2*" represent names of operating doctors. Their values might be helpful in a more general evaluation, but offer negligible relevance to the specific purposes of this study.
- The data includes 1912 out of 12311 cells with missing values (16%) after deletion of the redundant attributes (leaving 36 "meaningful" attributes). This is the same ratio as for the first site.
- As an example of numerical outlier values, the attribute "*PACK YRS*" has a big gap between the maximum value of 160, and the minimum value of 2. This will reduce the accuracy in any transformation process. Such outlier values will be replaced with more meaningful maximum and minimum values.
- The site does not include the scored values (*PS* and *OSS*) for the POSSUM and PPOSSUM systems. Moreover, the information in the data is insufficient to generate these scored values and so cannot be used with these risk prediction systems.

In summary the clinical data is noisy, contains many null values and is problematic for use with standard risk prediction models (Kuhan et al., 2001). This is typical of the challenges faced by researchers and workers who want to apply data mining techniques to clinical data. The naïve application of data mining techniques to raw data of this type typically provides poor results. Indeed clinicians availing themselves of data mining packages reported a disillusion with data mining on initially applying these packages to the data used in this study. The same may well be true for other domains.

Generic Clinical Risk Prediction Models

The Physiological and Operative Severity Score for the enUmeration of Mortality and Morbidity (POSSUM) and the Portsmouth POSSUM (PPOSSUM) (Prytherch et al., 2001) are generic clinical risk assessment systems which are widely used in the UK. When used over a database of patient records, they produce a classification of patients ranked in percentile groups. Neither can be used with a single patient record. This is problematic where clinicians want to compare a new patient with an existing group, or where only new patient data is available to the referring clinician.

Copeland (2002) originally assessed 48 physiological factors plus 14 operative and postoperative factors for each patient. Using multivariate analysis techniques these were reduced to 12 physiological and 6 operative factors based on the following key factors:

- Physiological status of the patient
- Disease process that requires surgical intervention
- Nature of operation
- Pre and post-operative support

POSSUM is a two stage process, where the 12 physiological factors give rise to a physiological score (PS), and the 6 operative factors are used to generate an operative severity score (OSS). These can then be used to generate a Mortality and Morbidity rate.

Mortality rate: $R_1 = 1/(1+e^{-x})$ (1)

where x = (0.16* physiological score) + (0.19* operative score) - 5.91.

Morbidity rate: $R_2 = 1/(1+e^{-y})$ (2)

where y = (0.13* physiological score) + (0.16* operative score) - 7.04.

The scalars in the above formulae were found using regression analysis in the work by Copeland, and are medical domain independent. POSSUM was evaluated by Prytherch et al. (2001) using 10,000 patients over a two year period, and found that POSSUM over predicted mortality. In an effort to counteract the perceived shortcoming of conventional POSSUM, Whitley et al. (1996) devised the similar PPOSSUM (Portsmouth Predictor) equation for mortality. The PPOSSUM equation uses the same physiological and operative severity scores to provide a risk-adjusted operative mortality rates, but generates a Predicted Death Rate:

Predicted Death Rate: $R_3 = 1/(1+e^{-z})$ (3)

where z = (0.1692 * PS) + (0.150 * OS) - 9.065.

Both POSSUM and PPOSSUM give a numeric measure of risk for groups of patients. A relatively naïve clinical model for assigning individual patients as High or Low risk, based on these numbers for Mortality, Morbidity or Death rate, is possible using the following heuristics:

Mortality Prediction: IF "Mortality Score" ≥ *Threshold* *THEN Patient ="High risk"*
Otherwise Patient = "Low risk"
Morbidity Prediction: IF "Morbidity Score" ≥ *Threshold* *THEN Patient ="High risk"*
Otherwise Patient = "Low risk"
Death Rate Prediction: IF "Death Rate Score" ≥ *Threshold* *THEN Patient ="High risk"*
Otherwise Patient = "Low risk"

The threshold used in these prediction heuristics will vary depending on the intended use of the prediction, but typically the *Threshold* is set to the mean score for the predictor in question.

Clinical Heuristic Models

A different form of risk prediction model are those that make use of the clinical expertise of practitioners in the domain. Such models arise from the daily use of data for clinical purposes, or result from research, which can involve practitioners from other fields (e.g. statisticians and computer scientists). Typically, the indicative attributes used in such models are those to be found in the POSSUM models, or deemed to be important by the clinicians based on their experience or found to significant when matched against outcomes in logistic regression studies. Many of these heuristic models use an aggregation of attributes from clinical records to form the outcome labels. The following models (or risk prediction rules) arose from exactly such studies. They either make use of the attributes used in the POSSUM (and PPOSSUM) models, attributes found to be highly related to the given output from logistic regression studies, or deemed to be important, by experienced clinicians, in attributing risk (Kuhan et al., 2001).

One clinical model in this study (heuristic model `CM1`) uses patient death within 30 days of an operation as the "`High Risk`" outcome, with other patients are labeled as "`Low Risk`". A further model (`CM2`) uses patient death or severe cardiovascular event (for example `Stroke` or `Myocardial Relapse` or `Cardio Vascular Arrest`) within 30 days of an operation as the "`High Risk"` outcome; other patients are labeled as "`Low Risk`". Both the `CM1` and `CM2` models use all attributes from the "cleaned" patient records, other than those aggregated to form the output labels, as inputs. Further models use only a limited set of attributes. Heuristic model `CM3a`, for example, uses 16 input attributes derived from the `CM1` and `CM2` models. These attributes are thought to be significant by experienced clinicians. Again the outcome label is based on an aggregation of attributes as described for `CM2`. Heuristic model `CM3b`, a variation on `CM3a,` uses four outcome labels; a variation on the four attributes used in the outcome labels of `CM1`, `CM2` and `CM3a`. Hence, given `Aggregate2` is `Stroke` or `Myocardial Relapse` or `Cardio Vascular Arrest` (all Boolean valued attributes), outcome for `CM3b` is determined by the following aggregation rules:

IF Status="Dead" AND Aggregate2="TRUE" *THEN Outcome = "Very High risk"*
Else IF Status="Dead" *THEN Outcome = "High risk"*
Else IF Aggegrate2="TRUE" *THEN Outcome = "Medium risk"*
Otherwise *Outcome = "Low risk"*

The remaining two models (CM4a and CM4b) have similar outcome variations to CM3a and CM3b (respectively) but with 15 input attributes, derived from a combination of clinical knowledge and those marked as significant in a logistic regression exercise using the complete data.

Like the heuristic rules used with the POSSUM models, patients can be assigned a risk prediction outcome that allows a grading of patients from low to high risk. However, unlike the POSSUM models, these heuristic models can be used to provide a qualitative labeling of patients, based on individual records and do not require a complete data set of cardiovascular patients to be available. This is an important point. The opening paragraph of this chapter stated that these risk prediction models should offer the means to aide selection from a general medical population, those patients that need referral to medical consultants and specialists. In many cases the referring clinician does not have a population of cardiovascular patients with which to compare a new patient. Indeed, in many cases, patient records are represented as single entry databases. In such situations the POSSUM type models are of limited use.

TESTING EXISTING RISK PREDICTION MODELS

The clinical and heuristic model outcomes described in the previous section were evaluated against data using a variety of supervised classifiers. A variety of performance measures were used; in particular, the Mean Square Error (*MSE*), the confusion matrix, sensitivity (*sen*) and specificity (*spec*) rates, and true positive (*tpr*) and false positive (*fpr*) rates as used in ROC (Receiver Operating Characteristics) graphs (Kononenko & Kukar, 2007).

Assume that the data domain has n input patterns x_i $(i=1,\ 2..n)$, each with a target pattern Y_i, for which the classifier produces the output y_i. The *MSE* is the averaged square of the error between the predicted and the target output, given by:

$$MSE = \sum_i (y_i - Y_i)^2 \Big/ n \tag{4}$$

Assume that the cardiovascular classifier output set includes two outcomes {High risk; Low risk}. Each pattern x_i $(i=1,\ 2..n)$ is allocated to one label from the set *{P, N}, Positive (P) = High Risk* or *Negative (N) = Low Risk.* Hence, each input pattern might be mapped into one of four possible classifier outcomes: *TP (True Positive- True High Risk); FP (False Positive- False High Risk); TN (True Negative- True Low Risk); or FN (False Negative- False Low Risk).* The set {*P, N*} and the predicted risk set are used to build a confusion matrix (Kohavi & Provost, 1998).

From the confusion matrix in Table 1 the number of correct or incorrect (misclassified) patterns is generated as a measure of classifier Accuracy, where:

$$Accuracy = \frac{TP + TN}{TP + TN + FP + FN} \tag{5}$$

Some related concepts, such as true positive rate (*tpr*), false positive rate (*fpr*), sensitivity (*sen*) and specificity (*spec*), can all be built from the confusion matrix. True positive rate (*tpr*) is the rate of the correct "*High risk*" number in the total correct prediction pattern number (including "*High risk*" and "*Low risk*"):

$$tpr = \frac{TP}{TP + TN} \tag{6}$$

Table 1. A confusion matrix

		Predicted classes	
		P (High risk)	N (Low risk)
Desired classes	P (High risk)	*TP*	*FP*
	N (Low risk)	*FN*	*TN*

Figure 1. An example ROC graph

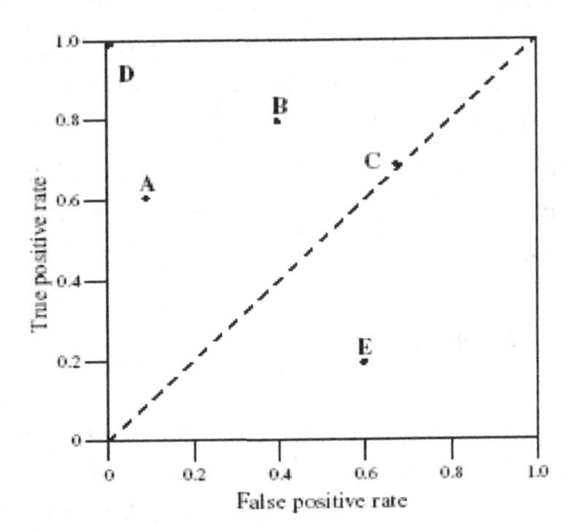

Conversely, false positive rate (*fpr*) is the rate of the incorrect "*High risk*" number in the total incorrect prediction pattern number:

$$fpr = \frac{FP}{FP + FN} \tag{7}$$

The sensitivity rate (*sen*) indicates the effectiveness at identifying the true positive cases, and is calculated as:

$$sen = \frac{TP}{TP + FN} \tag{8}$$

The specificity rate (*spec*) is the rate of correct "*Low risk*" number (*TN*) in the total of the *TN* and *FP* number:

$$spec = \frac{TN}{TN + FP} \tag{9}$$

ROC graphs (Swets, 1988; Tom, 2006) are two-dimensional graphs in which the true positive rate is plotted on the Y axis and the false positive rate is plotted on the X axis. An ROC graph depicts relative tradeoffs between benefits (*tpr*) and costs (*fpr*). Figure 1 shows an example ROC graph. The pair of (*fpr*, *tpr*) for each classifier is represented as a point in the ROC space. It shows the benefit and the cost results of 5 classifiers labeled as A, B, C, D, and E. The diagonal line in the ROC graph presents the strategy of randomly guessing a class. Any classifier (E) that appears in the lower right triangle performs worse than random; conversely good classifiers (A, B, D) appear above the diagonal. The classifier labeled as D is *perfect* because of its *tpr* =1 and *fpr* =0. This means all input patterns are classified correctly; i.e. the prediction risks are the same as the prior classified outcomes. The classifier labeled as C yields the point (0.7; 0.7) in the ROC graph, meaning it guesses "*High risk*" (*tpr=70%)* at the same rate as its "incorrect High risk" (*fpr=70%)*; in effect, equivalent to random.

POSSUM and PPOSSUM

Table 2 shows the confusion matrix, and classifier measures, for the two POSSUM risk scoring models, with the Mortality, Morbidity, and Death Rate Predictions from the models evaluated against the actuality from the patient data for individual patients. Note that the model data are derived from only one clinical site, and makes use of 499 records.

There is very little difference between the three models and overall, all the POSSUM model predictors give poor results, with the exception of the specificity rate; demonstrating their limited reliability as predictors of high risk patients.

Heuristic Models and Neural Nets

In this section three supervised neural net techniques, Multi-Layer Perceptrons (MLP), Radial Basis Functions (RBF), and Support Vector Machines (SVM) (Haykin, 1999; Bishop, 2006) are used with the heuristic models described above (CM1, CM2, CM3a, CM3b, CM4a and CM4b). The available data was prepared according to the attribute input list and output labeling as given by the various models. This resulted in six labeled data sets. Various training strategies were investigated, with varying parameters to identify the parameters that would result in the optimal neural classifier for these models. This experimentation determined that splitting the data into training, validation and test sets and then using bespoke neural net software gave no benefit over using 10-fold cross validation within a more general data mining package, WEKA (Witten & Eibe, 2005). Other data mining techniques, available within WEKA, were also investigated. These other classifiers, for example J48 Decision Tree or Naïve Bayesian classifier, offered no improvement on the supervised classifiers described in the rest of this chapter.

Table 2. Confusion matrix and classifier measures for POSSUM and PPOSSUM

Model	Risk	*High risk*	*Low risk*	*Total*	Sen	Spec	tp rate	fp rate
Mortality	*High risk*	10	**69**	79	0.4	0.85	0.13	0.16
	Low risk	15	405	420				
	Total	25	474	499				
Morbidity	*High risk*	15	64	79	0.38	0.86	0.19	0.15
	Low risk	24	396	420				
	Total	39	460	499				
Death rate	*High risk*	10	69	79	0.38	0.85	0.13	0.16
	Low risk	16	404	420				
	Total	26	473	499				

The data for `CM1` and `CM2` models includes 26 attributes with 839 patient records. Table 3 shows a confusion matrix for both models with the three supervised neural techniques. Overall, all classifiers give poor results especially in regard to the important *sensitivity* rates, with values typically less than 0.2. The classifier `CM2-SVM` has the poorest *sensitivity* rate (0.13), while `CM1-SVM` has the highest (0.27). Interestingly, all classifiers display very similar *specificity* rates (about 0.85). Specificity rates represent the outcomes labeled as "Low Risk", the negative risk prediction outcome in this domain. Both models, irrespective of the neural net used, give poorer Sensitivity but similar Specificity to the POSSUM models.

The clinical risk prediction models `CM3a` and `CM4a` are two outcome models based on 16 (`CM3a`) and 14 (`CM4a`) input attributes. Table 4 shows the use of the three neural techniques (MLP, RBF, and SVM) on the same patient records as for `CM1` and `CM2` in table 3. Overall, all classifiers display identical *specificity* rates (about 0.85) with poor *sensitivity* rates (on average 0.18). The best of these classifiers (`CM3a-SVM`) gives poorer *sensitivity* performance than the POSSUM models. Again, similarly to the `CM1` and `CM2` results, these classifiers and models offer poor prediction results for identifying high risk patients.

Table 5 shows the confusion matrix results from applying the neural techniques to clinical models `CM3b` and `CM4b`, using the same 839 patient records but with the expanded outcome scales as described above. It is clear that for many records the outcome labeled as "*Medium risk*" is misclassified as "*Low risk*". This might be due to the close distance between the classes labeled as "*Medium risk*" and "Low risk" in the prediction risk scales defined in the heuristic formulae.

Overall none of the existing risk prediction models, when combined with the supervised neural net techniques, offer sufficiently high sensitivity rates to be considered useful for regular clinical practice or investigated further in trial studies for that purpose. Experimentation with other supervised techniques,

Table 3. Confusion matrix for CM1 and CM2 models with NN techniques

Classifiers	Risk	*High risk*	*Low risk*	Total	Sensitivity	Specificity
CM1-MLP	*High risk*	19	107	126	0.15	0.86
	Low risk	45	668	713		
CM1-RBF	*High risk*	23	103	126	0.18	0.86
	Low risk	33	680	713		
CM1-SVM	*High risk*	34	92	126	0.27	0.86
	Low risk	99	614	713		
CM2-MLP	*High risk*	24	111	135	0.18	0.85
	Low risk	32	672	704		
CM2-RBF	*High risk*	24	111	135	0.18	0.85
	Low risk	32	672	704		
CM2-SVM	*High risk*	17	118	135	0.13	0.85
	Low risk	23	681	704		

Table 4. Confusion matrix for CM3a and CM4a models with NN techniques

Classifiers	Risk	High risk	Low risk	Total	Sen	Spec
CM3a-MLP	High risk	26	109	135	0.19	0.85
	Low risk	79	625	704		
CM3a-RBF	High risk	20	115	135	0.15	0.85
	Low risk	24	680	704		
CM3a-SVM	High risk	32	103	135	0.24	0.85
	Low risk	111	593	704		
CM4a-MLP	High risk	28	107	135	0.20	0.85
	Low risk	69	635	704		
CM4a-RBF	High risk	19	116	135	0.14	0.85
	Low risk	17	687	704		
CM4a-SVM	High risk	20	115	135	0.15	0.85
	Low risk	49	655	704		

such as the many Decision Tree or Naïve Bayesian classifiers within WEKA, showed no improvement; and in many cases poorer performance.

An issue that came to light when discussing the results with the cardiovascular clinicians is an inherent bias in the given data. This bias arises from an interpretation of raw data from handwritten patient records as it was entered into the database. Judgments on interpreting values were made at that point. Unfortunately access to the raw, uninterpreted data is not possible. Problems associated with the gathering of the data are discussed further in the final sections of this chapter.

The use of otherwise reliable neural net (and other supervised classifier) techniques suggest that the input attribute set does not match well to the outcome label for any of these models. It is argued that this failure is due, in part, to the poor outcome labeling rules in the heuristic model rules and the poor transfer from general clinical practice to this specific domain for the POSSUM and PPOSSUM models. It is suggested that the input attribute set when used with no coerced outcome label may be sufficient to produce more reliable predictions for clinical risk. To do this requires the use of unsupervised classifier or machine learning techniques, where the inherent structure of the data is used to produce more natural outcomes (or clusters).

The Self Organizing Map (Kohonen, 1995) is one of the most popular unsupervised neural network models (Haykin, 1999). It is a competitive unsupervised learning network that produces a low dimensional output space where the input topological properties remain. The SOM provides a topology preserving mapping from the high dimensional input space onto the output map units. The topology preserving property means the mapping preserves the relative distance between points near each other in the input space, and nearby map units in the SOM. Hence, SOM can serve as a cluster analyzing tool of high-dimensional data, with the ability to recognize and characterize the input data. The input attributes from model CM3b were used to create a SOM within Matlab, with a final U-matrix quantization error of *1.723*, and topographic error of *0.021*. The U-matrix was then sectioned into 4 (predetermined) clusters; each defined using final quantization error and topographic error. While this provided what appeared to

Table 5. Confusion matrix for CM3b and CM4b models with NN techniques

Classifiers	Risk	*Very High risk*	*High risk*	*Medium risk*	*Low risk*
CM3b-MLP	*Very High risk*	3	3	0	14
	High risk	2	13	0	91
	Medium risk	0	1	0	12
	Low risk	6	53	5	636
CM3b-RBF	*Very High risk*	1	3	0	16
	High risk	3	6	2	95
	Medium risk	0	0	0	13
	Low risk	3	19	5	673
CM3b-SVM	*Very High risk*	0	2	0	18
	High risk	1	18	0	87
	Medium risk	0	0	0	13
	Low risk	9	98	10	583
CM4b-MLP	*Very High risk*	1	3	0	16
	High risk	2	18	0	86
	Medium risk	0	1	0	12
	Low risk	7	52	2	639
CM4b-RBF	*Very High risk*	1	4	1	14
	High risk	3	7	2	94
	Medium risk	0	1	0	12
	Low risk	3	11	2	684
CM4b-SVM	*Very High risk*	2	5	0	13
	High risk	4	12	0	90
	Medium risk	0	0	0	13
	Low risk	13	49	10	628

be visually appropriate groupings, SOM offers an uncertainty as a clustering algorithm, as alternative runs might offer alternative clustering results. Furthermore specific cases could not be easily identified so negating the use of SOM for individual patient risk assessment. So alternative means of performing unsupervised learning (or clustering) were investigated. The following sections detail this.

CLUSTERING WITH KMIX

Partitioning is a fundamental operation in data mining for dividing a set of objects into homogeneous clusters. Clustering is a popular partitioning approach. A set of objects are placed into clusters such that objects in the same cluster are more similar to each other than objects in other clusters according to some defined criteria. The K-means algorithm (Kanungo et al., 2002) is well used for implementing this operation because of its efficiency in clustering large data sets. However, K-means only works on continuous values. This limits its use in medical domains where data sets often contain Boolean, categorical, and continuous data. The traditional approach to convert categorical data into numeric values does not necessarily produce meaningful results where categorical attributes are not ordered. KMIX, and later WKMIX, are improved from K-means in order to cluster mixed numerical and categorical data values. In the KMIX algorithm, a dissimilarity measure is defined that takes into account both numeric and categorical attributes via the Euclidean distance for numerical features and the number of mismatches of categorical values for discrete features. For example, assume that $d^N(X,Y)$ is the squared Euclidean distance between two objects X and Y over continuous features; and $d^C(X,Y)$ is the dissimilarity measure on categorical features in X, Y. The dissimilarity between two objects X, Y is given by the distance:

$$d(X,Y) = d^N(X,Y) + d^C(X,Y) \qquad (10)$$

The clustering process of the KMIX algorithm is similar to the K-means algorithm except that a new method is used to update the categorical attribute values of cluster. The motivation for proposing KMIX based on K-means is that KMIX can be used for large data sets, where hierarchical clustering methods are not efficient.

Clustering and Similarity Measures

Cluster analysis provides the means for the organization of a collection of patterns into clusters based on the similarity of these patterns, where each pattern is represented as a vector in a multidimensional space. Assume that X is a pattern (an observation or sample from a data set). X typically consists of m components, represented in multidimensional space as:

$$X = (x_1, x_2, \ldots, x_m) = (x_j) \quad j = 1, \ldots, m$$

Each component in multidimensional space is called a feature (attribute). A data set includes n patterns X_i where $i \in [1, n]$ and $X_i = (x_{i,1}, x_{i,2}, \ldots, x_{i,m})$; forming a $n \otimes m$ pattern matrix. Note that the m features here may include continuous and discrete valued features. Due to the variety of feature types and scales, the distance measure (or measures) must be chosen carefully (Jain, 1999; Bishop, 2006). It is most common to calculate the dissimilarity between two patterns using a distance measure defined on the feature space.

A similarity measurement is the strength of the relationship between two patterns in the same multidimensional space. It can be represented as some function of their observed values such as:

$$sim_{i,j} = sim(x_i, x_j), \quad i, j \in [1, n]$$

Similarity is regarded as a symmetric relationship requiring $sim(x_i, x_j) = sim(x_j, x_i)$ (Gower, 1988). However, the dissimilarity measure of patterns has been introduced as the complement of similarity measures. Gower provides a list of dissimilarity measures. For continuous features, the most common used measure is the Euclidean distance between two patterns. This is very dependent upon the particular scales chosen for the variables (Everitt, 1994). Typically all (numeric) features are transformed to the range [0, 1], so as to avoid feature bias.

The dissimilarity measure of two "continuous" patterns using Euclidean distance is given as:

$$dissim(x_i, x_j) = [D(x_i, x_j)]^2 = \sum_{k=1}^{m} (x_{ik} - x_{jk})^2, i, j \in [1, n_1], n_1 \le n \quad (11)$$

where D is the Euclidean distance between x_i and x_j.

This means the dissimilarity of two patterns x_i and x_j is the sum of the square of the feature distance between them.

For discrete features, the similarity measure between two patterns depends on the number of similar values in each categorical feature (Kaufman & Rousseeuw, 1990). This means the dissimilarity will be the number of different values between two patterns for each categorical feature. We can represent this dissimilarity in the following formula:

$$dissim(x_i, x_j) = d(x_i, x_j) = \sum_{k=1}^{m} \theta(x_{ik}, x_{jk}) \quad i, j \in [1, n_2], n_2 \le n \quad (12)$$

where $\theta(x_{ik}, x_{jk}) = \begin{cases} 0 & if\ x_{ik} = x_{jk} \\ 1 & if\ x_{ik} \ne x_{jk} \end{cases}, \quad k = 1, 2, ..m; i, j \in [1, n_2]$

For binary features, the dissimilarity measures are calculated as for either discrete (categorical) features or continuous (numeric) valued attributes dependent on the interpretation of the provided binary data.

Clusters and Centre Vectors

For each cluster to be produced, the cluster defining vector is referred to as the centre vector. Here, the centre vector will include two groups of continuous and discrete components as the data feature set includes both continuous and discrete features; binary features are treated as continuous or discrete dependent upon the interpretation of each binary-valued attribute. Assume that the data feature set includes *m* features, where the *p* first features are continuous features and the *m-p* remaining features are discrete. This means each pattern X_i in the space can be seen as:

$$X_i = (x_{i1}, x_{i2}, \ldots x_{ip}, x_{ip+1}, x_{ip+2}, \ldots x_{im})$$

Assume that Q_j is a centre vector for the data set cluster *C* (*C* is a sub set of whole data set). So Q_j can be represented as:

$$Q_j = (q_{j1}, q_{j2}, \ldots q_{jp}, q_{jp+1}, q_{jp+2}, \ldots, q_{jm})$$

The task is to find *p continuous* component values, and *m-p discrete* component values for vector Q_j. For *continuous* component values, $\{q_{jk}\}_{k=1,..p}$ defines the means of the kth feature in *C*. For *discrete* component values, $\{q_{jk}\}_{k=p+1,...,m}$ defines the set of $mode_k$, where $mode_k$ is the mode of the kth feature.

Definition 1: A vector *Q* is a mode vector of a data set:

$$C = (X_1, X_2, \ldots X_c), c \le n$$

if the distance from each vector X_i $(i \in [1,c])$ is minimized. This means:

$$d(C,Q) = \sum_{i=1}^{c} d(X_i, Q)$$

is minimized. Huan (1998) proved that this distance will be minimized only if the frequency of value $q_j \in Q$ is maximized. This means the frequency of each value q_j in data set C, considered in terms of feature j, needs to be greater or equal to the frequency of all different $x_{i,j}$ such that $x_{i,j} \neq q_j$ for the same feature $(j \in [1,m])$. Hence we can choose the mode vector for the m-p categorical components where each component value is the mode of that feature or the value which has biggest frequency value in that feature using:

$$\{q_{jk}\}_{k=p+1,\dots,m} = \text{mode}_k = \{\max \text{freq}(\text{Val}_{Ck})\}$$

The K-MIX Algorithm

The K-MIX algorithm is a four step process:

- **Step 1:** Initialise K clusters according to K partitions of data matrix.
- **Step 2:** Update K centre vectors in the new data set (for the first time the centre vectors are calculated):

  $$Q_j = (q_{j1}^N, q_{j2}^N, \dots, q_{jp}^N, q_{jp+1}^C, \dots, q_{jm}^C), j \in [1, K]$$
  where $\{q_{jk}^N\}(k \in [1, p]) = \{\text{mean}_{jk}^N\}$ (mean of kth feature in cluster j)
  and $\{q_{jk}^C\}(k \in [p+1, m]) = \{\text{mode}_{jk}^C\}$ (mode of kth feature in cluster j)

- **Step 3:** Update clusters. Calculate the distance between X_i in i^{th} cluster to K centre vectors:

  $$d(X_i,Q_j) = d^N(X_i,Q_j) + d^C(X_i,Q_j); j = 1,2,..k \quad (13)$$
  where $d^N(X_i,Q_j)$ is calculated according to (11)
  and $d^C(X_i,Q_j)$ is calculated according to (12)

  Allocate X_i into the nearest cluster such that $d(X_i,Q_j)$ is least.
  Do this for whole data set, and save them to the new interpretation of the data set with K new centre vectors.
- **Step 4:** Repeat step 2 and 3 until no change in the distance between X_i and new K centre vectors is seen.

Experiments with Standard Data Sets

Before running on the target data domain, many experiments were run with data derived from the UCI repository of databases as used by the machine learning community for the empirical analysis of machine learning algorithms (Merz & Murphy, 1996). The clustering accuracy for measuring the clustering results was computed as follows. Given the final number of clusters, K, clustering accuracy r was defined as:

$$r = \sum_{i=1}^{K} a_i \Big/ n$$

where n is the number of samples in the dataset, a_i is the number of data samples occurring in both cluster i and its corresponding class. Consequently, the clustering error is defined as $e= 1- r$. The lower value of e suggests the better clustering result.

The experimental data sets are Small Soybean data set (Michalski & Chilausky, 1980) with 47 samples and 35 attributes, in 4 class distributions, Votes data set (Jeff, 1987) containing 16 key attributes with all categorical data types in 435 records (included meaningful missing value records "?"), and 2 output classes labelled to 168 republicans and 267 democrats. This algorithm is also used for experiments with Zoo small data set (Merz & Murphy, 1996). It has 101 records distributed in 7 categories with 18 attributes (included 15 Boolean, 2 numerical, and 1 unique attribute(s)). The fourth experiment for KMIX is with the Wisconsin Breast Cancer data set (Merz & Murphy, 1996). It contains 683 records by removing 16 missing value records. The data set includes 9 numerical attributes divided into 2 class label of "2" or "4". The comparison results can be seen in Table 6.

From Table 6, KMIX performs as well as other published results for the Soy Bean[1] [Ohn et al., 2004); Votes[2,] (Shehroz & Shri, 2007), Votes[3] (Zengyou et al., 2005), and Wisconsin Breast Cancer[4] (Camastra & Verri, 2005) data sets. For the latter, the KMIX result of 0.03 compares favourably compared to 0.132[2] (Shehroz & Shri, 2007). Further more, this algorithm solves problems associated with the mixture of categorical and discrete data; a common feature of medical data domains.

Experiments in the Clinical Domain

The research project requires that a comparative audit of the data for different outcomes to be investigated. Patient parameters such as "`Patient Status`", and the combination of other risk outcomes, such as "`Heart Disease`" (`HD`), "`Diabetes`" (`D`), and "`Stroke`" (`St`) may all be used as outcome indicators for individual patients. Subsequently a new summary output attribute (`Risk`) is built based on the value for the combination of the main disease symptoms. For alternative outcomes the appropriate models are built based on different heuristic rules:

- Model 1 (`CM32`): Two outcome levels are defined as:
  Σ(Status, Combine) = 0 $\rightarrow$ Risk =Low
  Σ(Status, Combine) > 0 $\rightarrow$ Risk =High

Table 6. Comparison of KMIX to publication results on standard data sets (see text for explanation of labels)

Data set	Publication results	KMIX results
Soy Bean	0.11[1] ~	0.07
Votes	0.132[2,3]	0.141
Zoo small	0.166[2]	0.151
Wisconsin Breast Cancer	0.03[4]; 0.132[2]	0.03

- Model 2 (CM33): Similar to CM32 but divided into three levels of risk:
  Σ(Status, Combine) = 0 $\rightarrow$ Risk =Low
  Σ(Status, Combine) = 1 $\rightarrow$ Risk =Medium
  Σ(Status, Combine) > 1 $\rightarrow$ Risk=High

These outcomes will be used to provide meaningful names to the clusters generated using the KMIX algorithm, and its variation WKMIX.

The next experiment used the K-means algorithm for comparison with KMIX on the cardiovascular data. Inputs were defined as the attribute set from the heuristic model CM3a; the best performing of the existing models. Hence these experiments were run using 16 input attributes, with 341 patient records. The results, in Table 7, show the derived clusters compared to the existing outcomes, and so indicate the extent of agreement between the unsupervised clustering algorithms and the existing clinical outcomes. The sensitivity rates for the two algorithms are small (0.15, 0.25 for K-means, and KMIX), with high specificity rates. However Table 7 clearly shows the advantage of KMIX over K-means, with it also improving over the best of the supervised classifiers (*CM3a-SVM*) in Table 4.

It is possible using KMIX to define the number of clusters required. Again, the input attribute set from clinical model CM3 was used, with the algorithm allowed to generate a two cluster output (model CM32) and a three cluster output (model CM33). The records associated with each cluster were cross-referenced to the Low, High (for CM32) and Low, Medium, High outcomes (for model CM33) associated with the clinical models. Supervised neural network techniques, Support Vector Machine (SVM), and Multilayer Perceptron (MLP), were then trained on these machine generated outcomes. Tables 8 and Table 9 show the results.

From Tables 8 and 9 it can be deduced that the boundary for each cluster may be ambiguous. However in Table 9 no High Risk patients were placed in the cluster most closely associated with Low Risk patients (C3). Fortunately in the cardiovascular domain, and the given data mining task, the clinician's interest is primarily with the identification of both medium and high risk patients. These cases can be

Table 7. Clustering results of K-means and KMIX compared to Model CM3a outcomes

Algorithm	Risk	C1 (High)	C2 (Low)	Sensitivity	Specificity
K-means	High	36	21	0.15	0.82
	Low	168	116		
KMIX	High	35	22	0.25	0.89
	Low	107	177		

Table 8. Supervised NN results for KMIX generated CM32 outcomes

Classifier	Cluster	C1 (High)	C2 (Low)	Sensitivity	Specificity
MLP	C1H	121	21	0.90	0.90
	C2L	13	186		
SVM	C1H	120	22	0.85	0.89
	C2L	22	177		

reported in terms of the sensitivity rate. In both table 8 and 9 both sensitivity and specificity rates are over 0.90 except for the `CM32-SVM` classifier (0.85; 0.89 respectively). The clinicians have an accepted rate of 0.80 for the use of neural classifiers; all classifiers achieve this. This suggests that the KMIX clustering results show some promise for the identification of risk for individual patients in the cardiovascular data domain. To better these results, an improved version was developed as explained in the next section.

CLUSTERING WITH WKMIX

WKMIX (Weighted KMIX), an extension to the KMIX algorithm described above, makes use of an entropy based measure to weight the input attributes. In the previous section, KMIX was described working with inputs where the attribute set was defined using the existing, acknowledged as flawed, risk prediction models. An alternative approach is to take the complete dataset and determine what are the more appropriate attributes to use as classifier and clustering inputs.

Feature selection is a very important step in classification (Liu & Motoda, 1998). It can reduce the irrelevant and redundant features, which often degrade the performance of classification algorithms in both speed and prediction accuracy. Most feature selection methods use certain evaluation functions and search procedures to achieve their targets. The evaluation functions measure how good a specific feature subset is in discriminating between the classes (Dash & Liu, 1997). Here a variation on Mutual Information is used. In this work, features determined to be irrelevant, using MI, are automatically given a low (near zero) coefficient; so reducing their impact on the clustering dissimilarity measure. Experimentation has shown that this technique is as reliable as the more common Relief feature selection techniques (Kononenko, 2001).

Mutual Information

Mutual Information (MI) measures the arbitrary dependencies between random variables. It is suitable for assessing the "information content" of the attribute contributions to the outcome classes in data domain. In information theory, Shannon (1948) defined entropy or information entropy as a measure of the uncertainty associated with a discrete random variable. Equivalently, entropy is a measure of the

Table 9. Supervised NN results for KMIX generated CM33 outcomes

Classifier	Cluster	C1 (Medium)	C2 (High)	C3 (Low)	Sensitivity	Specificity
MLP	C1M	75	4	6	0.98	0.96
	C2H	5	112	0		
	C3L	4	0	135		
SVM	C1M	71	0	14	0.98	0.91
	C2H	8	109	0		
	C3L	3	1	135		

average information content the recipient is missing when they do not know the value of the random variable. Mathematically, entropy can be written as:

$$H(X) = -c\sum_{i=1}^{n} p_i(x)\log p_i(x) \qquad (14)$$

where $p_i(x)$ is probabilities of occurrence in a set of possible events X, and c is a positive constant (usually c=1).

Suppose there are two events *X* and *Y*. *H(X,Y)* is a joint entropy of two discrete variables *X* and *Y* with a joint distribution *p(x,y)*, and *H(X,Y)* can be written as the follows:

$$H(X,Y) = -c\sum_{i=1}^{n}\sum_{j=1}^{m} p_{i,j}(x,y)\log p_{i,j}(x,y) \qquad (15)$$

where $p_{i,j}(x,y)$ is the probability of the joint occurrence of x for the first and y for the second.

The Mutual Information (MI) between two discrete random variables *X* and *Y*, *MI(X,Y)*, is a measure of the amount of information in *X* that can be predicted when *Y* is known. Whereas entropy is a measure of the uncertainty in its distribution (Shannon, 1948), the relative entropy (Equation 16) is a measure of the statistical distance between two distributions. Originally introduced by Kullback and Leibler (1951), it is known as the Kullback Leibler distance, or Kullback Leibler divergence (Cover & Thomas, 1991).

$$K(p,q) = \sum_{x\in A} p(x)\log\left(\frac{p(x)}{q(x)}\right) \qquad (16)$$

where p(x), q(x) are probability density functions of x.

For the case where *X* and *Y* are discrete random variables, *MI(X,Y)* can be written as the follows:

$$MI(X,Y) = H(X) - H(X \mid Y) = \sum_{i}\sum_{j} p_{i,j}(x,y)\log[p_{i,j}(x,y) \mid p_i(x)p_j(y)] \qquad (17)$$

where H(X) is the entropy of X, which is a measure of its uncertainty, and H(X|Y) (or $H_X(Y)$) is the conditional entropy, which represents the uncertainty in X after knowing Y.

The concepts of entropy can be extended to the continuous random variables (Shannon, 1948; Cover & Thomas, 1991). So *MI(X,Y)* for the continuous valued case can be written as:

$$MI(X,Y) = H(X) - H(X \mid Y) = \int p_{i,j}(x,y)\log\left(p_{i,j}(x,y) \mid p_i(x)p_j(y)\right)dxdy \qquad (18)$$

Based on the Kullback Leibler divergence, in equation 16, equations 17 and 18 can be rewritten as:

$$MI(x,y) = K(P(x),P(x).P(y)) = \sum_{x\in X}\sum_{y\in Y} P(x,y).\log\frac{P(x,y)}{P(x).P(y)} \qquad (19)$$

and:

$$MI(x,y) = K(P(x),P(x).P(y)) = \int_{-\infty}^{\infty}\int_{-\infty}^{\infty} P(x,y).\log\frac{P(x,y)}{P(x).P(y)}dxdy \qquad (20)$$

The Weighted KMIX Algorithm (WKMIX)

This algorithm is improved from KMIX algorithm by putting the weight for each attribute during the cluster process in KMIX algorithm. The steps of the algorithm are the same as the KMIX algorithm described above, and equation 13 is rewritten as:

$$d(X_i,Q_j) = W_{iN}d^N(X_i,Q_j) + W_{iC}d^C(X_i,Q_j); j=1,2,..k \tag{21}$$

where W_{iN}, W_{iC} are the MI of each numerical, or categorical attribute, and all the ith,j^{th}, and k^{th} remain unchanged in their meaning.

The MI for Equation 20 is calculated as in Equation 22:

$$MI(C,x_j) = \sum_{i=1}^{c} \sum_{k=1}^{s} p_{ijk} \log\left(\frac{p_{ijk}}{q_i.r_{jk}}\right) \tag{22}$$

where:

$p_{ijk} = \frac{sum_{ijk}}{sum}$ with sum_{ijk} the number of patterns in class C_i with attribute x_j in state k.

$q_i = \frac{sum_i}{sum}$ where sum_i is number of patterns belong to class C_i

$r_{jk} = \frac{sum_{jk}}{sum}$ where sum_{jk} is number of patterns with attribute x_j in the kth state.

Hence Equation 21 is finally rewritten as:

$$d(X_i,Q_j) = MI_{iN}d^N(X_i,Q_j) + MI_{iC}d^C(X_i,Q_j); j=1,2,..k \tag{23}$$

The experimental data used here is identical to that used in comparing the K-Means and KMIX algorithms, using the inputs attributes from risk prediction model CM3a. The results from the weighted KMIX algorithm (WKMIX) are compared to the KMIX algorithm from Table 7 (for the CM3a model), and given in Table 10. The WKMIX outcome models are then derived from the clustering results. These models are then investigated with the use of supervised NN techniques.

General speaking, Table 10 shows that the experimental performance of using an Information Theory based weight in clustering is higher than without it. In particular, the sensitivity and specificity rates for using weights (WKMIX) are the highest of any model and classifier combination in this study (1, 0.96). They better the use of the clustering algorithm without attribute weight (KMIX: 0.25, 0.89), and higher than the rate from clinical expert's advice (about 80%).

Table 10. The results of alternative weights for CM3a model

Algorithm	Output	High risk	Low risk	Sensitivity	Specificity
WKMIX	*High risk*	48	9	1	0.96
	Low risk	0	284		
KMIX	*High risk*	35	22	0.25	0.89
	Low risk	107	177		

The new clustering model (CM3aC) is built with new outcomes derived from the clusters produced using the WKMIX algorithm. The NN techniques applied here are Support Vector Machine (SVM); Radial Basis Function (RBF); and MultLayer Perceptron (MLP). More over the decision tree technique J48 is also applied to this new model. The results can be seen in Table 11. This shows that there are no errors in the classification process (MSE =0.00) except with the use of the RBF technique (0.08). Moreover, all classifiers achieve very high *sensitivity* and *specificity* rates.

Looking at the confusion matrix in Table 11, it is clear that all techniques classified the risks the same as the clustering results except RBF with 2 mis-classed "*High risk*" and 1 mis-classed "*Low risk*" respectively. Interestingly, from Table 11 the sensitivity and specificity rates achieve ideal results except for the Radial Basis Function net (0.97 and 0.99 respectively). This means the neural techniques (SVM and MLP) and the decision tree method (J48) achieve 100% accuracy.

Although this study achieves ideal results from a data mining perspective, its acceptance as a clinical risk model is problematic. The use of MI values as algorithm weights achieves a high performance in the case study, albeit on attributes associated with an existing clinical heuristic model. An extended investigation with an expanded data set is required, allowing an increased number of attributes and patterns. Such a study is perhaps best undertaken in closer collaboration with the consultant clinicians within the aegis of a clinical study to derive a more reliable, medically acceptable, risk prediction model.

DISCUSSION

The paucity of the current risk prediction models, in cardiovascular medicine, are made evident in this case study, with none of the existing individual patient risk prediction models being able to better 27% sensitivity (Support Vector Machine classifier with clinical model CM1 in Table 3), although many of the models present 85% Specificity. The POSSUM and PPOSSUM models better this but with the disadvantage of losing single patient risk prediction capability. The clinicians working in this field of medicine are well aware of these limitations in their current models (Kuhan et al, 2001). However the clustering algorithms which use the input attribute sets from these models (and WKMIX in particular) manage to produce very much higher Sensitivity and Specificity. This suggests that the outcome models

Table 11. The results of alternative techniques for the CM3aC clustering model

Classifier	Risk	High risk	Low risk	MSE	Sens	Spec	Accuracy
SVM	High risk	48	0	0.00	1	1	100%
	Low risk	0	293				
RBF	High risk	46	2	0.08	0.97	0.99	99%
	Low risk	1	292				
MLP	High risk	48	0	0.00	1	1	100%
	Low risk	0	293				
J48	High risk	48	0	0.00	1	1	100%
	Low risk	0	293				

in the existing clinical risk prediction models are inadequate. Furthermore it suggests that much better risk prediction models are possible and that the present attributes offer sufficient inherent patterns, as detected using these clustering algorithms, to support much better risk prediction rules.

The proposed algorithm KMIX compares favourably to publicised results on standard machine learning data sets. Furthermore, because this algorithm was developed for use with a specific medical data domain, it meets the requirement to work with data that contains a mixture of numerical, categorical and Boolean data types. By using the clustering algorithm, new outcomes are generated for input attributes associated with the heuristic CM32 and CM33 risk models. These new models are evaluated through the use of the neural network techniques, such as MLP and SVM. From Table 8 and 9 we can see that the boundary of each cluster is not clear. For example, in Table 8, a number of high risk patients (C1H) fell in clusters C1 and C2. However no high risk patients were placed in the cluster most closely associated with low risk patients (C3 in Table 9). Fortunately in the cardiovascular domain, the clinician's interest is in the rate of potential risk of patients (medium and high risk). Further work on improving this algorithm allowed weights to be applied in order to indicate the level of importance for attributes in the feature set for the data domain. This algorithm gives near ideal classifier performance on the given clinical data. However, alternative data domains need to be investigated to determine the usefulness of this algorithm for medical data domains in general.

The history of expert and knowledge base systems contains many examples of intelligent decision systems used in medical domains (Davies & Owen, 1990; Shortliffe, 1990). More recently decision support tools that make use of data mining techniques have been developed for medicine (Groselj, 2002; Lavrač & Zupan, 2005). The combination of clinical knowledge and the approach adopted in this case study via fuzzy set theory might produce a realistically more intelligent tool for the risk prediction process (Negnevitsky, 2004). Moreover, the use of neuro-fuzzy classification techniques might enhance the results; enabling multiple models to be used to suit the needs of the clinician, and make for more reliable risk prediction in a clinical situation. For this to happen, a number of important and time-consuming hurdles, relating to clinical trials, have to be met. Most of these hurdles are the constraints imposed by a highly regulated health system. Some are the results of ill-informed clinical data practices. The latter are particularly problematic where paper based data collection (i.e. patient records) are prevalent. In an effort to simplify subsequent human decision making, much data is interpreted as it is transferred to computer record. This means that instead of access to raw data (and many meaningful data values), many clinical attributes are reduced to a small number of clinical interpretations. The interpretation can vary from one region to another and between clinicians, according to their school of thought on best medical practice. This form of interpretation introduces a bias into the data model that cannot be overcome by any data mining technique, other than collection of the original raw values. Such a bias in the data will cause problems for even the most intelligent of decision systems.

CONCLUSION

This case study showed the advantages of using Pattern Recognition techniques in producing risk models. However, these techniques are poor in providing a visualization of the data domain. Although the Self Organising Feature Map (SOM) showed its ability to visualize the data, its clustering was limited. Further research with a combination of KMIX or WKMIX and SOM might provide meaningful insights into the nature of the data, cluster models and medical outcomes.

The concept of MI is introduced and discussed in depth. From there, a combination of Bayes theorem and MI produced a new formula to calculate the MI between the attributes and the outcome classes (Equation 22). This idea has been used for alternative data mining purposes (water quality ascription) as a measurement for SOM clustering (O'Connor & Walley, 2000). Here it is used for ranking the significance of attributes in the cardiovascular data domain. The rewriting of the KMIX algorithm by using the MI weights provides a new clustering algorithm. Although its results show a very high performance level, more investigation was needed. The use of MI values as the weights in the clustering algorithm (WKMIX) has given better initial results. However, more experiments with alternative sources of data need to be investigated. The building of an independent feature selection algorithm using MI is another further task. This will be one of the required tools for the classification process, in particular with the current data domain.

This research has shown how Pattern Recognition and Data Mining techniques (both supervised and unsupervised) can better the current risk prediction models in cardiovascular data. The research can be seen as setting the base knowledge, with a set of practical decision metrics, for a complete decision support tool in the cardiovascular area. The research limitations for its use require a more complete ontology for the medical domain, involving general medical knowledge. Furthermore, it cannot be used in trials for clinical diagnosis, without ethical clearance. So, the supervised and unsupervised results in these case studies can not, as yet, be used to support the clinicians in their decision making for individual cardiovascular patients. There needs to be further collaborative research, between clinicians and computer scientists, to build a more complete decision support tool for the cardiovascular area. A complete decision tool is one that encompasses every stage of the decision process from the collection of raw data to feedback on predictions. Making the clinicians aware of their data gathering practices, and the effect it has on subsequent computer based decision making is an issue that will have a great impact on the feasibility of such collaborations. Hopefully, the move to collecting raw data directly onto computer databases rather than relying on the interpretation of data in paper based systems may help to reduce clinical bias. The same is probably true for many other clinical domains. Given this proviso, the future for data mining domain improving risk prediction in medical domains looks very promising.

ACKNOWLEDGMENT

The majority of the work reported here is undertaken in conjunction with PhD thesis research at the Computer Science Department in The University of Hull. Funding for the PhD studentship to Ms Nguyen is from the Government of Vietnam, with further travel bursaries from The Clinical Biosciences Institute, University of Hull. We are grateful for the clinical input from cardiovascular consultants, Dr Ganesh Kuhan and Professor Peter McCollum of the Hull Royal Infirmary.

REFERENCES

Bishop, C. M. (2006). *Pattern Recognition and Machine Learning.* Springer.

Camastra, F., & Verri, A. (2005). A novel Kernel Method for Clustering. *IEEE Transaction on Pattern Analysis and Machine Intelligence (PAMI), 27(5),* 801-805.

Copeland, G. P. (2002). The POSSUM system of surgical audit. *Archives of Surgery, 137*, 15-19.

Cover, T., & Thomas, J. (1991). *The Elements of Information Theory*. NewYork: Plenum Press.

Dash, M., & Liu, H. (1997). Feature selection for classification. *Intelligent Data Analysis, 1(3).*

Davies, M., & Owen, K. (1990). Complex uncertain decisions: medical diagnosis. Case Study 10 in *Expert System Opportunities from the DTI's Research Technology Initiative*, HMSO.

Everitt, B. S. (1994). *Cluster Analysis*, 3rd ed. John Wiley & Son, New York.

Gower, J. C. (1988). Classification, geometry and data analysis. In H.H. Bock, (Ed.), *Classification and Related Methods of Data Analysis. Elsevier*, North-Holland, Amsterdam.

Groselj, C. (2002). Data Mining Problems in Medicine. *15th IEEE Symposium on Computer-Based Medical Systems (CBMS'02)*. Maribor, Slovenia.

Haykin, S. (1999). *Neural networks: A comprehensive foundation*, 2/e, Macmillan College Publishing Company, Inc.

Huan, Z. (1998). Extensions to the K-Means Algorithm for Clustering Large Data Sets with Categorical Values. *Data Mining and Knowledge Discovery, 2(3).* Kluwer Academic Publishers

Jain, A. K. (1999). Data clustering: A review. *ACM Computing Surveys, 31(3).*

Janet, F. (1997). Artificial Neural Networks Improve Diagnosis of Acute Myocardial Infarction. *Lancet, 350(9082)*, 935.

Jeff, S. (1987). *Concept acquisition through representational adjustment.* Doctoral dissertation, Department of Information and Computer Science, University of California, Irvine, CA

Kanungo, T., Mount, D. M., Netanyahu, N., Piatko, C., Silverman, R. & Wu, A. Y. (2002). An efficient K-Means clustering algorithm: Analysis and implementation. *IEEE Trans. Pattern Analysis and Machine Intelligence, 24*, 881-892.

Kaufman, L., & Rousseeuw, P. J. (1990). *Finding Groups in Data—An Introduction to Cluster Analysis.* Wiley.

Kohavi, R., & Provost, F. (1998). Glossary of Terms. *Machine Learning, 30(2/3)*, 271-274.

Kohonen, T. (1995). *Self-Organizing Maps.* Springer, Berlin, Heidelberg.

Kononenko, I. (2001). Machine Learning for Medical Diagnosis: History, State of the Art and Perspective. *Artificial Intelligent Medicine. 23(1)*, 89-109.

Kononenko, I., & Kukar, M. (2007). *Machine Learning and Data Mining.* Horwood Publishing Ltd.

Kuhan, G., Gadiner, E. D., Abidia, A. F., Chetter, I. C., Renwick, P. M., Johnson, B. F., Wilkinson, A. R., & McCollum, P. T. (2001). Risk Modelling study for carotid endatorectomy. *British Journal of Surgery, 88*, 1590-1594.

Kullback, S., & Leibler, R. A. (1951). On information and sufficiency. Annals *of Mathematical Statistics, 22*, 79-86.

Lavrač, N., & Zupan, B. (2005). Data Mining in Medicine. In O. Maimon & L. Rokach (Eds.). *Data Mining and Knowledge Discovery Handbook*, Springer US.

Lisboa, P. J. G. (2002). A review of evidence of health benefit from artificial neural networks in medical intervention. *Neural Network, 15*, 11-39.

Liu, H., & Motoda, H. (1998). *Feature Selection for Knowledge Discovery and Data Mining.* Kluwer Academic, Norwell, MA USA.

Merz, C. J. & Murphy, P. (1996). UCI *Repository of Machine Learning Database*. Available: http://www.ics.uci.edu/~mlearn/MLRepository.html

Michalski, R. S. & Chilausky, R. L. (1980). Learning by Being Told and Learning from Examples: An Experimental Comparison of the Two Methods of Knowledge Acquisition in the Context of Developing an Expert System for Soy- bean Disease Diagnosis. *International Journal of Policy Analysis and Information Systems, 4(2)*, 125-161.

Negnevitsky, M. (2004). Design of a hybrid neuro-fuzzy decision-support system with a heterogeneous structure. *Proceedings IEEE International Conference on Fuzzy Systems, 2,* 1049-1052.

O'Connor, M. A., & Walley, W. J. (2000). An information theoretic self-organising map with disaggregation of output classes. *2nd Int. Conf. on Environmental Information systems, Stafford, UK.* 108-115. ISBN 9 72980 501 6.

Ohn, M. S., Van-Nam, H., & Yoshiteru, N. (2004). An alternative extension of the K-means algorithm for clustering categorical data. *International Journal Mathematic Computer Science, 14(2),* 241-247.

Prytherch, D. R., Sutton, G. L., & Boyle, J. R. (2001). Portsmouth POSSUM models for abdominal aortic aneurysm surgery. *British Journal of Surgery, 88(7),* 958-63.

Rowan, K. M., Kerr, J. H., Major, E., McPherson, K., Short, A., & Vessey, M. P. (1994). Intensive Care Society's Acute Physiology and Chronic Health Evaluation (APACHE II) study in Britain and Ireland: a prospective, multicenter, cohort study comparing two methods for predicting outcome for adult intensive care patients. *Critical Care Medicine, 22,* 1392-1401.

Shannon, C. E. (1948). A mathematical theory of communication. *Bell System Technical Journal, 27,* 379-423 and 623-656.

Shehroz, S. K., & Shri, K. (2007). Computation of initial modes for K-modes clustering algorithm using evidence accumulation. *20th International Joint Confference on Artificial Intelligence (IJCAI-07),* India.

Shortliffe, E. H. (1990). Clinical decision-support systems. In Shortliffe, E.H., Perreault, L. E.,Wiederhold, G., & Fagan, L. M. (Eds.). *Medical informatics - Computer Applications in Health Care*, Addison-Wesley, Reading, M.A.

Swets, J. (1988). Measuring the accuracy of diagnostic systems. *Science, 240,* 1285-1293.

Tom, F. (2006). An introduction to ROC analysis. *Pattern Recognition Letters, 27.* Science Direct, Elsevier.

Witten, I. H. & Eibe, F. (2005). *Data Mining: Practical Machine Learning Tools and Techniques with Java Implementations.* Morgan Kaufmann, 2/e.

Yii, M. K., & Ng, K. J. (2002). Risk-adjusted surgical audit with the POSSUM scoring system in a developing country. *British Journal of Surgery, 89*, 110-113.

Zengyou, H., Xiaofei, X., & Shengchun, D. (2005). TCSOM: Clustering Transactions Using Self-Organizing Map. *Neural Processing Letters, 22*, 249–262.

KEY TERMS

Centre Vectors: For each cluster to be produced, the cluster defining vector (the idealized data entry for that cluster) is referred to as the centre vector.

Clustering: Clustering is a popular partitioning approach, whereby a set of objects are placed into clusters such that objects in the same cluster are more similar to each other than objects in other clusters according to some defined criteria.

Confusion Matrix: A confusion matrix or table details the number of correct and incorrect (or misclassified) patterns generated by a classifier. It gives rise to measures such as accuracy, true positive rate, false positive rate, sensitivity and specificity.

Mutual Information: Mutual Information measures the arbitrary dependencies between random variables. It arises from information theory, where Shannon (1948) defined entropy or information entropy as a measure of the uncertainty associated with a discrete random variable.

Partitioning: Partitioning is a fundamental operation in data mining for dividing a set of objects into homogeneous clusters, or sets of data that are more similar to each other than other data. A partition can be hierarchical in nature.

Risk Prediction: Risk prediction models offer the means to aide selection from a general medical population, those patients that need referral to medical consultants and specialists.

Sensitivity: The sensitivity rate indicates the effectiveness of a classifier at identifying the true positive cases, i.e. those cases that are of most interest.

Specificity: The specificity rate indicates the effectiveness of a classifier at identifying the true negative cases, i.e. those cases that are the complement of those categories of most interest.

Supervised Classifier: A classifier that learns to associate patterns in data with a-priori (given) labels for each pattern. Examples include multi-layer perceptrons and decision trees.

Chapter X
Management of Medical Website Quality Labels via Web Mining

Vangelis Karkaletsis
National Center of Scientific Research "Demokritos", Greece

Konstantinos Stamatakis
National Center of Scientific Research "Demokritos", Greece

Pythagoras Karampiperis
National Center of Scientific Research "Demokritos", Greece

Martin Labský
University of Economics, Prague, Czech Republic

Marek Růžička
University of Economics, Prague, Czech Republic

Vojtěch Svátek
University of Economics, Prague, Czech Republic

Enrique Amigó Cabrera
ETSI Informática, UNED, Spain

Matti Pöllä
Helsinki University of Technology, Finland

Miquel Angel Mayer
Medical Association of Barcelona (COMB), Spain

Dagmar Villarroel Gonzales
Agency for Quality in Medicine (AquMed), Germany

ABSTRACT

The World Wide Web is an important channel of information exchange in many domains, including the medical one. The ever increasing amount of freely available healthcare-related information generates, on the one hand, excellent conditions for self-education of patients as well as physicians, but on the other hand, entails substantial risks if such information is trusted irrespective of low competence or even bad intentions of its authors. This is why medical Web site certification, also called quality labeling, by renowned authorities is of high importance. In this respect, it recently became obvious that the labelling process could benefit from employment of Web mining and information extraction techniques, in combination with flexible methods of Web-based information management developed within the Semantic Web initiative. Achieving such synergy is the central issue in the MedIEQ project. The AQUA (Assisting Quality Assessment) system, developed within the MedIEQ project, aims to provide the infrastructure and the means to organize and support various aspects of the daily work of labelling experts.

INTRODUCTION

The number of health information websites and online services is increasing day by day. It is known that the quality of these websites is very variable and difficult to assess; we can find websites published by government institutions, consumer and scientific organizations, patients associations, personal sites, health provider institutions, commercial sites, etc. (Mayer et.al., 2005). On the other hand, patients continue to find new ways of reaching health information and more than four out of ten health information seekers say the material they find affects their decisions about their health (Eysenbach, 2000; Diaz et.al., 2002). However, it is difficult for health information consumers, such as the patients and the general public, to assess by themselves the quality of the information because they are not always familiar with the medical domains and vocabularies (Soualmia et.al., 2003).

Although there are divergent opinions about the need for certification of health websites and adoption by Internet users (HON, 2005), different organizations around the world are working on establishing standards of quality in the certification of health-related web content (Winker et.al., 2000; Kohler et.al., 2002; Curro et.al., 2004; Mayer et.al., 2005). The European Council supported an initiative within eEurope 2002 to develop a core set of "Quality Criteria for Health Related Websites" (EC, 2002). The specific aim was to specify a commonly agreed set of simple quality criteria on which Member States, as well as public and private bodies, may build upon for developing mechanisms to help improving the quality of the content provided by health-related websites. These criteria should be applied in addition to relevant Community law. As a result, a core set of quality criteria was established. These criteria may be used as a basis in the development of user guides, voluntary codes of conduct, trust marks, certification systems, or any other initiative adopted by relevant parties, at European, national, regional or organizational level.

This stress on content quality evaluation contrasts with the fact that most of the current Web is still based on HTML, which only specifies how to layout the content of a web page addressing human readers. HTML as such cannot be exploited efficiently by information retrieval techniques in order to provide visitors with additional information on the websites' content. This "current web" must evolve in the next years, from a repository of human-understandable information, to a global knowledge repository, where information should be machine-readable and processable, enabling the use of advanced knowledge management technologies (Eysenbach, 2003). This change is based on the exploitation of *semantic web* technologies. The Semantic Web is "an extension of the current web in which information is given a well-defined meaning, better enabling computers and people to work in cooperation" based on metadata (i.e. semantic annotations of the web content) (Berners-Lee et.al., 2001). These metadata can be expressed in different ways using the Resource Description Framework (RDF) language. RDF is the key technology behind the Semantic Web, providing a means of expressing data on the web in a structured way that can be processed by machines.

In order for the medical quality labelling mechanisms to be successful, they must be equipped with semantic web technologies that enable the creation of machine-processable labels as well as the automation of the labelling process. Among the key ingredients for the latter are *web crawling* techniques that allow for retrieval of new unlabelled web resources, or *web spidering and extraction* techniques that facilitate the characterization of retrieved resources and the continuous monitoring of labeled resources alerting the labelling agency in case some changes occur against the labelling criteria.

The *AQUA* (Assisting QUality Assessment) system[1], developed within the MedIEQ project[2], aims to provide the infrastructure and the means to organize and support various aspects of the daily work of labelling experts by making them computer-assisted. AQUA consists of five major components (each, in turn, incorporating several specialized tools): Web Content Collection (WCC), Information Extraction (IET), Multilingual Resources Management (MRM), Label Management environment (LAM), and Monitor Update Alert (MUA). While WCC, IET and MUA together constitute the web data analysis engine of AQUA, MRM provides them access to language-dependent medical knowledge contained in terminological resources, and LAM handles the generation, storage and retrieval of resulting labels. The user interface of AQUA allows for both entirely manual labelling and labelling based on the results of automatic analysis. In this chapter we will describe the challenges addressed and results achieved by applying the WCC and IET tools to raw web data, as well as the subsequent processes of quality label handling by LAM.

CATEGORIES AND QUALITY OF MEDICAL WEB CONTENT: A SURVEY

In order to investigate what types of Medical Web Content exist, at the beginning of the project we conducted a survey on a set of Greek health-related websites, classifying them into the following categories: "government organization", "healthcare service provider", "media and publishers", "patient organization / self support group", "pharmaceutical company / retailer", "private individual" and "scientific or professional organization". Apart from the categorization of these websites, we also collected additional information for them in order to construct a *medical web map*. The extra fields of information were the following: "last update", "language(s)", "title", "location", "description" and "keywords" of the website but also "trust marks: are they present or not", "trustworthiness (a first estimation on the quality of the medical content: is it reliable?)", "advertisements: are they present or not?".

We first collected a few thousands of URLs with the assistance of a *search engine wrapper*. The wrapper queried the Google search engine with several sets of health related keywords, in both Greek and English languages, and collected the resulting websites. From the English keywords' results we only kept those corresponding to websites originated from Greece. On the resulting Greek URLs' list, an automated filtering procedure was applied, where duplicates, overlapping and other irrelevant URLs were removed. 1603 URLs remained. Checking manually the remaining URLs, 723 websites were selected for having health-related content. These were then categorized according to the categories mentioned above. The *crawling software*, developed for the purposes of the project, based on machine learning and heuristic methods, extracted the machine detectable information, which is "last update", "language(s)", "title", "location", "description" and "keywords".

Apparently, the 723 sites examined do not cover the totality of the Greek medical web content. However, they comprise a fair sample of that, which allowed us to make some useful observations with regard to this content.

Table 1. Categorization of Medical Web Content under review

Categories	*URLs*	*Percentage (%)*
Government organizations	15	2%
Healthcare service providers	211	28%
Media and publishers	64	9%
Patient organizations/ self support groups	33	5%
Pharmaceutical companies/ retailers	51	7%
Private individuals	199	28%
Scientific or professional organizations	110	15%
Universities/ research institutions	40	6%
Total	**723**	**100%**

The majority of websites belong to the *healthcare service provider* category (211 URLs) and to the *private individual* category (199 URLs). This fact reveals that in Greek medical web, the private sector is dominant (which seems reasonable), while the websites coming from the public sector like government organizations and universities/research institutions are a minority (54 URLs). Furthermore, it is remarkable that a great portion (110 URLs) of the Greek medical web belongs to scientific/professional organizations.

We also noticed that, at the time of the survey, only three websites had a *quality seal*, namely, HON Code (HON, 2001) and all of them belong to the *scientific or professional organization* category. We could argue that the non-conformance to trust mark quality criteria characterizes the Greek medical web as a whole, which demonstrates that Greek online medical content providers are not familiar with the quality labelling aspect. Thus, the quality of the content of Greek medical websites appears to be doubtful. To support this, note that the HTML tags for "description" and "keywords" (which the crawler reads automatically), were found as either empty or containing misleading information in most Greek medical pages, while, for example, a quick look into a portion of the German medical web showed the opposite. Concluding, only few Greek medical websites conform to the biggest part of the selected criteria as to be considered of good quality.

We also conducted analogous but less elaborate studies for other 'less-spoken' languages that are involved in the MedIEQ project but not covered by the partner labelling agencies, namely Czech and Finnish. The first observations of the Czech and Finnish medical web maps seem to confirm the hypotheses formed based on the analysis of Greek websites detailed above.

Thus, the establishment of mechanisms/infrastructures for the quality certification of health related websites is quite critical. Its positive role would amount to forcing health content providers to the following directions:

- For *existing* online medical content: conform to generally accepted quality criteria defined by experts. For online medical content *planned* to be published: adapt to specific standards (presence of detailed information on the content provider, authorship information, last update, contact data, etc.).
- *High-quality* websites, already trusted by health information consumers, would clearly boost the opinion that the web is not an advertising-oriented or dangerous space, but a powerful source of

information and must be considered as such. In the same direction, the national medical sector could be motivated to develop web resources of quality, extending the usefulness of the medium and eventually attracting a larger amount of users.

The MedIEQ project aims to directly contribute to this direction.

STATE OF THE ART IN HEALTH WEB QUALITY LABELLING

Two major approaches currently exist concerning the labelling of health information in the internet: a) *filtering portals* (organizing resources in health topics and providing opinions from specialists on their content) and b) *third-party certification* (issuing certification trustmarks or seals once the content conforms to certain principles). In general, and in both approaches, the labelling process comprises three tasks that are carried out entirely or partially by most labelling agencies:

- *Identification* of new web resources: this could happen either by active web searching or on the request of the information provider, i.e. the website responsible actively asks for the review in order to get a certification seal.
- *Labelling* of the web resources: this could be done with the purpose of awarding a certification seal or in order to classify and index the web resources in a filtering portal.
- *Re-reviewing* or *monitoring* the labeled web resources: this step is necessary to identify changes or updates in the resources as well as broken links, and to verify if a resource still deserves to be awarded the certification seal.

This is the general case; eventually, any particular agency can integrate additional steps which may be necessary in its work. The two labelling agencies participating in MedIEQ, Agency for Quality in Medicine – AQuMed (http://www.aezq.de) and Web Mèdica Acreditada - WMA (http://wma.comb.es), represent the two approaches mentioned above: AQuMed maintains a filtering portal while WMA acts as a third-party certification agency.

The indexing and labelling process in AQuMed consists of five steps:

1. *Inclusion of a new resource.* There are two ways through which a new resource can be identified for indexing in AQuMed database. The first one is through internet search and the second one is through a direct request from the information provider. The websites are selected according to general criteria: content, form and presentation should be serious, authorship, sponsorship and creation/update date should be clear, and only websites without commercial interest should be indexed.
2. *Website classification.* Previously unlabelled websites are classified into four groups: treatment information, background information, medical associations/scientific organizations and self-help/counseling organizations. Only the sites with treatment information proceed to the next step.
3. *Evaluation.* Sites with treatment information are evaluated using the DISCERN (DISCERN, 2008) and Check-In (Sanger, 2004) instruments. DISCERN is a well-known user guidance instrument, and Check-In was developed by AQuMed in collaboration with the "Patient Forum" of the German

Medical Association. Check-In is based on DISCERN and the AGREE (AGREE, 2004) instrument for critical evaluation of medical guidelines.

4. *Confirmation.* The database administrator has to confirm the result of the evaluation. It can be modified, erased, or simply confirmed.
5. *Feedback to the information provider.* AQuMed sends an e-mail with the result of the evaluation in the case of sites with treatment information and with the information about the admission into the AQuMed database in the case of other categories.

AQuMed's database is periodically populated through new internet searches and is regularly examined for broken links. The evaluated web resources are also periodically re-reviewed in order to identify changes against the criteria or other updates.

Similarly, the complete certification process in WMA consists of the following four steps:

1. The person in charge of a website sends a (voluntary) request to WMA in order to initiate the process. Using the online application form, the interested party provides certain information to WMA and has the chance to auto-check the WMA criteria based on the Code of Conduct and the Ethical Code;
2. The WMA Standing Committee assesses the website based on the WMA criteria (medical authorship, updating, web accessibility, rules in virtual consultation, etc.), and issues recommendations;
3. WMA sends a report to the person in charge who implements the recommendations;
4. When the recommendations have been implemented, it is possible to obtain the seal of approval. In such a case, WMA sends an HTML seal code to be posted on the accredited website. In addition, WMA includes the site's name and URL to the index of accredited websites and an RDF file is generated.

EXPERIMENTAL COLLECTION OF LABELLING CRITERIA

In the MedIEQ project we decided to develop a representative collection of *labelling criteria*, which would reflect the needs of the *labelling agencies* involved in the project consortium and at the same time provide an adequate proof of concept for our general methodology for computer-assisted labelling. It is important to stress that the methodology and software tools are to a large degree independent of the concrete criteria and thus could be easily adapted to different criteria used by various agencies. Such adaptation is also eased by the fact that the criteria specification was also influenced by the analysis of criteria used by other organizations such as HON, and thus has significant overlap with them.

The set of labelling criteria used in MedIEQ (36 in total, organized in 10 different categories) is shown in Table 2. For each of these criteria, the AQUA system aims to identify and extract relevant information to be proposed to the expert (i.e. automatically provide information otherwise searched for manually within the site). The expert can accept or modify AQUA's suggestions and generate a quality label on the fly.

Table 2. The set of criteria examined in MedIEQ

ID	Criterion Name	Description
1. Resource Defining Information		
1.1	Resource URI	Includes information identifying/describing the resource. Concerning the resource URI: a) whether the resource's URI is valid or not and b) in case it redirects to external domains, are these domains between those specified when the resource was added? The rest is information like the resource's last update, its title and the language(s) in which content is provided.
1.2	Resource title	
1.3	Resource last update	
1.4	Resource language(s)	
2. Ownership / Creatorship		
2.1	Organization name(s) (owner)	The user should know who is behind the resource in order to judge by himself the credibility of the provided information. Therefore, information like the name(s) of the organization(s) providing the information and the type of this(these) organization(s) should be available. At the same time, the name(s), title(s) (e.g. MD, PhD, Dr, etc.) and contact details of website responsible(s), to contact in case of questions on health related issues, as well as the name(s) and contact details of the webmaster(s) should be available.
2.2	Organization type(s) (owner)	
2.3	Responsible name(s)	
2.4	Responsible title(s)	
2.5	Responsible(s) contact details	
2.6	Webmaster name(s)	
2.7	Webmaster(s) contact details	
3. Purpose / mission		
3.1	Purpose / mission of the resource provided	It has to be clear for the user which is the goal and motivation of the provided information and for what kind of users it was created e.g. adults, children, people with diabetes, etc.
3.2	Purpose / mission of the owner(s) provided	
3.3	Target / intended audience(s)	
3.4	Statement declaring limitation of the provided information	
4. Topics / Keywords		
4.1	Topics / Keywords (UMLS)	Mapping of the resource's content to concepts from the UMLS Metathesaurus.
5. Virtual consultation		
5.1	VC service available	A virtual consultation (VC) service is an online service allowing the user to ask questions and/or send/upload information on health related issues asking for advice. The name(s) and details of the person(s) responsible(s) for this service should also be clearly mentioned. Moreover, a declaration that VC is only a supporting means that cannot replace a personal consultation with a physician should be provided.
5.2	VC responsible name(s)	
5.3	VC responsible(s) contact details	
5.4	Statement declaring limitation of the VC service	
6. Funding / Advertising		
6.1	Statement declaring sources of funding (sponsors, advertisers, etc.)	Health web resources should disclose possible conflicts of interest. For this reason it is important to know how and by whom a web resource is funded. If there are any sponsors, it has to be clear who they are. Furthermore, it should be stated that sponsors do not have any influence on the content. Additionally, it has to be known whether the web resource hosts or not advertising material in whatever format. In case that happens, such material should be clearly distinguished from informative material. Furthermore, information on resource's policy with regard to advertising must be easily accessible and clear.
6.2	Name(s) of funding (sponsoring) organization(s)	
6.3	Statement declaring limitation of influence of sponsors on content	
6.4	Advertising present	
6.5	Are advertisements clearly separated from editorial content?	
6.6	Policy with regard to advertisement	

continued on the following page

Table 2. (continued)

7. Other Seal or Recommendation		
7.1	Other seal(s) present	Are there other seals identified in the resource? Indicates that the resource already conforms to other, known quality criteria. Identifiers for other seals: a) Real seals: WMA, HONcode, pWMC, URAC, eHealth TRUST-E, AFGIS, b) Filtering health portals (a resource is recommended by): AQUMED, Intute, WHO ("Vaccine Safety Net")
7.2	Which other seal(s)?	
8. Information Supporting Scientific Content		
8.1	References, bibliography (with links to literature)	Regarding the provided specialized health information (scientific parts of the resource) it is relevant to know if it is based on scientific books, medical journal articles, etc. For this, scientific articles or documents should include a references or bibliography section. Additionally, it is important to know if such information is up-to-date (publication and last modification dates are required) and who is the author of such content (author(s) name(s) and contact details are required for pages/documents providing scientific information).
8.2	Publication / creation date	
8.3	Last revision / modification date	
8.4	Author name(s)	
8.5	Author(s) contact details	
8.6	Editorial policy	
9. Confidentiality / privacy policy		
9.1	Explanation on how personal data (visitor coordinates, e-mail messages, etc.) is handled	Internet users are much concerned about protection of their privacy and personal data. For this reason the resource should provide a confidentiality/ privacy policy ensuring that personal data (visitor coordinates, e-mail messages, etc.) is safely handled, describing how these data are handled.
10. Accessibility		
10.1	Accessibility level	The resource is examined upon various accessibility criteria and information on its accessibility level (whether the resource is of level A, AA or AAA) is deduced.

THE AQUA SYSTEM OVERVIEW

Development Objectives

Taking into account WMA and AQuMed approaches, the AQUA tool (Stamatakis et. al., 2007) was designed to support the main tasks in their labelling processes, more specifically:

1. Identification of unlabelled resources having health-related content
2. Visit and review of the identified resources
3. Generation of content labels for the reviewed resources
4. Monitoring the labeled resources

Compared to other approaches that partially address the assessment process (Griffiths et. al., 2005; Wang & Liu, 2006), the AQUA system is an integrated solution. AQUA aims to provide the infrastructure and the means to organize and support various aspects of the daily work of labelling experts by making them computer-assisted. The steps towards this objective are the following:

- **Step 1:** Creating machine readable labels by:
    - Adopting the use of the RDF model (W3C, 2004) for producing machine-readable content labels; at the current stage, the RDF-CL model (W3C, 2005) is used. In the final version of

AQUA, another model called POWDER, introduced by the recently initiated W3C Protocol for Web Description Resources (POWDER) working group (W3C, 2007), will be supported.
- Creating a vocabulary of criteria, consolidating on existing ones from various Labelling Agencies; this vocabulary is used in the machine readable RDF labels.
- Developing a label management environment allowing experts to generate, update and compare content labels.

- **Step 2:** Automating parts of the labelling process by:
  - Helping in the identification of unlabelled resources.
  - Extracting from these resources information relative to specific criteria.
  - Generating content labels from the extracted information.
  - Facilitating the monitoring of already labeled resources.
- **Step 3:** Putting everything together; AQUA is implemented as a large-scale, enterprise-level, web application having the following three tiers:
  - The user tier, including the user interfaces for the labelling expert and the system administrator.
  - The application tier where all applications run.
  - The storage tier consisting of the MedIEQ file repository and the MedIEQ database.

System Architecture

AQUA addresses a complex task. However, various design and implementation decisions helped MedIEQ partners keep AQUA extensible and easy to maintain. The main characteristics of its implementation include:

a. Open architecture
b. Accepted standards adopted in its design and deployment
c. Character of large-scale, enterprise-level web application
d. Internationalization support

AQUA incorporates several subsystems (see the application level in Figure 1) and functionalities for the labelling expert. The *Web Content Collection* (WCC) component identifies, classifies and collects online content relative to the criteria proposed by the labelling agencies participating in the project. The *Information Extraction Toolkit* (IET) analyses the web content collected by WCC and extracts attributes for MedIEQ-compatible content labels. The *Label Management* (LAM) component generates, validates, modifies and compares the content labels based on the schema proposed by MedIEQ. The *Multilingual Resources Management* (MRM) gives access to health-related multilingual resources; input from such resources is needed in specific parts of the WCC, IET and LAM toolkits. Finally, *Monitor-Update-Alert* (MUA) handles auxiliary but important jobs like the configuration of monitoring tasks, the MedIEQ database updates, or the alerts to labelling experts when important differences occur during the monitoring of existing content labels.

While the first prototype, made operational in autumn 2007, only addresses the certification of new resources and covers two languages (English and Spanish), the full version of the system will also enable monitoring of already labeled resources and will cover 7 languages in total.

Figure 1 shows all the possible data flows in AQUA (dashed arrows): a) From WCC to IET: pages collected by WCC, once undergone a first-level extraction by WCC (extraction of metadata 1), are then

Figure 1. Architecture of the AQUA system

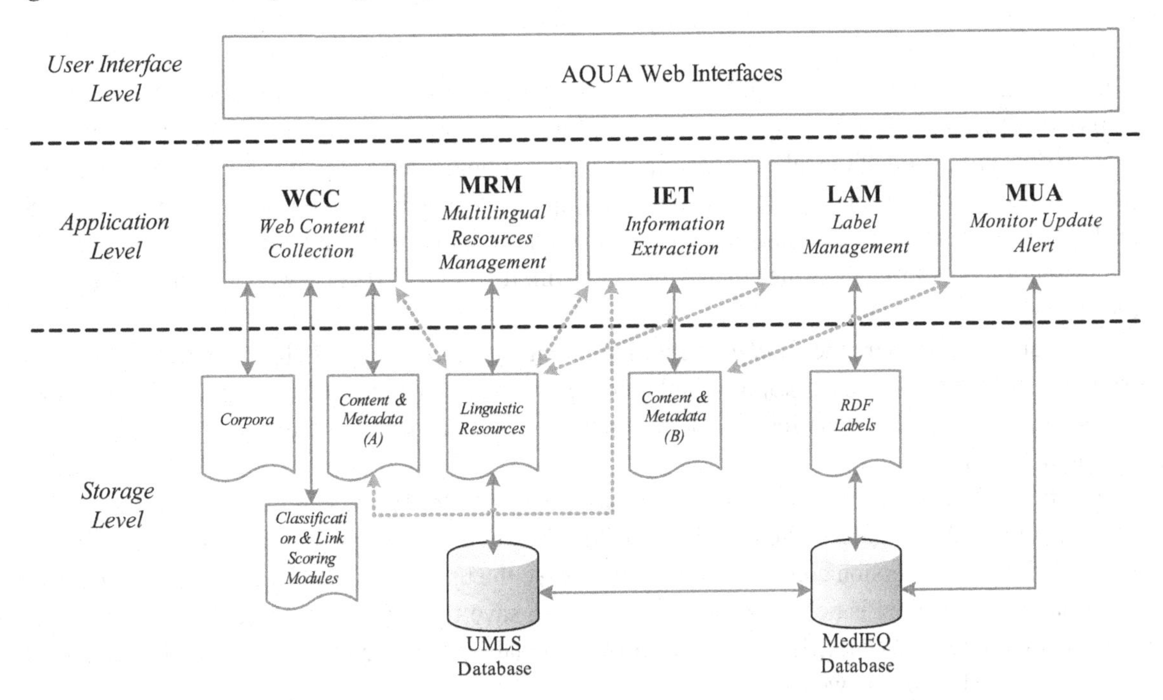

forwarded to IET for further processing (extraction of metadata 2); b) From IET to MUA: MUA takes all metadata collected by both WCC and IET and updates the MedIEQ database; c) From MRM to WCC, IET, LAM: custom vocabularies, generated by the MedIEQ users through MRM interface, can be accessed from other toolkits (WCC, IET, LAM), where the user may need them.

The following two sections are devoted to a more detailed description of AQUA, namely of its (manual) label management components and of its automated labelling support components.

AQUA LAM COMPONENT: CREATING MACHINE-READABLE LABELS

Representation Formalism for Machine-Readable Labels

To make content labels machine-readable the use of the RDF model is adopted. At the current stage, the RDF-CL model is used. The RDF-CL model was issued by the EC-funded project Quality Assistance and Content Description (QUATRO) (www.quatro-project.org); it is currently being refined by the W3C Protocol for Web Description Resources (POWDER) working group (W3C, 2007). POWDER is expected to be completed before the end of the MedIEQ project and the plan is to use it in the final version of AQUA.

User Interaction with the Label Management Environment

The *label management* interface and associated tools, together called LAM, allows experts to generate, update and compare content labels. From within the LAM user interface the user is able to a) generate new RDF labels from information automatically extracted by other AQUA tools, b) manually fill the relevant fields and generate new RDF labels, c) edit and update existing RDF labels, and d) compare RDF labels among themselves.

The user interface to generate/edit a label is a *web form* (see Figure 2) with input boxes, single and multiple select boxes, links and buttons. It is split into two distinct areas. The first part lets the user *constrain* the application of the label to certain hosts by explicitly declaring the host URIs or by adding regular expressions that properly identify them. Multiple hosts can be defined. Regular expressions for more fine-grained addressing can be defined as well. These definitions can be combined via the union and intersection operators and thus create rules that link different parts of a web resource with different labels.

The second part is where the *label properties* are assigned *values*. The label properties are the actual descriptors of a web resource, mapping the labelling criteria. A set of label descriptors can be linked with a set of host restrictions defined in the first part. Related properties are grouped to make the user filling them easier.

Once the user has filled the label metadata, restrictions and properties, s/he can *save* the label. There is a notification field that alerts the user if the label already exists in the system, and its changes are tracked by the AQUA version control system. In this case the user can save the label as a *revision* of an existing label. If the label is new, the user just selects to save the label. In both cases the user has the option to download an RDF/XML serialized form of the label. This serialized label can be assigned to the web resource by the site webmaster.

AQUA WCC+IET: AUTOMATING PARTS OF THE LABELLING PROCESS

Locating Unlabeled Web Resources

The AQUA *crawling* mechanism is part of the *web content collection* environment (WCC) (Stamatakis et. al., 2007). Its AQUA interface is shown in Figure 3. The Crawler searches the Web for health-related content that does not have a content label yet (at least not a label found in MedIEQ records). It is a meta-search engine that exploits results returned from known search engines and directory listings from known Web directories. All collected URLs from all sources are merged and filtered, and a pre-final URLs list is returned. The merging / filtering process: a) removes possible duplicates, b) ignores sub-paths of URLs already in list, and c) removes URLs already having a content label (the Crawler consults the MedIEQ database for this).

The crawling process becomes even more focused with the aid of a *content classifier*, inductively trained to distinguish health content from non-health content. This classification component visits every URL from the merged / filtered pre-final URL list and checks its contents, thus filtering out some more entries.

The current version of the AQUA Crawler queries Google and Yahoo! *search engines* (with terms proposed by the user) and explores Web directories (again proposed by the user). By merely using general-purpose search engines, the Crawler inevitably inherits their shortcomings. Therefore, aiming to further enhance our Crawler, we also include two search mechanisms specialized to the *health domain*: one provided by HON (www.hon.ch) and another by Intute's Health and Life Sciences branch (www.intute.ac.uk). The Crawler interface is shown in Figure 3.

Figure 2. The AQUA label management environment (LAM) interface

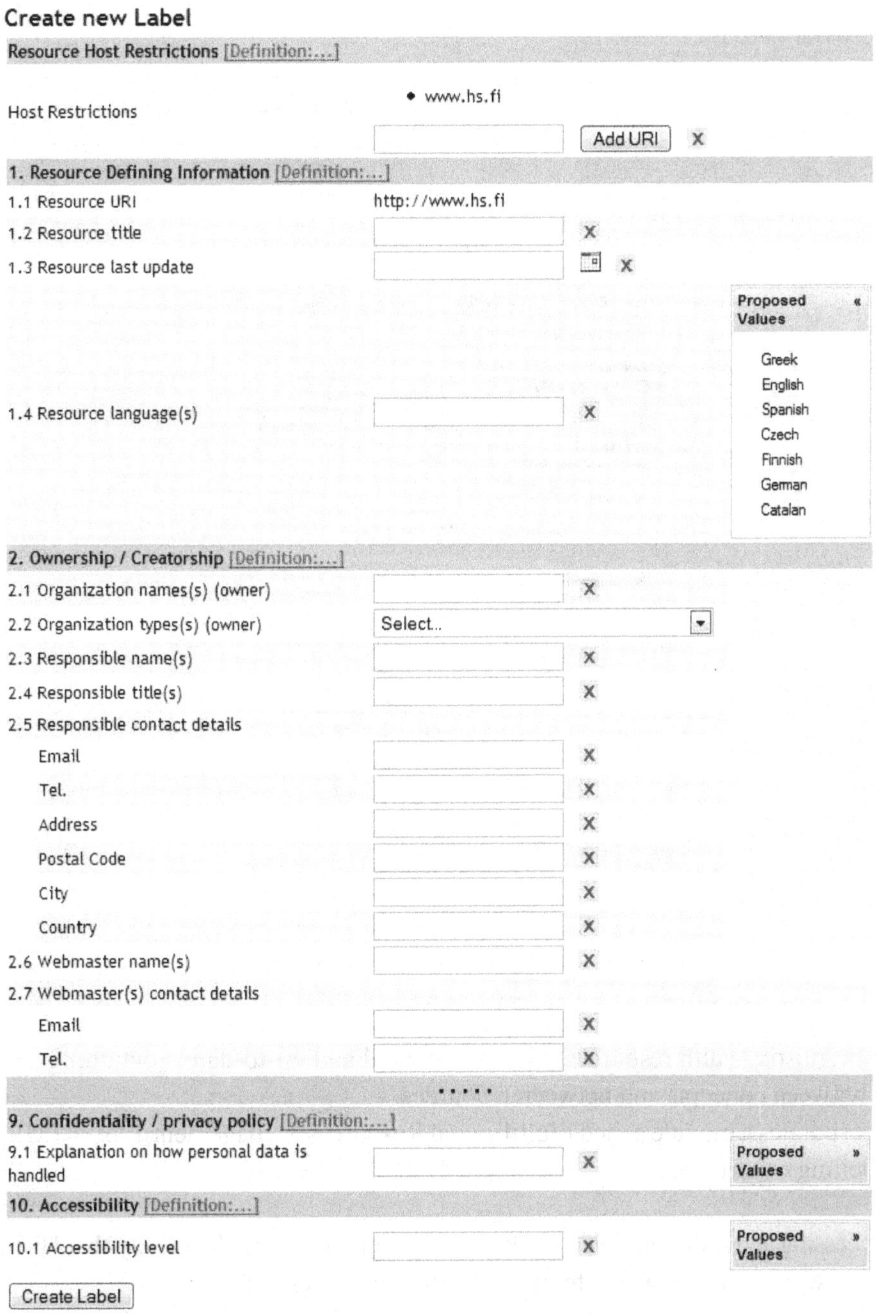

Create new Label

Resource Host Restrictions [Definition:...]

Host Restrictions
- www.hs.fi

Add URI X

1. Resource Defining Information [Definition:...]

1.1 Resource URI http://www.hs.fi
1.2 Resource title X
1.3 Resource last update X
1.4 Resource language(s) X

Proposed Values «
Greek
English
Spanish
Czech
Finnish
German
Catalan

2. Ownership / Creatorship [Definition:...]

2.1 Organization names(s) (owner) X
2.2 Organization types(s) (owner) Select..
2.3 Responsible name(s) X
2.4 Responsible title(s) X
2.5 Responsible contact details
Email X
Tel. X
Address X
Postal Code X
City X
Country X
2.6 Webmaster name(s) X
2.7 Webmaster(s) contact details
Email X
Tel. X

.....

9. Confidentiality / privacy policy [Definition:...]

9.1 Explanation on how personal data is handled X Proposed Values »

10. Accessibility [Definition:...]

10.1 Accessibility level X Proposed Values »

Create Label

Browsing Medical Knowledge Sources

One of the main requirements when working with medical web resources, is to identify and classify them based on standardized medical terms. Such terms (knowledge sources) have been globally defined by the Unified Medical Language System (UMLS) (www.nlm.nih.gov/ research/umls/). UMLS provides

Figure 3. Configuring the MedIEQ Crawler from the AQUA interface

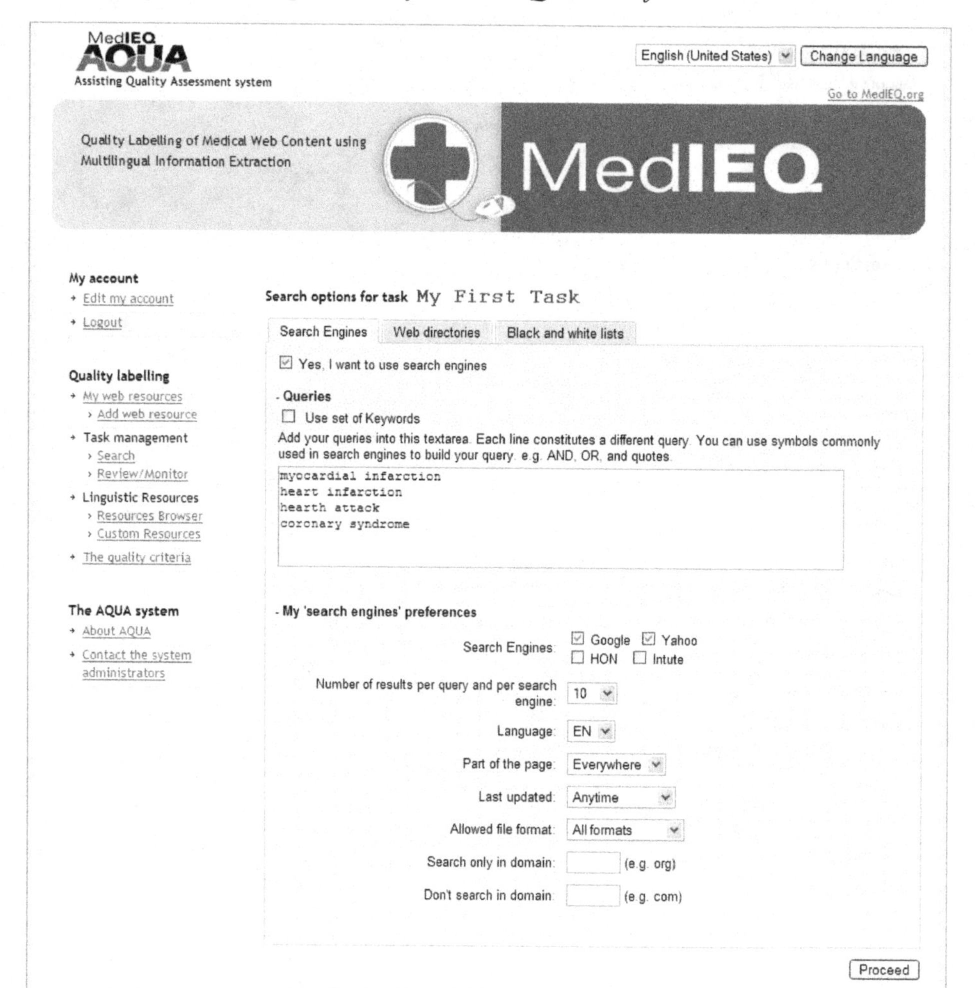

a wide set of linguistic health resources, well maintained and up-to-date, containing health concepts and relations between concepts and between resources.

AQUA incorporates a module called Multilingual Resources Management Toolkit (MRM) that aims to support labelling experts in:

- Easily accessing and browsing selected “knowledge sources” form the variety that UMLS provides
- Creating new, custom resources, to better support the labelling process

MRM is an environment from which linguistic resources, either UMLS-supported or not (custom or user generated) in different languages can be managed. MRM provides a user-friendly environment for accessing and managing both UMLS “knowledge sources” and custom resources (see Figure 4).

Spidering the Website

While the Crawler proceeds from the initial user's content collection requirement to the identification of a relevant website as a whole, the *Spider*, in turn, examines individual pages of the site. The sites whose URLs are obtained from the Crawler are processed by the Spider one-by-one in several independent threads. Unreachable sites/pages are revisited in next run.

Since not all the pages of a web site are interesting for the labelling process, the Spider utilizes a content classification component that consists of a number of *classification modules* (statistical and heuristic ones). These modules decide which pages contain interesting information. Each of them relies on a different classification method according to the classification problem on which it is applied. Pages identified as belonging to classes relevant to the labelling criteria are stored locally in order to be exploited by the Information Extraction subsystem.

One of the main classification modules of the Spider is the "UMLS/MeSH categoriser", called POKA. POKA (http://www.seco.tkk.fi/tools/poka/) is a tool for automatic extraction of ontological resources (RDF, OWL, SKOS) from text documents. In the MedIEQ framework, POKA is used to find relations between medical web content and medical vocabularies such as MeSH to facilitate categorization of web resources. The POKA system is used as a component of the web spidering tool where the spider traverses health web sites by gathering internal links and visiting the corresponding web pages one by one. POKA is then harnessed to find medical terminology inside these pages by matching content with the MeSH vocabulary.

Figure 4. Browsing medical knowledge sources with AQUA

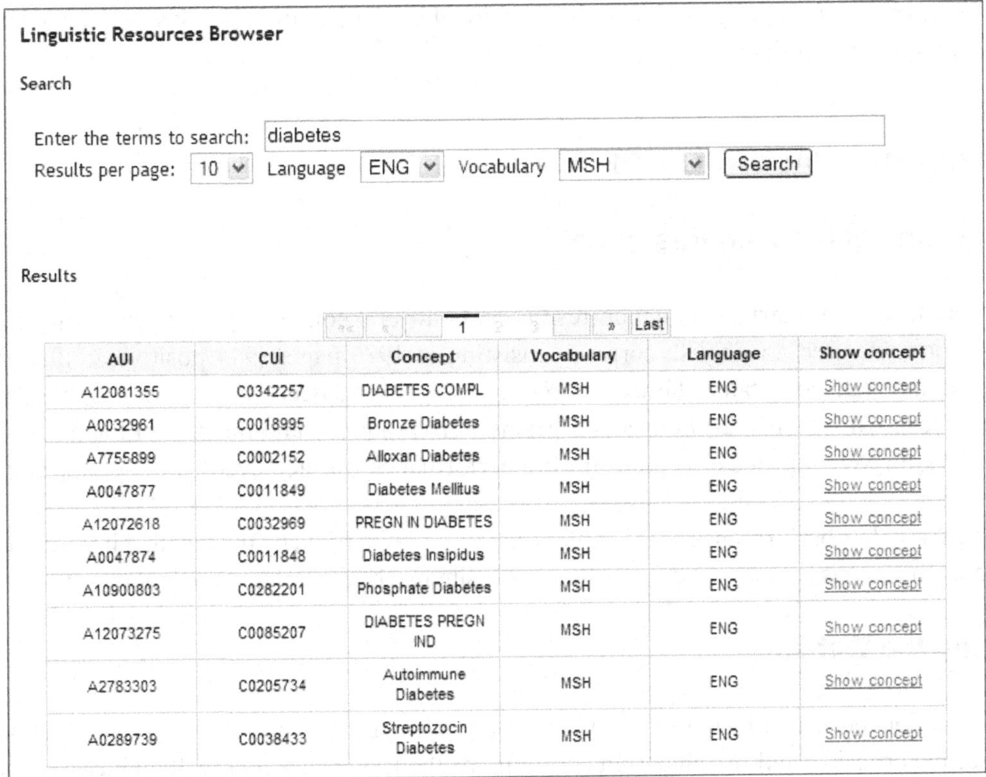

AUI	CUI	Concept	Vocabulary	Language	Show concept
A12081355	C0342257	DIABETES COMPL	MSH	ENG	Show concept
A0032961	C0018995	Bronze Diabetes	MSH	ENG	Show concept
A7755899	C0002152	Alloxan Diabetes	MSH	ENG	Show concept
A0047877	C0011849	Diabetes Mellitus	MSH	ENG	Show concept
A12072618	C0032969	PREGN IN DIABETES	MSH	ENG	Show concept
A0047874	C0011848	Diabetes Insipidus	MSH	ENG	Show concept
A10900803	C0282201	Phosphate Diabetes	MSH	ENG	Show concept
A12073275	C0085207	DIABETES PREGN IND	MSH	ENG	Show concept
A2783303	C0205734	Autoimmune Diabetes	MSH	ENG	Show concept
A0289739	C0038433	Streptozocin Diabetes	MSH	ENG	Show concept

Extracting Information Relative to Criteria

MedIEQ continues and builds upon the work of previous projects in the area of *information extraction* (IE) (Karkaletsis et.al. 2004; Rainbow, 2005; Labsky & Svatek, 2006). The AQUA IE toolkit (IET) employs a set of components responsible for the extraction of elementary information items found in each document and for the integration of these items into a set of semantically meaningful objects called *instances*. An instance (of certain general class) can be for example the set of contact information about a health provider or the set of bibliographic information about a scholarly resource referred to on the website.

The core IE engine currently used within IET is the *Ex* system (Labsky et al., 2007), which relies on combination of so-called *extraction ontologies* with exploiting local *HTML formatting regularities* and the option of embedding *trainable classifiers* to perform selected extraction subtasks. IET is built as a generic information extraction toolkit that supports changes and additions to the utilized labelling schemes. In this way, IET can also be used for IE using third-party labelling schemes and within other domains.

Monitoring of Already Described Resources

Another part of AQUA, called MUA (from Monitor-Update-Alert), handles problems such as the *configuration* of *monitoring tasks*, the necessary MedIEQ *repository updates* and the *alerts* to labelling experts when important differences (relative to the quality criteria) occur during the monitoring of previously labeled sites. MUA thus extends the functionality of the content collection and extraction toolkits by shifting from a one-shot scenario to that of continuous monitoring.

MUA is currently in its design phase. Fully functional implementation is envisaged in the late phase of the MedIEQ project (mid-2008).

PRELIMINARY EVALUATION OF AQUA

Locating Unlabeled Web Resources

In this section, we summarize evaluation results on Crawler's content classification component. For this evaluation, we used an English corpus, consisting of 1976 pages (944 positive & 1032 negative samples), all manually annotated. Three different classifiers have been tested (SMO, Naïve Bayes and Flexible Bayes). All 1-grams, 2-grams and 3-grams were produced and the best of them according to information gain were selected (see Table 3). Best performance was achieved with 1-grams and HTML tags removed.

The relatively low performance of the content classifiers is justified by the fact that it is difficult, even for humans, in various cases to assess whether a website has health-related content or not.

Spidering the Website

The classification mechanism our Spider exploits has been examined using statistical classification techniques, for the criteria listed in Table 4. In addition, for the last criterion, a method based on heuristic detection was examined.

Table 3. Classification performance results for content classification

	1-grams (Tags removed)		
	Prec.	**Rec.**	**Fm.**
NB	0.75	0.63	**0.68**
FB	0.73	0.55	**0.62**
SMO	0.75	0.61	**0.67**

Table 4. The MedIEQ criteria upon which our classification components were evaluated

Criterion	*MedIEQ approach*
The target audience of a website	Classification among three possible target groups: adults, children and professionals
Contact information of the responsible of a website must be present and clearly stated	Detection of candidate pages during the spidering process and forwarding for information extraction
Presence of virtual consultation services	Detection of parts of a website that offer such services during the spidering process
Presence of advertisements in a website	Detection of parts of a website that contain advertisements during the spidering process

Several learning schemes, decision trees, naive Bayes and supported vector machines (SMO) were tested. The performance of the SMO classifier, which provides the best results, is presented in Table 5. As expected, the most difficult criterion for classification purposes is the target audience, being a highly subjective one.

Extracting Information Relative to Criteria

Table 6 shows preliminary results for extraction of *contact information*. Data sets were collected through website crawling and spidering, contact pages were identified and manually annotated for English (109 HTML pages), Spanish (200) and Czech (108). The collections contained roughly 7000, 5000 and 11000 named entities, respectively. The *contact extraction* ontologies (one per language with shared common parts) were developed based on seeing 30 randomly chosen documents from each dataset and evaluated using the remaining documents. Extraction ontologies utilize nested regular patterns at word, character and HTML tag level. They also refer to gazetteers such as lists of city names, common first names and surnames. Each ontology contained about 100 textual patterns for the context and content of attributes and also for the single extracted 'contact' class, attribute length and data type constraints and several axioms. For the results below we did not exploit trainable classifiers; their meaningful combination with the manually authored extraction knowledge is still work-in-progress, and when applied standalone, their results were so far slightly inferior to those achieved via extraction ontologies. We attribute this observation to small amount and large heterogeneity of training data.

The effort spent on developing and tuning the ontologies was about 2-3 person-weeks for the initial, English ontology, and 1-2 person weeks for its customization to Spanish and Czech. In the strict mode of evaluation, only exact matches are considered to be successfully extracted. In the loose mode, partial credit is also given to incomplete or overflown matches; e.g. extracting 'John Newman' where 'John

Table 5. SMO performance

	English			Spanish		
Category	**Precision**	**Recall**	**Fm**	**Precision**	**Recall**	**Fm**
Contact Info	0.84	0.96	0.90	0.80	0.65	0.72
Advertisements	0.87	0.80	0.83	0.77	0.72	0.75
Virtual Consultation	0.87	0.87	0.87	0.75	0.58	0.65
Adults	0.78	0.75	0.77	0.65	0.64	0.65
Children	0.80	0.78	0.79	-	-	-
Professional	0.77	0.81	0.79	0.62	0.63	0.62

Table 6. Results of IET for contact information[3]

	English			Spanish			Czech		
Attribute	**Precision**	**Recall**	**Fm**	**Precision**	**Recall**	**Fm**	**Precision**	**Recall**	**Fm**
Degree/Title	71/78	82/86	76/82	-	-	-	87/89	88/91	88/90
Name	66/74	51/56	58/64	71/77	81/86	76/81	74/76	82/83	78/80
Street	62/85	52/67	56/75	71/93	46/58	56/71	78/83	66/69	71/75
City	47/48	73/76	57/59	48/50	77/80	59/61	67/75	69/79	68/77
Zip	59/67	78/85	67/75	88/91	91/94	89/93	91/91	97/97	94/94
Country	58/59	89/89	70/71	67/67	78/78	72/72	64/66	87/96	74/78
Phone	97/99	84/87	90/93	84/89	91/96	87/92	92/93	85/85	88/89
Email	100/100	99/99	100/100	94/95	99/99	96/97	99/99	98/98	98/98
Company	57/81	37/51	44/63	-	-	-	-	-	-
Department	51/85	31/45	38/59	-	-	-	-	-	-
Overall	70/78	62/68	66/72	71/76	81/86	76/80	81/84	84/87	82/84

Newman Jr.' was supposed to be extracted will count as a 66% match (based on overlapping word counts). Table 6 shows results in 'strict/loose' order. Some of the performance numbers below may be impacted by a relatively low inter-annotator agreement (English and Spanish datasets are still being cleaned to remove inconsistencies).

AQUA Usability Evaluation

The 1st AQUA prototype was also evaluated by the labelling organizations participating in the MEDIEQ project (namely, WMA and AQUMED). The primary goal of this evaluation was to conclude with a functional prototype that has the potential to be fully integrated within the day-to-day activities of a labelling organization. To this end, a parallel technical improvement action took place, refining given functionalities. The main objective of the extra technical improvement action was to enhance the overall system workflow, so as to better match the day-to-day practice. The specifications for these technical refinements were given by an iterative feedback process with the MedIEQ labelling organizations, during the evaluation. It must be noted that the current interim version of AQUA was well received by both labelling organizations participating in the Usability Evaluation testing, and that they expressed their confidence that AQUA will be fully integrated within their day-to-day labelling activities.

CONCLUDING REMARKS

Other attempts to automatically assess health information in the internet exist but address the assessment process only partially. The Automated Quality Assessment procedure (AQA) (Griffiths et. al., 2005) ranks depression websites merely according to their evidence-based quality. The Automatic Indicator Detection Tool (AIDT), presented in a recent study (Wang & Liu, 2006), is suggested as a complementary instrument for the assessment of health information quality. AIDT is evaluated upon the automatic detection of pre-defined indicators that correspond to a number of technical quality criteria. However, AIDT focuses on a narrow scope of extraction techniques only, and does not address the assessment process as a whole. In contrast, the AQUA approach seems to be unique in covering the whole workflow of labelling agencies and employing a comprehensive and flexible collection of automated tools.

Assessing the quality of health-related information published on the internet is a task with great importance for the quality of the healthcare itself, due to a large proportion of patients as well as medical practitioners nowadays using the internet as a high-coverage information resource. It is at the same time a complex task as it has to examine the conjunction of a number of different aspects. Various initiatives around the world have attempted to codify these aspects into criteria, principles, codes of conduct, etc. Health specialists review online health resources and label them, either by issuing certification trustmarks or by including them in a thematic health portal. However this work can be proven quite tedious even for experienced users. Additionally, as it currently relies on manual effort, the labelling process is very time-consuming. Instruments to assist certain parts of the work exist; they however focus on specific problems only and none of them addresses the assessment process as a whole. In this context, efforts such as the MedIEQ project will bring wide reusability to content labels in the health domain by giving them machine-readable semantics and by providing services, such as those of the AQUA system, for creating and exploiting these machine-readable labels.

From the knowledge technology research viewpoint, the added value of MedIEQ is in employing existing technologies in a novel application: the automation of the labelling process in health-related web content. These technologies are *semantic web* technologies for describing web resources and *web search* (crawling and spidering) *and mining* (classification and information extraction) technologies for collecting domain-specific web content and extracting information from it. Experimental results for the mining components, investigating the performance of different inductive-learning-based as well as knowledge-engineering-based methods, are promising.

REFERENCES

AGREE, Appraisal of Guidelines Research and Evaluation (AGREE), 2004. Available Online at: http://www.agreecollaboration.org/instrument/

Berners-Lee, T., Hendler, J., & Lassila, O. (2001). The Semantic Web. *Scientific American*, May 2001.

Curro, V., Buonuomo, P. S., Onesimo, R., Vituzzi, A., di Tanna, G. L., & D'Atri, A. (2004). A quality evaluation methodology of health web-pages for non-professionals. *Med Inform Internet Med,* 29(2), 95-107.

Diaz, J. A., Griffith, R. A., Ng, J. J., Reinert, S. E., Friedmann, P. D., & Moulton, A. W. (2002). Patients´use of the Internet for medical Information. *J Gen Intern Med,* 17(3), 180-5.

DISCERN (2008). *DISCERN: Quality criteria for consumer health information.* Retrieved from http://www.discern.org.uk/.

European Commission. (2002). *eEurope 2002: Quality Criteria for Health related Websites.* Retrieved from http://europa.eu.int/information_society/eeurope/ehealth/ doc/communication_acte_en_fin.pdf.

Eysenbach, G. (2000). Consumer health informatics. *BMJ,* 320 (4), 1713-16.

Eysenbach, G. (2003). The Semantic Web and healthcare consumers: A new challenge and opportunity on the horizon? *J Health Techn Manag,* 5, 194-212.

Griffiths, K. M., Tang, T. T., Hawking, D., & Christensen, H. (2005) Automated assessment of the quality of depression Web sites. *J Med Internet Res.,*7(5), e59.

HON, Health on the Net Foundation (2001). *HONCode.* Retrieved from http://www.hon.ch

HON, Health on the Net Foundation. (2005). *Analysis of 9th HON Survey of Health and Medical Internet Users Winter 2004-2005.* Retrieved from http://www.hon.ch/Survey/Survey2005/res.html

Karkaletsis, V., Spyropoulos, C. D., Grover, C., Pazienza, M. T., Coch, J., & Souflis, D. (2004) A Platform for Crosslingual, Domain and User Adaptive Web Information Extraction. In *Proceedings of the European Conference in Artificial Intelligence* (ECAI), Valencia, Spain; p. 725-9.

Kohler, C., Darmoni, S. D., Mayer, M. A., Roth-Berghofer, T., Fiene, M., & Eysenbach, G. (2002). MedCIRCLE – The Collaboration for Internet Rating, Certification, Labelling, and Evaluation of Health Information. Technology and Health Care, Special Issue: Quality e-Health. *Technol Health Care, 10*(6), 515.

Labsky, M., & Svatek, V. (2006, June) Information Extraction with Presentation Ontologies. In: ESWC'06 *Workhshop on Mastering the Gap: From Information Extraction to Semantic Representation,* Budva, Montenegro.

Labsky, M., Svatek, V., Nekvasil, M., & Rak D. (2007). The Ex Project: Web Information Extraction using Extraction Ontologies. In: *Proc. PriCKL'07, ECML/PKDD Workshop on Prior Conceptual Knowledge in Machine Learning and Knowledge Discovery.* Warsaw, Poland, October 2007.

Mayer, M. A., Leis, A., Sarrias, R., & Ruíz, P. (2005). Web Mèdica Acreditada Guidelines: realiability and quality of health information on Spanish-Language websites. In Engelbrecht R et al. (ed.). *Connecting Medical Informatics and Bioinformatics.* Proc of MIE2005, 1287-92.

Rainbow, University of Economics Prague, Knowledge Engineering Group. (2005). *Reusable Architecture for Intelligent Brokering Of Web information access (Rainbow).* Retrieved from: http://rainbow.vse.cz/descr.html

Sanger, S (ed.) (2004). *Check-In.* Retrieved from http://www.patienten-information.de/content/ informationsqualitaet/informationsqualitaet/images/check_in.pdf

Soualmia, L. F, Darmoni, S. J., Douyère, M., & Thirion, B. (2003). Modelisation of Consumer Health Information in a Quality-Controled gateway. In Baud R et al. (ed.). *The New Navigators: from Professionals to Patients.* Proc of MIE2003, 701-706.

Stamatakis, K., Chandrinos, K., Karkaletsis, V., Mayer, M. A, Gonzales, D. V, Labsky, D.V, Amigó, E., & Pöllä, M. (2007) AQUA, a system assisting labelling experts assess health Web resources. In *Proceedings of the 12th International Symposium for Health Information Management Research* (iSHIMR 2007), Sheffield, UK, 18-20 July, 75-84.

Stamatakis, K., Metsis, V., Karkaletsis, V., Ruzicka, M., Svátek, V., Amigó, E., & Pöllä, M. (2007). Content collection for the labelling of health-related web content. In *Proceedings of the 11th Conference on Artificial Intelligence in Medicine* (AIME 07), LNAI 4594, Amsterdam, 7-11 July, 341-345.

W3C. (2004). *Resource Description Framework (RDF).* Retrieved from http:// www.w3.org/TR/rdf-schema/

W3C. (2005). *RDF-Content Labels (RDF-CL).* Retrieved from http://www.w3.org/ 2004/12/q/doc/content-labels-schema.htm

W3C. (2007). *Protocol for Web Description Resources (POWDER).* Retrieved from http://www.w3.org/2007/powder/

Wang, Y., & Liu, Z. (2006, May 31). Automatic detecting indicators for quality of health information on the Web. *Int J. Med Inform.*

Winker, M. A., Flanagan, A., Chi-Lum, B. (2000). Guidelines for Medical and Health Information Sites on the Internet: principles governing AMA Web sites. American Medical Association. *JAMA, 283*(12), 1600-1606.

KEY TERMS

Crawling: A web crawler is a program or automated script which browses the World Wide Web in a methodical, automated manner. This process is called web crawling. Web crawlers are mainly used to create a copy of all the visited pages for later processing.

Information Extraction: Automatic assignment of meaning to elementary textual entities and possibly more complex structured objects.

Metadata: Data that describes information about either online or offline data. Information that characterizes the who, what, where, and how related to data collection. Often, the information refers to special tagged fields in a document that provide information about the document to search engines and other computer applications. Web pages often include metadata in the form of meta tags. Description and keywords meta tags are commonly used to describe the Web page's content. Most search engines use this data when adding pages to their search index.

Resource Description Framework (RDF): Resource Description Framework (RDF) is a family of World Wide Web Consortium (W3C) specifications originally designed as a metadata data model, but which has come to be used as a general method of modeling information through a variety of syntax formats. The RDF metadata model is based upon the idea of making statements about Web resources in the form of subject-predicate-object expressions, called triples in RDF terminology. The subject denotes the resource, and the predicate denotes traits or aspects of the resource and expresses a relationship between the subject and the object.

Semantic Web: The Semantic Web is an evolving extension of the World Wide Web in which the semantics of information and services on the web is defined, making it possible for the web to understand and satisfy the requests of people and machines to use the web content. It derives from W3C director Tim Berners-Lee's vision of the Web as a universal medium for data, information, and knowledge exchange. At its core, the semantic web comprises a set of design principles, collaborative working groups, and a variety of enabling technologies. Some elements of the semantic web are expressed as prospective future possibilities that have yet to be implemented or realized. Other elements of the semantic web are expressed in formal specifications.

Spidering: A web spider is a complementary mechanism/tool to a web crawler. Web crawlers are mainly used to create a copy of all the visited pages for later processing, whereas, web spiders are used to gather specific types of information from Web pages. Many sites, in particular search engines, use spidering as a means of providing up-to-date data.

Web Mining: Web mining is the application of data mining techniques to discover patterns from the Web. According to analysis targets, web mining can be divided into three different types, which are Web usage mining, Web content mining and Web structure mining. Web usage mining is the application that uses data mining to analyse and discover interesting patterns of user's usage data on the web. Web content mining is the process to discover useful information from the content of a web page. The type of the web content may consist of text, image, audio or video data in the web. Web structure mining is the process of using graph theory to analyse the node and connection structure of a web site.

ENDNOTES

1. http://www.medieq.org/aqua/welcome.seam
2. http://www.medieq.org
3. At the time of writing, degrees were not annotated as part of the Spanish collection and results for company and department names for Spanish and Czech were still work in progress.

Chapter XI
Two Case-Based Systems for Explaining Exceptions in Medicine

Rainer Schmidt
University of Rostock, Germany

ABSTRACT

In medicine, a lot of exceptions usually occur. In medical practice and in knowledge-based systems, it is necessary to consider them and to deal with them appropriately. In medical studies and in research, exceptions shall be explained. In this chapter, we present two systems that deal with both sorts of these situations. The first one, called ISOR-1, is a knowledge-based system for therapy support. It does not just compute therapy recommendations, but it especially investigates therapy inefficacy. The second system, ISOR-2, is designed for medical studies or research. It helps to explain cases that contradict a theoretical hypothesis. Both systems are working in close co-operation with the user, who is not just considered as knowledge provider to build the system but is incorporated as additional knowledge source at runtime. Within a dialogue between the doctor and the system solutions respectively explanations are searched.

INTRODUCTION

Very often doctors are confronted with exceptions. This does not only happen in medical practise but also in medical research. Systems that are intended to support doctors have to take such situations into account. This does not hold only for knowledge-based systems but also for systems for supporting medical research studies. In knowledge-based systems exceptions have to be considered and dealt with appropriately. In rule-based systems this can lead to a huge amount of exceptional rules. In medical studies, statisticians are usually quite happy when a statistical test significantly supports a hypothesis. However, when the number of cases contradicting the hypothesis is rather big, physicians are often not satisfied with significant test results but additionally wish to get explanations for the exceptional cases.

In this chapter, we present two systems that deal with both sorts of these situations. The first one, called ISOR-1, especially investigates therapy inefficacy in the course of a dialogue with the user. The second system, ISOR-2, helps to explain cases that contradict a theoretical hypothesis.

These two systems are presented separately in this chapter, one after the other, first ISOR-1, subsequently ISOR-2.

ISOR-1: INVESTIGATING THERAPY INEFFICACY

In medical practice, therapies prescribed according to a certain diagnosis sometimes do not give desired results. Sometimes therapies are effective for some time but then suddenly stop helping any more. There are many possible reasons. A diagnosis might be erroneous, the state of a patient might have changed completely, or the state might have changed just slightly but with important implications for an existing therapy. Furthermore, a patient might have caught an additional disease, some other complication might have occurred, a patient might have changed his/her lifestyle (e.g. started a diet) and so on.

For long-term therapy support, especially in the endocrine domain and in psychiatry, we have developed a Case-Based Reasoning (CBR) system, named ISOR-1, which not only performs typical therapeutic tasks but also especially deals with situations where therapies have become ineffective. Therefore, it first attempts to find causes for inefficacy and subsequently computes new therapy recommendations that should perform better than those administered before.

ISOR-1 is a medical Case-Based Reasoning system that deals with the following tasks:

- Choose appropriate (initial) therapies
- Compute doses for chosen therapies
- Update dose recommendations according to laboratory test results
- Establish new doses of prescribed medicine according to changes in a patient's medical status or lifestyle
- Find out probable reasons why administered therapies are not as efficient as they should be
- Test obtained reasons for inefficacy and make sure that they are the real cause
- Suggest recommendations to avoid inefficacy of prescribed therapies

ISOR-1 deals with long-term diseases, e.g. psychiatric diseases, and with diseases even lasting for a lifetime, e.g. endocrine malfunctions.

For psychiatric diseases some Case-Based Reasoning systems have been developed, which deal with specific diseases or problems, e.g. with Alzheimer's disease (Marling and Whitehouse 2001) or with eating disorders (Bichindaritz 1994). Since we do not want to discuss various psychiatric problems but intend to illustrate ISOR by understandable examples, in this chapter we mainly focus on some endocrine and psychiatric disorders, namely on hypothyroidism and depressive symptoms. Inefficacy of pharmacological therapy for depression is a widely known problem (e.g. Hirschfeld, 2002; Cuffel, 2003). There are many approaches to solve this problem. Guidelines and algorithms have been created (e.g. Alacorn, 20008; Osser, Patterson, 1998). ISOR gives reference to a psychopharmacology algorithm (Osser, Patterson, 1998) that is available on the website htp://mhc.com/Algorithms/Depression.

In this section, we firstly introduce typical therapeutic tasks, subsequently we present the architecture of ISOR-1 and finally we illustrate how it works by three examples.

Methods: Typical Therapeutic Tasks

Based on our experiences with ICONS (Schmidt, Gierl, 2001), a system for antibiotic therapy advice, and with therapy support programs for hypothyroidism (Schmidt, Vorobieva, 2006), we believe that for medicinal therapies mainly four tasks exist. The first one means computing an initial therapy, secondly an initial dose has to be determined, later on dose updates may be necessary, and finally interactions with further diseases, complications, and especially with already administered therapies have to be considered.

In the following we illustrate these four tasks by our programs that deal with therapy support for hypothyroid patients. The antibiotics therapy adviser ICONS deals only with two of these tasks: computing initial therapies and initial doses.

Computing an initial therapy. Probably, the most important task for therapies is the computation of initial therapies. The main task of ICONS is to compute promising antibiotic therapies even before the pathogen that caused the infection is determined in the laboratory. However, for hypothyroidism ISOR-1 does not compute initial therapies but only initial doses, because for hypothyroidism only one therapy is available: it is thyroid hormone, usually in form of levothyroxine.

Computing an initial dose. In ICONS the determination of initial doses is a rather simple task. For every antibiotic a specific calculation function is available and has to be applied.

For hypothyroidism the determination of initial doses is much more complicated. A couple of guidelines exist that have been defined by expert commissions (Working group 1998). The assignment of a patient to a fitting guideline is obvious because of the way these guidelines have been defined. With the help of these guidelines a range for good doses can be calculated. To compute a dose with best expected impact we retrieve similar cases whose initial doses are within the calculated ranges. Since cases are described by few attributes and since our case-base is rather small, we use a sequential measure of dissimilarity, namely the one proposed by Tversky (1977). On the basis of those retrieved cases that had best therapy results an average initial therapy is calculated. Best therapy results can be determined by values of a blood test after two weeks of treatment with the initial dose. The opposite idea to consider cases with bad therapy results does not work here, because bad results can have various other reasons.

To compute optimal dose recommendations, we apply two forms of adaptation. First, a calculation of ranges according to guidelines and patients attribute values. Second, we use compositional adaptation. That means, we take only similar cases with best therapy results into account and calculate the average dose for these cases, which has to be adapted to the data of the query patient by another calculation.

Updating the dose in a patient's lifetime. For monitoring a hypothyroidism patient, three basic laboratory blood tests (TSH, FT3, FT4) have to be undertaken. Usually, the results of these tests correspond to each other. Otherwise, it indicates a more complicated thyroid condition and additional tests are necessary. If the results of the basic tests show that the thyroid hormone level is normal, it means that the current levothyroxine dose is OK. If the tests indicate that the thyroid hormone level is too low, the current dose has to be increased by 25 or 50 μg, if it is too high, the dose has to be decreased by 25 or 50 μg (DeGroot, 1994). So, for monitoring, adaptation means a calculation according to some rules, which are based on guidelines. Since an overdose of levothyroxine may cause serious complications for a patient, a doctor cannot simply consider test results and symptoms that indicate a dose increase but additionally has to investigate reasons why the current dose is not appropriate any more. In ISOR-1 this situation is described as a problem of therapy inefficiency. In most cases the solution is obvious, e.g. puberty, pregnancy and so on. These situations are covered by adaptation rules. Sometimes cases are observed in which the hypothyroidism syndromes are unexplained. For these cases ISOR-1 uses the problem solving program.

Additional diseases or complications. It often occurs that patients do not only have hypothyroidism, but they suffer from further chronic diseases or complications. Thus, a levothyroxine therapy has to be checked for contraindications, adverse effects and interactions with additionally existing therapies. Since no alternative is available to replace levothyroxine, if necessary additionally existing therapies have to be modified, substituted, or compensated (DeGroot, 1994).

ISOR-1 performs three tests. The first one checks if another existing therapy is contraindicated to hypothyroidism. This holds only for very few therapies, namely for specific diets like soybean infant formula, which is the most popular food for babies who do not get enough mother's milk but it prevents the effect of levothyroxine. Such diets have to be modified. Since no exact knowledge is available to explain how to accomplish this, just a warning is issued, which says that a modification is necessary.

The second test considers adverse effects. There are two ways to deal with them. A further existing therapy has either to be substituted or it has to be compensated by another drug. Such knowledge is available, and we have implemented corresponding rules for substitutional and compensational adaptation.

The third test checks for interactions between both therapies. We have implemented some adaptation rules, which mainly attempt to avoid the interactions. For example, if a patient has heartburn problems that are treated with an antacid, a rule for this situation states that levothyroxine should be administered at least four hours after or before an antacid. However, if no adaptation rule can solve such an interaction problem, the same substitution rules as for adverse effects are applied.

ISOR-1's Architecture

ISOR-1 is designed to solve typical therapy problems, especially inefficacy of prescribed therapies that can arise in many medical domains. Therefore most algorithms and functions are domain independent. Another goal is to cope with situations where important patient data are missing and/or where theoretical domain knowledge is controversial.

ISOR-1 does not generate solutions itself. Its task is to help users by providing all available information and to support them when they search for optimal solutions. Users shall be doctors, maybe even together with a patient.

In addition to the typical Case-Based Reasoning knowledge, namely former already solved cases, ISOR-1 uses further knowledge components, namely medical histories of query patients themselves and prototypical cases (prototypes). Furthermore, ISOR-1's knowledge base consists of therapies, conflicts, instructions etc. The idea of combining case-bases with different knowledge courses was, for example, already used in Creek (Aamodt, 2004).

Medical Case Histories

Ma and Knight (2003) have introduced a concept of case history in Case-Based Reasoning. Such an approach is very useful when we deal with chronic patients, because often the same complications occur again, former successful solutions can be helpful again, and former unsuccessful solutions should be avoided.

The case history is written in the patient's individual base in form of a sequence of records. A patient's base contains his/her whole medical history, all medical information that is available: diseases, complications, therapies, circumstances of his/her life, and so on. Each record describes an episode in a patient's medical history. Episodes often characterise a specific problem. Since the case-base is problem oriented, it contains just episodes and the same patient can be mentioned in the case-base a few times, even concerning different problems.

Information from the patient's individual base can be useful for a current situation, because for patients with chronic diseases very similar problems often occur again. If a similar situation is found in the patient's history, it is up to the user to decide whether to start retrieval in the general case-base or not.

In endocrinology, case histories are designed according to a standard scheme, one record per visit. Every record contains the results of laboratory tests and of an interrogatory about symptoms, complaints and physiological conditions of a patient. Therefore the retrieval of former similar situations from the individual base of an endocrine patient is easy to organise.

For psychiatric patients, case histories are often unsystematic and they can be structured in various forms. A general formalisation of psychiatric cases and their histories is not achieved yet. The design of case histories is problem dependent.

In both domains, we first search in the query patient's history for similar problems and for similar diagnoses.

Knowledge Base, Case-Base, and Prototypes

The knowledge base contains information about problems and their solutions that are possible according to the domain theory. It has a tree structure and it consists of lists of diagnoses, corresponding therapies, conflicts, instructions, and medical problems (including solutions) that can arise from specific therapies. The knowledge base also contains links to guidelines, algorithms and references to correspondent publications (Alacorn, 2000; Osser, Patterson, 1998).

The case-base is problem oriented. Thus a case in the case-base is just a part of a patient's history, namely an episode that describes a specific problem that usually has a solution too. So, the case-base represents decisions of doctors (diagnosis, therapies) for specific problems, and their generalisations and their theoretical foundations (see the examples in the following section). A solution is called "case solution". Every case solution has (usually two) generalisations, which are formulated by doctors. The first one is expressed in terms of the knowledge base and it is used as a keyword for searching in the knowledge base. Such a generalisation is called "knowledge base solution". The second generalisation of a solution is expressed in common words and it is mainly used for dialogues. It is called "prompt solution".

Former cases (attribute value pairs) in the case-base are indexed by keywords. Each case contains keywords that have been explicitly placed by an expert. For retrieval three main key words are used: a code of the problem, a diagnosis, and a therapy. Further key words such as age, sex and so on can be used optionally.

Prototypes (generalized cases) play a particular role. Prototypes help to select a proper solution from the list of probable or available solutions. A prototype may help to point out a reason of inefficacy of a therapy or it may support the doctor's choice of a drug.

Retrieval, Adaptation, and Dialogue

For retrieval keywords are used. Since ISOR-1 is problem oriented, the first keyword is a code that implies a specific problem. The second one is the diagnosis and the other ones are retrieved from the knowledge base.

Adaptation takes place as a dialogue between the doctor and the system. The idea of dialogue interaction with the user is similar to conversational CBR (Gupta, 2002). The system presents different solutions, versions of them, and asks questions to manifest them. The doctor answers and selects suggestions, while the patient himself suggests possible solutions that can be considered by the doctor and by ISOR-1.

We differentiate between two steps of adaptation. The first one occurs as a dialogue between ISOR-1 and the user. Usually, doctors are the users. However, sometimes even a patient may take part in this dialogue. The goal of these dialogues is to select probable solutions from all information sources mentioned in the sections above. Pieces of information are retrieved by the use of keywords. Specific menus support the retrieval process. The first step of adaptation can be regarded as partly user based, because ISOR-1 presents lists of probable solutions and menus of keywords, the user selects the most adequate ones. The second adaptation means proving obtained solutions. This proving is rule based and it includes further dialogues, laboratory test results, and consultations with medical experts. While the procedures supporting the first adaptation step are domain independent, the adaptation rules of the second step are mainly domain dependent.

Examples

By three examples we illustrate how ISOR-1 works. The first and the second example are from the endocrine domain, the third one deals with a psychiatric problem.

Inefficacy of Levothyroxine Therapy

Every morning a mother gives her 10 year-old boy not only the prescribed Levothyroxine dose but also vitamin pills. These pills have not been prescribed but they are healthy and have lately been advertised on TV. Part of this medication is sodium hydrocarbonate (cooking soda) that causes problems with Levothyroxine.

Problem: Levothyroxine does not help any more.

Individual base. The same problem, inefficacy of Levothyroxine therapy, is retrieved from the patient's history. The solution of the former problem was that the boy did not take the drug regularly. This time it must be a different cause, because the mother controls the intake.

Knowledge base. It has a tree structure that is organised according to keys. One main key is *therapy* and the keyword is *Levothyroxine*. Another keyword is *instructions*. These instructions are represented in form of rules that concern the intake of Levothyroxine. For Levothyroxine a rather long list of instructions exists. Since the idea is that the boy may break an instruction rule, this list is sorted according to the observed frequency of offences against them in the case-base.

Concerning these instructions a couple of questions are asked, e.g. whether the boy takes sodium hydrocarbonate together with Levothyroxine. Since the mother is not aware of the fact that Sodium hydrocarbonate is contained in the vitamin pills, she gives a negative answer and no possible solution can be established by the knowledge base. However, *soda* is generated as one keyword for retrieval in the case-base.

Eventually, three general solutions are retrieved from the knowledge base: sodium hydrocarbonate, soy, and estrogen. Since estrogen does not fit for the boy, it is eliminated.

Case-base. Using the keyword *soda* eight cases with seven individual solutions are retrieved.

Thus we get a list of drugs and beverages that contain sodium hydrocarbonate. All of them belong to the generalised solution "soluble" (Figure 1).

Solution. The boy admits to take Levothyroxine together with an instantiation of the generalised solution "soluble", namely soluble vitamin.

Recommendation. The boy is told to take vitamin four hours later than Levothyroxine. Additionally, further interactions between vitamin and Levothyroxine must be checked, because it might be necessary to adjust the Levothyroxine dose.

Improving the Efficacy by Dose Updates

Figure 2 shows an example of a case study. We compared the decisions of an experienced doctor with the recommendations of ISOR-1. The decisions are based on basic laboratory tests and on lists of observed symptoms. Intervals between two visits are approximately six months. In this example, there are three

Figure 1. Dialogue for the first example

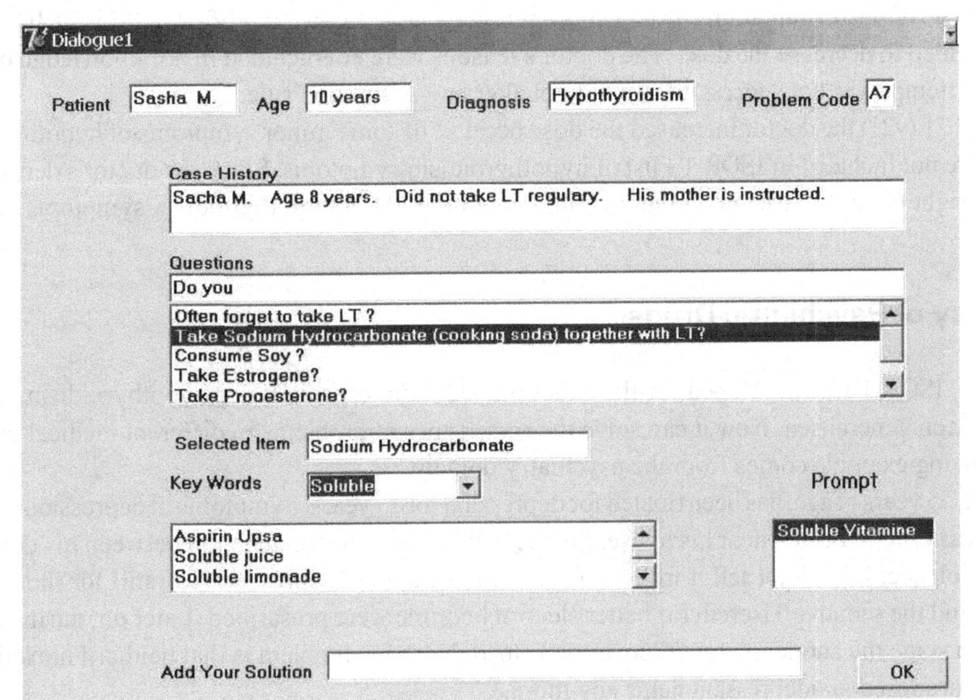

Figure 2. Dose updates recommended by our program compared with doctor's decision. V1 means the first visit, V2 the second visit etc.

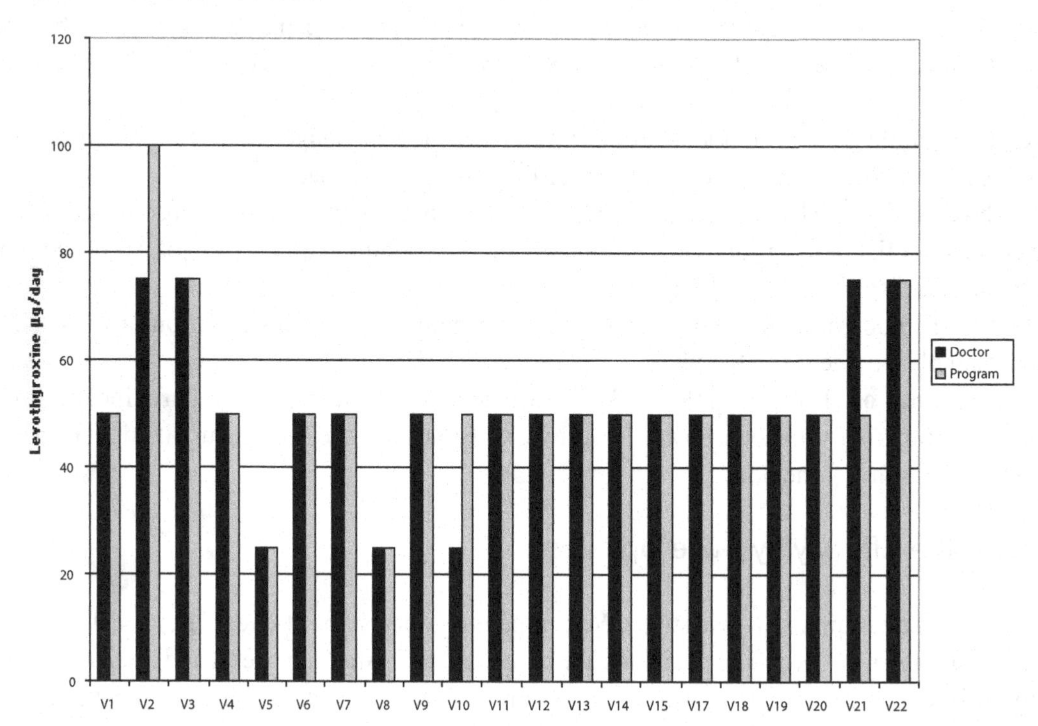

deviations between the doctor's and ISOR-1's decisions, usually there are less. At the second visit (v2), according to laboratory results the Levothyroxine should be increased. ISOR-1 recommended a too high increase. The applied adaptation rule was not precise enough. So, we modified it. At visit 10 (v10) the doctor decided to decrease the dose. The doctor's reasons were not included in our knowledge base and since his attempt was not successful, we did not alter any adaptation rule.

At visit 21 (v21) the doctor increased the dose because of some minor symptoms of hypothyroidism, which were not included in ISOR-1's list of hypothyroidism symptoms. Since the doctor's decision was probably right (visit 22), we added these symptoms to the list of hypothyroidism symptoms of ISOR-1.

Inefficacy of Psychiatric Drugs

Originally, ISOR-1 was developed for the endocrine domain, especially for hypothyroidism, but later on it has been generalised. Now it can solve the same types of problems in different medical domains. The following example comes from the psychiatry domain.

A man, 55 years of age, has been treated for depression for 15 years. Symptoms of depression appeared after he was cruelly beaten near his house. Since he did not see any connection between his depression and the violence, he did not tell it to his doctor. At first, the antidepressant Tofranil for intake in the morning and the sedative Tisercin for better sleep at bedtime were prescribed. Later on, during another depression stage the antidepressant Fluoxetine helped. Now, his problem is that neither Fluoxetine, nor any other proposed antidepressant helps any more.

Retrieval. Keywords are used to retrieve information from all data sources. Since optional keywords about a patient's feeling (e.g. *feeling worse*) are used for retrieval in the patient's medical history, even biographical events of a patient can be retrieved.

Individual base. Since the problem of inefficacy of an antidepressant never arose in the patient's past, no solution can be found. However, indirect information was retrieved. The keyword *feeling better* provided a trip to Switzerland, while the result of the keyword *feeling worse* provided a trip to Israel, where the latest very severe depression began:

- *Feeling better:* A trip to Switzerland
- *Feeling worse:* A trip to Israel

The knowledge base contains information about depression, anxiety and other psychiatric diseases, possible complications and references to their theoretical grounds (e.g. Davidson 1991; Gelder 2000). References to similar problems are retrieved, the most remarkable one is a link to the algorithm for psychopharmacology of depression (Osser and Patterson 1998). Though the idea of the algorithm is to solve the problem of non-response to an antidepressant, it does not really fit here, because it does not cover the situation that a therapy helped for some time and then stopped having an effect.

Case-base. Eleven cases with similar depression problems are retrieved. Three of them are characterised by the general idea *depression is secondary to anxiety resulting from a psychical trauma.* These three cases are:

- Case solution 1: A severe stress during World War 2 (a woman)
- Case solution 2: A bad experience in jail (a young man)
- Case solution 3: Sexual assault in childhood (a woman)

All other cases have solutions that are generalised to *changes in therapy.*

Adaptation. ISOR-1 displays retrieved information pieces. In this case, two strategies are offered. The first one suggests trying some other therapy. This strategy is supported by the majority of the retrieved cases and partly by theoretical recommendations. The second strategy means to check the diagnosis. This strategy is supported by the three retrieved cases mentioned above and by the patient's medical history. The choice between both strategies is up to the user. In this example, the doctor chooses to attempt the second strategy at first, because various therapy changes have already been attempted in the past – without success. Furthermore, the doctor is especially led by the patient's medical history, because Switzerland is usually associated with a safe life (especially in comparison to life in Russia), while living in Israel is considered as unsafe. Additionally, this strategy is supported by the general situation that some sedative drugs (Neuroleptics) had helped for some time (e.g. Tisercin at the beginning).

ISOR-1 offers a list of questions for the favoured strategy and as a result the doctor concludes that in this case depression is in fact only second to anxiety. The man is permanently afraid of possible violence and anxiety is based on strong fear that occurred long ago.

Explaining remarks. Diagnosing anxiety needs good medical skills, because patients try to suppress traumatic events from their memory (Stein, 2003). In this example, depression even served as a mechanism of suppression. The accepted case-based solution spared the patient unnecessary experiments with other psychopharmacological drugs.

So, the first problem is solved, a new diagnosis is ascertained.

The next problem is prescription of a therapy. According to the domain theory and to our knowledge base anxiety implies Neuroleptics (Gelder, 2000; Kalinowsky, Hippius, 1969). Many of them are available but a good choice is not trivial.

Individual base. From the patient's history those sedatives (Neuroleptics) are retrieved that he took in his lifetime and that had positive effects on his psychical condition: Tisercin and Paxil, which is a drug that has both sedative and antidepressive effects.

Prototype. Among those prototypes that have been defined by doctors (based on their long experience with cases) the prototypical solution Paxil is retrieved.

Adaptation. Before described, every drug must be checked for conflicts with the patient's additional diseases and already existing therapy. Though the query patient has already taken Paxil in the past, ISOR-1 checks all possible conflicts. If necessary, adaptation has to be performed. In this case no conflicts are discovered and Paxil is prescribed.

ISOR-2: INCREMENTAL DEVELOPMENT OF AN EXPLANATION MODEL FOR EXCEPTIONAL DIALYSE PATIENTS

In ISOR-1, we demonstrated advantages of CBR in situations where a theoretically approved medical decision does not produce the desired and usually expected results.

ISOR-2 is a logical continuation. It is still the same system and the same structure of dialogues, but ISOR-2 deals with situations where neither a well-developed theory nor reliable knowledge nor a proper case-base is available. So, instead of reliable theoretical knowledge and intelligent experience, just a theoretical hypothesis and a set of measurements are given. In such situations the usual question is, how do measured data fit to a theoretical hypothesis. To statistically confirm a hypothesis it is necessary, that the majority of cases fit the hypothesis. Mathematical statistics determines the exact quantity of necessary confirmation (Kendall, Stuart, 1979). However, usually a few cases do not fit the hypothesis. We examine these exceptional cases to find out why they do not satisfy the hypothesis. ISOR-2 offers a dialogue to guide the search for possible reasons in all components of the data system.

This approach is justified by a certain mistrust of statistical models by the doctors, because modelling results are usually unspecific and "average oriented" (Hai, 2002), which means a lack of attention to individual "imperceptible" features of concrete patients.

The usual Case-Based Reasoning assumption is that a case-base with complete solutions is available. Our approach starts in a situation where such a case-base is not available at the beginning but has to be set up incrementally (Figure 3). So, we must:

1. Construct a model
2. Point out the exceptions
3. Find causes why the exceptional cases do not fit the model
4. Set up a case-base

Case-Based Reasoning is combined with a model, in this specific situation with a statistical one. The idea to combine CBR with other methods is not new. Care-Partner, for example, resorts to a multi-modal reasoning framework for the co-operation of CBR and Rule-based Reasoning (RBR) (Bichindaritz, 1998).

Figure 3. The general program scheme of ISOR-2

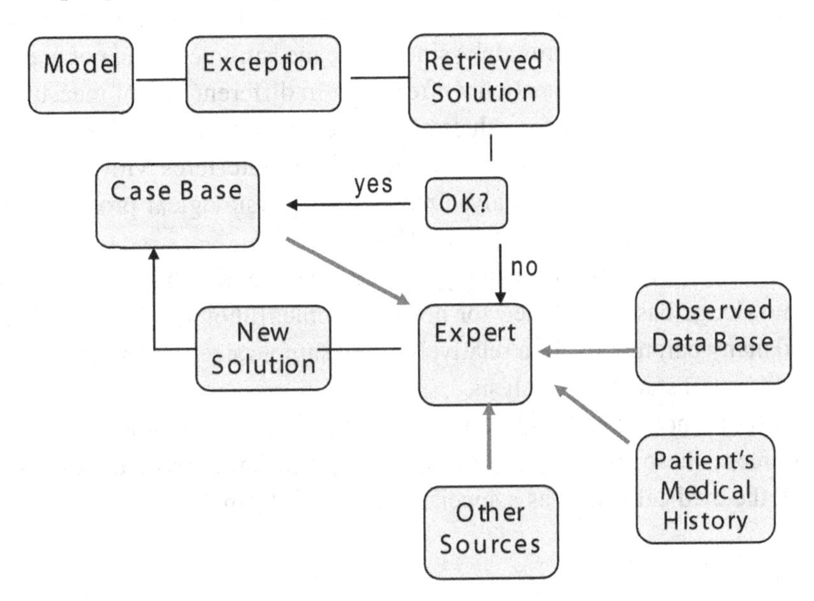

Another way of combining hybrid rule bases with CBR is discussed by Prentzas and Hatzilgeroudis (2002). The combination of CBR and model-based reasoning is discussed in (Shuguang 2000). Statistical methods are used within CBR mainly for retrieval and retention (e.g. Corchado, 2003; Rezvani, Prasag, 2003). Arshadi proposes a method that combines CBR with statistical methods like clustering and logistic regression (Arshadi, Jurisica, 2005).

Dialyse and Fitness

Hemodialyse means stress for a patient's organism and has significant adverse effects. Fitness is the most available and relative cheap way of support. It is meant to improve the physiological condition of a patient and to compensate negative dialyse effects.

One of the intended goals of this research is to convince the patients of the positive effects of fitness and to encourage them to make efforts and to go in for sports actively. This is important because dialyse patients usually feel sick, they are physically weak, and they do not want any additional physical load (Davidson, 2005).

At the University clinic in St. Petersburg, a specially developed complex of physiotherapy exercises including simulators, walking, swimming etc. was offered to all dialyse patients but only some of them actively participated, whereas some others participated but were not really active.

Data

For each patient a set of physiological parameters is measured. These parameters contain information about burned calories, maximal power achieved by the patient, his oxygen uptake, his oxygen pulse (volume of oxygen consumption per heart beat), lung ventilation and others. There are also biochemical parameters like haemoglobin and other laboratory measurements. More than 100 parameters were measured for every patient.

Parameters are supposed to be measured four times during the first year of participating in the fitness program. There is an initial measurement followed by a next one after three months, then after six months and finally after a year. Unfortunately, since some measurements did not happen, many data are missing. Therefore the records of the patients often contain different sets of measured parameters.

It is necessary to note that parameter values of dialyse patients essentially differ from those of non-dialysis patients, especially of healthy people, because dialyse interferes with the natural, physiological processes in an organism. In fact, for dialyse patients all physiological processes behave abnormal. Therefore, the correlation between parameters differs too.

For statistics, this means difficulties in applying statistical methods based on correlation and it limits the usage of a knowledge base developed for normal people. Inhomogeneity of observed data, many missing data, and many parameters for a relatively small sample size, all this makes the data set practically impossible for usual statistical analysis.

Since the data set is incomplete, additional or substitutional information has to be found in other available data sources. These are databases – the already existent individual base, the sequentially set up case-base, and the medical expert as a special source of information.

Setting up a Model

We start with a medical problem that has to be solved based on given data. In this application it is: "Does special fitness improve the physiological condition of dialyse patients?" More formal, physical conditions of active and non-active patients have to be compared. The patients are divided into two groups, depending on their activity, active patients and non-active ones.

According to our assumption active patients should feel better after some months of fitness, whereas non-active ones should feel rather worse. The meaning of "feeling better" and "feeling worse" has to be defined in this context. A medical expert selects appropriate factors from ISOR's menu. The expert selected the following main factors:

- **F1:** O2PT - oxygen pulse by training
- **F2:** MUO2T - maximal uptake of oxygen by training
- **F3:** WorkJ – performed work (joules) during control training

Subsequently the "research time period" has to be determined. Initially, this period was planed to be twelve months, but after a while some patients tend to give up the fitness program. This means, the longer the time period, the more data are missing. Therefore, we have to make a compromise between time period and sample size. A period of six months has been chosen.

The next question is whether the model shall be quantitative or qualitative? The observed data are mostly quantitative measurements. The selected factors are of quantitative nature too. On the other side, the goal of this research is to find out whether physical training improves or worsens the physical condition of the dialyse patients.

It is not necessary to compare one patient with another patient. Instead, each patient has to be compared with his own situation some months ago, namely just before the start of the fitness program. The success shall not be measured in absolute values, because the health statuses of patients are very different. Thus, even a modest improvement for one patient may be as important as a great improvement of another. Therefore, the development is simply classified in two categories: "better" and "worse". Since the usual tendency for dialyse patients is to worsen in time, those few patients, where no changes could be observed, are added to the category "better".

The three main factors are supposed to describe the changes of the physical conditions of the patients. The changes are assessed depending on the number of improved factors:

- Weak version of the model: At least one factor has improved
- Medium version of the model: At least two factors have improved
- Strong version of the model: All three factors have improved

The final step means to define the type of model. Popular statistical programs offer a large variety of statistical models. Some of them deal with categorical data. The easiest model is a 2x2 frequency table. The "better/ worse" concept fits this simple model very well. The results are presented in Table 1.

Unfortunately, the most popular Pearson Chi-square test is not applicable here because of the small values "2" and "3" in Table 1. But Fisher's exact test (Kendall, Stuart, 1979) can be used. In the three versions shown in Table 1, a very strong significance can be observed. The smaller the value of p is, the more significant the dependency.

So, the performed Fisher test confirms the hypothesis that patients doing active fitness achieve better physical conditions than non-active ones. However, there are exceptions, namely active patients whose health conditions did not improve.

Exceptions should be explained. Incrementally, explained exceptions build the case-base. According to Table 1, the stronger the model, the more exceptions can be observed and have to be explained. Every exception is associated with at least two problems. The first one is "Why did the patient's condition get worse?" Of course, "worse" is meant in terms of the chosen model. Since there may be some factors that are not included in the model but have changed positively, the second problem is "What

Table 1. Results of Fisher's Exact Test, performed with an interactive Web-program: http://www.matforsk.noIola/fisher.htm

Improvement mode	Patient's physical condition	Active	Non-active	Fisher Exact p
Strong	Better	28	2	< 0.0001
	Worse	**22**	21	
Medium	Better	40	10	< 0.005
	Worse	**10**	12	
Weak	Better	47	16	< 0.02
	Worse	**3**	6	

has improved in the patient's condition?" To solve this problem, significant factors, where the values improved, have to be found.

In the following section we explain the set-up of a case-base on the strongest model version.

Setting up a Case-Base

We intend to solve both problems (mentioned above) by means of CBR. So, a case-base has to be set up sequentially. That means, as soon as an exception is explained, it is incorporated into the case-base and can help to explain further exceptional cases. A random order is chosen for the exceptional cases. In fact, they are taken in alphabetical order.

The retrieval of already explained cases is performed by keywords. The main keywords are the usual ISOR ones, namely "problem code", "diagnosis", and "therapy". Here, the instantiations of these keywords are "adverse effects of dialysis" (diagnosis), "fitness" (therapy), and two specific problem codes.

Besides the main ISOR-2 keywords additional problem specific ones are used. Here, the additional keyword is the number of worsened factors. Further keywords are optional. They are just used when the case-base becomes bigger and retrieval is not simple any longer.

However, ISOR-2 does not only use the case-base as knowledge source but further sources are involved, namely the patient's individual base (his medical history) and observed data (partly gained by dialogue with medical experts). Since in the domain of kidney disease and dialyse the medical knowledge is very detailed and much investigated but still incomplete, it is unreasonable to attempt to create an adequate knowledge base. Therefore, a medical expert, observed data, and just a few rules serve as medical knowledge sources.

Expert Knowledge and Artificial Cases

Expert's knowledge can be used in many different ways. It can be used to acquire rules, to select appropriate items from the list of retrieved solutions, to propose new solutions, and last but not least – to create artificial cases.

Initially, an expert creates artificial cases, afterwards they can be used in the same way as real cases. They are created in the following situation. An expert points out a factor F as a possible solution for a query patient. Since many values are missing, it can happen that just for the query patient values of factor F are missing. In this case, the doctor's knowledge can not be applied. However, it is sensible to save it anyway. Principally, there are two different ways to do this. The first one means to generate a correspondent rulc and to insert it into ISOR-2's algorithms. Unfortunately, this is very complicated, especially to find an appropriate way for inserting such a rule. The alternative is to create an artificial case. Instead of a patient's name an artificial case number is generated. The other attributes are either inherited from the query case or declared as missing. The retrieval attributes are inherited within the dialogue (see the fields eleven and twelve of figure 5). ISOR-2's algorithms remain intact. Artificial cases can be treated in the same way as real cases, they can be revised, deleted, generalised and so on.

Solving the Problem "Why did Some Patients Conditions Became Worse?"

As results we obtain a set of solutions of different origin and different nature. There are three solution categories: additional factor, model failure, and wrong data (Figure 4).

Figure 4. Resulting tree of solutions concerning the model and the example

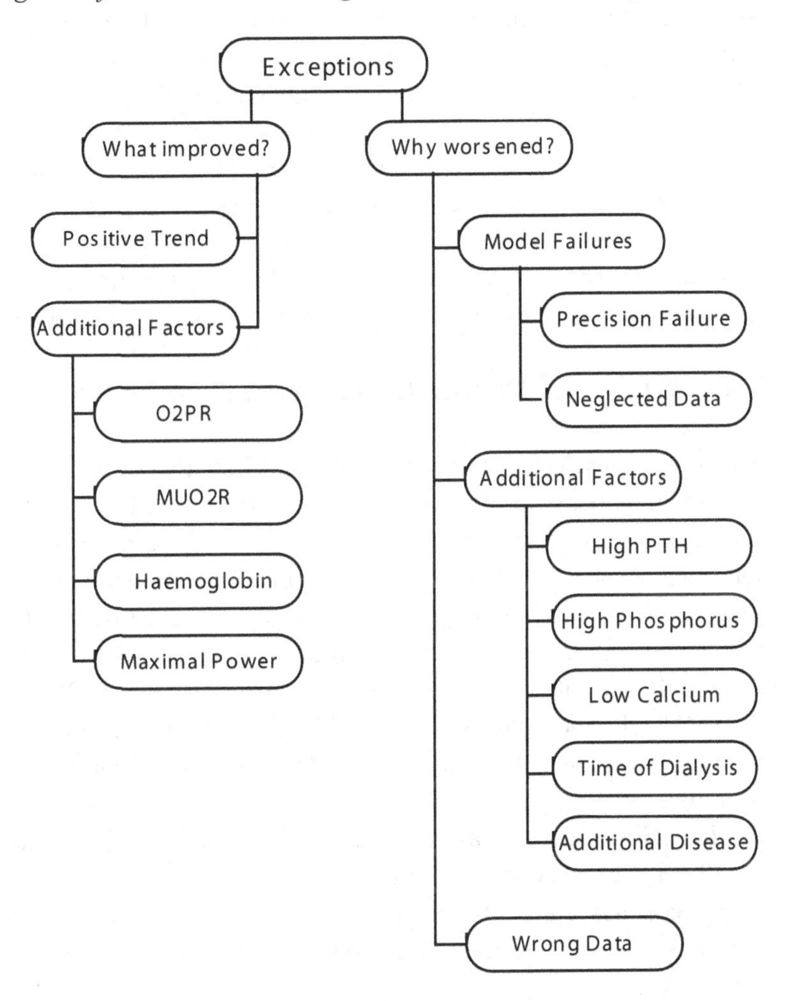

Additional factor. The most important and most frequent solution is the influence of an additional factor. Only three main factors are obviously not enough to describe all cases. Unfortunately, for different patients different additional factors are important. When ISOR-2 has discovered an additional factor as explanation for an exceptional case, the factor has to be confirmed by the expert before it can be accepted as a solution. One of these factors is Parathyroid Hormone (PTH). An increased PTH level sometimes can explain a worsened condition of a patient (Osser, Patterson, 1998). PTH is a significant factor, but unfortunately it was measured only for some patients.

Another additional factor solution is a phosphorus blood level. We use the principle of artificial cases to introduce the factor phosphorus as a new solution. One patient's record contains many missing data. The retrieved solution means high PTH, but PTH data in the current patient's record is missing too. The expert proposes an increased phosphorus level as a possible solution. Since data about phosphorus data are also missing, an artificial case is created, who inherits all retrieval attributes of the query case whereas the other attributes are recorded as missing. According to the expert, high phosphorus can explain the solution. Therefore it is accepted as an artificial solution or a solution of an artificial case.

Model failure. We regard two types of model failures. One of them is deliberately neglected data. As a compromise we just consider six months as research period but later data of a patient might be important. In fact, three of the patients did not show an improvement in the considered six months period but in the following six months. So, they are wrongly classified and shall really belong to the "better" category.

The second type of model failure is based on the fact that the two-category model is not precise enough. Some exceptions can be explained by a tiny and not really significant change in one of the main factors.

Wrong data are usually due to a technical mistake or to data that has not really been proved. One patient, for example, was reported as actively participating in the fitness program but really was not.

Solving the Problem "What in a Patient's Condition Became Better?"

There are at least two criteria to select factors for the model. First, a factor has to be significant, and second there must be enough patients for which this factor was measured at least for six months. So, some principally important factors are initially not taken into account because of missing data.

The list of solutions includes these factors (Figure 4): haemoglobin, maximal power (watt) achieved during control training. Oxygen pulse and oxygen uptake were measured in tow different situations, namely during the training under loading and before training in a state of relax. Therefore we have two pairs of factors: oxygen pulse in state of relax (O2PR) and during training (O2PT); maximal oxygen uptake in state of relax (MUO2R) and during training (MUO2T). Measurements made in a state of relax are more indicative and significant than those made during training. Unfortunately, most measurements were made during training. Only for some patients correspondent measurements in relax state exist. Therefore O2PT and MUO2T are accepted as main factors and are taken into the model. On the other side, O2PR and MUO2R serve as solutions for the current problem.

In the case-base every patient is represented by a set of cases, every case represents a specific problem. This means that a patient is described from different points of view and accordingly different problem keywords are used for retrieval.

Illustration of ISOR-2's Program Flow

Figure 5 shows the main dialogue of ISOR-2. For illustration purposes, we have numbered the fields of the menu. At first, the user sets up a model (fields one to four), subsequently he/she gets the result (field 5) and an analysis of the model (fields six to eight), and then he/she attempts to find explanations for the exceptions (fields nine and ten). Finally, the case-base is updated (fields eleven and twelve). Now the steps are explained in detail.

At first, the user has to set up a model. To do this, he has to select a grouping variable. In the example of figure 5, CODACT is chosen. It stands for "activity code" and means that active and none active patients are to be compared. Provided alternatives are the sex and the beginning with the fitness program (within the first year of dialyse or later). In another menu, the user can define further alternatives. Furthermore, the user has to select a model type (alternatives are "strong", "medium", and "weak"), the length of the research period (3, 6, or 12 months), and the main factors have to be selected. The list contains all factors from the observed database. In the example of figure 5, three factors are chosen: O2PT (oxygen pulse by training), MUO2T (maximal oxygen uptake by training), and WorkJ (work in joules during the test training). In the menu list, the first two factors have alternatives: "R" instead of "T", where "R" stands for state of rest and "T" stands for state of training.

When the user has selected these items, the program calculates the table. "Better" and "worse" are meant in the sense of the chosen model, in the example the strong model has been chosen. ISOR-2 does not only calculate the table but additionally extracts the exceptional patients from the observed database. In the menu, the list of exceptions shows the code names of the patients. In the example of Figure 5, patient "D5" is selected" and all further data belong to this patient. The goal is to find an explanation for this exceptional case "D5". In field seven of the menu it is shown that all selected factors worsened (-1), and in field eight the values according to different time intervals are depicted. All data for the twelve months measurements are missing (-9999).

The next step means creating an explanation for the selected patient "D5". From the case-base ISOR-2 retrieves general solutions. The first retrieved one, the PTH factor, denotes that the increased Parathyroid hormone blood level may explain the failure. Further theoretical information (e.g. normal values) about a selected item can be received by pressing the button "show comments". The PTH value of patient "D5" is missing (-9999). From menu field ten the expert user can select further probable solutions. In the example, an increased phosphorus level (P) is suggested. Unfortunately, phosphorus data

Figure 5. ISOR-2's program flow

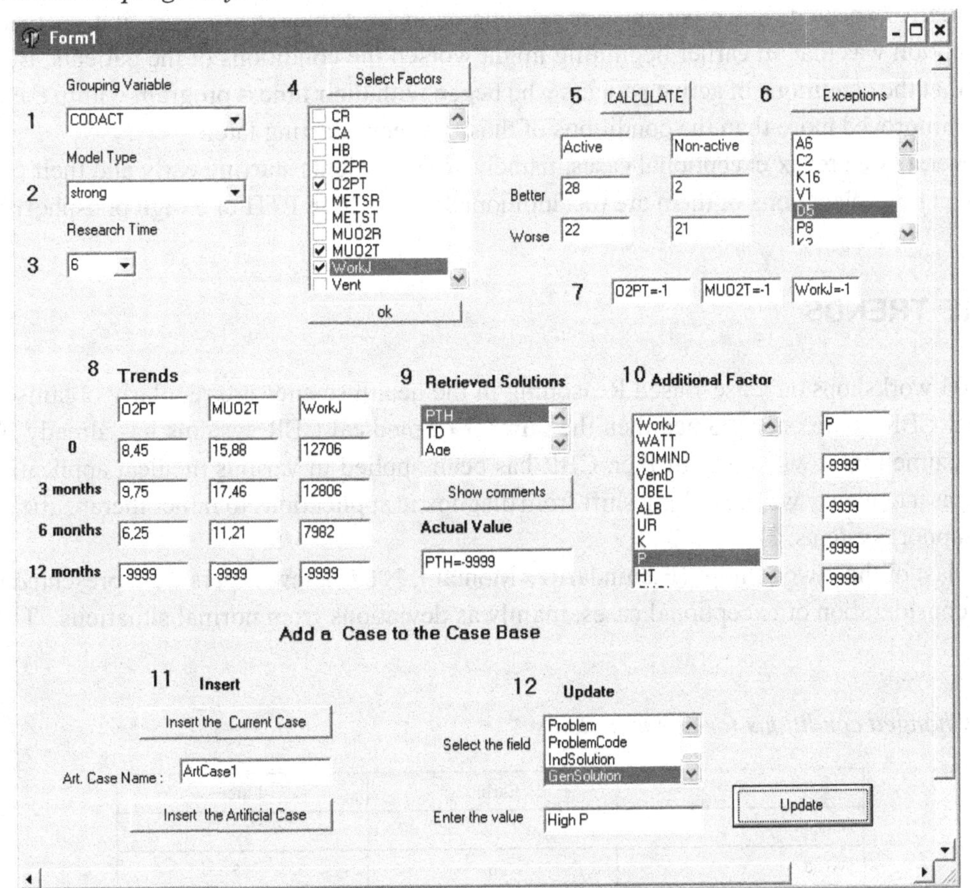

are missing too. However, the idea of an increased phosphorus level as a possible solution shall not be lost. So, an artificial case can be generated.

The final step means inserting new cases into the case-base. There are two sorts of cases, query cases and artificial cases. Query cases are stored records of real patients from the observed database.

Artificial cases inherit the key attributes from the query cases (field seven in the menu). Other data may be declared as missing, by the update function data can be inserted. In the example, the generalised solution "High P" is inherited, it may be retrieved as a possible solution (field nine of the menu) for future cases.

Example: A Different Problem

Above we described just one of many problems that can arise and that can be solved and analysed by ISOR-2. Another interesting research question is "Does is make sense to begin with the fitness program during the first year of dialyse?" The question arises because the conditions of the patients are considered to be unstable during their first year of dialyse. The question can be expressed in this way "When shall patients begin with the fitness program, earlier or later?" The term "earlier" is defined as "during the first year of dialyse". The term "later" means that they begin with their program after at least one year of dialyse. To answer this question, two groups of active patients are considered, those who began their training within the first year of dialyse and those who began it later (Table 2).

According to Fisher's Exact Test dependence can be observed, with $p < 0.05$. However, it is not as it was initially expected. Since patients are considered as unstable during their first year of dialyse, the assumption was that an earlier beginning might worsen the conditions of the patients. But the test revealed that the conditions of active patients who began with their fitness program within the first year of dialyse improved more than the conditions of those patients starting later.

However, there are six exceptional cases, namely active patients starting early and their conditions worsened. The explanations of them are the additional factors high PTH or a high phosphorus level.

FUTURE TRENDS

Since 2003 workshops on Case-Based Reasoning in the health science are regularly organised within the annual CBR conferences. Since then the number of medical CBR systems has already increased and we assume that it will grow further. CBR has been applied in various medical application areas. However, as a tendency we see a slight shift from diagnostic applications to rather therapeutic and other sorts of support systems.

At the last of these workshops (Bichindaritz, Montani, 2007) a few papers were presented that deal with the consideration of exceptional cases, mainly as deviations from normal situations. Though we

Table 2. Changed conditions for active patients

	Earlier	Later
Better	18	10
Worse	6	15

are dealing with exceptional cases more explicitly than the other approaches, we believe that this is just the current situation and that a future trend even in medical knowledge-based systems in general might be a more extensive consideration of exceptional cases.

For many years knowledge-based applications have been developed, where medical experts are just considered as knowledge providers. Their knowledge is incorporated in systems that for given input compute results that are presented to the users as output. From our experience, doctors have seldom been happy with such systems, because they especially want to know why and how a system draws conclusions.

We see a new direction emerge, namely conversational systems. The idea is to find solutions within a dialogue between the user (a doctor) and a knowledge-based system. Of course, domain knowledge still has to be incorporated in such a system before it starts. Additionally, further knowledge shall be added at run-time. This is a dialogue process in which both participants (system and doctor) should stimulate each other. By both ISOR systems presented in this chapter we have shown steps into this direction.

Within the CBR community the first workshop on conversational systems was organised in 2003 (Aha, 2003). For medical applications, first steps were undertaken even earlier (McSherry, 2001). However, just recently it seems that it is becoming a more popular idea (e.g. McSherry, 2007, Vorobieva, Rumyantsev, Schmidt, 2006).

CONCLUSION

In medical practise and in medical research, doctors very often are confronted with exceptions. Every system that is developed to support doctors shall take this into account. In knowledge-based systems exceptions have to be considered, which may lead to a huge amount of exceptional rules.

In medical studies, statisticians are usually quite happy when a statistical test significantly supports a hypothesis. However, when the number of cases contradicting the hypothesis is rather big, physicians often are not satisfied with significant test results but additionally wish to get explanations for the exceptional cases.

In this chapter, we have presented two systems that deal with both sorts of these situations. The first one, called ISOR-1, especially investigates therapy inefficacy by a dialogue with the user. The second system, ISOR-2, helps to explain cases that contradict a theoretical hypothesis.

First, we have presented ISOR-1, a CBR system designed to help doctors to solve therapeutic problems, particularly to investigate causes of inefficacy of therapies. At present, it deals with two application areas. In the endocrine domain a strong theory exists and therefore usually a lot of solutions are theoretically possible. So, here the task is to reduce a set of possible solutions as much as possible.

ISOR-1 includes different knowledge containers, namely a case-base, a knowledge base, prototypes, and individual bases of patients that reflect their medical histories. Information retrieved from these containers is arranged in form of dialogues. The case-base plays a central role in the dialogue forming process. It serves as a kind of filter when the knowledge base suggests too many possible solutions for the problem (as in the first example). In this situation the most typical cases are retrieved from the case-base. When a solution from the knowledge base is not convincing or when it is hardly adaptable, the case-base may provide better alternatives (as in the example from the psychiatry domain). Generalisations, keywords and references to other knowledge components belong to the case-base. The adaptation program uses them to create dialogues.

ISOR-1 is designed to solve problems from different medical domains. Specific, domain dependant features are mainly attributed to the individual base, because every domain requires a special design of case histories. The knowledge base in ISOR-1 is domain-oriented, but all algorithms and functions are completely domain independent.

Second in this paper, we have proposed to use CBR in ISOR-2 to explain cases that do not fit a statistical model. Since for the dialyse and fitness problem too many parameters exist (nearly 100), the idea is to select three main ones to set up a model and to search subsequently for better parameters to explain the exceptional cases.

The statistical model we presented for ISOR-2 is one of simplest ones but here it is relatively effective because it demonstrates statistically significant dependence between fitness activity and health improvement of dialyse patients. For the strong alternative, the model covers about two thirds of the cases, whereas the remaining one third of them has to be explained by the help of CBR. According to table 1, the stronger the model, the more exceptional cases have to be explained. This means more work for CBR but with a stronger model the confidence in the result of the data analysis increases.

Seven of the exceptional cases seemed to be wrongly classified. After the expert's consultation their classification has been changed. Two kinds of model faults are observed. First, just six months are chosen as relevant time period, whereas for a couple of patients the health condition improved later on. Second, with the choice of qualitative categories, better and worse, it is not possible to assess the amount of the change. So, it cannot be distinguished between small and big changes of the health conditions.

ACKNOWLEDGMENT

We especially thank Olga Vorobieba, Sechenov Institute of Evolutionary Physiology and Biochemistry in St.Petersburg, and Prof. Alexander Rumyantsev, Pavlov Medical State University in St. Petersburg, for their close cooperation.

We thank Dr. Monika Mix, Children's Hospital of the University Clinic of Rostock, and Prof. Nikolai Nikolaenko, Sechenov Institute of Evolutionary Physiology and Biochemistry in St.Petersburg, for their data and for their help and time during our consultations.

Furthermore, we thank Professor Aleksey Smirnov, director of the Institute for Nephrology of Saint-Petersburg Medical University and we thank Natalia Korosteleva, researcher at the Institute for Nephrology of St.-Petersburg Medical University for collecting and managing the data.

REFERENCES

Aamodt, A. (2004). Knowledge-Intensive Case-Based Reasoning in CREEK. In: Funk, P., Gonzalez Calero, P.A. (eds.): *Proceedings European Conference on Case-Based Reasoning*, ECCBR 2004, Springer-Verlag, Berlin 5- 15.

Aha, D. (2003). Workshop – Mixed-Initiative Case-Based Reasoning. In McGinty, L. (ed.): *ICCBR'03 Workshop Proceedings*, Trondheim 127-209.

Alacorn, R. D., Glover, S., Boyer, W., & Balon, R. (2000). Proposing an algorithm for the pharmacological treatment of posttraumatic stress disorder. *Ann Clin Psychiatry, 12*(4) 239-246.

Arshadi, N., & Jurisica, I. (2005). Data Mining for Case-based Reasoning in high-dimensional biological domains. *IEEE Transactions on Knowledge and Data Engineering, 17*(8), 1127-1137.

Bichindaritz, I. (1994). A case-based assistant for clinical psychiatry expertise. *Journal of the American Medical Informatics Association*, Symposium Supplement, 673-677.

Bichindaritz, I., Kansu, E., & Sullivan, K. M. (1998). Case-based Reasoning in Care-Partner. In: Smyth, B., Cunningham, P. (eds.): *Proceedings European Workshop on Case-based Reasong*, EWCBR-98, Springer-Verlag, Berlin, 334-345.

Bichindaritz, I., & Montani, S. (2007). Workshop – Case-Based Reasoning in the Health Science. In Wilson, D.C., Khemani, D. (eds.): *ICCBR- Workshop Proceedings*, Belfast 257-368.

Corchado, J. M., Corchado, E. S., Aiken, J., Fyfe, C., Fernandez, F., & Gonzalez, M. (2003). Maximum likelihood Hebbian learning based retrieval method for CBR systems. In Ashley, K. D., Bridge, D. G. (eds.): *Proceedings International Conference on Case-based Reasoning*, ICCBR 2003, Springer-Verlag, Berlin 107-121.

Cuffel, B. J. (2003). Remission, residual symptoms, and nonresponse in the usual treatment of major depression in managed clinical practice. *J Clin Psychiatry, 64*(4) 397-402.

Davidson, A. M., Cameron, J. S., & Grünfeld, J.-P. (eds.) (2005). *Oxford Textbook of Nephrology, 3.* Oxford University Press

Davidson, R. J. (1991). Cerebral asymmetry and affective disorders: A developmentalperspective. In: Cicchetti, D., Toth, S.L. (eds.) *Internalizing and externalizing expressions of dysfunction.* Rochester Symp. on Developmental Psychopathology 2, Hillsdale 123-133.

DeGroot, L. J. (1994). Thyroid Physiology and Hypothyroidsm. In Besser, G.M., Turner, M. (eds.) *Clinical endocrinilogy.* Wolfe, London Chapter 15.

Gelder, M. G., Lopez-Ibor, U., & Andeasen, N.C. (eds.) (2000). *New Oxford Textbook of Psychiatry.* Oxford University Press, Oxford.

Gupta, K. M., Aha, D. W., & Sandhu, N. (2002). Exploiting Taxonomic and Causal Realations in Conversational Case Retrieval. In Craw, S., Preeece, A. (eds.): *Proceedings European Conference on Case-Based Reasoning*, ECCBR 2002, Springer-Verlag, Berlin 133-147.

Hai, G. A. (2002). Logic of diagnostic and decision making in clinical medicine. Politheknica publishing, St. Petersburg.

Hirschfeld, R. M. (2002). Partial response and nonresponse to antidepressant therapy: Current approaches and treatment options. *J Clin Psychiatry, 63*(9) 826-37.

Kalinowsky, L., & Hippius, H. (1969). *Pharmacolological, convulsive and other somatic treatments in psychiatry.* Grunee&Stratton, New York London.

Kendall, M. G., & Stuart, A. (1979). *The advanced theory of statistics.* 4 ed. New York: Macmillan publishing, New York.

Ma, J., & Knight, B. A. (2003). Framework for Historical Case-Based Reasoning. In 5th *International Conference on Case-Based Reasoning,* Springer Berlin 246-260.

Marling, C., & Whitehouse, P. (2001). Case-Based Reasoning in the care of Alzheimer's disease patients. In: Aha, D.W., Watson, I. (eds.): *Case-Based Reasoning Research and Development,* Springer Berlin, 702-715.

McSherry, D. (2001). Interactive Case-Based Reasoning in Sequential Diagnosis. *Applied Intelligence* 14, 65-76.

McSherry, D. (2007). Hypothetico-Deductive Case-Based Reasoning. In: (Bichindaritz, Montani, 2007) 315-324.

Osser, D. N., & Patterson, R. D. (1998). Algorithms for the pharmacotherapy of depression, parts one and two. *Directions in Psychiatry,* 18, 303-334.

Prentzas, J., & Hatzilgeroudis, I. (2002). Integrating Hybrid Rule-Based with Case-Based Reasoning. In Craw, S., Preeece, A. (eds.): *Proceedings European Conference on Case-Based Reasoning,* ECCBR 2002, Springer-Verlag, Berlin, 336-349.

Rezvani, S., & Prasad, G. (2003). A hybrid system with multivariate data validation and Case-based Reasoning for an efficient and realistic product formulation. In Ashley, K.D., Bridge, D.G. (eds.): *Proceedings International Conference on Case-based Reasoning,* ICCBR 2003, Springer-Verlag, Berlin 465-478.

Schmidt, R., & Gierl, L. (2001). Case-based Reasoning for Antibiotics Therapy Advice: An Investigation of Retrieval Algorithms and Prototypes. *Artificial Intelligence in Medicine,* 23 (2), 171-186.

Schmidt, R., & Vorobieva, O. (2006). Case-Based Reasoning Investigation of Therapy Inefficacy. *Knowledge-Based Systems,* 19(5), 333-340.

Shuguang, L., Qing, J., & George, C. (2000). Combining case-based and model-based reasoning: a formal specification. In *Seventh Asia-Pacific Software Engineering Conference,* APSEC'00 416.

Stein, M. B. (2003). Attending to anxiety disorders in primary care. *J Clin Psychiatry,* 64(suppl 15), 35-39.

Vorobieva, O., Rumyantsev, A., & Schmidt, R. (2006). Incremental Development of an Explanation Model for Exceptional Dialysis Patients. In Bichindaritz, I., Montani, S. (Eds.) *Workshop on CBR in the Health Sciences,* ECCBR'06 Workshop Proceedings, University of Trier Press, 170-178.

Tversky, A. (1977). Features of similarity. *Psychological review,* 84, 327-352.

Working group for paediatric endocrinology of the German society for endocrinology and of the German society for children and youth medicine (1998) 1-15.

KEY TERMS

Adaptation: Adjusting a retrieved case to fit the given problem situation. Simple adaptation processes concern the proportional adjustment of parameters, whereas more complex ones can require problem specific rules (see: adaptation rules) or can include the recombination of solutions from several cases (see: compositional adaptation).

Adaptation Rules: Complex adaptation usually requires domain specific rules, which have to be acquired by expert consultation. These rules state how differences between a retrieved case and the query case have to be considered, that mainly means how a solution of a retrieved case has to be altered to fit for the query case.

Case-Based Reasoning (CBR): It is an AI method that mainly uses experiences expressed in form of cases. The underlying principle is expressed by the assumption that "similar problems have similar solutions". The method consists of two main steps, namely the search for similar cases or problems in the case-base, called retrieval, and for the intelligent reuse of similar problem solutions, called adaptation.

Compositional Adaptation: It is a domain independent adaptation method that does not consider just one retrieved case but a couple of cases. The solutions of these cases are used to find a solution for the query, which is often done by calculating an average value.

Explanation: In this chapter explanation is used in the context of exceptional cases (exceptions). It is meant as the reasons why cases behave exceptional.

Prototype: Since single cases are very specific. In Case-Based Reasoning, often an abstraction occurs. The result is an abstracted or more general case. A prototype or prototypical case is a general case that contains the typical features of the cases that belong to this prototype.

Retrieval: Searching for similar cases in the case-base, and providing the found case(s). Many methods and algorithms exist for this task, including explicit similarity measures and algorithms in which the similarity measure, e.g. indexing and case retrieval nets.

Solution: In Case-Based Reasoning, cases are supposed to be expressed in form of a case problem and a case solution. In this chapter the term solution is used as an explanation for an exceptional case.

Section III
Specific Cases

Chapter XII
Discovering Knowledge from Local Patterns in SAGE Data

Bruno Crémilleux
Université de Caen, France

Arnaud Soulet
Université François Rabelais de Tours, France

Jiři Kléma
Czech Technical University in Prague, Czech Republic

Céline Hébert
Université de Caen, France

Olivier Gandrillon
Université de Lyon, France

ABSTRACT

The discovery of biologically interpretable knowledge from gene expression data is a crucial issue. Current gene data analysis is often based on global approaches such as clustering. An alternative way is to utilize local pattern mining techniques for global modeling and knowledge discovery. Nevertheless, moving from local patterns to models and knowledge is still a challenge due to the overwhelming number of local patterns and their summarization remains an open issue. This chapter is an attempt to fulfill this need: thanks to recent progress in constraint-based paradigm, it proposes three data mining methods to deal with the use of local patterns by highlighting the most promising ones or summarizing them. Ideas at the core of these processes are removing redundancy, integrating background knowledge, and recursive mining. This approach is effective and useful in large and real-world data: from the case study of the SAGE gene expression data, we demonstrate that it allows generating new biological hypotheses with clinical applications.

INTRODUCTION

In many domains, such as gene expression data, the critical need is not to generate data, but to derive knowledge from huge and heterogeneous datasets produced at high throughput. It means that there is a great need for automated tools helping their analysis. There are various methods, including global techniques such as hierarchical clustering, K-means, or co-clustering (Madeira & Oliveira, 2004) and approaches based on local patterns (Blachon et al., 2007). In the context of genomic data, a local pattern is typically a set of genes displaying specific expression properties in a set of biological situations. A great interest of local patterns is to capture subtle relationships in the data which are not detected by global methods and leading to the discovery of precious nuggets of knowledge (Morik et al., 2005). But, the toughness of extraction of various local patterns is a substantial limitation of their use (Ng et al.,1998; Bayardo, 2005). As the search space of the local patterns exponentially grows according to the number of attributes (Mannila &Toivonen, 1997), this task is even more difficult in *large* datasets (i.e., datasets where objects having a large number of columns).This is typically the case in gene expression data: few biological situations (i.e., objects) are described by ten of thousands of gene expressions values (i.e., attributes) (Becquet et al. 2002). In such situations, naive methods or usual level-wise techniques are unfeasible (Pan et al.,2003; Rioult et al., 2003). Nevertheless, especially in the context of transactional data, the recent progress in constraint-based pattern mining (see for instance (Bonchi & Lucchese, 2006; De Raedt et al., 2002) enable to extract various kind of patterns even in large datasets (Soulet et al., 2007). But, this approach has still a limitation: it tends to produce an overwhelming number of local patterns. Pattern flooding follows data flooding: the output is often too large for an individual and global analysis performed by the end-user. This is especially true in noisy data,such as genomic data where the most significant patterns are lost among too many trivial, noisy and redundant information. Naive techniques such as tuning parameters of methods (e.g., increasing the frequency threshold) limit the output but only lead to produce trivial and useless information.

This paper tackles this challenge. Relying on recent progress in constraint-based paradigm, it presents three data mining methods to deal with the use of local patterns by highlighting the most promising ones or summarizing them. The practical usefulness of these methods are supported by the case study of the SAGE gene expression data (introduced in the next section). First, we provide a method to mine the set of the simplest characterization rules while having a controlled number of exceptions. Thanks to their property of minimal premise, this method limits the redundancy between rules. Second, we describe how to integrate in the mining process background knowledge available in literature databases and biological ontologies to focus on the most promising patterns only. Third, we propose a recursive pattern mining approach to summarize the contrasts of a dataset: only few patterns conveying a trade-off between significance and representativity are produced. All of these methods can be applied even on large data sets. The first method comes within the general framework of removing redundancy and providing lossless representations whereas the two others propose summarizations (all the information cannot be regenerated but the most meaningful features are produced). We think that these two general approaches are complementary. Finally, we sum up the main lessons coming from mining and using local patterns on SAGE data, both from the data mining and the biological points of view. It demonstrates the practical usefulness of these approaches enabling to infer new relevant biological hypotheses.

This paper abstracts our practice of local patterns discovery from SAGE data. We avoid technical details (references are given for in-depth information), but we emphasize the main principles and results and we provide a cross-fertilization of our "in silico" approaches for discovering knowledge in gene expression data from local patterns.

MOTIVATIONS AND CONTEXT

Motivations

There is a huge research effort to discover knowledge from genomics data and mining local patterns such as relevant synexpression groups or characterization rules is requested by biologists. It is a way to better understand the role and the links between genes. Elucidating the association between a set of co-regulated genes and the set of biological situations that gives rise to a transcription module is a major goal in functional genomics. Different techniques including microarray (DeRisi et al., 1997) and SAGE (Velculescu et al., 1995) enable to study the simultaneous expression of thousands of genes in various biological situations. The SAGE technique aims to measure the expression levels of genes in a cell population. Analyzing such data is relevant since this SAGE data source has been largely under-exploited as of today, although it has the immense advantage over micro-arrays to produce datasets that can be directly compared between libraries without the need for external normalization. In our work, we use publicly available human serial analysis of gene expression SAGE libraries. We built a 207x11082 data set made up of 207 biological situations described by 11,082 gene expressions (i.e., a set of genes identified without ambiguous tags which will be useful for the techniques integrating the background knowledge) and a 90x27679 data set gathering 90 biological situations for 27,679 gene expressions (i.e., all the available transcriptomic information from these libraries).

As said in introduction, local pattern discovery has become a rapidly growing field (Blachon et al., 2007) and a range of techniques is available for producing extensive collections of patterns. Because of the exhaustive nature of most such techniques, the so-called local patterns provide a fairly complete picture of the information embedded in the database. But, as these patterns are extracted on the basis of their individual merits, this results in large sets of local patterns, potentially highly redundant. Moreover, the collections of local patterns represent fragmented knowledge and their huge size prevents a manual investigation. A major challenge is their combination and summarization for global modeling and knowledge discovery. It is a key issue because a useful global model, such a classifier or a co-clustering, is often the expected result of a data mining process. As well as their exhaustive nature and their ability to catch subtle relationships, summarizations of local patterns can capture their joint effect and reveal a knowledge not conveying by the usual kinds of patterns. The next section provides a few attempts in this general direction.

Related Work

Several approaches have been proposed to reduce the number of local patterns irrespective of their subsequent use. Examples include condensed representations (Calders et al., 2005), compression of the dataset by exploiting the Minimum Description Length Principle (Siebes et al., 2006) or the constraint-based paradigm (Ng et al., 1998; De Raedt et al., 2002). Constraints provide a focus that allows to reduce the number of extracted patterns to those of a potential interest given by the user. Unfortunately, even if these approaches enable us to reduce the number of produced patterns, the output still remains too large for an individual and global analysis performed by the end-user. Recently, two approaches appeared in the literature, which explicitly have the goal of combining and selecting patterns on the basis of their usefulness in the context of the other selected patterns: these pattern set discovery methods are constraint-based pattern set mining (De Raedt & Zimmermann, 2007), and pattern teams (Knobbe

& Ho, 2006). Constraint-based pattern set mining is based on the notion of constraints defined on the level of pattern sets (rather than individual patterns). These constraints capture qualities of the set such as size or representativeness. In the pattern team approach, only a single subset of patterns is returned. Pattern sets are implicitly ranked on the basis of a quality measure, and the best-performing set (the pattern team) is reported. Even if these approaches explicitly compare the qualities of patterns between them, they are mainly based on the reduction of the redundancy.

On the other hand, we think that it should be a pity to consider the summarization of local patterns only from the point of view of the redundancy. Local patterns can be fruitfully gathered for global modeling and knowledge discovery. Interestingly, such global models or patterns can capture the joint effect of local patterns such as co-classification performs. This approach is a way of conceptual clustering and provides a limited collection of bi-clusters. These bi-clusters are linked for both objects (i.e., biological situations) and attributes (i.e., genes). Tackling genomic data, Pensa et al. (Pensa et al., 2005) show that the bi-clusters of the final bi-partition are not necessary elements of the initial set of the local patterns. The bi-partition may come from a reconstruction of the biological situations and genes defining the local patterns. Except for particular kinds of local patterns (e.g., closed patterns (Blachon et al., 2007)), due to their large number of attributes, there are few works on discovery knowledge from SAGE data (Kléma et al.).

Constraint-Based Pattern Mining

As said in introduction, methods presented in this paper stem from recent progress in constraint-based paradigm. A constraint is a way to express a potential interest given by the user. Due to the huge search space of candidate patterns, a challenge is to push constraints in the core of the mining process by automatically inferring powerful and safe pruning conditions in order to get patterns satisfying a constraint. At least in transactional domains, there are now generic approaches to discover *local patterns* under constraints (De Raedt et al., 2002; Soulet & Crémilleux, 2005) even in large datasets (Soulet et al., 2007). A survey of the primitive-based framework (Soulet & Crémilleux, 2005) is provided below. This framework is at the basis of our method integrating background knowledge. We give now basic definitions used among the paper.

Let I be a set of distinct literals called *items*, an itemset (or pattern) corresponds to a non-null subset of I. These patterns are gathered together in the language L_I: $L_I = 2^I \backslash \varnothing$. A transactional dataset is a multi-set of patterns (i.e., transactions) of L_I. Each *transaction* is a database entry. More generally, transactions are called *objects* and items *attributes*. For instance, Table 1 gives a transactional dataset D with 8 objects $o_1,\ldots, o_8$ (e.g., biological situations) described by 6 items $A,\ldots, F$ (e.g., gene expressions). This is a toy example which will be used throughout this paper. A value 1 for a biological situation and a gene expression means that this gene is over-expressed in this situation. In the SAGE data, each situation belongs to a class value (cancer versus no cancer) according to the biological origin of the tissue of the situation. For that reason, we divide D in two datasets D_1 and D_2 and a situation is labeled by the item C_1 (i.e., it belongs to D_1) or C_2 (i.e., it belongs to D_2).

Local patterns are regularities that hold for a particular part of the data. Let X be a pattern. We recall that the support of X in D denoted by $supp(X, D)$ is the proportion of objects in D containing X (we omit D when this data set is used by default). For instance, $supp(AB) = 3/8$. The constraint-based pattern mining framework D aims at discovering all the patterns of L_I satisfying a given predicate q, named *constraint*, and occurring in D. A well-known example is the *frequency* constraint focusing on

Table 1. Example of a transactional dataset

$\mathcal{D}$

	Gene expressions							
Situations	A	B	C	D	E	F		
o_1			1				C_1	$\mathcal{D}_1$
o_2	1	1		1		1	C_1	$\mathcal{D}_1$
o_3	1			1	1		C_1	$\mathcal{D}_1$
o_4	1	1		1			C_1	$\mathcal{D}_1$
o_5	1			1			C_2	$\mathcal{D}_2$
o_6	1	1	1			1	C_2	$\mathcal{D}_2$
o_7		1	1	1			C_2	$\mathcal{D}_2$
o_8			1		1		C_2	$\mathcal{D}_2$

patterns having a support exceeding a given minimal threshold *minsupp* > 0: *supp*(X, D) ≥ *minsupp*. For instance, AB is a frequent pattern with *minsupp* = 0.2. We will also use an absolute definition of the support, the frequency of X denoted *freq*(X) (*freq*(X, D) = *supp*(X,D) x |D|). As previously, we omit D when this data set is used by default. For instance, *freq*(AB) = 3. The frequency of the rule $X \rightarrow Y$ is *freq*(XY) and its *confidence* is *supp*(XY)/*supp*(X).

There are a lot of various constraints to evaluate the relevance of local patterns (Ng et al., 1998; Soulet & Crémilleux, 2005). The constraint-based paradigm also includes interestingness measures (the frequency is an example) to select local patterns. In the following, we will use the area of a pattern *area*(X): it is the frequency of a pattern times its length (i.e., *area*(X) = *freq*(X) x *count*(X) where *count*(X) denotes the cardinality of X. The area can be seen as the translation in the constraint paradigm of a synexpression group. For instance, the pattern AB (or ABD) satisfies the constraint *area*(X) ≥ 6 (as previously, if no data set is specified, it means that D is used). Emerging patterns (EPs) are another example. They are at the core of the summaries presented in the following. An EP is a pattern whose support strongly varies between two parts of a dataset (i.e., two classes),enabling to characterize classes (Dong & Li, 1999). The growth rate of X is $gr_i(X) = supp(X, D_i)/supp(X, D \backslash D_i)$. More formally, if we consider the two cancer and no cancer classes, a frequent emerging pattern X satisfies the constraint $supp(X,D) \geq minsupp \wedge (gr_{cancer}(X) \geq mingr \vee gr_{no\ cancer}(X) \geq mingr)$.

MINING A SYNTHESIS OF CLASSIFICATION RULES

There is an intense need of classification and classes characterization techniques to perform data mining tasks required on real-world databases. For instance, the biological situations in SAGE data are divided into two classes (cancer and no cancer) and biologists would like to better understand the relationships between the genes and these classes. For that purpose, we use the characterization rules previously introduced in (Crémilleux & Boulicaut, 2002). Thanks to a property of minimal premises, these characterization rules provide a kind of synthesis of the whole set of classification rules (i.e., all the rules concluding on a class value). This result stems from the property of specific patterns, the δ-free patterns which are made of attributes without frequency relations between them (Boulicaut et al., 2003). Experiments (Crémilleux & Boulicaut, 2002) show that the number of characterization rules is at least an order of magnitude lower than the number of classification rules. Unfortunately, the method given in (Crémilleux & Boulicaut, 2002) does not run on large datasets such as the SAGE data. For that reason we have proposed a new method (Hébert et al., 2005) based on the extension of patterns (the extension of a pattern X is the maximal set of the objects containing X), because the extension has few objects in large databases. We give now a formal definition of these characterization rules (X and Y are patterns and C_i is an item referring to a class value).

Definition 1 (characterization rules): *Let minfreq be a frequency threshold, δ be an integer, a rule* $X \rightarrow C_i$ *is a characterization rule if there is no rule* $Y \rightarrow C_i$ *with* $Y \subset X$ *and a confidence greater than or equal to 1-(δ/minfreq).*

Given a frequency threshold *minfreq*, this definition means that we consider only the minimum sets of attributes (i.e., the minimal premises) to end up C_i, the uncertainty being controlled by δ. For instance, in our running example (Table 1), with δ = 1 and *minfreq* = 2, $C \rightarrow C_2$ is a characterization rule (there is one exception), but $CD \rightarrow C_2$ is not a characterization rule (it is covered by the previous rule). We argue that this property of minimal premise is a fundamental issue for classification. Not only it prevents from over-fitting but also it makes the characterization of an example easier to explain. It provides a feedback on the application domain expertise that can be reused for further analysis.

The value of δ is fundamental to discover relevant rules. With δ = 0, every rule must have a confidence value of 1 (i.e., *exact* rule). In many practical applications, such as the SAGE data, there are generally very few exact rules due to the non-determinism of the phenomena. We have to relax the condition on δ to accept exceptions (the more δ raises, the more the confidence decreases).

We developed the FTCminer prototype which extracts the sound and complete collection of frequent characterization rules (Hébert et al., 2005). FTCminer follows the outline of a level-wise algorithm (Mannila & Toivonen, 1997). Its originality is the use of the extension of patterns and that there is no generation phase of all the candidates at a given level since the candidates are generating one at a time. Thanks to these techniques, we are able to mine characterization rules even in large data sets whereas it was impossible before (Becquet at al., 2002; Hébert et al., 2005). Main results on SAGE data are given in the section on experiments.

INTEGRATING INFORMATION SOURCES SYNTHESIZING BACKGROUND KNOWLEDGE

This section sketches our approach to integrate background knowledge (BK) in the mining process to focus on the most plausible patterns consistent with pieces of existing knowledge. For instance, biologists are interested in constraints both on synexpression groups and common characteristics of the descriptions of the genes and/or biological situations under consideration. BK is available in relational and literature databases, ontological trees and other sources. Nevertheless, mining in a heterogeneous environment allowing a large set of descriptions at various levels of detail is highly non-trivial. There are various ways to interconnect the heterogeneous data sources and express the mutual relations among the entities they address. We tackle this issue with the constraint paradigm. We think it is a promising way for such a work, the constraints can effectively link different datasets and knowledge sources (Soulet et al., 2007).

Our approach is based on the primitive-based constraints (Soulet & Crémilleux, 2005). There are no formal properties required on the final constraints and they are freely built of a large set of primitives. The primitives have to satisfy solely a property of monotonicity according to their variables (when the others remain constant). We showed that the whole set of primitive-based constraints constitutes a super-class of monotone, anti-monotone, succinct and convertible constraints (Soulet & Crémilleux, 2008). Consequently, the proposed framework provides a flexible and rich constraint (query) language. For instance, the product of two primitives *count*(*X*) x *freq*(*X*) may address the patterns having a certain minimum length (i.e., containing a minimum number of genes) and frequency (i.e., covering a minimum number of situations). We referred to it as *area*(*X*) above.

Furthermore, this framework naturally enables to integrate primitives addressing external data. Let us consider the transcriptomic mining context given in Figure 1. The involved data include a transcriptome dataset also called internal data as in our running example. External data - a similarity matrix and textual resources - summarize BK that contains various information on genes. Each field of the triangular matrix $s_{ij} \in [0,1]$ gives a similarity measure between the genes *i* and *j*. The textual dataset provides a description of genes. Details on the processing of textual resources within this approach and primitives tackling external data are given in another chapter of this book (Kléma & Zelezny). The mined patterns are composed of genes of the internal data, the corresponding objects are usually also noted (and possibly analyzed). The external data are used to further specify constraints in order to focus on meaningful patterns. In other words, the constraints may stem from all the datasets. The user can iteratively develop complex constraints integrating various knowledge types.

A real example of a constraint *q*(*X*) is given in Figure 1. The first part (a) of *q* addresses the internal data and means that the biologist is interested in patterns satisfying a minimal area. The other parts deal with the external data: (b) is used to discard ribosomal patterns (one gene exception per pattern is

Figure 1. Example of a toy (transcriptomic) mining context and a constraint

Internal data

Boolean matrix $\mathcal{D}$

	Gene expressions					
Situations	*A*	*B*	*C*	*D*	*E*	*F*
o_1			1			
o_2	1	1		1		1
o_3	1			1	1	
o_4	1	1		1		

External data

Similarity matrix

	A	*B*	*C*	*D*	*E*	*F*
A		.07	?	?	.2	0
B			.06	?	?	0
C				.07	.05	.04
D					.03	.1
E						?

Textual data

A	'metal ion binding' 'transcription factor'
B	'serine-type peptidase activity' 'proteolysis'
C	'DNA binding' 'metal ion binding'
D	'ATP binding' 'nucleotide binding'
E	'proteolysis'
F	'ATP binding' 'metal ion binding'

↕ ***freq, count,...*** ↕ ***sumsim, svmsim,...*** ↕ ***regexp***

$$
\begin{aligned}
q(X) \equiv\ & freq(X) \times count(X) \geq 24 && \text{(a)} \\
& \wedge length(regexp(X, '*ribosom*', \texttt{TEXT\_terms})) \leq 1 && \text{(b)} \\
& \wedge svsim(X, \texttt{TEXT})/(svsim(X, \texttt{TEXT}) + mvsim(X, \texttt{TEXT})) \geq 0.7 && \text{(c)} \\
& \wedge sumsim(X, \texttt{TEXT})/svsim(X, \texttt{TEXT}) \geq 0.025 && \text{(d)}
\end{aligned}
$$

allowed), (c) avoids patterns with prevailing items of an unknown function and (d) is to ensure a minimal average gene similarity. The usefulness of such a constraint is shown in the section on experiments.

We have proposed a general prototype Music-dfs which discovers soundly and completely all the patterns satisfying the specified set of constraints (Soulet et al., 2007). Its efficiency lies in its depth-first search strategy and a safe pruning of the pattern space by pushing the constraints. Extractions in large data sets such as the SAGE data are feasible. Section on experiments demonstrates that our procedure leads to a very effective reduction of the number of patterns, together with an "interpretation" of the patterns.

RECURSIVE PATTERN MINING

This section outlines the recursive pattern mining framework and the discovery of the recursive emerging patterns (Soulet, 2007). The key idea is to repeat the pattern mining process on output to reduce it until few and relevant patterns are obtained. The final recursive patterns bring forward information coming from each mining step.

As often in mining constraint-based local patterns, the so-called collections of frequent emerging patterns (EPs) are huge and this hinders their uses. Several works address methods to reduce these collections by focusing on the most expressive ones (Bailey et al., 2002) (which are only present in one class) or by mining a lossless condensed representation (Li et al., 2007; Soulet et al., 2004). Nevertheless, these approaches do not reduce enough the number of mined patterns. Moreover, setting thresholds (i.e., *minsupp* or *mingr*) is often too subtle. Both the quantity and the quality of desired patterns are unpredictable. For instance, a too high threshold may generate no answer, a small one may generate thousands of patterns. Increasing thresholds to diminish the number of output patterns may be counter-productive (see the example with the area constraint in the section on experiments). Mining recursive patterns aims at solving these pitfalls.

In this work, we deal with frequent emerging patterns. Recursive emerging patterns (REPs) are the EPs which frequently occur within the outputted EPs according to the classes. The assumption is that these EPs are significant because the recursive mining process enables to synthesize and give prominence to the most meaningful contrasts of a dataset. A recursive emerging pattern *k*-summary (a REP *k*-summary, see Definition 2) provides a short description of the dataset constituted at most *k* REPs summarizing the contrasts according to the classes. It is produced by the generic recursive pattern mining framework: for each step, the previous mined patterns constitute the new transactional dataset. A first step mines all the frequent emerging patterns, as usual in the constraint-based pattern mining framework. Then the outputted EPs are joined to form a new dataset $D^2 = D^2_{cancer} \cup D^2_{no\ cancer}$. The EPs concluding on the class cancer (or no cancer) constitute the new sub-dataset D^2_{cancer} (or $D^2_{no\ cancer}$) and the process is repeated. This recursive process is ended as soon as the result becomes stable. At the end, we get at most *k* patterns brought forward information coming from each mining step. They summarize the main contrasts repeated through the outputs. From an abstract point of view, REPs can be seen as generalizations of emerging patterns. Main features on the method, (e.g., the theoretical convergence of recursive mining, number of steps) are given in (Soulet, 2007) and are not developed here because they are not crucial in practice.

For example, Table 2 depicts the mining of REPs from D (cf. Table 1) with *minsupp*=0.1 and *mingr*=2. Obviously, the datasets D^2_1 and D^2_2 are exactly the EPs in $D = D^1$ with *minsupp*=0.1 and *mingr*=2. At the

Table 2. REPs mined from D with minsupp = 0.1 and mingr = 2

$\mathcal{D}_1^2$

A	B	D	E	F
A			E	
A		D	E	
A		D		F
A	B	D		F
A		D		
A	B	D		
A	B			
		D	E	
		D		F
	B	D		F
	B	D		

$\mathcal{D}_2^2$

A	B	C	D	E	F
A		C			
A	B	C			
A	B	C			F
A		C			F
		C			
		C		E	
		C			F
	B	C			F
		C	D		
	B	C	D		
	B	C			

$\mathcal{D}_1^3$

A	B	D	E	F
A		D		
			E	
		D		F
	B	D		
		D		

$\mathcal{D}_2^3$

A	B	C	F
A		C	
		C	F
	B	C	
		C	

Table 3. REP 10-summary of D with mingr = 2

REPs of $\mathcal{D}_1$

REP	*supp*	gr_1
AD	0.5	3
E	0.25	1
DF	0.125	∞
BD	0.375	2
D	0.625	1.5

REPs of $\mathcal{D}_2$

REP	*supp*	gr_2
AC	0.125	∞
CF	0.125	∞
BC	0.25	∞
C	0.5	3

next mining step, the number of REPs (i.e., union of D^3_1 and D^3_2 : 9 patterns) is lower than the number of EPs (i.e., union of D^2_1 and D^2_2 : 22 patterns). In this example, EPs in D^4 are exactly the patterns of D^3 and then the collection of frequent REPs is stable: final REPs come from D^3. We define below a REP *k*-summary which straightforwardly stems from REPs:

Definition 2 (REP *k*-summary): *A REP k-summary (according to mingr) is the whole collection of REPs obtained with minsupp=1/k and mingr.*

We argue that a REP *k*-summary is a compact collection of EPs having a good trade-off between significance and representativity. We proved (Soulet, 2007) that the size of a REP *k*-summary is bounded according to *minsupp*: to get at most *k* patterns in a REP *k*-summary, it is enough to fix *minsupp* = 1/*k*. For instance, the 10-summary in Table 3 contains 9 patterns (we have $9 \leq 10$ with *k*=10=1 /*minsupp* = 1/0.1). Moreover, we claim that it is easier for a user to fix a maximal value for the number of patterns than the support threshold.

Besides a REP *k*-summary covers a large part of the dataset D: most objects support at least one EP of the summary. This is due to REPs are frequent patterns in the dataset of each step. Thus, they are representative of the original dataset D, but also of all the emerging patterns from D. Table 3 recalls the REP 10-summary with *mingr*=2 from our running example. Supports (column *supp*) and growth rates (column gr_i) in the initial dataset D are added. As *minsupp*=1/10, this summary is exactly the REPs given in Table 2. Interestingly, we note that the growth rates of the REPs may be lower than *mingr* (e.g., $gr_1(D,D)$=1.5 whereas *mingr* = 2). This avoids the crisp effect of a threshold where a promising pattern is deleted only because its value for the measure is just under the threshold. The power of the recursive mining approach relies on the summarization: most of the REPs have a significative growth rate and all the objects (except o_1 and o_5) are covered by a REP concluding to their class values. Clearly, o_1 is closer to the objects of D_2 than objects of D_1, this explains why o_1 is not characterized by a REP. A similar reasoning can be done with o_5.

The tunable concision of REPs favours users' interpretation. Each REP can be individually interpreted as usual EPs, providing a qualitative and quantitative information. Appropriately, the small collection of REPs offers a global and complementary description of the whole dataset.

LESSONS FROM MINING SAGE DATA

The section outlines the main results achieved on SAGE data thanks to the previous data mining methods. Then, we synthesize the major lessons both from the data mining and the biological points of view.

A Sketch of Biological Results

To fully understand the results of experiments, we have to precise that each attribute of a SAGE data set is a *tag*. The identification of genes is closely related to the tags and biologists are able to associate genes and tags. In the case of the 207x11082 data set, each tag is unambiguously identified. This property is very useful to link together the information coming from several sources of BK.

Gene expressions are quantitative values and we must identify a specific gene expression property to get binary value and run the data mining methods depicted above. In principle, several properties per gene could be encoded, e.g. over-expression and under-expression. In our studies, we decided to focus on over-expression (over-expression has been introduced in the beginning of the paper). Several ways exist for identifying gene over-expression (Becquet et al., 2002). Results given in this paper are performed by using the mid-range method: the threshold is fixed w.r.t. the maximal value (*max*) observed for each tag. All the values which are greater than (100 - X%) of *max* are assigned to 1, 0 for the others (here, $X = 25$). For the 90x27679 data set, the values of tags vary from 0 to 26021. The percentage of tags which values are different from 0 is 19.86% and the arithmetic mean is around 4. As already said, the biological situations are divided into two classes (cancer and no cancer). 59 situations are labelled by cancer and 31 by no cancer (i.e., normal).

Characterization rules. We give the mean features on our work on mining characterization rules on SAGE data (more experiments and details are provided in (Hébert et al., 2005). In this paper, we only deal with the classes cancer and no cancer. More fruitful further biological investigations will require to use sub-groups of these classes, such sub-groups being defined according to biological criteria (e.g., a cancer type).

Table 4 presents a selection of rules with at least two tags in their body and a rather high confidence and frequency with *minfreq* and δ=1. Table 5 provides the description of tags (identification number, sequence and description) only for the tags which appear the most frequently in our results. Some tags are identified by several genes: their identifications are separated by ";".

Few tags (e.g., 4602, 8255, 11115, 22129) clearly arise in many rules concluding on cancer. They may have an influence on the development of this disease. It is interesting to note that the frequencies of these tags strongly varies from one class to another. For example, the tag 11115 appears 28.7 times more in rules characterizing cancer than no cancer. The tag 11115 is identified as GPX1. The expression of GPX1 has been found in various studies to be correlated with cancerous situations (Korotkina et al., 2002; Nasr et al., 2004). On the contrary, the tag 22129 appears 22 times more in rules concluding on no cancer than concluding on cancer. It might mean that this tag is related to normal development. We will come back on this tag below, with regard to the interestingness of biological results.

Table 4. Examples of potential relevant rules with minfreq = 4 and δ= 1

Premise	Conclusion	Exceptions	Frequency	Confidence
11115 19811	cancer	1	13	0.92
5961 11115	cancer	0	12	1
8279 23600	cancer	1	12	0.92
10960 11115	cancer	1	12	0.92
11115 20766	cancer	1	12	0.92
4602 7259 18882	cancer	1	10	0.9
4602 7259 24686	cancer	1	10	0.9
8255 11115 19811	cancer	1	10	0.9
4602 7259 20461	cancer	1	9	0.89
4602 7259 25202	cancer	1	9	0.89
4602 18882 24686	cancer	1	9	0.89
4287 4602 7818	cancer	1	8	0.88
4287 4602 19811	cancer	1	8	0.88
4602 7259 19734	cancer	1	8	0.88
4602 24686 25202	cancer	1	8	0.88
4602 25128 25202	cancer	1	8	0.88
7259 12667 16807	cancer	1	8	0.88
8255 11115 13642	cancer	0	8	1
8255 11115 26846	cancer	1	8	0.88
8255 19811 26846	cancer	1	8	0.88
22619 25202 26846 27358	cancer	1	5	0.8
16786 26715	no cancer	1	7	0.86
22129 25356	no cancer	1	7	0.86
22129 27414	no cancer	1	7	0.86
22647 25356	no cancer	1	7	0.86
1722 25202 26715	no cancer	1	6	0.83

Table 5. Characteristics of potential relevant tags

Number	Sequence	Description
4287	AGCTCTCCCT	RPL17 ribosomal protein L17
4602	AGGCTACGGA	Similar to ribosomal protein L13a, 60S ribosomal protein L13a, 23 kD highly basic protein
8255	CATCCAAAAC	HNRPH1 Heterogeneous nuclear ribonucleoprotein H1 (H)
11115	CTCTTCGAGA	GPX1 Glutathione peroxidase 1
19811	GTTGCTGCCC	NIFIE14 Seven transmembrane domain protein
22129	TCAGAGAATA	SLC25A22 Solute carrier family 25 (mitochondrial carrier: glutamate), member 22; IRS2 Insulin receptor substrate 2
25202	TGTGCTAAAT	RPL34 Ribosomal protein L34

Integrating BK. A highly valuable biological knowledge comes from the patterns that concern genes with interesting common features (e.g., process, function, location, disease) whose synexpression is observed in a homogeneous biological context (i.e., in a number of analogous biological situations). We give now an example of such a context with the set of medulloblastoma SAGE libraries discovered from constrained patterns taking into account the BK. We use the 207x11082 data set because each tag is unambiguously identified. This property is very useful to link together the information coming from several sources of BK.

The area constraint is the most meaningful constraint on the internal data for the search of such synexpression groups. On the one hand, it products large patterns (the more genes they contain, the better ; the higher the frequency is, the better). On the other hand, it enables exceptions on genes and/or biological situations contrary to the maximal patterns (Rioult et al., 2003; Blachon et al., 2007) (i.e., formal concepts) which require that all the connected genes are over-expressed. In domains such as gene expressions where the non-determinism is intrinsic, this lead to a fragmentation of the information embedded in the data and a huge number of patterns covering very few genes or biological situations.

We fix the area threshold thanks to statistical analysis of random datasets having the same properties as the original SAGE data. We obtain a value of 20 as an optimal area threshold to distinguish between spurious (i.e., occurring randomly) and meaningful patterns (first spurious patterns start to appear for this threshold area). Unfortunately, we get too many (several thousands) candidate patterns. Increasing the threshold of the area constraint to get a reasonable number of patterns is rather counterproductive. The constraint $area \geq 75$ led to a small but uniform set of 56 patterns that was flooded by the ribosomal proteins which generally represent the most frequent genes in the dataset. Biologists rated these patterns as valid but useless.

The most valuable synexpression groups expected by biologists have non-trivial size containing genes and situations whose characteristics can be generalized, connected, interpreted and thus transformed into knowledge. To get such patterns, constraints based on the external data have to be added to the minimal area constraint just like in the constraint q given in the section on integration of information sources synthetizing BK. It joins the minimal area constraint with background constraints coming from the NCBI (cf. http://www.ncbi.nlm.nih.gov) textual resources (gene summaries and adjoined PubMed abstracts). There are 46671 patterns satisfying the minimal area constraint (the part (a) of the constraint q), but only 9 satisfy q. This shows the efficiency of reduction of patterns brought by the BK. One of these patterns is of biological interest (Kléma et al.). It consists of 4 genes (KHDRBS1 NONO TOP2B FMR1) over-expressed in 6 biological situations (BM_P019 BM_P494 BM_P608 BM_P301 BM_H275 BM_H876), BM stands for brain medulloblastoma. A cross-fertilization with other external data was obviously attractive. So, we define a constraint q' which is similar to q, except that the functional Gene Ontology (cf. http://www.geneontology.org/) is used instead of NCBI textual resources. Only 2 patterns satisfy q'. Interestingly, the previous pattern that was identified by the expert as one of the "nuggets" provided by q' is also selected by q'. The constraints q and q' demonstrate two different ways to reach a compact and meaningful output that can be easily human surveyed.

REP summaries. Following our work to study the relationships between the genes and the type of biological situations according to cancer and no cancer, we computed REP summaries from the SAGE data. We use the same binary data set as in the characterization rules task.

Table 6 depicts the REP 4-summary with $mingr$=2. We observe that all patterns describe the class cancer. Using other values for the parameters k and $mingr$ also leads to only characterize cancer. Interestingly, the 3 extracted genes characterize 40% of biological situations and even 61% of cancerous situations. We will see below that this REP summary confirms the results obtained with characterization rules. Nevertheless, a great interest of the approach based on the summarization is to directly isolate genes without requiring a manual inspection of rules.

A Breakthrough on Mining and Using Local Pattern Methods

A first challenge in discovery knowledge from local patterns in SAGE data is to perform the local pattern extractions. Recalling that few years ago it was impossible to mine such patterns in large datasets and only association rules with rather a high frequency threshold were used (Becquet et al., 2002). Relying on recent progress in constraint-based paradigm, we have proposed efficient data mining methods to mine local patterns solving the problem due to the size of the search space. Key ideas are the use of

Table 6. REP 4-summary of SAGE data with mingr = 2

Sequence (tag)	Description (gene)	*supp*	*gr*
	cancer		
CATCCAAAAC	HNRPH1 Heterogeneous nuclear ribonucleoprotein H1 (H)	0.28	2.10
CTCTTCGAGA	GPX1 Glutathione peroxidase 1	0.32	3.28
GTTGCTGCCC	NIFIE14 Seven transmembrane domain protein	0.26	2.50

Class coverage : 40% / Running-time: 1.37s

the extension of patterns and depth-first search. Thanks to the constraint-based mining approach, the user can handle a wide spectrum of constraints expressing a viable notion of interestingness. We deal with characterization rules, emerging patterns, minimal area (which is the translation in the constraint paradigm of a synexpression group), but many other possibilities are offered to the user.

A second challenge is to deal with the (huge) collections of local patterns. We claim that we propose fruitful methods to eliminate redundancy between patterns and highlighting the most promising ones or summarizing them. Integrating BK in a data mining process is a usual work for the biologist, but he did it manually. To the best of our knowledge, there is no other constraint-based method to efficiently discover patterns from large data under a broad set of constraints linking BK distributed in various knowledge sources. Recursive mining is a new and promising way which ensures to produce very few patterns summarizing the data. These summaries can easily be inspected by the user.

Interestingness of Biological Results

A first result is that most of the extracted patterns were harboring (or even composed only of) genes encoding ribosomal proteins, and proteins involved in the translation process. This is for example the case for the vast majority of the characterization rules concluding on cancer (see Tables 4 and 5). Such an overexpression has been documented in various contexts ranging from prostate cancer (Vaarala et al., 1998) to v-erbA oncogene over-expression (Bresson et al., 2007). The biological meaning of such an over-expression is an open question which is currently investigated in the CGMC lab.

As a second lesson, we demonstrated that mining local patterns discovers promising biological knowledge. Let us come back on the pattern highlighted by the BK (see above). This pattern can be verbally characterized as follows: it consists of 4 genes that are over-expressed in 6 biological situations, it contains at most one ribosomal gene, the genes share a lot of common terms in their descriptions as well as they functionally overlap, at least 3 of the genes are known (have a non-empty record) and all of the biological situations are medulloblastomas which are very aggressive brain tumors in children. This pattern led to an interesting hypothesis regarding the role of RNA-binding activities in the generation and/or maintenance of medulloblastomas (Kléma et al.).

Finally, our data mining approaches enable a cross-fertilization of results, indicating that a relatively small number of genes keeps popping up throughout various analysis. This is typically the case of the GPX1 gene highlighted both on characterization rules and REP summaries to have an influence on the development of cancer. This gene encodes a cytosolic glutathione peroxidase acting as an antioxidant by detoxifying hydroperoxides (Brigelius-Flohe, 2006). It is known that exposition to an oxidative stress is a factor that favors development of different types of tumors (Halliwell, 2007). It is therefore reasonable to suggest that this gene is over-expressed to respond to an oxidative stress to which cells have been exposed. It would be of interest to verify its expression level by RT-PCR in normal versus cancerous samples in human.

CONCLUSION

There are now a few methods to mine local patterns under various sets of constraints even in large data sets such as gene expression data. Nevertheless, dealing with the huge number of extracted local patterns is still a challenge due to the difficult location of the most interesting patterns. In this chapter, we have presented several methods to reduce and summarize local patterns. We have shown the potential impact of these methods on the large SAGE data. By highlighting few patterns, these approaches are precious in domains such as genomics where a manual inspection of patterns is highly time consuming. Our methods provide qualitative information (e.g., biological situations associated to genes, text resources) but also quantitative information (e.g., growth rate or other measures). Such characteristics are major features in a lot of domains with noisy data and non-deterministic phenomena for knowledge discovery. We think that our results on SAGE data illustrate the power of local patterns to highlight gene expression patterns appearing through very different conditions, and that such patterns would not be captured by global tools such as hierarchical clustering.

A future issue is the combination of these methods: how to ensure to build non redundant optimal recursive patterns? how to integrate BK in recursive mining? Another way is to design new kinds of constraints to directly mine global patterns as sets of local patterns or produce models.

ACKNOWLEDGMENT

This work has mainly been done within the Bingo project framework (http://www.info.unicaen.fr/~bruno/bingo). The work of Jiři Kléma was funded by the Czech Ministry of Education in terms of the research programme Transdisciplinary Research in the Area of Biomedical Engineering II, MSM 6840770012. The authors thank all members of the

Bingo project and especially Sylvain Blachon for generating the SAGE gene expression matrices and Jean-François Boulicaut for fruitful discussions. This work is partly supported by the ANR (French Research National Agency) funded project Bingo2 ANR-07-MDCO-014 (http://bingo2.greyc.fr/), which is a follow-up of the first Bingo project and the Czech-French PHC Barrande project "Heterogeneous Data Fusion for Genomic and Proteomic Knowledge Discovery".

REFERENCES

Bailey, J., Manoukian, T., & Ramamohanarao, K. (2002). Fast algorithms for mining emerging patterns. *Proceedings of the Sixth European Conference on Principles Data Mining and Knowledge Discovery (PKDD'02)* (pp. 39-50). Helsinki, Finland: Springer.

Bayardo, R. J. (2005). The hows, whys, and whens of constraints in itemset and rule discovery. *Proceedings of the workshop on Inductive Databases and Constraint Based Mining* (pp. 1-13) Springer.

Becquet, C., Blachon, S., Jeudy, B., Boulicaut, J.-F., & Gandrillon, O. (2002). Strong association rule mining for large gene expression data analysis: a case study on human SAGE data. *Genome Biology, 3.*

Blachon, S., Pensa, R. G., Besson, J., Robardet, C., Boulicaut, J.-F., & Gandrillon, O. (2007). Clustering formal concepts to discover biologically relevant knowledge from gene expression data. *Silico Biology, 7.*

Bonchi, F., & Lucchese, C. (2006). On condensed representations of constrained frequent patterns. *Knowledge and Information Systems, 9*, 180-201.

Boulicaut, J.-F., Bykowski, A., & Rigotti, C. (2003). Free-sets: A condensed representation of boolean data for the approximation of frequency queries. *Data Mining and Knowledge Discovery journal, 7*, 5-22. Kluwer Academics Publishers.

Bresson, C., Keime, C., Faure, C., Letrillard, Y., Barbado, M., Sanfilippo, S., Benhra, N., Gandrillon, O., & Gonin-Giraud, S. (2007). Large-scale analysis by sage reveals new mechanisms of v-erba oncogene action. *BMC Genomics, 8.*

Brigelius-Flohe, R. (2006). Glutathione peroxidases and redox-regulated transcription factors. *Biol Chem, 387*, 1329-1335.

Calders, T., Rigotti, C., & Boulicaut, J.-F. (2005). A survey on condensed representations for frequent sets. *Constraint-Based Mining and Inductive Databases* (pp. 64-80). Springer.

Crémilleux, B., & Boulicaut, J.-F. (2002). Simplest rules characterizing classes generated by delta-free sets. *Proceedings 22nd Int. Conf. on Knowledge Based Systems and Applied Artificial Intelligence* (pp. 33-46). Cambridge, UK.

De Raedt, L., Jäger, M., Lee, S. D., & Mannila, H. (2002). A theory of inductive query answering. *Proceedings of the IEEE Conference on Data Mining* (ICDM'02) (pp. 123-130). Maebashi, Japan.

De Raedt, L., & Zimmermann, A. (2007). Constraint-based pattern set mining. *Proceedings of the Seventh SIAM International Conference on Data Mining.* Minneapolis, Minnesota, USA: SIAM.

DeRisi, J., Iyer, V., & Brown, P. (1997). Exploring the metabolic and genetic control of gene expression on a genomic scale. *Science, 278*, 680-686.

Dong, G., & Li, J. (1999). Efficient mining of emerging patterns: discovering trends and differences. *Proceedings of the Fifth International Conference on Knowledge Discovery and Data Mining (ACM SIGKDD'99)* (pp. 43-52). San Diego, CA: ACM Press.

Halliwell, B. (2007). Biochemistry of oxidative stress. *Biochem Soc Trans, 35*, 1147-1150.

Hand, D. J. (2002*). ESF exploratory workshop on pattern detection and discovery in data mining, 2447 of Lecture Notes in Computer Science.* Chapter Pattern detection and discovery, 1-12. Springer.

Hébert, C., Blachon, S., & Crémilleux, B. (2005). Mining delta-strong characterization rules in large sage data. *ECML/PKDD'05 Discovery Challenge on gene expression data co-located with the 9th European Conference on Principles and Practice of Knowledge Discovery in Databases (PKDD'05)* (pp. 90-101). Porto, Portugal.

Kléma, J., Blachon, S., Soulet, A., Crémilleux, B., & Gandrillon, O. (2008). Constraint-based knowledge discovery from sage data. *Silico Biology, 8*(0014).

Kléma, J., & Zelezny, F. In P. Berka, J. Rauch and D. J. Zighed (Eds.), *Data mining and medical knowledge management: Cases and applications, chapter Gene Expression Data Mining Guided by Genomic Background Knowledge*. IGI Global.

Knobbe, A., & Ho, E. (2006). Pattern teams. *Proceedings of the 10th European Conference on Principles and Practice of Knowledge Discovery in Databases (PKDD'06)* (pp. 577-584). Berlin, Germany: Springer-Verlag.

Korotkina, R. N., Matskevich, G. N., Devlikanova, A. S., Vishnevskii, A. A., Kunitsyn, A. G., & Karelin, A. A. (2002). Activity of glutathione-metabolizing and antioxidant enzymes in malignant and benign tumors of human lungs. *Bulletin of Experimental Biology and Medicine, 133*, 606-608.

Li, J., Liu, G., & Wong, L. (2007). Mining statistically important equivalence classes and delta-discriminative emerging patterns. *Proceedings of the 13th ACM SIGKDD international conference on Knowledge discovery and data mining (KDD'07)* (pp. 430-439). New York, NY, USA: ACM.

Madeira, S. C., & Oliveira, A. L. (2004). Biclustering algorithms for biological data analysis: A survey. IEEE/ACM Trans. Comput. *Biology Bioinform., 1*, 24-45.

Mannila, H., & Toivonen, H. (1997). Levelwise search and borders of theories in knowledge discovery. *Data Mining and Knowledge Discovery, 1*, 241-258.

Morik, K., Boulicaut, J.-F., & (eds.), A. S. (Eds.). (2005). *Local pattern detection, 3539* of *LNAI*. Springer-Verlag.

Nasr, M., Fedele, M., Esser, K., & A, D. (2004). GPx-1 modulates akt and p70s6k phosphorylation and gadd45 levels in mcf-7 cells. *Free Radical Biology and Medicine, 37*, 187-195.

Ng, R. T., Lakshmanan, V. S., Han, J., & Pang, A. (1998). Exploratory mining and pruning optimizations of constrained associations rules. *Proceedings of ACM SIGMOD'98* (pp. 13-24). ACM Press.

Pan, F., Cong, G., Tung, A. K. H., Yang, Y., & Zaki, M. J. (2003). CARPENTER: finding closed patterns in long biological datasets. *Proceedings of the 9th ACM SIGKDD international conference on Knowledge discovery and data mining (KDD'03)* (pp. 637-642). Washington, DC, USA: ACM Press.

Pensa, R., Robardet, C., & Boulicaut, J.-F. (2005). A bi-clustering framework for categorical data. *Proceedings of the 9th European Conference on Principles and Practice of Knowledge Discovery in Databases (PKDD'05)* (pp. 643-650). Porto, Portugal.

Rioult, F., Boulicaut, J.-F., Crémilleux, B., & J., B. (2003). Using transposition for pattern discovery from microarray data. *Proceedings of the 8th ACM SIGMOD Workshop on Research Issues in Data Mining and Knowledge Discovery (DMKD'03)* (pp. 73-79). San Diego, CA.

Siebes, A., Vreeken, J., & Van Leeuwen, M. (2006). Item sets that compress. *Proceedings of the Sixth SIAM International Conference on Data Mining.* Bethesda, MD, USA: SIAM.

Soulet, A. (2007). Résumer les contrastes par l'extraction récursive de motifs. Conférence *sur l'Apprentissage Automatique (CAp'07)* (pp. 339-354). Grenoble, France: Cépaduès Edition.

Soulet, A., & Crémilleux, B. (2005). An efficient framework for mining flexible constraints *Proceedings 9th Pacific-Asia Conference on Knowledge Discovery and Data Mining (PAKDD'05)* (pp. 661-671). Hanoi, Vietnam: Springer.

Soulet, A., & Crémilleux, B. (2008). Soulet A., Crémilleux B. Mining constraint-based patterns using automatic relaxation. *Intelligent Data Analysis, 13*(1). IOS Press. To appear.

Soulet, A., Crémilleux, B., & Rioult, F. (2004). Condensed representation of emerging patterns. *Proceedings 8th Pacific-Asia Conference on Knowledge Discovery and Data Mining (PAKDD'04)* (pp. 127-132). Sydney, Australia: Springer-Verlag.

Soulet, A., Kléma, J., & Crémilleux, B. (2007). *Post-proceedings of the 5th international workshop on knowledge discovery in inductive databases in conjunction with ECML/PKDD 2006 (KDID'06), 4747 of Lecture Notes in Computer Science, chapter Efficient Mining under Rich Constraints Derived from Various Datasets*, 223-239. Springer.

Vaarala, M. H., Porvari, K. S., Kyllonen, A. P., Mustonen, M. V., Lukkarinen, O., & Vihko, P. T. (1998). Several genes encoding ribosomal proteins are over-expressed in prostate-cancer cell lines: confirmation of l7a and l37 over-expression in prostate-cancer tissue samples. *Int. J. Cancer, 78*, 27-32.

Velculescu, V., Zhang, L., Vogelstein, B., & Kinzler, K. (1995). Serial analysis of gene expression. *Science, 270*, 484-487.

KEY TERMS

Background Knowledge: Information sources or knowledge available on the domain (e.g., relational and literature databases, biological ontologies).

Constraint: Pattern restriction defining the focus of search. It expresses a potential interest given by a user.

Functional Genomics: Functional Genomics hints at understanding the function of genes and other parts of the genome.

Local Patterns: Regularities that hold for a particular part of the data. It is often required that local patterns are also characterized by high deviations from a global model (Hand, 2002).

Recursive Mining: Repeating the pattern mining process on output to reduce it until few and relevant patterns are obtained.

SAGE Method: SAGE produces a digital version of the thanscriptome that is made from small sequences derived from genes called "tags" together with their frequency in a given biological situation.

Chapter XIII
Gene Expression Mining Guided by Background Knowledge

Jiří Kléma
Czech Technical University in Prague, Czech Republic

Filip Železný
Czech Technical University in Prague, Czech Republic

Igor Trajkovski
Jožef Stefan Institute, Slovenia

Filip Karel
Czech Technical University in Prague, Czech Republic

Bruno Crémilleux
Université de Caen, France

Jakub Tolar
University of Minnesota, USA

ABSTRACT

This chapter points out the role of genomic background knowledge in gene expression data mining. The authors demonstrate its application in several tasks such as relational descriptive analysis, constraint-based knowledge discovery, feature selection and construction or quantitative association rule mining. The chapter also accentuates diversity of background knowledge. In genomics, it can be stored in formats such as free texts, ontologies, pathways, links among biological entities, and many others. The authors hope that understanding of automated integration of heterogeneous data sources helps researchers to reach compact and transparent as well as biologically valid and plausible results of their gene-expression data analysis.

INTRODUCTION

High-throughput technologies like microrarrays or SAGE are at the center of a revolution in biotechnology, allowing researchers to simultaneously monitor the expression of tens of thousands of genes. However, gene-expression data analysis represents a difficult task as the data usually show an inconveniently low ratio of samples (biological situations) against variables (genes). Datasets are often noisy and they contain a great part of variables irrelevant in the context under consideration. Independent of the platform and the analysis methods used, the result of a gene-expression experiment should be driven, annotated or at least verified against genomic background knowledge (BK).

As an example, let us consider a list of genes found to be differentially expressed in different types of tissues. A common challenge faced by the researchers is to translate such gene lists into a better understanding of the underlying biological phenomena. Manual or semi-automated analysis of large-scale biological data sets typically requires biological experts with vast knowledge of many genes, to decipher the known biology accounting for genes with correlated experimental patterns. The goal is to identify the relevant "functions", or the global cellular activities, at work in the experiment. Experts routinely scan gene expression clusters to see if any of the clusters are explained by a known biological function. Efficient interpretation of this data is challenging because the number and diversity of genes exceed the ability of any single researcher to track the complex relationships hidden in the data sets. However, much of the information relevant to the data is contained in publicly available gene ontologies and annotations. Including this additional data as a direct knowledge source for any algorithmic strategy may greatly facilitate the analysis.

This chapter gives a summary of our recent experience in mining of transcriptomic data. The chapter accentuates the potential of genomic background knowledge stored in various formats such as free texts, ontologies, pathways, links among biological entities, etc. It shows the ways in which heterogeneous background knowledge can be preprocessed and subsequently applied to improve various learning and data mining techniques. In particular, the chapter demonstrates an application of background knowledge in the following tasks:

- Relational descriptive analysis
- Constraint-based knowledge discovery
- Feature selection and construction (and its impact on classification accuracy)
- Quantitative association rule mining

The chapter starts with an overview of genomic datasets and accompanying background knowledge analyzed in the text. Section on relational descriptive analysis presents a method to identify groups of differentially expressed genes that have functional similarity in background knowledge. Section on genomic classification focuses on methods helping to increase accuracy and understandability of classifiers by incorporation of background knowledge into the learning process. Section on constraint-based knowledge discovery presents and discusses several background knowledge representations enabling effective mining of meaningful over-expression patterns representing intrinsic associations among genes and biological situations. Section on association rule mining briefly introduces a quantitative algorithm suitable for real-valued expression data and demonstrates utilization of background knowledge for pruning of its output ruleset. Conclusion summarizes the chapter content and gives our future plans in further integration of the presented techniques.

GENE-EXPRESSION DATASETS AND BACKGROUND KNOWLEDGE

The following paragraphs give a brief overview of information resources used in the chapter. The primary role of background knowledge is to functionally describe individual genes and to quantify their similarity.

Gene-Expression (Transcriptome) Datasets

The process of transcribing a gene's DNA sequence into the RNA that serves as a template for protein production is known as gene expression. A gene's expression level indicates an approximate number of copies of the gene's RNA produced in a cell. This is considered to be correlated with the amount of corresponding protein made.

Expression chips (DNA chips, microarrays), manufactured using technologies derived from computer-chip production, can now measure the expression of thousands of genes simultaneously, under different conditions. A typical gene expression data set is a matrix, with each column representing a gene and each row representing a class labeled sample, e.g. a patient diagnosed having a specific sort of cancer. The value at each position in the matrix represents the expression of a gene for the given sample (see Figure 1). The particular problem used as an example in this chapter aims at distinguishing between acute lymphoblastic leukemia (ALL) and acute myeloid leukemia (AML) (Golub, 1999). The gene expression profiles were obtained by the Affymetrix HU6800 microarray chip, containing probes for 7129 genes, the data contains 72 class-labeled samples of expression vectors. 47 samples belong to the ALL class (65%) as opposed to 25 samples annotated as AML (35%).

SAGE (Serial Analysis of Gene Expression) is another technique that aims to measure the expression levels of genes in a cell population (Velculescu, 1995). It is performed by sequencing tags (short sequences of 14 to 21 base pairs (bps) which are specific of each mRNA). A SAGE library is a list of transcripts expressed at one given time point in one given biological situation. Both the identity (assessed through a tag-to-gene complex process, (Keime, 2004)) and the amount of each transcript is recorded. SAGE, as a data source, has been largely under-exploited as of today, in spite of its important advantage over microarrays. In fact, SAGE can produce datasets that can be directly compared between libraries without the need for external normalization. The human transcriptome can be seen as a set of libraries that would ideally be collected in each biologically relevant situation in the human body. This is clearly out of reach at the moment, and we deal in the present work with 207 different situations ranging from embryonic stem cells to foreskin primary fibroblast cells. Unambiguous tags (those that enable unequivocal gene identification) were selected leaving a set of 11082 tags/genes. A 207x11082 gene expression matrix was built.

Figure 1. The outcome of a microarray or SAGE experiment

	gene 1	gene 2	...	gene n	target
sample/situation 1	Values of gene expression (binary, symbolic, integer or real)				T_1
sample/situation 2					T_2
...	Sample expression signatures in rows, gene expression profiles in columns				...
sample/situation m					T_m

The biological situations embody various tissues (brain, prostate, breast, kidney or heart) stricken by various possible diseases (mainly cancer, but also HIV and healthy tissues). As the main observed disorder is carcinoma, a target binary attribute Cancer was introduced by the domain expert. The class value is 0 for all the healthy tissues and also the tissues suffering by other diseases than cancer (77 situations in total, 37.2%). It is equal to 1 for all the cancerous tissues (130 situations, 62.8%). The dataset was also binarized to encode the over-expression of each gene using the MidRange method described in (Becquet, 2002). For each gene it takes its highest value (max), the lowest value (min), and calculates the mid-range as (max-min)/2. Values above the threshold are given a boolean value of 1; all others are given a value of 0.

Background Knowledge

In this chapter, the term genomic background knowledge refers to any information that is not available in a gene-expression dataset but it is related to the genes or situations contained in this dataset. The richest body of background knowledge is available for genes. Gene datatabases such as Entrez Gene (NCBI website: http://www.ncbi.nlm.nih.gov/) offer a large scale of gene data – general information including a short textual summary of gene function, cellular location, bibliography, interactions and further links with other genes, memberships in pathways, referential sequences and many other pieces of information. Having a list of genes (i.e. colums in Figure 1), the information about all of the genes from the list can be collected automatically via services such as Entrez Utils (NCBI website: http://www.ncbi.nlm.nih.gov/). Similarly, annotations of the biological samples (i.e. rows in Figure 1) contained in the gene-expression dataset are available. In the simplest case, there is at least a brief description of the aim of the experiment where the sample was used.

Two forms of external knowledge require special attention during data pre-processing. These are freetexts and gene ontologies (GOs). We use them in two principal ways. The first way of utilization extracts all the relevant keywords for each gene, the main purpose is to **annotate**. In the second way we aim to **link** the genes. We introduce a quantitative notion of gene similarity that later on contributes to the cost-efficient reduction of computational costs across various learning and data mining algorithms. In the area of freetexts we have been inspired mainly by (Chaussabel, 2002; Glenisson, 2003). Both of them deal with the term-frequency vector representation which is a simple however prevailing representation of texts. This representation allows for an annotation of a gene group as well as a straightforward definition of gene similarity. In the area of gene ontologies we mostly rely on (Martin, 2004), the gene similarity results from the genes' positions in the molecular functional, biological process or cellular component ontology.

However, alternative sources can also be used, e.g., (Sevon, 2006) suggests an approach to discover links between entities in biological databases. Information extracted from available databases is represented as a graph, where vertices correspond to entities and edges represent annotated relationships among entities. A link is manifested as a path or a sub-graph connecting the corresponding vertices. Link goodness is based on edge reliability, relevance and rarity. Obviously, the graph itself or a corresponding similarity matrix based on the link goodness can serve as an external knowledge source.

Free Texts and Their Preprocessing

To access the gene annotation data for every gene or tag considered, probe identifiers (in the case microarrays) or Reference Sequence (RefSeq) identifiers (for SAGE) were translated into Entrez Gene

Identifiers (Entrez Ids) using the web-tool MatchMiner (http://discover.nci.nih.gov/ matchminer/). The mapping approached 1 to 1 relationship. Knowing the gene identifiers, the annotations were automatically accessed through hypertext queries to the EntrezGene database and sequentially parsed (Klema, 2006). Non-trivial textual records were obtained for the majority of the total amount of unique ids. The gene textual annotations were converted into the vector space model. A single gene corresponds to a single vector, whose components correspond to the frequency of a single vocabulary term in the text. This representation is often referred to as bag-of-words (Salton, 1988). The particular vocabulary consisted of all stemmed terms (Porter stemmer, http://www.tartarus.org/~martin/ PorterStemmer/) that appear in 5 different gene records at least. The most frequent terms were manually checked and insufficiently precise terms (such as gene, protein, human etc.) were removed. The resulting vocabulary consisted of 17122 (ALL/AML), respectively 19373 terms (SAGE). The similarity between genes was defined as the cosine of the angle between the corresponding term-frequency inverse-document-frequency (TFIDF) (Salton, 1988) vectors. The TFIDF representation statistically considers how important a term is to a gene record.

A similarity matrix *s* for all the genes was generated (see Figure 2). Each field of the triangular matrix $s_{ij} \in \langle 0,1 \rangle$ gives a similarity measure between the genes *i* and *j*. The underlying idea is that a high value of two vectors' cosine (which means a low angle among two vectors and thus a similar occurrence of the terms) indicates a semantic connection between the corresponding gene records and consequently their presumable connection. This model is known to generate false positive relations (as it does not consider context) as well as false negative relations (mainly because of synonyms). Despite this inaccuracy, bag-of-words format corresponds to the commonly used representation of text documents. It enables efficient execution of algorithms such as clustering, learning, classification or visualization, often with surprisingly faithful results (Scheffer, 2002).

Gene Ontology

One of the most important tools for the representation and processing of information about gene products and functions is the Gene Ontology (GO). It provides a controlled vocabulary of terms for the description of cellular components, molecular functions, and biological processes. The ontology also identifies those pairs of terms where one **is a** special case of the other. Similarly, term pairs are identified where

Figure 2. Gene similarity matrix – the similarity values lie in a range from 0 (total mismatch between gene descriptions) to 1 (pertfect match), n/a value suggests that at least one of the gene tuple has no knowledge attached

	gene 1	gene 2	gene 3	gene 4	...	gene n
gene 1	1	0.05	n/a	n/a	...	0.63
gene 2		1	0.01	0.33	...	0.12
gene 3			1	n/a	...	n/a
gene 4				1	...	n/a
...	...	...	...	...	...	...
gene n						1

one term refers to a **part of** the other. Formally this knowledge is reflected by the binary relations "**is a**" and "**part of**".

For each gene we extracted its ontological annotation, that is, the set of ontology terms relevant to the gene. This information was transformed into the gene's background knowledge encoded in relational logic in the form of Prolog facts. For example, part of the knowledge for particular gene SRC, whose EntrezId is 6714, is as follows:

```
function(6714,'ATP binding').
function(6714,'receptor activity').
process(6714,'signal complex formation').
process(6714,'protein kinase cascade').
component(6714,'integral to membrane').
...
```

Next, using GO, in the gene's background knowledge we also included the gene's generalized annotations in the sense of the "**is a**" relation described above. For example, if one gene is functionally annotated as: "zinc ion binding", in the background knowledge we also included its more general functional annotations such as e.g. transition metal ion binding or metal ion binding.

The genes can also be functionally related on the basis of their GO terms. Intuitively, the more GO terms the genes share, and the more specific the terms are, the more likely the genes are to be functionally related. (Martin, 2004) defines a distance based on the Czekanowski-Dice formula, the methodology is implemented within the GOProxy tool of GOToolBox http://crfb.univ-mrs.fr/GOToolBox/). A similarity matrix of the same structure as shown in Figure 2 can be generated.

Gene Interactions

The similarity matrix described in the previous paragraphs is one specific way to represent putative gene interactions. Besides, public databases also offer the information about pairs of genes for which there is traced experimental evidence of mutual interaction. In this case we use a crisp declarative representation of the interaction, in the form of a Prolog fact. The following example represents an interaction between gene SRC (EntrezId 6714) and genes ADRB3 (EntrezId 155) and E2F4 (EntrezId 1874):

```
interaction(6714,155).
interaction(6714,1874).
```

RELATIONAL DESCRIPTIVE ANALYSIS

This section presents a method to identify groups of differentially expressed genes that have functional similarity in background knowledge formally represented by gene annotation terms from the gene ontology (Trajkovski, 2006). The input to the algorithm is a multidimensional numerical data set, representing the expression of the genes under different conditions (that define the classes of examples), and an ontology used for producing background knowledge about these genes. The output is a set of gene groups whose expression is significantly different for one class compared to the other classes. The distinguishing property of the method is that the discovered gene groups are described in a rich, yet human-readable language. Specifically, each such group is defined in terms of a logical conjunction of features, that each member of the group possesses. The features are again logical statements that describe gene properties using gene ontology terms and interactions with other genes.

Medical experts are usually not satisfied with a separate description of every important gene, but want to know the processes that are controlled by these genes. The presented algorithm enables to find these processes and the cellular components where they are "executed", indicating the genes from the pre-selected list of differentially expressed genes which are included in these processes.

These goals are achieved by using the methodology of Relational Subgroup Discovery (RSD) (Lavrac, 2002). RSD is able to induce sets of rules characterizing the differentially expressed genes in terms of functional knowledge extracted from the gene ontology and information about gene interactions.

Fundamental Idea

The fundamental idea of learning relational descriptions of differentially expressed gene groups is outlined in Figure 3 (Trajkovski 2008). First, a set of differentially expressed genes, $G_C(c)$, is constructed for every class $c \in C$ (e.g. types of cancer). These sets can be constructed in several ways. For example: $G_C(c)$ can be the set of k ($k > 0$) most correlated genes with class c, for instance computed by Pearson's correlation. $G_C(c)$ can also be the set of best k single gene predictors, using the recall values from a microarray/SAGE experiment (absent/present/marginal) as the expression value of the gene. These predictors can acquire the form such as:

If $gene_i$ = present Then class = c

In our experiments, $G_C(c)$ was constructed using a modified version of the t-test statistics. The modification lies in an additional condition ensuring that each selected gene has at least twofold difference in its average expression for the given class with respect to the rest of the samples. The second step aims at improving the interpretability of G_C. Informally, we do this by identifying subgroups of genes in $G_C(c)$ (for each $c \in C$) which can be summarized in a compact way. Put differently, for each $c_i \in C$ we search for

Figure 3. An outline of the process of gene-expression data analysis using RSD

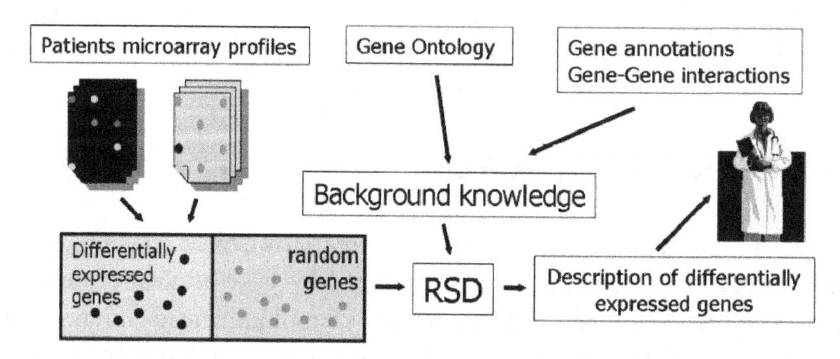

compact descriptions of gene subgroups with expression strongly correlating (positively or negatively) with c_i and weakly with all $c_j \in C$; $j \neq i$.

Searching for these groups of genes, together with their description, is defined as a supervised machine learning task. We refer to it as the secondary mining task, as it aims to mine from the outputs of the primary learning process in which differentially expressed genes are searched. This secondary task is, in a way, orthogonal to the primary discovery process in that the original attributes (genes) now become training examples, each of which has a class label "differentially expressed" and "not differentially expressed". Using the gene ontology information, gene annotation and gene interaction data, we produce background knowledge for differentially expressed genes on one hand, and randomly chosen genes on the other hand. The background knowledge is represented in the form of Prolog facts. Next, the RSD algorithm finds characteristic descriptions of the differentially expressed genes. Finally, the discovered descriptions can be straightforwardly interpreted and exploited by medical experts.

Relational Subgroup Discovery

The RSD algorithm proceeds in two steps. First, it constructs a set of relational features in the form of first-order logic atom conjunctions. The entire set of features is then viewed as an attribute set, where an attribute has the value true for a gene (example) if the gene has the feature corresponding to the attribute. As a result, by means of relational feature construction we achieve the conversion of relational data into attribute-value descriptions. In the second step, interesting gene subgroups are searched, such that each subgroup is represented as a conjunction of selected features. The subgroup discovery algorithm employed in this second step is an adaptation of the popular propositional rule learning algorithm CN2 (Clark, 1989).

The feature construction component of RSD aims at generating a set of relational features in the form of relational logic atom conjunctions. For example, the informal feature *"gene g interacts with another gene whose functions include protein binding"* has the relational logic form:

interaction(g,B), function(B,'protein binding')

where upper cases denote variables, and a comma between two logical literals denotes a conjunction. The user specifies mode declarations which syntactically constrain the resulting set of constructed features and restrict the feature search space. Furthermore, the maximum length of a feature (number of contained literals) is declared. RSD proceeds to produce an exhaustive set of features satisfying the declarations. Technically, this is implemented as an exhaustive depth-first backtrack search in the space of all feature descriptions, equipped with certain pruning mechanisms. Finally, to evaluate the truth value of each feature for each example for generating the attribute-value representation of the relational data, the first-order logic resolution procedure is used, provided by a standard Prolog language interpreter.

Subgroup discovery aims at finding population subgroups that are statistically "most interesting", e.g., are as large as possible and have the most unusual statistical characteristics with respect to the target class. To discover interesting subgroups of genes defined in terms of the constructed features, RSD follows a strategy stemming from the popular rule learner CN2. See (Zelezny, 2006) for details on this procedure.

Experiments

In ALL, RSD has identified a group of 23 genes, described as a conjunction of two features: component(G,'nucleus') AND interaction(G,B),process(B,'regulation of transcription, DNA-dependent'). The products of these genes, proteins, are located in the nucleus of the cell, and they interact with genes that are included in the process of regulation of transcription. In AML, RSD has identified several groups of overexpressed genes, located in the membrane, that interact with genes that have 'metal ion transport' as one of their function.

Subtypes of ALL and AML can also be distinguished, in a separate subgroup discovery process where classes are redefined to correspond to the respective disease subtypes. For example, two subgroups were found with unusually high frequency of the BCR (TEL, respectively) subtype of ALL. The natural language description of BCR class derived from the automatically constructed subgroup relational description is the following: *genes coding for proteins located in the integral to membrane cell component, whose functions include receptor activity.* This description indeed appears plausible, since BCR is a classic example of a leukemia driven by spurious expression of a fusion protein expressed as a continuously active kinase protein on the *membrane* of leukemic cells. Similarly, the natural language description for the TEL class is: genes coding for proteins located in the nucleus whose functions include protein binding and whose related processes include transcription. Here again, by contrast to BCR, the TEL leukemia is driven by expression of a protein, which is a transcription factor active in the *nucleus.*

A statistical validation of the proposed methodology for discovering descriptions of differentially expressed gene groups was also carried out. The analysis determined if the high descriptive capacity pertaining to the incorporation of the expressive relational logic language incurs a risk of descriptive overfitting, i.e., a risk of discovering subgroups whose bias toward differential expression is only due to chance. The discrepancy of the quality of discovered subgroups on the training data set on one hand and an independent test set on the other hand was measured. It was done through the standard 10-fold stratified cross-validation regime. The specific qualities measured for each set of subgroups produced for a given class are average precision (PRE), recall (REC) and area under ROC (AUC) values among all subgroups in the subgroup set. In ALL/AML dataset, RSD showed PRE 100(±0)%, REC 16% and AUC 65% in training data and PRE 85(±6)%, REC 13% and AUC 60% in independent testing data. The results demonstrate an acceptable decay from the training to the testing set in terms of both PRE and REC, suggesting that the discovered subgroup descriptions indeed capture the relevant gene properties. In terms of total coverage, in average, RSD covered more then 2/3 of the preselected differentially expressed genes, while 1/3 of the preselected genes were not included in any group. A possible interpretation is that they are not functionally connected with the other genes and their initial selection through the t-test was due to chance. This information can evidently be back-translated into the gene selection procedure and used as a gene selection heuristic.

GENOMIC CLASSIFICATION WITH BACKGROUND KNOWLEDGE

Traditional attribute-value classification searches for a mapping from attribute value tuples, which characterize instances, to a discrete set whose elements correspond to classes. When dealing with a large number of attributes and a small number of instances, the resulting classifier is likely to fit the training data solely by chance, rather than by capturing genuine underlying trends. Datasets are often noisy and they contain a great part of variables irrelevant in the context of desired classification.

In order to increase the predictive power of the classifier and its understandability, it is advisable to incorporate background knowledge into the learning process. In this section we study and test several simple ways to improve a genomic classifier constructed from gene expression data as well as textual and gene ontology annotations available both for the genes and the biological situations.

Motivation

Decision-tree learners, rule-based classifiers or neural networks are known to often overfit gene expression data, i.e., identify many false connections. A principal means to combat the risk of overfitting is feature selection (FS); a process aiming to filter irrelevant variables (genes) from the dataset prior to the actual construction of a classifier. Families of classifiers are available, that are more tolerant to abundance of irrelevant attributes than the above mentioned traditional methods. Random forests (Breiman, 2001; Diaz-Uriarte, 2006) or support vector machines (Furey, 2000; Lee, 2003) exemplify the most popular ones. Still, feature selection remains helpful in most gene expression classification analyses. Survey studies (such as (Lee, 2005)) stress that the choice of feature selection methods has much effect on the performance of the subsequently applied classification methods.

In the gene expression domain, feature selection corresponds to the task of finding a limited set of genes that still contains most of the information relevant to the biological situations in question. Many gene selection approaches create rankings of gene relevance regardless of any knowledge of the classification algorithm to be used. These approaches are referred to as filter methods. Besides general filter ranking methods (different modifications of the t-test, information gain, mutual information), various specific gene-selection methods were published. The signal-to-noise (S2N) ratio was introduced in (Golub, 1999), significance analysis of microarrays (SAM) appeared in (Tusher, 2001). (Tibshirani, 2002) proposed and tested nearest shrunken centroids (NSC). The wrapper methods can be viewed as gene selection methods which directly employ classifiers. Gene selection is then guided by analyzing the embedded classifier's performance as well as its result (e.g. to detect which variables proved important for classification). Recursive Feature Elimination (RFE) based on absolute magnitude of the hyperplane elements in a support vector machine is discussed in (Guyon, 2002). (Uriarte, 2006) selects genes according to the decrease of the random forest classification accuracy when values of the gene are permuted randomly.

Here we consider feature selection techniques in a different perspective. All of the above-mentioned methods rely on gene expression data itself. No matter whether they apply a single-variate or multivariate selection criteria, they disregard any potential prior knowledge on gene functions and its true or potential interactions with other genes, diseases or other biological entities. Our principal aim is to exploit background knowledge such as literature and ontologies concerning genes or biological situations as a form of evidence of the genes' relevance to the classification task.

The presented framework uses the well-known CN2 (Clark, 1989) rule learning algorithm. In fact, rule-based classification exhibits a particular weakness when it comes to gene expression data classification. This is due to their small resistance to overfitting, as commented above. As such, a rule learning algorithm is a perfect candidate to evaluate the possible assets of background knowledge. Thus, the main goal is not to develop the best possible classifier in terms of absolute accuracy. Rather, we aim to assess the relative gains obtained by integrating prior knowledge. The evaluated gains pertain to classification accuracy, but also to the comprehensibility of the resulting models.

Feature Selection

We first consider the widely accepted dogma that feature selection helps improve classification accuracy and test it in the gene expression domain. A single-variate gain ratio (GR) (Quinlan, 1986) evaluation criterion was used. The criterion is information-based and disregards apriori knowledge. The graphs in Figure 4 show that indeed: 1) FS improves classification accuracy (SAGE dataset – the average accuracy grows from 67.1% for 5052 features to 72.8% for 50 features, ALL/AML dataset – the average accuracy grows from 86.9% for 7129 features to 92.4% for 10 features), 2) informed FS outperforms the random one.

Next, we want to design a mechanism which could guide feature selection using available apriori knowledge. The main idea is to promote the genes whose description contains critical keywords relevant to the classification objective. For example, SAGE classification tries to distinguish among cancerous and non-cancerous tissues. Consequently, the genes that are known to be active in cancerous tissues may prove to be more important than they seem to according to their mutual information with the target (expressed in terms of entropy, gain ratio or mutual information itself). These genes should be promoted into the subset of selected features. Auxiliary experiments proved that there are large gene groups whose mutual information with the target differs only slightly. As a consequence, even an insignificant difference then may decide whether the gene gets selected. To avoid this threshold curse, one may favor multi-criteria gene ranking followed by gene filtering.

The way in which we rank genes with respect to their textual and/or ontological description depends on the amount of information available for biological situations. In the SAGE dataset, each situation contains a brief textual annotation. The frequent words from these annotations serve to create a list of relevant keywords. In the ALL/AML dataset, there are descriptions of the individual classes and the list of keywords is made of the words that characterize these classes. In order to calculate gene importance, the list of keywords is matched with the bag-of-words that characterizes the individual genes. A gene is rated higher if its description contains a higher proportion of situation keywords. Let us show the following simple example:

Figure 4. Gain ratio - development of classification accuracy with decreasing number of features/ genes

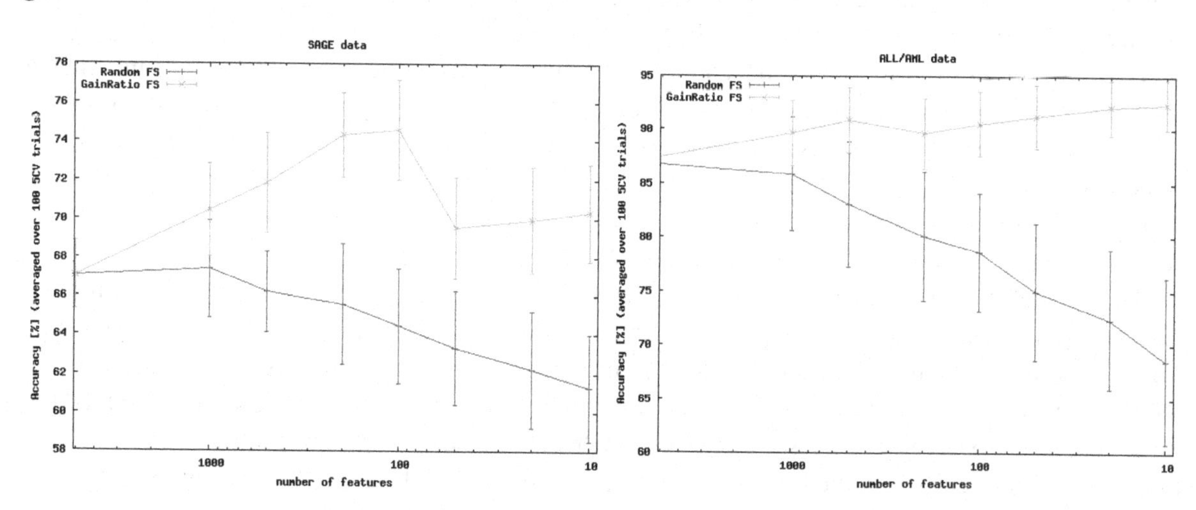

Keywords (characterize the domain): carcinoma, cancer, glioblastoma
Bag of words (characterize the gene): bioactive, cancer, framework, glioblastoma
gene1: 1, 3, 4, 2, gene2: 0, 0, 2, 0 (the word bioactive appears 3 times in gene1 annotations etc.)
gene1 scores (1+4)/(1+3+4+2)=0.5, gene2 scores 0/2=0

We refer to this process as the apriori-based FS. The graphs in Figure 5 compare the apriori-based FS with the random one. In the SAGE dataset, the list of apriori genes is better than random, although the margin is not as distinct as for the information-based criterion used in Figure 4. In the ALL/AML dataset, the apriori-based genes proved to have similar predictive power as randomly selected genes. A likely explanation for this is that the list of keywords was too short. The gene ranking was too rough to correlate with the real gene importance. A great portion of genes scored 0 as they never co-occur with any keyword.

We next tackle the question whether one can cross-fertilize the information-based and apriori-based FS. Two different FS procedures were implemented – conditioning and combination. Conditioning FS keeps the gain ratio ranking but removes all the genes scoring less than a threshold on the apriori-based ranking scale. When asked for X best genes, it takes the X top genes from the reduced list. Combination FS takes the best genes from top of both the lists. When asked for X best genes it takes X/2 top genes from the gain ratio list and X/2 top genes from the apriori list. The result is shown in Figure 6. In spite of better than random quality of apriori-based FS in SAGE dataset, neither conditioning nor combination outperforms gain ratio. The apriori list seems to bring no additional strong predictors. In the ALL/AML dataset, conditioning gives the best performance. It can be explained by the good informativeness of the set of 1000 top genes from the apriori list, which enriches the original gain-ratio list.

In general, the experiments proved that usability of apriori-based FS strongly depends on the domain and the target of classification. The amount of available keywords and their relevance make the crucial issue.

Figure 5. Apriori-based feature selection - development of classification accuracy with decreasing number of features/genes

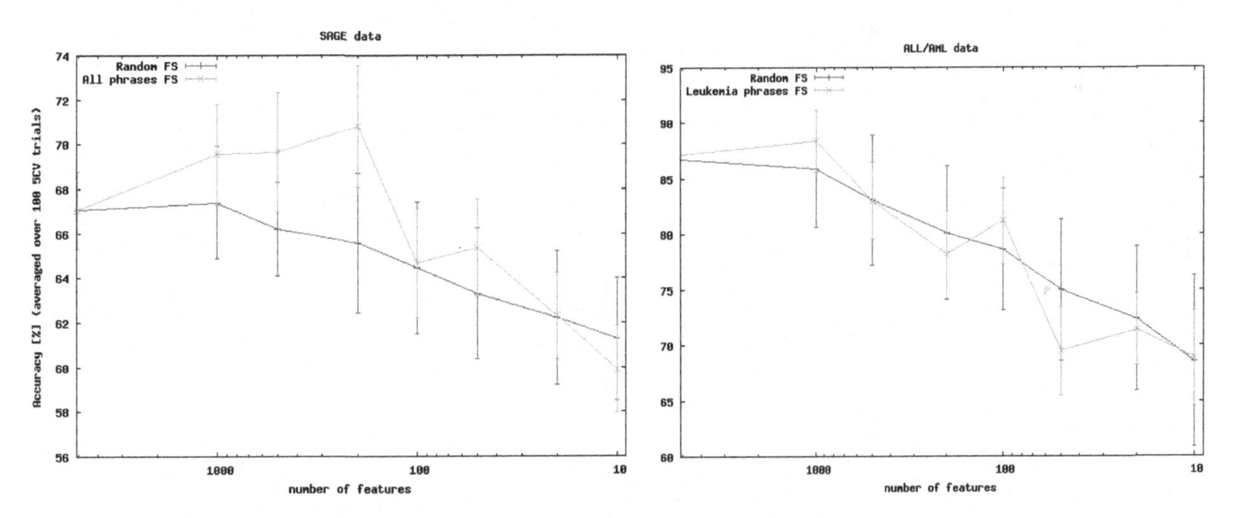

Feature Extraction

The curse of feature space dimensionality can also be overcome or in the least reduced by feature extraction (FE). It is a procedure that transforms the original feature space by building new features from the existing ones. (Hanczar, 2003) proposed a prototype-based feature extraction that consists of two simple steps: 1) identify equivalence classes inside the feature space, 2) extract feature prototypes that represent the classes invented in step 1. In practice, the features are clustered and each cluster is represented by its mean vector – the prototype. The prototypes are used to learn a classifier and to classify new biological situations.

An interesting fact is that equivalence classes can be derived from the gene expression profiles as well as from the known gene functions or any other biologically relevant criteria. The gene similarity matrix based on gene-expression profiles can be combined with the gene-similarity matrices inferred from the background knowledge. Although the prototypes did not prove to increase classification accuracy either in the ALL/AML or the SAGE task, the prototypes can increase understandability of the resulting classifier. The classifier does not treat the individual genes but it reports the equivalence classes whose interpretability is higher as they are likely to contain "similar" genes.

Another idea is to inject background knowledge into the learning algorithm itself. In case of CN2, the algorithm implements a laplacian heuristic that drives rule construction. As mentioned earlier, the algorithm is likely to overfit the data as it searches a large feature space, verifies a large number of simple conditions and randomly finds a rule with a satisfactory heuristic value. Background knowledge can complement the laplacian criteria in the following way: 1) promote short rules containing genes with apriori relevance to the target (a kind of late feature *selection* conditioned by rule length and heuristic value), 2) promote the rules with interacting genes (a kind of late feature *extraction* with the same conditioning). This form of background knowledge injection was implemented and evaluated in (Trna, 2007). The main benefit of this method is the understandability of the resulting classifier.

Figure 6. Combined feature selection - development of classification accuracy with decreasing number of features/genes

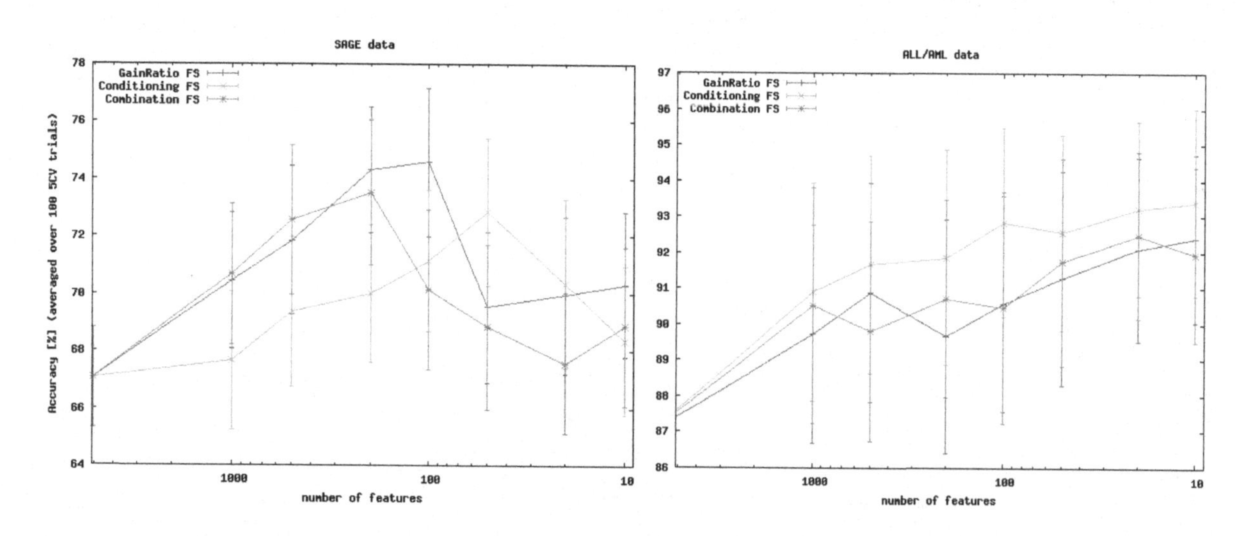

CONSTRAINT-BASED KNOWLEDGE DISCOVERY

Current gene co-expression analyses are often based on global approaches such as clustering or bi-clustering. An alternative way is to employ local methods and search for patterns – sets of genes displaying specific expression properties in a set of situations. The main bottleneck of this type of analysis is twofold – computational costs and an overwhelming number of candidate patterns which can hardly be further exploited by a human. A timely application of background knowledge can help to focus on the most plausible patterns only. This section discusses various representations of BK that enables the effective mining and representation of meaningful over-expression patterns representing intrinsic associations among genes and biological situations.

Constraints Inferred from Background Knowledge

Details on knowledge discovery from local patterns are given in another chapter of this book (Cremilleux, 2008). This section focuses on processing, representation and utilization of BK within the constraint-based framework presented ibid. In the domain of constraint-based mining, the constraints should effectively link different datasets and knowledge types. For instance, in the domain of genomics, biologists are interested in constraints both on co-expression groups and common characteristics of the genes and/or biological situations concerned. Such constraints require to tackle transcriptome data (often provided in a transactional format) and external databases. This section provides examples of a declarative language enabling the user to set varied and meaningful constraints defined on transcriptome data, similarity matrices and textual resources.

In our framework, a constraint is a logical conjunction of propositions. A proposition is an arithmetic test such as $C > t$ where t is a number and C denotes a *primitive* or a *compound*. A primitive is one of a small set of predefined simple functions evaluated on the data. Such primitives may further be assembled into compounds.

We illustrate the construction of a constraint through an example. A textual dataset provides a description of genes. Each row contains a list of phrases that characterize the given gene. The phrases can be taken from gene ontology or they can represent frequent relevant keywords from gene bibliography:

Gene 1: 'metal ion binding' 'transcription factor activity' 'zinc ion binding'
Gene 2: 'hydrolase activity' 'serine esterase activity' 'cytoplasmic membrane-bound vesicle'
...
Gene n: 'serine-type peptidase activity' 'proteolysis' 'signal peptide processing'

In reference to the textual data, *regexp(X,RE)* returns the items among *X* whose phrase matches the regular expression *RE*.

As concerns the similarity matrices, we deal with primitives such as *sumsim(X)* denoting the similarity sum over the set of items *X* or *insim(X,min,max)* for the number of item pairs whose similarity lies between *min* and *max*. As we may deal with a certain portion of items without any information, there are primitives that distinguish between *zero* similarity and *missing value* of similarity. The primitive *svsim(X)* gives the number of item pairs belonging to *X* whose mutual similarity is valid and *mvsim(X)* stands for its counterpart, i.e., the missing interactions when one of the items has an empty record within the given similarity representation. The primitives can make compounds. Among many others, *sumsim(X)/svsim(X)* makes the average similarity, *insim(X,thres,1)/svsim(X)* gives a proportion of the strong interactions (similarity higher than the threshold) within the set of items, *svsim(X)/(svsim(X)+mvsim(X))* can avoid patterns with prevailing items of an unknown function.

Relational and logical operators as well as other built in functions enable to create the final constraint, e.g., $C_1 \geq thres_1$ and $C_2 \neq thres_2$ where C_i stands for an arbitrary compound or primitive. Constraints can also be simultaneously derived from different datasets. Then, the dataset makes another parameter of the primitive. For example, the constraint *length(regexp(X,'*ribosom*', TEXT))>1* returns all the patterns that contain at least 2 items involving "ribosom" in any of their characteristic phrases within the TEXT dataset.

Internal and External Constraints to Reach a Meaningful Limited Pattern Set

Traditional pattern mining deals with constraints that we refer to as internal. Truth values of such constraints are fully determined by the transcriptome dataset. The most meaningful internal constraints usually are the *area*, i.e. the product of the number of genes in the pattern (gene set), and the frequency of the pattern (number of transactions where the set is contained). This is because the main goal is usually to identify large gene sets that tend to co-occur frequently. For these constraints to apply, one must consider a *binarized* expression dataset enabling to state whether or not a gene is expressed in a given situation. Verifying the area constraints means checking whether the area is larger than a certain threshold.

However, the area constraint is not a panacea for distinction between meaningful patterns and spurious ones, i.e., the patterns occurring randomly. Indeed, the largest area patterns often tend to be trivial, bringing no new knowledge. In SAGE, the increase of the area threshold in order to get a reasonable number of patterns leads to a small but uniform set that is flooded by the ribosomal genes which represent the most frequently over-expressed genes in the dataset. On the other hand, if the area threshold is decreased, the explosion of patterns may occur. It has been experimentally proven that the number of potentially large patterns is so high that they cannot be effectively surveyed by a human expert.

The described deficiency may be healed by augmenting internal constraints by further constraints, called *external*. An external constraint is one whose truth value is determined exclusive of the transcriptome dataset. Such constraints are for example *interestingness or expressiveness*, i.e., the future interpretability by a biologist. The interesting patterns are those exhibiting a general characteristic common for the genes and/or samples concerned (or at least their sub-sets). The more internal functional links in the pattern the more interesting the pattern.

Selectivity of selected external constraints in SAGE dataset is shown in Figure 7. The constraints capture the amount of similarity in given patterns through the measurement of the similarity of all gene pairs within that given pattern as well as they can avoid patterns with prevailing tags of an unknown function. The pruning starts with 46671 patterns that are larger than 3 genes and more frequent than 5 samples. The graphs depict that if both similarity (sumsim or insim) and existence (svsim) are thresholded, very compact sets of patterns can be reached. (Klema, 2006) gives a demonstration that these sets also gather biologically meaningful patterns.

Figure 7. Pattern pruning by the external constraints - simultaneous application of internal and external constraints helps to arbitrarily reduce the number of patterns while attempting to conserve the potentially interesting ones. The figures show the decreasing number of patterns with increasing threshold of selected external constraints. The effect of six different constraints of various complexity is shown

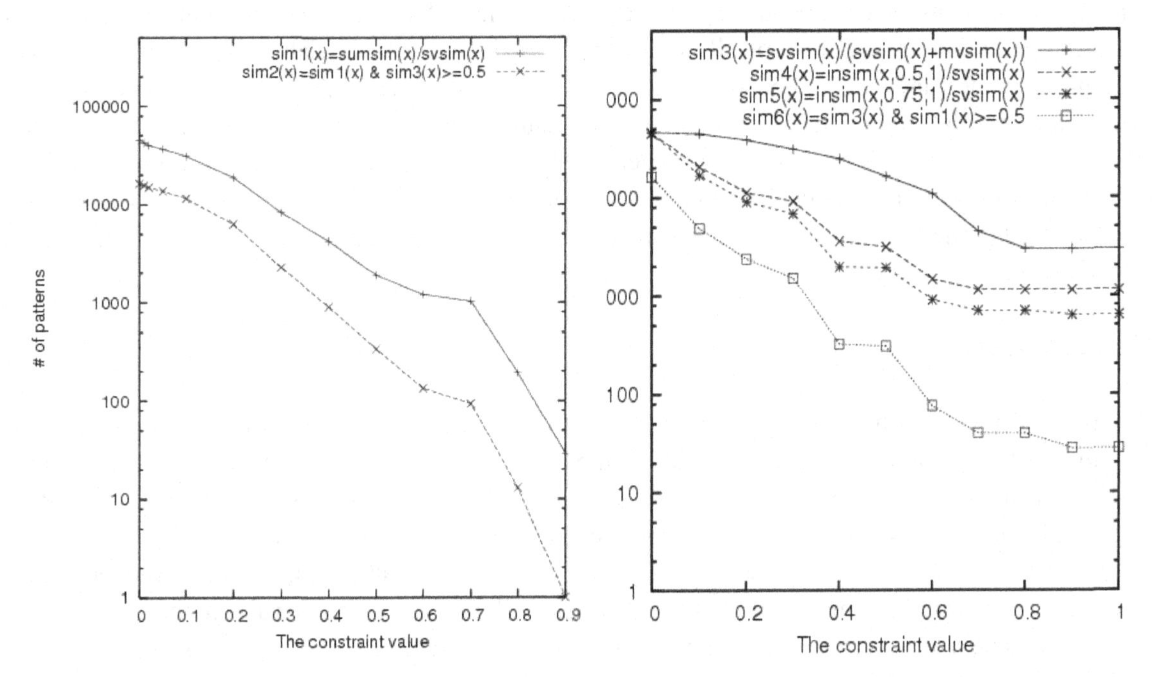

QUANTITATIVE ASSOCIATION RULE MINING IN GENOMICS USING BACKGROUND KNOWLEDGE

Clustering is one of the most often used methods of genomic data mining. The genes with the most similar profiles are found so that the similarity among genes in one group (cluster) is maximized and similarity among particular groups (clusters) is minimized. While clustering arguably is an elegant approach to provide effective insight into data, it does have drawbacks as well, of which we name three (Becquet, 2002):

1. One gene has to be clustered in one and only one group, although it functions in numerous physiological pathways.
2. No relationship can be inferred between the different members of a group. That is, a gene and its target genes will be co-clustered, but the type of relationship cannot be rendered explicit by the algorithm.
3. Most clustering algorithms will make comparisons between the gene expression patterns in all the conditions examined. They will therefore miss a gene grouping that only arises in a subset of cells or conditions.

Admittedly, drawback 1 is tackled by soft-clustering and drawback 2 is tackled by conceptual clustering. We are not aware of a clustering algorithm void of all the three deficiencies.

Association rule (AR) mining can overcome these drawbacks, however transcriptomic data represent a difficult mining context for association rules. First, the data are high-dimensional (typically contain several thousands of attributes), which asks for an algorithm scalable in the number of attributes. Second, expression values are typically quantitative variables. This variable type further increases computational demands and moreover may result in an output with a prohibitive number of redundant rules. Third, the data are often noisy which may also cause a large number of rules of little significance. In this section we discuss the above-mentioned bottlenecks and present results of mining association rules using an alternative approach to quantitative association rule mining. We also demonstrate a way in which background genomic knowledge can be used to prune the search space and reduce the amount of derived rules.

Related Work

One of the first thorough studies of AR mining on genomic data sets was provided in (Becquet, 2002). To validate the general feasibility of association rule mining in this data domain, the authors of (Becquet, 2002) have applied it to a freely available data set of human serial analysis of gene expression (SAGE). The SAGE data was first normalized and binarized as to contain only zeros and ones. These values stand for underexpression and overexpression of a given gene in a given situation, respectively. The authors selected 822 genes in 72 human cell types and generated all frequent and valid rules in the form of 'when gene a and gene b are overexpressed within a situation, then often gene c is over expressed too'.

To avoid this discretization step, authors in (Georgii, 2005) investigate the use of *quantitative association rules*, i.e., association rules that operate directly on numeric data and can represent the cumulative effects of variables. Quantitative association rules have the following form:

If the weighted sum of some variables is greater than a threshold, then, with high probability, a different weighted sum of variables is greater than second threshold.

An example of such rule can be:

$0.99 \times gene1 - 0.11 \times gene2 > 0.062 \rightarrow 1.00 \times gene3 > -0.032.$

This approach naturally overcomes the discretization problem; on the other hand it is quite hard to understand the meaning of the rule. This algorithm does not exhaustively enumerate all valid and strong association rules present in the data, it uses an optimization approach.

An analysis of a microarray data-set is presented in (Carmona-Saez, 2006). The authors bring external biological knowledge to the AR mining by setting a specific language bias In particular, only gene ontology terms are allowed to appear in the antecedent part of the rule. Annotated gene expression data sets can thus be mined for rules such as:

cell cycle → [+]condition1, [+]condition2, [+]condition3, [−]condition6 which means that a significant number of the genes annotated as 'cell cycle' are over-expressed in condition 1, 2 and 3 and under-expressed in condition 6, where the conditions here correspond to time interval <T1..T7>. A proviso for this method is, of course, that ontology annotations are available for all genes in question.

Time Complexity of Association Rule Mining

Time complexity is a serious issue in association rule mining, as it is an exponential function of sample dimensionality. To get a glimpse of the problem size, consider a binarized gene-expression dataset. Here, the number of possible itemsets is $2^{1000} \approx 10^{300}$ Although algorithms such as APRIORI use effective pruning techniques to dramatically reduce the search space traversed, the time complexity bound remains exponential.

With quantitative association rules, things get even worse. Consider the discretization into three bins, when each gene takes three values: 1 – gene is underexpressed, 2 – gene is averagely expressed, 3 – gene is overexpressed. Number of possible conditions (itemsets) grows to $5^{1000} \approx 10^{700}$, because now there are **five** possibilities for gene's value {1; 2; 3; 1..2; 2..3}. Any complete search-based algorithm becomes unfeasible even if it is completed by pruning or puts restrictions on the number of attributes on the left-hand and right-hand side (LHS, RHS). Clearly, the strong restrictions mentioned above have to be complemented by other instruments.

Background Knowledge Experiments in Association Rule Mining

In order to increase noise robustness, focus and speed up the search, it is vital to have a mechanism to exploit BK during AR generation. In the following we employ BK in the form of a similarity matrix as defined earlier. In particular, the similarity matrix describes how likely the genes are functionally related based on the GO terms they share. The experiments are carried out in the frame of the SAGE dataset.

BK is employed in pruning. The pruning takes a following form: generate a rule only if the similarity of the genes contained in the rule is above some defined threshold'. Similarly to constraint-based learning, this condition reduces the search space and helps to speed up the algorithm. It also provides us with results, which could be better semantically explained and/or annotated.

The QAR mining algorithm presented in (Karel, 2006) was used for experiments on SAGE dataset. The QAR algorithm uses a modified procedure of rule generation – it constructs compound conditions using simple mathematical operations. Then it identifies areas of increased association between LHS and RHS. Finally, rules are extracted from these areas of increased association. The procedure is incomplete as it does not guarantee that all the rules satisfying the input conditions are reported. Although the algorithm differs in principle from traditional AR mining, it outputs association rules in the classical form.

The numbers of rules as well as the numbers of candidate rule verifications were examined during the experiments, since the number of rules quantifies the output we are interested in and the number of verifications determinates time complexity of the algorithm.

The SAGE dataset is sparse – a great portion of gene-expression values equal to zero. The distribution of zeroes among genes is very uneven. So called housekeeping genes are expressed (nearly) in all the tissues; however there is a reasonable amount of genes having zero values in almost all situations.

A total of 306 genes having more than 80% non-zero values were used in the experiment. The raw data were preprocessed and discretized into three bins using K-means discretization.

While the right hand side of rules can take arbitrary forms within the language bias, we do fix it to only refer to the target variable *cancer*, as this variable is of primary interest. Additional restrictions needed to be introduced to keep time complexity in reasonable limits. The maximum number of LHS genes was bounded. The results of experiments are summarized in Table 1.

The theoretical number of verifications is computed without considering a *min_supp* pruning, because it is hard to estimate the reached reduction. Numbers of rules and verifications using background knowledge depend on the BK pruning threshold.

A vector *gene_appearance* was generated for the purpose of overall analysis of the results; the value $gene\_appearance_i$ is equal to the number of corresponding gene appearances in generated rules. Spearman rank correlation coefficient among *gene_appearance* vectors of all results was computed, see Table 2.

As we can see using background knowledge we receive most similar rules. Surprising is negative correlation between results with 2 LHS genes with background knowledge and 3 LHS genes without background knowledge. Background knowledge influences not only number of rules generated but also the character of the rules. Some concrete examples of generated rules can be found in Table 3.

Table 1. The number of rules and verifications for 2 and 3 antecedent genes. The settings were following: 2 gene thresholds: min_supp = 0.3, min_conf = 0.7 and min_lift = 1.3, 3 gene thresholds: min_supp = 0.15, min_conf = 0.8 and min_lift = 1.3

algorithm	number of LHS genes	number of rules	number of verifications
complete search (theoretical)	2	n/a	2 318 000
QAR algorithm (without BK)		530	76 747
QAR algorithm (with BK)		92	12 770
complete search (theoretical)	3	n/a	591 090 000
QAR algorithm (without BK)		7 509	14 921 537
QAR algorithm (with BK)		243	699 444

Table 2. Spearman rank correlation coefficients for vectors describing number of genes' appearances in generated rules

	2-ant with BK	2-ant without BK	3-ant with BK	3-ant without BK
2-ant with BK	1	0.04	0.29	-0.25
2-ant without BK	0.04	1	0.09	0.17
3-ant with BK	0.29	0.09	1	0.26
3-ant without BK	-0.25	0.17	0.26	1

Table 3. Examples of generated association rules. For gene expression levels it holds 1 – underexpressed, 2 – averagely expressed, 3 – overexpressed. Consequent condition stands for binary class cancer (0 – cancer did not occur, 1 – cancer did occur).

nr.	antecedent genes and their values	antecedent genes full name	cons. condition	conf	supp	lift
1	RPL31 = 1..2 NONO = 2..3	ribosomal protein L31 non-POU domain containing, octamer-binding	1	0.83	0.35	1.32
2	NONO = 2..3 FKBP8 = 1	non-POU domain containing, octamer-binding FK506 binding protein 8, 38kDa	1	0.81	0.31	1.29
3	MIF = 1..2 CDC42 = 2..3	macrophage migration inhibitory factor (glycosylation-inhibiting factor) cell division cycle 42 (GTP binding protein, 25kDa)	1	0.79	0.30	1.25
4	PHB2 = 2 PGD = 1 LGALS1 = 1	prohibitin 2 phosphogluconate dehydrogenase lectin, galactoside-binding, soluble, 1 (galectin 1)	1	0.94	0.15	1.50
5	COPA = 1..2 CDC42 = 2..3 NDUFS3 = 2..3	coatomer protein complex, subunit alpha cell division cycle 42 (GTP binding protein, 25kDa) NADH dehydrogenase (ubiquinone) Fe-S protein 3, 30kDa (NADH-coenzyme Q reductase)	1	0.90	0.17	1.43
6	PCBP1 = 2..3 ZYX = 1..1 ATP5B = 1..1	poly(rC) binding protein 1 zyxin ATP synthase, H+ transporting, mitochondrial F1 complex, beta polypeptide	1	0.88	0.18	1.40

Discussion

A heuristic QAR approach reduces the number of verifications and thus time costs. The usage of AR mining is extended beyond boolean data and can be applied on genomic data sets, although the number of attributes in the conditions has still to be restricted. The number of generated rules was also reduced by other means – there were at most two rules for each gene tuple. Consequently, the output is not flooded by quantities of rules containing the same genes having only small changes in their values.

Background knowledge was incorporated into QAR mining. BK provides a principled means to significantly reduce the search space and focus on plausible rules only. In general, the genes with prevalence of 'n/a' values in the similarity matrices are discriminated from the rules when using BK. However, a gene without annotation can still appear in a neighbourhood of 'a strong functional cluster' of other genes. This occurrence then signifies its possible functional relationship with the given group of genes and it can initiate its early annotation. On the other hand, the genes with extensive relationships to the other genes may increase their occurrence in the rules inferred with BK.

CONCLUSION

The discovery of biologically interpretable knowledge from gene expression data is one of the hottest contemporary genomic challenges. As massive volumes of expression data are being generated, intelligent analysis tools are called for. The main bottleneck of this type of analysis is twofold – computational costs and an overwhelming number of candidate hypotheses which can hardly be further post-processed exploited by a human expert. A timely application of background knowledge available in literature, databases, biological ontologies and other sources, can help to focus on the most plausible candidates only. We illustrated a few particular ways how background knowledge can be exploited for this purpose.

Admittedly, the presented approaches to exploiting background knowledge in gene expression data mining were mutually rather isolated, despite their common reliance on the same sources of external genomic knowledge. Intuition suggests that most effective results could be obtained by their pragmatic combination. For example, gene-gene similarity has so far been computed on the sole basis of gene ontology or textual term occurrences in the respective annotations. This definition admittedly may be overly shallow. Here, the RSD mechanism of constructing non-trivial relational logic features of genes may instead be used for computing similarity: two genes would be deemed functionally similar if they shared a sufficient number of the relational logic features referring to gene functions. The inverse look at the problem yields yet another suggestion for combining the methods. The similarity matrix computed from gene ontology term occurrences can be used as a part of background knowledge which RSD uses to construct features. Technically, a new predicate *similar(A,B)* would be introduced into the feature language, while its semantics for two genes *A* and *B* would be determined in the obvious way from the precomputed similarity matrix. These ideas form grounds for our future explorations.

ACKNOWLEDGMENT

Jiří Kléma, Filip Železný and Filip Karel have been supported by the grant 1ET101210513 "Relational Machine Learning for Analysis of Biomedical Data" funded by the Czech Academy of Sciences. Thc Czech-French travels were covered by Czech-French PHC Barrande project "Fusion de données hétérogenes pour la découverte de connaissances en génomique". The Czech-USA travels were covered by Czech Ministry of Education through project ME910 "Using Gene Ontologies and Annotations for the Interpretation of Gene Expression Data through Relational Machine Learning Algorithms". We thank Olivier Gandrillon and his team at the Centre de Génétique Moléculaire et Cellulaire for helpful and stimulating biological discussions and providing us with the SAGE dataset. We are grateful to Arnaud Soulet for providing us with his tool MUSIC applied in constraint-based knowledge discovery.

REFERENCES

Becquet, C., Blachon, S., Jeudy, B., Boulicaut, J. F. & Gandrillon O. (2002). Strong Association Rule Mining for Large Gene Expression Data Analysis: A Case Study on Human SAGE Data. *Genome Biology*, 3(12):531-537.

Breiman, L. (2001) Random Forests. *Machine Learning*, 45(1), 5–32.

Carmona-Saez, P., Chagoyen, M., Rodriguez, A., Trelles, O., Carazo, J. M., & Pascual-Montano, A. (2006). Integrated analysis of gene expression by association rules discovery. BMC *Bioinformatics*, *7*, 54.

Chaussabel, D., & Sher, A. (2002). Mining microarray expression data by literature profiling. *Genome Biology, 3*.

Clark, P., & Niblett, T. (1989). The CN2 induction algorithm. *Machine Learning*, 261–283.

Cremilleux, B., Soulet, A., Klema, J., Hebert, C., & Gandrillon, O. (2009). Discovering Knowledge from Local Patterns in SAGE data. In P. Berka, J. Rauch and D. J. Zighed (Eds.), *Data mining and medical knowledge management: Cases and applications*. Hershey, PA: IGI Global.

Diaz-Uriarte, R., & Alvarez de Andres, S. (2006). Gene selection and classification of microarray data using random forest. *BMC Bioinformatics*, *7*(3).

Furey, T.S., Cristianini, N., Duffy, N., Bednarski, D.W., Schummer, M. & Haussler, D. (2000). Support vector machine classifcation and validation of cancer tissue samples using microarray expression data. *Bioinformatics*, *16*, 906–914.

Georgii, E., Richter, L., Ruckert, U., & Kramer S. (2005) Analyzing Microarray Data Using Quantitative Association Rules. *Bioinformatics*, 21(Suppl. 2), ii123–ii129.

Glenisson, P., Mathys, J., & Moor, B. D. (2003) Meta-clustering of gene expression data and literature-based information. *SIGKDD Explor. Newsl.* 5(2), 101–112.

Golub, T., Slonim, D., Tamayo, P., Huard, C., Gaasenbeek, M., Mesirov, J., Coller, H., Loh, M., Downing, J., Caligiuri, M., Bloomfield, C., & Lander, E. (1999). Molecular classification of cancer: Class discovery and class prediction by gene expression monitoring. *Science*, 531–537.

Hanczar, B., Courtine, M., Benis, A., Hennegar, C., Clement, C. & Zucker, J. D. (2003). Improving classification of microarray data using prototype-based feature selection. *SIGKDD Explor. Newsl.*, *5*(2), 23--30. ACM, NY, USA.

Karel, F. (2006) Quantitative and ordinal association rules mining (QAR mining). In *Knowledge-Based Intelligent Information and Engineering Systems*, 4251, 195–202. Springer LNAI.

Karel, F., & Klema, J. (2007). Quantitative Association Rule Mining in Genomics Using Apriori Knowledge. In Berendt, B., Svatek, V. Zelezny, F. (eds.), Proc. of The *ECML/PKDD Workshop On Prior Conceptual Knowledge in Machine Learning and Data Mining*. University of Warsaw, Poland, (pp. 53-64).

Keime, C., Damiola, F., Mouchiroud, D., Duret, L. & Gandrillon, O. (2004). Identitag, a relational database for SAGE tag identification and interspecies comparison of SAGE libraries. *BMC Bioinformatics*, *5*(143).

Klema, J., Soulet, A., Cremilleux, B., Blachon, S., & Gandrilon, O. (2006). Mining Plausible Patterns from Genomic Data. *Proceedings of Nineteenth IEEE International Symposium on Computer-Based Medical Systems*, Los Alamitos: IEEE Computer Society Press, 183-188.

Klema, J., Soulet, A., Cremilleux, B., Blachon, S., & Gandrilon, O. (submitted). Constraint-Based Knowledge Discovery from SAGE Data. Submitted to *In Silico Biology.*

Lavrac, N., Zelezny, F., & Flach, P. (2002). RSD: Relational subgroup discovery through first-order feature construction. In *Proceedings of the 12th International Conference on Inductive Logic Programming*, 149–165.

Lee, J. W., Lee, J. B., Park, M., & Song, S. H. (2005). An extensive evaluation of recent classification tools applied to microarray data. *Computation Statistics and Data Analysis*, *48*, 869-885.

Lee, Y., & Lee, Ch. K. (2003) Classification of Multiple Cancer Types by Multicategory Support Vector Machines Using Gene Expression Data. *Bioinformatics*, *19*(9), 1132-1139.

Martin, D., Brun, C., Remy, E., Mouren, P., Thieffry, D., & Jacq, B. (2004). GOToolBox: functional investigation of gene datasets based on Gene Ontology. *Genome Biology* *5*(12), R101.

Quinlan, J.R. (1986) Induction of decision trees. *Machine Learning*, *1*, 81-106.

Salton, G., & Buckley, C. (1988). Term-weighting approaches in automatic text retrieval. *Information Processing Management*, *24*(5), 513–523.

Scheffer, T., & Wrobel, S. (2002). Text Classification Beyond the Bag-of-Words Representation. Proceedings of the *International Conference on Machine Learning (ICML) Workshop on Text Learning.*

Sevon, P., Eronen, L., Hintsanen, P., Kulovesi, K., & Toivonen, H. (2006). Link discovery in graphs derived from biological databases. In *3rd International Workshop on Data Integration in the Life Sciences* (DILS'06), Hinxton, UK.

Soulet, A., Klema J., & Cremilleux, B. (2007). Efficient Mining Under Rich Constraints Derived from Various Datasets. In Džeroski, S., Struyf, J. (eds.), *Knowledge Discovery in Inductive Databases*, LNCS,4747, 223-239. Springer Berlin / Heidelberg.

Tibshirani, R., Hastie, T., Narasimhan, B., & Chu, G. (2002). Diagnosis of multiple cancer types by shrunken centroids of gene expression. Proc. *Natl Acad. Sci.*, 99(10), 6567-6572.

Trajkovski, I., Zelezny, F., Lavrac, N., & Tolar, J. (in press). Learning Relational Descriptions of Differentially Expressed Gene Groups. *IEEE Trans. Sys Man Cyb C, spec. issue on Intelligent Computation for Bioinformatics.*

Trajkovski, I., Zelezny, F., Tolar, J., & Lavrac, N. (2006) Relational Subgroup Discovery for Descriptive Analysis of Microarray Data. In *Procs 2nd Int Sympos on Computational Life Science*, Cambridge, UK 9/06. Springer Lecture Notes on Bioinformatics / LNCS.

Trna, M. (2007) *Klasifikace s apriorni znalosti.* CTU Bachelor's Thesis, In Czech.

Tusher, V.G., Tibshirani, R. & Chu G. (2001) Significance analysis of microarrays applied to the ionizing radiation response. Proc. *Natl Acad. Sci.*, 98(9). 5116–5121.

Velculescu, V., Zhang, L., Vogelstein, B. & Kinzler, K. (1995). Serial Analysis of Gene Expression. *Science, 270*, 484–7.

Zelezny, F., & Lavrac, N. (2006) Propositionalization-Based Relational Subgroup Discovery with RSD. *Machine Learning, 62*(1-2), 33-63.

KEY TERMS

ALL, AML: Leukemia is a form of cancer that begins in the blood-forming cells of the bone marrow, acute leukemias usually develop suddenly (whereas some chronic varieties may exist for years before they are diagnosed), acute myeloid leukemia (AML) is the most frequently reported form of leukemia in adults while acute lymphoblastic leukemia (ALL) is largely a pediatric disease.

Association Rule: A rule, such as implication or correlation, which relates elements co-occurring within a dataset.

Background Knowledge: Information that is essential to understanding a situation or problem, knowledge acquired through study or experience or instruction that can be used to improve the learning process.

Classifier: A mapping from unlabeled instances (a discrete or continuous feature space X) to discrete classes (a discrete set of labels Y), a decision system which accepts values of some features or characteristics of a situation as an input and produces a discrete label as an output.

Constraint: A restriction that defines the focus of search, it can express allowed feature values or any other user's interest.

DNA, RNA, mRNA: Deoxyribonucleic acid (DNA) is a nucleic acid that contains the genetic instructions used in the development and functioning of all known living organisms, ribonucleic acid (RNA) is transcribed from DNA by enzymes, messenger RNA (mRNA) is the RNA that carries information from DNA to the ribosome sites of protein synthesis (translation) in the cell, the coding sequence of the mRNA determines the amino acid sequence in the protein that is produced.

Functional Genomics: A field of molecular biology that attempts to make use of the vast wealth of data produced by genomic projects to describe gene and protein functions and interactions.

Gene Expression: The process of transcribing a gene's DNA sequence into the RNA that serves as a template for protein production.

Gene Ontology: A controlled vocabulary to describe gene and gene product attributes in any organism.

Knowledge Discovery: The nontrivial process of identifying valid, novel, potentially useful, and ultimately understandable patterns in data.

RefSeq: Non-redundant curated data representing current knowledge of a known gene.

Relational Data Mining: Knowledge discovery in databases when the database has information about several types of objects.

SRC: V-src sarcoma (Schmidt-Ruppin A-2) viral oncogene homolog (avian) – a randomly taken gene to illustrate knowledge representation format.

Chapter XIV
Mining Tinnitus Database for Knowledge

Pamela L. Thompson
University of North Carolina at Charlotte, USA

Xin Zhang
University of North Carolina at Pembroke, USA

Wenxin Jiang
University of North Carolina at Charlotte, USA

Zbigniew W. Ras
University of North Carolina at Charlotte, USA

Pawel Jastreboff
Emory University School of Medicine, USA

ABSTRACT

This chapter describes the process used to mine a database containing data, related to patient visits during Tinnitus Retraining Therapy. The original collection of datasets containing diagnostic and treatment data on tinnitus patients and visits was collected by P. Jastreboff. This sparse dataset consisted of eleven tables primarily related by patient id, number, and date of visit. First, with the help of P. Jastreboff, we gained an understanding of the domain knowledge spanning different disciplines (including otology and audiology), and then we used this knowledge to extract, transform, and mine the constructed database. Complexities were encountered with temporal data and text mining of certain features. The researchers focused on analysis of existing data, along with automating the discovery of new and useful features in order to improve classification and understanding of tinnitus diagnosis.

INTRODUCTION

Tinnitus, commonly called "ringing in the ears", affects a significant portion of the population and is difficult to treat. Tinnitus is a phantom auditory perception (Jastreboff, 1999; 2004) and needs to be distinguished from sounds produced by a body - somatosounds. Tinnitus Retraining Therapy (TRT) (Jastreboff, 1995, 2004) is based on the neurophysical model of tinnitus, and is aimed at inducing and sustaining habituation of tinnitus-evoked reactions and tinnitus perception. TRT has provided relief for many patients. Extensive patient data are collected during evaluation of the patients to be treated with TRT and during the treatment. We used this data for related knowledge extraction and its analysis. The goal of the authors is to determine unknown yet potentially useful attributes related to tinnitus research and treatment.

This chapter will focus on the basic domain knowledge necessary to understand TRT; the features present in the original tinnitus database; the extraction, transformation, and loading of the data for analysis including new feature generation; the data mining and exploration process; and a summary of the process along with recommendations for future work,

DOMAIN KNOWLEDGE

The domain knowledge for tinnitus involves many disciplines, primarily including otology and audiology. Tinnitus appears to be caused by a variety of factors including exposure to loud noises, head trauma, and a variety of diseases. An interesting fact is that tinnitus can be induced in 94% of the population by a few minutes of sound deprivation (Heller & Bergman, 1953).

Decreased sound tolerance frequently accompanies tinnitus and can include symptoms of hyperacucisis (an abnormal enhancement of signal within the auditory pathways), misophonia (a strong dislike of sound) or phonophobia (a fear of sound) (Jastreboff, 2004). Past approaches to treatment tend to have been based on anecdotal observations and treatment often focused on tinnitus suppression. Currently a wide variety of approaches are utilized, ranging from sound use to drugs or electrical or magnetical stimulation of the auditory cortex.

Jastreboff (1995) offers an important new model (hence treatment) for tinnitus that focuses on the phantom aspects of tinnitus with tinnitus resulting exclusively from activity within the nervous system that is not related to corresponding activity with the cochlea or external stimulation. The model furthermore stresses that in cases of clinically-significant tinnitus, various structures in the brain, particularly the limbic and autonomic nervous system, prefrontal cortex, and reticular formations play a dominant role with the auditory system being secondary.

Tinnitus Retraining Therapy (TRT), developed by Jastreboff, is a treatment model with a high rate of success (over 80% of the cases) and is based on the neurophysical model of tinnitus. Neurophysiology is a branch of science focusing on the physiological aspect of nervous system function (Jastreboff, 2004). Tinnitus Retraining Therapy "cures" tinnitus-evoked reactions by retraining its association with specific centers throughout the nervous system, particularly the limbic and autonomic systems.

The limbic nervous system (emotions) controls fear, thirst, hunger, joy and happiness and is involved in learning, memory, and stress. The limbic nervous system is connected with all sensory systems. The autonomic nervous system controls functions of the brain and the body over which we have limited control, e.g., heart beating, blood pressure, and release of hormones. The limbic and autonomic nervous systems are involved in stress, annoyance, anxiety etc. When these systems become activated by tinnitus-related neuronal activity (tinnitus signal) negative symptoms are evoked (Jastreboff, 2004). Unfortunately, many patients seeking treatment other than TRT are often told that nothing can be done about their tinnitus. This can have the negative effect of enhancing the limbic nervous system reactions, which then can cause strengthening of the negative effect of the tinnitus on a patient (see Figure 1: Block diagram of the neurophysiological model of tinnitus (Jastreboff, 2004)).

Tinnitus Retraining Therapy combines medical evaluation, counseling and sound therapy to successfully treat a majority of patients. TRT is aimed at evoking and sustaining habituation of tinnitus-evoked reactions and tinnitus perception. Degree of habituation determines treatment success, yet greater understanding of why this success occurs and validation of the TRT technique will be useful (Baguley, 2006). The ultimate goal is to lessen or eliminate the impact of tinnitus on the patient's life (Jastreboff, 2004). Dr. Jastreboff has observed statistically significant improvement after 3 months and treatment lasts approximately 12-18 months.

Data Collection During Tinnitus Retraining Therapy

A preliminary medical evaluation of patients is required before beginning TRT. Sensitive data from the medical evaluation is not contained in the tinnitus database presented to the authors (Dr. Jastreboff maintains this data). Much of this data would contain information subject to privacy concerns, a consideration of all researchers engaged in medical database exploration. Some medical information, however, is included in the tinnitus database such as a list of medications the patient may take and other conditions that might be present, such as diabetes.

Patient categorization is performed after the completion of the medical evaluation, the structured interview guided by special forms (Jastreboff 1999) and audiological evaluation. This interview collects data on many aspects of the patient's tinnitus, sound tolerance, and hearing loss. The interview also helps determine the relative contribution of hyperacusis and misophonia. A set of questions relate to activities prevented or affected (concentration, sleep, work, etc.) for tinnitus and sound tolerance, levels of severity, annoyance, effect on life, and many others. All responses are included in the database. As

Figure 1. Block diagram of the neurophysiological model of tinnitus

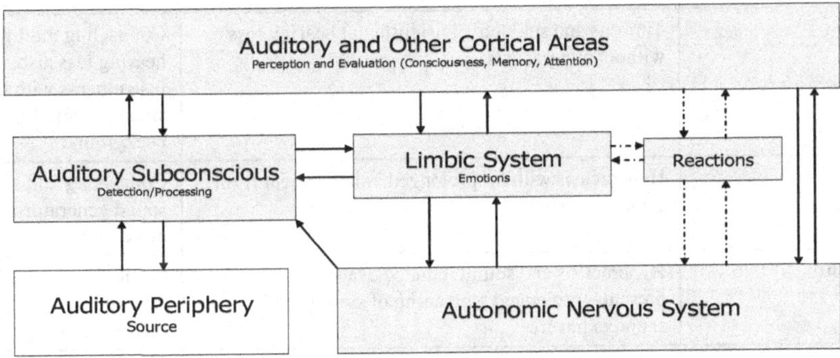

a part of audiological testing, left and right ear pitch, loudness discomfort levels, and suppressibility are determined.

Based on all gathered information a patient category is assigned (see Table 1) (Jastreboff et al., 2003). The category is included in the database, along with a feature that lists problems in order of severity (Ex. TH is Tinnitus first, then Hyperacusis).

Counseling begins immediately and all information on patients is tied to a patient identification number, and visit date. During initial and subsequent visits, patients complete a questionnaire assessing tinnitus severity referred to as a Tinnitus Handicap Inventory (THI), as well as undergo a structured interview. Instruments (table top sound generator, ear-level sound generator, combination instruments, hearing aids) are assigned, when appropriate, and tracked.

ORIGINAL DATABASE FEATURES

A tinnitus patient database of ten tables and 555 patient tuples was prepared at Emory University School of Medicine. All identifying information related to the patient had been removed from the database. Figure 2 shows all tables and original attributes and will be used as a basis for discussion of the original database features.

The database is an unnormalized relational database, and the metadata is enhanced to include a comment on each attribute explaining the contents.

The demographic table contains features related to gender, date of birth, state and zip. The tuples of the demographic table are uniquely identified by patient id, and one tuple per patient exists. Additionally, three text attributes are present that contain information on how and when the tinnitus and hyperacusis were induced, and a comments attribute that contains varied information that may be of interest to research. Text fields such as these required some work before they can be used. In the original state, they were not useful as the information was hidden in the narrative. Further complications existed due to misspellings, missing values, and inconsistencies in the way information was represented. For example,

Table 1. Patient categories

Category	Impact on Life	Description	Treatment
0	Low	Mild or recent symptoms of Tinnitus	Abbreviated counseling
1	High	Tinnitus alone, no hyperacusis, subjectively important hearing loss or worsening of symptoms following noise exposure	Counseling and sound generators set at mixing point
2	High	Tinnitus and subjectively significant hearing loss without hyperacusis	Counseling modified to address hearing loss also, combination instruments with hearing aid with stress on enrichment of the auditory background
3	High	Hyperacusis without prolonged enhancement from sound exposure	Counseling and sound therapy with sound generators set above threshold of hearing
4	High	Hyperacusis and sound induced exacerbation present – prolonged worsening of symptoms by sound exposure	Counseling and sound generators set at threshold of sound, very slow increase of sound level

it is of interest in continuing research to separate patients whose tinnitus was induced by a noise. A new Boolean feature was developed that shows if the tinnitus was induced in this way or not. In order to create this attribute, the T-induced, H-induced, and Comments attributes from the Demographic table needed to have the text mined while looking for key words that are derived from the domain knowledge. Key words for this task include "loud noise", "concert", "military explosion", etc. If these words are present, the Loud Noise Boolean attribute contains the value "true". Other text mining applications show

Figure 2. Original database description (from Access)

Demographic
PK THC #
Date
G
DOB
State
Zip
Country
T Induced
H Induced
Comments

Neuman_Q
PK,I1 THC #
PK Date
v #
F-1
F-2
E-3
F-4
C-5
E-6
F-7
C-8
F-9
E-10
C-11
F-12
F-13
E-14
F-15
E-16
E-17
F-18
C-19
F-20
E-21
E-22
C-23
F-24
E-25
Sc F
Sc E
Sc C
Sc T
Comments

Questionaires_tin
PK,I1 THC #
PK Date
v #
Prob
C
Ms
CC
Instr
Where
>
Fluc
Sleep h
Sleep desc
Conc
Sleep
QRA
Work
Rest
Sprt
Soc
Oth
oth_des
Aw% T
An% T
Tch
T Sv
T An
T EL
On perc
On prbl
On G/S
On assoc
Bad D
Freq
As Freq
As Bad
Eff snd
How Ing
Treatm
Why prob
Comments

Questionaires_HL
PK,I1 THC #
PK Date
v #
Hp
HA
HAt
HAr
Com
Out
T pr
H pr
HL pr
Pr
Ret
Recom
Next v
Next t
Comments

REM
THC #
date
Freg RE
Th R SPL
Mix R SPL
Mix R SL
Tol R SPL
Tol R SL
Max R SPL
Max R SL
Freg LE
Th L SPL
Mix L SPL
Mix L SL
Tol L SPL
Tol L SL
Max L SPL
Max L SL
Category
Instruments
Comments

Questionaires_DST
PK,I1 THC #
PK Date
v #
DST
Phys
Desc
Concert
shopp
Mov
Wrk
Rest
Drv
Sport
Church
House
Child
Soc
Oth
Oth_des
H Sv
H An
H EL
Bad D
Freq
As Freq
As Bad
Eff snd
How Ing
Prot
%T
When
Treatm
Why prob
Comments

Pharmacology
PK,I1 THC #
PK v #
PK Med #
Medication
Generic
Dose
Duration
Cat chem
Action
application
Usual
MAxim
T side
Comments

Instruments
PK,I2 TH#
PK Date
v #
Ins
Type
Model
I1 ID
Comments

Audiological
PK,I1 THC #
PK Date
v #
R TD 1
R TD f2
R TD 2
R TD f3
R TD 3
L TD 1
L TD f2
L TD 2
L TD f3
L TD 3
R25
R50
R1
R2
R3
R4
R6
R8
R10
R12
L25
L50
L1
L2
L3
L4
L6
L8
L10
L12
T PR
T Rm
T LR
Th R
T RLs
T PL
T Lm
T LL
Th L
T Ls
WNR
WNL
MRR
MRL
MRB
MLR
MLL
MLB
MBR
M BL
M BB
R SD
L SD
LR50
LR1
LR2
LR3
LR4
LR6
LR8
LR12
LRTP
LL50
LL1
LL2
LL3
LL4
LL6
LL8
LL12
LLTP
Comments

Miscel
I1 ID
v #
Ed Deg
Occup
Work
Comments

promise, and can be used to generate new rules. The occupation of the patient appears in the Comments attribute and extracting this information may be relevant to new rule generation. Keywords to use in knowledge mining will need to be developed, and may be used to create an additional Boolean field related to whether the patient is in a professional type position or not. Additionally, medications that the patient has or is taking show interest as they affect the treatment process and success.

The Neumann-Q table stores the data from the Tinnitus Handicap Inventory. This inventory is extremely important to assessing the severity of tinnitus and mapping treatment progress. Information stored in the table represents patients responses to questions related to their tinnitus effect on their functioning (F), emotions (E), how catastrophic it is (C), and then a total score (T) is calculated by adding the F, E, and C scores. The total score (T score) is important as it is a measure of tinnitus severity. A THI score of 0 to 16 represents slight severity, 18 to 36 is mild, 38 to 56 is moderate, 58 to 76 is severe, and 78 to 100 is catastrophic (Jastreboff, M. M.). The Tinnitus Handicap Inventory is completed during each patient visit and stored with Patient ID, Visit Number and Date. These attributes can be used in a relationship to other tables.

The Pharmacology table once again uniquely identifies attributes by Patient ID, Visit Number and Visit Date. This table stores information on medications taken by the patient. All information is stored in text form and may be used in later research.

Three tables are used to store information from the preliminary and follow-up questionnaire: Questionnaires-DST, Questionnaires-HL, and Questionnaires-Tin. Questionnaires-DST provides the information from the questionnaire related to sound tolerance, questionnaires-HL relates to hearing loss and general assessment of all problems, and questionnaires-Tin is related to tinnitus. These tables contain a tremendous amount of information and a patient will have an entry in each table at the beginning of treatment, with additional questionnaires represented every time there is subsequent contact (i.e., office visit or telephone follow ups). The information in the tables is identified by Patient ID, Visit Number and Date. The Visit Number is sometimes recorded as -1, meaning the questionnaire was completed before the first visit, with zero denoting the first visit. Another useful attribute is Prob which shows problems in order of importance: T represents tinnitus, H represents hyperacusis, L represents hearing loss; and if no problem the letter is omitted. For example an entry "TL" meaning the patient's primarily problem is Tinnitus, followed by Hearing Loss; "HTL" will denote the situation when hyperacusis is the main problem, followed by tinnitus and hearing loss.

The Instruments table contains information on the type of instrument prescribed to the patient. The data is incomplete, however, and is not particularly useful to this research.

The Audiological table contains information from the various audiological tests performed during treatment. The tuples in the table are identified by Patient ID, Visit Number and Visit Date.

Much time was spent in understanding tinnitus, the treatment process, and capture of data. Data tables in the tinnitus database had to be thoroughly analyzed and understood in order to make the data mining process relevant.

EXTRACTION, TRANSFORMATION AND LOADING

Useful features from the original database deemed pertinent to data mining were extracted and transformed in preparation for analysis. The goal was to extract those features that described the situation of the patient based on the behavior of the attributes over time, and to transform, discretize and classify them in new ways where useful, resulting in one table that could then be used in mining. Many algorithms exist for discretization, yet in this research the expert domain knowledge provided the basis for many of the discretization algorithms. This section will identify the resulting features along with a description of the transformation performed.

The patient id was standardized across tables. Patient id, along with visit number and date, is an important identifier for individual tuples and varied slightly in type and length in different tables. This was relatively easy to identify and correct. The visit number and visit data were transformed to total visits (representing number of visits) and length of visit, a continuous temporal feature that determined time span in number of days between first and last visits.

Patient data related to visits includes a determination of the problem in order of importance, stored as various combinations of the letters "T" for tinnitus, "H" for Hyperacusis, and L for "Loudness Discomfort". Only the first and last of these (First P and last P) are stored in two separate attributes in the analysis table related to first and last visit. Using the first and last gives the researchers information on problem determination at the beginning of the treatment cycle, and at the end when the patient should have moved toward category 0, indicating successful treatment.

Patient category represents the classification of the patient and is represented twice: first by original category as diagnosed, and second by category of treatment followed by a patient. To review, this feature is represented by a range of scores from 0 to 4 where 0 represents tinnitus as a minimal problem or very recent tinnitus (less than 4-6 weeks), 1 represents tinnitus only as a significant problem, 2 represents tinnitus as a significant problem and hearing loss, a significant problem for patient life, 3 represents dominant significant hyperacusis with tinnitus and hearing difficulties (if present) being secondary, and 4 with tinnitus or hyperacusis exhibiting prolonged exacerbation as a result of sound exposure (Jastreboff & Jastreboff, 2003). Two patient categories are stored in the final table (features C and Cc), the first category assigned representing the diagnosis and the last category assigned representing the category of the treatment followed by a patient. Assigning the patient to a category is important to treatment success, and a successfully treated patient will move gradually toward category 0 (Jastreboff, 2004). Some analysis was performed based on this feature.

The total Tinnitus Handicap Inventory score (T Score) was discretized based on the domain knowledge. Lower T scores are better. The T score ranges from 0 to 100, with a decrease of THI by 20 points from first to last visit showing statistical significance. The difference in T score from first to last visit was calculated and discretized into three bins: Bin A represents differences greater than or equal to 20, Bin B represents differences ranging from 0 up to 20, Bin C represents differences less than 0 representing a worsening of the condition. This feature is stored as category of T score.

The standard deviation of audiological testing features related to loudness discomfort levels (LDLs) was derived and stored in various attributes in the analysis table. Loudness discomfort level is related to a decreased sound tolerance as indicated by hyperacusis or dislike of sound - misophonia, and phonophobia - fear of sound. Loudness discomfort levels change with treatment and patient improvement, unlike other audiological features. For this reason the audiological data related to loudness discomfort levels is included in the analysis. Decreased values of LDLs are not necessary for a decreased sound tolerance but they are always lower in case of hyperacusis. In this research the relationship between LDLs and decreased sound tolerance was investigated.

Finally, information on instruments and models of equipment used by the patient is stored in text format in the analysis table.

Dirty data, such as patients with missing values in key features and patients with conflicting values in visit dates, were removed from the original database. After cleansing and extraction, the resulting database contained 253 unique patient tuples.

TEXT EXTRACTION AND MINING

Many of the features in the original database that are stored in text format may contain important information which may have correlation to the new feature tinnitus recovery rate, and to the overall evaluation of treatment method. Some preliminary work has been done in this area with several text fields that indicate the cause or origination of tinnitus.

Text mining (also referred to as text classification) involves identifying the relationship between application domain categories and the text data (words and phrases). This allows the discovery of key terms in text data and facilitates automatic identification of text that is "interesting". The authors used SQL Server 2005 Integration Services to extract terms from the text columns of T-induced, H-induced, and Comments of the Demographic table. The goal was to create a new Boolean feature that indicates if tinnitus was induced by exposure to a loud noise. When performing extraction on data entered in text format it is important to recognize that the data may have been entered in a non-systematic manner and may have been entered by multiple individuals. The authors are making the assumption that careful text mining is worthwhile on the tinnitus database in many of the comment style attributes. The following are the text mining steps that were used:

1. Term extraction transformation was used which performs such tasks as Tokenizing Text, Tagging Words, Stemming Words, and Normalizing Words. By this transformation, 60 frequent terms were determined from the T-induced feature (which is a text feature that describes how tinnitus was induced).
2. After reviewing these terms, some terms were determined to be inconsequential in the domain. These terms were classified as noise words as they occurred with high frequency. These terms were then added to the exclusion terms list which is used as a reference table for the second run of the Term extraction transformation.
3. The second term extraction transformation resulted in 14 terms which are related to the tinnitus induced reason of "noise exposure". The terms included in the dictionary table are 'concert', 'noise', 'acoustic', 'exposure', 'music', 'loud', 'gun', 'explosion', 'pistol', 'band', 'headphone', 'firecracker', 'fireworks', and 'military'.
4. Fuzzy Lookup transformation was applied which uses fuzzy matching to return close matches from the dictionary table to extract keywords/phrases into the new Boolean feature "IsNoiseExposure". This attribute indicates whether the induced reason for tinnitus is related to exposure to a noise of some type. As mentioned previously, it is well recognized that noise in general and impulse noise in particular are the most common factors evoking tinnitus.

After adding this new attribute to the table, data mining algorithms (Decision Tree) were applied in order to produce relevant rules. Twenty-nine patients have the value of true for the new attribute "IsNoiseExposure", and these will be identified by Patient ID. The patients identified by this process can be considered clearly to have tinnitus induced by noise exposure. The main purpose of the text mining process is to add extra information to the study in order to improve the accuracy of the prediction model. While not perfect, expanding the dictionary table will help improve the knowledge gained. Relaxation of the rules used for text extraction may serve to enhance the rate of positive responses. This will be addressed in future work, along with other text attributes such as patient occupation, prescription medications, and others.

TEMPORAL FEATURE DEVELOPMENT FOR CONTINUOUS DATA

Types of learning desired include classification learning to help with classifying unseen examples, association learning to determine any association among features (largely statistical) and clustering to seek groups of examples that belong together.

Temporal features have been widely used to describe subtle changes of continuous data over time in various research areas, such as stream tracer study (Waldon, 2004), music sound classification (Zhang, 2006), and business intelligence (Povinelli, 1998). It is especially important in the light of the tinnitus treatment process because examining the relationship of patient categorization, THI scores, and audiological test results over time may be beneficial to gaining new understanding of the treatment process. Evolution of sound loudness discomfort level parameters in time is essential for evaluation of treatment outcome for decreased sound tolerance, but irrelevant for tinnitus; therefore it should be reflected in treatment features as well. The discovered temporal patterns may better express treatment process than static features, especially considering that the standard deviation and mean value of the sound loudness discomfort level features can be very similar for sounds representing the same type of tinnitus treatment category, whereas changeability of sound features with tolerance levels for the same type of patients makes recovery of one type of patients dissimilar. New temporal features include: sound level Centroid *C,* sound level spread *S*, and recovery rate *R*, where sound level is the audiometric threshold of hearing.

1. **Sound level Centroid *C*:** A feature of center of gravity of an audiology therapy parameter over a sequence of visits. It is defined as a visit-weighted centroid:

$$\left\{ V \in \varphi \mid C = \frac{\sum_{n=1}^{length(T)} n / length(T) \cdot V(n)}{\sum_{n=1}^{length(T)} V(n)}) \right\}$$

   where φ represents the group of audiological features in the therapy, *C* is the gravity center of the sound-audiology level feature-parameter V, *V(n)* is a sound level feature *V* in the nth visit, *T* is the total number of visits.

2. **Sound level Spread *S*:** A feature of the Root of Mean Squared deviation of an audiology therapy parameter over a sequence of visits with respect to its center of gravity:

$$\left\{ V \in \varphi \mid S = \sqrt{\frac{\sum_{n=1}^{length(T)} (n / length(T) - C)^2 \cdot V(n)}{\sum_{n=1}^{length(T)} V(n)}} \right\}$$

where φ represents the group of audiological features in the therapy, S is the spread of the sound-audiology level feature-parameter V, $V(n)$ is a sound level feature V in the nth visit, T is the total number of visits:

$$\left\{ V \in \varphi \mid R = \frac{V_0 - V_k}{T_k - T_0}, k \in \min\{V_i\}, i \in [0, N] \right\}$$

3. **Recovery Rate *R*:** (see Figure 3). Describes the recovery over time, where V represents the total score from the Tinnitus Handicap Inventory in a patient visit. V_o is the first score recorded from the Inventory during the patient initial visit. V_k represents the minimum total score which is the best out of the vector of the scores across visits. V_o should be greater meaning the patient is worse based on the Inventory from the first visit. T_k is the date that has the minimum total score, T_o is the date that relates to V_o.

A large recovery rate score can mean a greater improvement over a shorter period of time. XY scatter plots were constructed using recovery rate compared against patient category, and recovery rate compared against treatment category in order to determine interesting patterns and relationships in the data among those dimensions.

FEATURE DEVELOPMENT FOR CATEGORICAL DATA

During a period of medical treatment, a doctor may change the treatment from one category to another based on the specifics of recovery of the patients. Also, the symptoms of a patient may vary as a result of the treatment; therefore, the category of patient may change over time. Other typical categorical features

Figure 3. Recovery rate

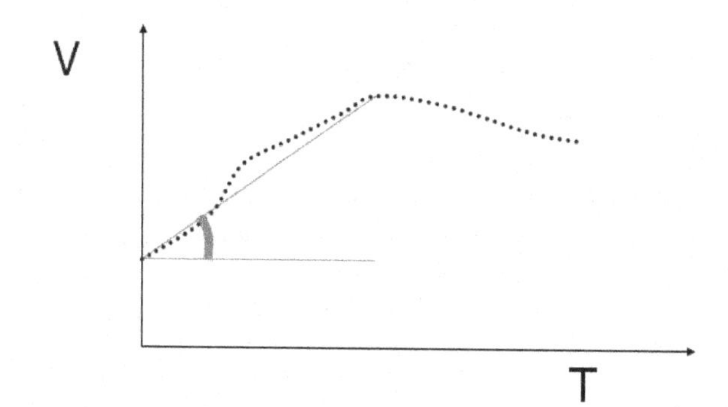

in our database include instruments in each treatment as well as visit dates. Statistical and econometric approaches to describe categorical data have been well discussed by Daniel Powers and Yu Xie, 1999. In our database, statistical features such as the most frequent pattern, the first pattern and the last pattern were used to describe the changes of categorical data over time.

Most frequent pattern MFP counts the pattern which occurred most frequently for a particular patient. First and last pattern FP/LP represents the initial and final state of a categorical attribute respectively.

DATA MINING

Decision tree study was performed using C4.5, a system that incorporates improvements to the ID3 algorithm for decision tree induction. C4.5 includes improved methods for handling numeric attributes and missing values, and generates decision rules from the trees (Witten, 2005). In this study C4.5 was used in order to evaluate the recovery rate by all of the attributes in our tinnitus database and to learn patient recovery by loudness discomfort levels, new temporal features and problem types.

Experiment and Results

In this research, we performed two different experiments: Experiment#1 explored Tinnitus treatment records of 253 patients and applied 126 attributes to investigate the association between treatment factors and recovery; Experiment#2 explored 229 records and applied 16 attributes to investigate the nature of tinnitus with respect to hearing measurements. All classifiers were 10-fold cross validation with a split of 90% training and 10% testing. We used WEKA for all classifications.

Preliminary research results show several interesting rules resulting from decision tree analysis.

Experiment #1

- **Rule 1.** When the category of treatment is 1, the sound level R50 of right ear is greater than 12.5, and the sound level R3 of the right ear is less than 15, the improvement of the symptoms tends to be neutral. The support of the above rule is 10, the accuracy is 90.9%.
- **Rule 2.** When the category of treatment is 2, the improvement of the symptoms tends to be significant. The support of the rules is 44, the accuracy is 74.6%.
- **Rule 3.** When the category of treatment is 3, and the instrument model is BTE, the improvement of the symptoms tends to be significant. The support of the rules is 17, the accuracy is 100.0%.

Experiment #2

- **Rule 4.** When the loudness discomfort level-50 of the right ear is between 19 and 40, Tinnitus tends to be a minor symptom for a patient most time. The support of the rules is 27, the accuracy is 100.0%.

Scatter plot analysis in Figure 4 shows when recovery rate is compared to patient and treatment category in XY scatter plot analysis, both patient and treatment category 4 shows a smaller rate of recovery value possibly indicating slower or reduced treatment success.

Figure 4. Scatter plot analysis

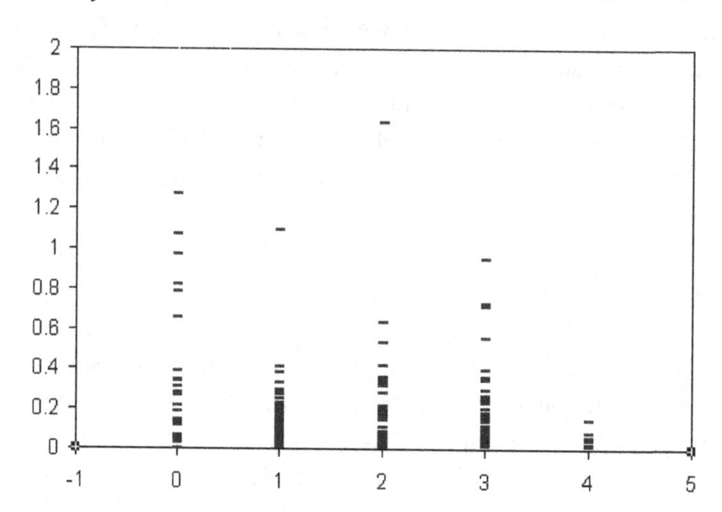

SUMMARY

Data mining is a promising and useful technique for the discovery of new knowledge related to tinnitus causes and cures. Challenges are represented in several areas, including acquiring domain knowledge, applying this knowledge to the data preparation and analysis process, and ensuring continued cooperation among domain experts and researchers. Data represented in text fields is rich yet presents some challenges for mining purposes. Continued research should provide additional learning as the data is more thoroughly analyzed and transformed for mining purposes. Data collection techniques can be analyzed and improved to facilitate data mining operations.

RECOMMENDATIONS FOR FUTURE WORK

This research is in the early stages, and many possibilities exist for further analysis and learning. The data set can be expanded to include medical data related to patients, yet considerations for privacy must be taken into account. Additional textual features need to be classified and discretized in order to be used in discovery, as mentioned previously. Text fields related to the cause of tinnitus, medications, occupation, and others provide promise for learning.

Questions related to the relationships among loudness discomfort levels, tinnitus and decreased sound tolerance with respect to treatment progress and success will be further explored.

The feedback loop with the autonomic and nervous systems and the ties to emotions represent additional possibilities for continued research. The Tinnitus Handicap Inventory tracks the effect of the tinnitus on patients' lives. During habituation therapy, prescribed sound protocols facilitate process of habituation and the rate of tinnitus recovery. A determination of additional features that can be tied to emotions will be useful in analysis.

REFERENCES

Baguley, D. M. (2006). What progress have we made with tinnitus? In *Acta Oto-Laryngologica*, 126(5).

Heller, M. F., & Bergman, M. (1953). Tinnitus in normally hearing persons. In *Ann. Otol.*

Henry, J. A., Jastreboff, M. M., Jastreboff, P. J., Schechter, M. A., & Fausti, S. (2003). Guide to conducting tinnitus retraining therapy initial and follow-up interviews. In *Journal of Rehabilitation Research and Development*, 40(2),159-160.

Jastreboff, M. M., Payne, L., & Jastreboff, P. J. (1999). *Effectiveness of tinnitus retraining therapy in clinical practice.* (Presentation).

Jastreboff, M. M., Payne, L., & Jastreboff, P. J. (2003). Tinnitus and hyperacusis. In *Ballenger's Otorhinolaryngology Head and Neck Surgery* (Eds. Snow Jr, J.B., Ballenger, J.J.), BC Decker Inc., pp. 456-475.

Jastreboff, P. J. (1995). Tinnitus as a phantom perception: theories and clinical implications, in *Mechanisms of Tinnitus,* Vernon, J. and Moller, A.R. (Eds), Boston, MA, Allyn & Bacon., pp. 73-94.

Jastreboff, P. J., & Hazell, J. W. (2004). *Tinnitus retraining therapy,* Cambridge, United Kingdom, Cambridge University Press.

Povinelli, R. J., & Feng, X. (1998). Temporal pattern identification of time series data using pattern wavelets and genetic algorithms, in *Artificial Neural Networks in Engineering*, Proceedings, pp. 691-696.

Powers, D., & Xie, Y. (2007). *Statistical methods for categorical data analysis*, Elsevier.

Waldon, M.G. (2004). Estimation of average stream velocity. In *Journal of Hydrologic Engineering, 130*(11), 1119-1122.

Witten, I. H., & Frank, E. (2005). *Data Mining: practical machine learning tools and techniques*. Morgan Kaufmann Publishers

Zhang, X., & Ras, Z. W. (2006). Differentiated harmonic feature analysis on music information retrieval for instrument recognition, in *Proceedings of IEEE International Conference on Granular Computing (IEEE GrC 2006)*, IEEE, pp. 578-581.

KEY TERMS

Autonomic Nervous System: Part of the nervous system that acts as a control system and maintains homeostasis in the body. This system primarily functions without conscious control.

C4.5: An algorithm developed by Ross Quinlan and used to generate a decision tree that can be used for classification.

Classification Learning: Learning where items are placed into groups based on quantitative information on one or more characteristics present in the items. These characteristics are often called traits, features, variables, etc. and are based on a training set of similar items.

Discretization: The process of transforming continuous values to discrete values.

Habituation: A progressive lessening of reactions to a stimulus. In Tinnitus Retraining Therapy, the goal of habituation is to reduce the reaction to tinnitus.

Hyperacussis: Increased sensitivity to sound. Can accompany tinnitus.

Limbic System: Part of the nervous system that supports a variety of functions including emotions, memory, and learning.

Misophonia: Dislike of sound or sounds. Can accompany tinnitus.

Phonophobia: Fear of sound or sounds. Can accompany tinnitus.

Recovery Rate: A new temporal feature related to Tinnitus Retraining Therapy. A large recovery rate score can mean a greater improvement for a patient over a shorter period of time.

Sound Level Centroid: A new temporal feature related to Tinnitus Retraining Therapy. It is the center of gravity of an audiology parameter over a sequence of visits.

Sound Level Spread: A new temporal feature related to Tinnitus Retraining Therapy. It is the root of means squared deviation of an audiology parameter over visits. It is a description of the spread of the audiology parameter over time.

Temporal Feature: A feature that has a time based component.

Tinnitus: The definition used for this research is a condition resulting exclusively from activity within the nervous system that is not related to corresponding activity with the cochlea or external stimulation, i.e., a phantom auditory perception. This definition was developed by Dr. Jastreboff and is associated with Tinnitus Retraining Therapy and the Neurophysical Model.

Tinnitus Handicap Inventory: A questionnaire used to assess severity of tinnitus. The THI is used for any kind of treatment.

Tinnitus Retraining Therapy: A highly successful treatment method for tinnitus developed by Dr. Pawel J. Jastreboff, Emory University, Atlanta, Georgia.

Chapter XV
Gaussian-Stacking Multiclassifiers for Human Embryo Selection

Dinora A. Morales
University of the Basque Country, Spain

Endika Bengoetxea
University of the Basque Country, Spain

Pedro Larrañaga
Universidad Politécnica de Madrid, Spain

ABSTRACT

Infertility is currently considered an important social problem that has been subject to special interest by medical doctors and biologists. Due to ethical reasons, different legislative restrictions apply in every country on human assisted reproduction techniques such as in-vitro fertilization (IVF). An essential problem in human assisted reproduction is the selection of suitable embryos to transfer in a patient, for which the application of artificial intelligence as well as data mining techniques can be helpful as decision-support systems. In this chapter we introduce a new multi-classification system using Gaussian networks to combine the outputs (probability distributions) of standard machine learning classification algorithms. Our method proposes to consider these outputs as inputs for a superior-level and to apply a stacking scheme to provide a meta-level classification result. We provide a proof of the validity of the approach by employing this multi-classification technique to a complex real medical problem: The selection of the most promising embryo-batch for human in-vitro fertilization treatments.

INTRODUCTION

In-vitro fertilization (IVF) and intra cytoplasmic sperm injection (ICSI) are assisted reproduction techniques that enable infertile couples to achieve successful pregnancy under certain conditions. Intensive research is being done in this field in order to improve both the techniques and treatments applied to maximize implantation rate while limiting the number of multiple pregnancies[1]. Success of the treatment is considered when pregnancy is proved by ultrasound study.

Even if these treatments have a history of several years, the success rate of pregnancy still remains very limited, around 29 % and 38 % in most of the cases (ESHRE, 2007). Success rates of IVF vary depending on many factors including causes of infertility and treatment approaches, and as an example of very optimistic results some clinics in France and the USA have reported pregnancy rates of up to 40%.

In order to improve this success rate, it is essential to select the most promising batch of embryos to be transferred in a patient, although there are also additional important features that need to be taken into account since they affect the final outcome of the treatment. Among the latter we can mention age, presence of oocyte dimorphism's, sperm quality, fertilization rate, cleavage rate and number of embryos transferred, endometrial thickness and number of previous cycles of treatment. Apart from the selection of the most suitable embryos, embryologists need to consider several possibilities when deciding which type of treatment to apply, among them the number of embryos to transfer, pre-implantation genetic diagnosis, the type of assisted reproduction technique, and the composition of culture media.

Infertility research trends include developments in medical technology on assisted human reproduction in aspects such as medical treatments, equipment technology, and also on the application of artificial intelligence. The latter combines both advances on clinician and embryologist expertise together with data mining techniques, by providing classification models able to be applied as decision-support systems. The final aim is to classify each of the possible embryos for transfer and select the ones that would have the highest probability to implant successfully.

Since it is very unlikely that a single classification paradigm performs best for all types of problems regarding the complexity and the quality of the databases available, one of the trends nowadays is to combine multiple algorithms to improve the overall classification performance. This carries out the application of different classification models from the same knowledge (e.g. data), with a posterior technique that gathers all the information and provides a prediction. When using this approach, the basic classification models are called *base-level classifiers* and the classification technique that gathers all inputs and provides an overall conclusion is referred to as *meta-level classifier.*

Actually, the way of combining the output scores of the different base-level classifiers in order to build a meta-level classifier is a major problem in the combination of different classification systems, and the literature provides examples of several approaches in which voting systems or weights are applied for this aim (Kuncheva, 2004). Stacking (Wolpert, 1992) is an alternative approach of combining base-level classifiers that is characterized by its ability to take into account the class probability distributions of base-level classifiers. This method has been very successfully applied in general classification domains and that has been applied only very recently to medical classification problems (Sierra et al, 2001). Due to the capability of stacking to further combine the knowledge represented in each classifier, in this Chapter we focus on an extension introduced by Wolpert (1992) called stacked generalization, and we propose to improve it applying a Gaussian meta-learning method to the supervised classification framework.

In brief, this chapter investigates the performance of the stacking schema improved with Gaussian networks to provide meta-learning from predictions of base-level multi-classifiers, particularly for the concrete application to the real complex problem of the selection of the most promising in-vitro human embryos, in order to improve the success rate (e.g. implantation rate) of in-vitro fertilization treatments.

The outline of this Chapter is the following: Section 2 introduces a brief description of some of the most representative classification models and provides the background on conditional Gaussian networks. Section 3 introduces a review of variant of the basic stacking algorithms and describes how it can be applied as an improvement of the stacking method. Section 4 describes the real complex problem of selecting the human embryos to be transferred on in-vitro treatments, which will serve as an example to present the validity of our approach for biomedical classification problems. Section 5 shows our experimental results when applying base-level classifiers independently, and confronts them with the combination of a Gaussian meta-level multiclassification. Finally, the last Section presents our conclusions and future work.

CLASSIFICATION PARADIGMS

In this section, we revise briefly some of the most representative supervised classification models in machine learning, focusing mainly on Bayesian classifiers as a concrete paradigm for supervised classification that has not been applied to medical problems until relatively later than other classical methods.

Particularly in the case of medical applications, the transparency in the outputs of the classification results is very important in order to prove to clinicians and other experts the support and extent in which they can trust. Therefore, classifiers are described in this section from this perspective.

Before reviewing supervised classification methods, we revise in the next subsection some basic concepts in supervised classification that apply to any classification paradigm: feature subset selection, and filter/wrapper approaches.

Feature Subset Selection and Filter/Wrapper Approaches in Supervised Classification

In medical domains as well as in other research fields, it is common to have general information about a specific problem, without all being relevant to resolve that problem. This implies that such predictor variables could be discarded resulting in a problem with a smaller complexity to be solved. Predictor variables that can be discarded when building the classification model are usually differentiated between irrelevant and redundant variables[2].

Before constructing a classifier, an induction algorithm can select a subset of features of the training data and discard some of all the irrelevant and redundant variables. This process is known as Feature Subset Selection (FSS). In some algorithms FSS produces little benefit in the improvement of the performance of a classifier, and in others it provides a major improvement in accuracy. A deep revision of FSS is not under the scope of this Chapter, the interested reader can find more information on Kohavi, R., & John, G. (1997).

Typically, supervised classification algorithms are divided between filter and wrapper types depending on the technique in which the FSS is applied. *Filter approaches* take into account the intrinsic characteristics of the data, filtering out the irrelevant features before the induction process by applying e.g. mutual information as the measure for feature selection. In this feature selection process, a subset of variables is chosen to induce the classification model. In filter approaches the search process is guided by conditional independence tests as score. On the other hand, *wrapper approaches* generate a subset of candidate features where the search is guided by the classification goodness measure as a score; this feature subset selection process is implicit into the procedure of inducing the model.

The filter and wrapper approaches for feature selection can be combined with any induction algorithm to in crease its learning rate in domains with irrelevant attributes.

Classical Supervised Classification Methods

In supervised classification problems we apply classification models learned from a database of previous cases whose outcome (class value, e.g. implanted or not) is already known, and the aim is to predict the class to which a new unseen instance belongs to. To accomplish this, a single variable is chosen to be the class variable.

More formally, if we denote by $\boldsymbol{x} = (x_1,\ldots,x_n)$ the vector of features, our task is to classify a new instance to one of the classes of a class-variable $C = \{c_1, c_2, \ldots, c_m\}$, where $c_1, c_2, \ldots, c_m$ are all the possible classes. We can regard a classifier as a function $\gamma : (x_1,\ldots,x_n) \rightarrow \{c_1, c_2, \ldots, c_m\}$ that assigns labels to observations. This function is learned from training data, and then it is applied to new cases.

The challenge of supervised classification is to design a classifier to learn a conditional density estimator $p(c|\boldsymbol{x})$ that minimizes the total misclassification cost by a cost function, assigning the case $\boldsymbol{x} = (x_1,\ldots,x_n)$ to the class with minimum total cost, that is:

$$\gamma(x) = \operatorname{argmin}_k \sum_{c=1}^{m} cost(k,c) p(c \mid x_1,\ldots,x_n) \quad (1)$$

where *cost(k,c)* is the cost matrix expressing the cost of assigning label *k* to an example whose true label is *c*. When a loss of 1 is assumed for every misclassified case (either a false positive or a false negative) and a 0 is considered for every correctly-classified one, the symmetric cost function is known as the *0/1 loss*.

In classical supervised learning, the usual measure of success to evaluate the performance of classifier is the proportion of test cases correctly classified –the *accuracy*. The accuracy is calculated from the confusion matrix which gives the results of classification process (e.g. true positive, false positive, true negative and false negative) by $Accuracy = (TP + TN) / N$ where *TP* is the true positive case classification, *TN* is the true negative case classified and N is the total of cases classified.

We revise next very briefly different supervised classification paradigms that can be applied to create a classifier in that form.

Nearest Neighbor

Among the various methods of supervised statistical pattern recognition, the nearest neighbor classifier is an intuitive method. It involves a training set of both positive and negative cases. A new case or instance is classified by calculating the distance to the nearest training case, assigning it to that class. The classification function implemented by this classifier will in general be a jagged, piece-wise linear function therefore it is influenced by each case in the training set.

Nearest Neighbor or k-nearest neighbor (k-NN) classifier is a simple instance-based classifier that applies what is referred to as lazy learning, since it stores all of the training samples and does not build a classifier until a new sample needs to be classified. In machine learning the opposed to lazy learning is called eager learning. Eager learning algorithms put significant effort in abstracting from the training instances by creating condensed representations (e.g. this is the case of Bayesian networks, decision trees, rule sets, hyper planes, etc.) during the learning phase.

k-NN classifies a new instance by assigning the same class as its nearest stored instance if the class is the same; or otherwise by calculating the Euclidean distance to find the training instance closest to the given test instance, and the predicted class is determined by majority if multiple instances have the same distances to the test instance .

IB1 is a variant of a lazy learning algorithm (Aha & Kibler, 1991) based on the k-nearest-neighbor method but in the case where multiples instances have the same Euclidean distances, this algorithm assigning the first one found is used.

The K* is an instance-based classifier where a new instance is classified by votes weighted according to similarity of the class to those training instances similar to it (Cleary & Trigg, 1995).

Decision Trees

Decision trees are directed trees which are also called classification trees (Quinlan, 1993). In the tree model, the top node is known as the root of the tree. The root node is connected by successive and directional arcs or branches to the other nodes until a leaf node is reached. A decision tree is induced by a sequence of questions about the testing instances which are represented by nodes and following the probability distribution of class predicted for the instances is represented as a leaf node. The classification tree will progressively split the set of training labeled data into smaller and smaller subsets.

As an classical example of decision trees, J48 classifier is a decision tree model based on C4.5 algorithm (Quinlan, 1993), which is basically an off line approach –e.g. the tree must be designed again if new data is provided.

Decision Tables

Decision tables (Kohavi, 1995) are tabular forms that present a set of conditions and their corresponding actions. Decision tables apply decision rule algorithms such as if-then-else and switch-case statements, which associate conditions with actions to perform. Each decision corresponds to a variable, relation, or predicate whose possible values are listed among the condition alternatives. Given an unlabeled instance, the decision table classifier searches for exact matches in the decision table using only the features in the set of features included in the table. If no instances are found, the majority class of the decision table is returned; otherwise, the majority class of all matching instances is assigned to the analyzed new instance.

Support Vector Machines

Vapnik (1995) introduced support vector machines as learning algorithms that can perform binary classification. When the input data are linearly separable, they find a linear separating hyper plane which discerns positive examples from negative ones. The split is chosen to have the largest distance from the hyper plane to the nearest of the positive and negative examples. When the input data are not linearly separable, it non-linearly maps the n-dimensional input space into a high dimensional feature space, leading to the assumption that the input data are linearly separable. Training an SVM requires the solution of a very large quadratic programming (QP) optimization problem.

The *Sequential Minimal Optimization* algorithm (SMO) was introduced by Platt (1999) to train a support vector classifier. The SMO algorithm surpasses the large QP problem into a series of smallest possible QP problems. These small QP problems are solved analytically, which avoids using a time-consuming numerical QP optimization as an inner loop. The SMO algorithm maps SVM outputs into posterior probabilities. It also normalizes all attributes by default and globally replaces all missing values and transforms nominal attributes into binary ones.

Naive Bayes

The *Naive Bayes* classifier (Minsky,1961) is a classical classifier based on the assumption that all predictor variables are conditionally independent given the class. According to the Bayes theorem, this classifier computes for each unseen instance $\boldsymbol{x} = (x_1,...,x_n)$ the a posteriori probability $p(c|\boldsymbol{x}) = p(c)\prod_{i=1}^{n} p(x_i|c)$ for all $c \in C$, and the and the new instance is assigned to the class with highest probability $p(c|\boldsymbol{x})$.

The literature presents a lot of improvements of the classical Naive Bayes classifier from its initial publication showing approximations and improvements to better adapt to concrete characteristics of the problems to which it is applied. As an example, we have the alternative of constructing the naive Bayes classifier is the fact of computing the likelihood for patterns of continuous features needed for probabilistic inference in a Bayesian network classifier by kernel density estimation (KDE), letting every pattern influence the shape of the probability density. This method, called *Naive Bayes KDE*, reduces a high-dimensional density estimation task to one-dimensional kernel density estimation. Although usually leading to accurate estimation, the Naive Bayes KDE algorithm suffers from computational cost making it no practical in many real-world applications.

Naive Bayes is the simplest Bayesian classifier, which is a paradigm that has been object of important improvements in the last years. This chapter focuses especially on this topic, that it is revised more deeply next.

BAYESIAN CLASSIFIERS

Probabilistic graphical models are especially well suited to handle uncertainty, which is very common in many real life problems such as medical ones. This characteristic, together with the fact that their visual representation in the form of a graph that expresses conditional dependencies between the different variables of a problem, has demonstrated to be very intuitive and effective for modeling real problems, which explains why physicians are using it in a broad range of medical applications (Sierra et al., 2001; Morales et al., 2008).

Bayesian networks are a concrete type of probabilistic graphical models characterized by being represented as directed acyclic graphs, where nodes represent variables and arcs represent conditional (in)dependence relations between the variables. In Bayesian networks each random variable follows a conditional probability function in discrete domains given a specific value of its parents.

Gaussian networks are also probabilistic graphical models, similarly as Bayesian networks although these containing continuous variables. In continuous domains, a common approach is to assume that predictor variables follow Gaussian distributions, instead of multinomial distributions.

There is a concrete type of Bayesian and Gaussian networks that are used for supervised classification, which are characterized by having an additional node *C* which is not a predictor variable but the variable representing the class to which each instance could belong to. This *C* node is known as the *class-node*. These classifiers –known as Bayesian classifiers– can be applied for both discrete and continuous domains. In this Chapter we consider only Bayesian classifiers whose discrete class variable C is the root of the graph, that is, the structure of Bayesian networks in which the class-variable C is the parent of all continuous predictor variables $(X_1,...,X_n)$.

Bayesian classifiers are presented in the form of probabilistic graphical models, that is, in the form of Bayesian networks when we have discrete domains. On the alternative case of supervised classification problems with continuous predictor variables and discrete class variable, *Conditional Gaussian networks* (Lauritzen, 1996) are applied. These have the ability to handle discrete and continuous variables assuming that each of the continuous variables follow a Gaussian distribution. Bayesian classifiers are based on encoding the joint distribution $p(x_1,...,x_n,c)$ between all predictor variables.

The complete structures of Bayesian classifiers can be defined as the factorization $P(c,\mathbf{x}) = P(c)p(\mathbf{x} \mid c)$. From the definition of conditional probability the posteriori probability is computed as:

$$p(c \mid \mathbf{x}) \propto p(c,\mathbf{x}) = p(c)\prod_{i=1}^{n} p(x_i \mid c) \tag{2}$$

where $p(x_i|c)$ represents the conditional probability of X given that C = c.

The Naive Bayes classifier revised in the previous section can be regarded as the concrete case of the simplest Bayesian classifier, in which the structure of the graph is fixed and only a posteriori probabilities $p(c|\mathbf{x}) = p(c)\prod_{i=1}^{n} p(x_i|c)$ need to be computed. This section presents a revision of Bayesian classifiers which require additionally to Naive Bayes a structural learning. For instance, in the learning process of inducing the model structure of a Bayesian classifier, all predictor variables are taken into account. However, due to an important feature selection process that is usually applied, decision to exclude some of them in the final structure might be taken.

In this work we present some conditional Gaussian networks-based classifiers, adapted by Perez et al. (2006) to the naive Bayes (Minsky, 1961), selective naive Bayes (Kononenko,1991), semi naive Bayes (Pazzani, 1997), tree augmented naive Bayes (Friedman, Geiger & Goldsmidt, 1997) and k-dependence Bayesian classifier (Sahami, 1996). These Bayesian classifiers were designed specifically for supervised classification problems. Figure 1 illustrates some of the classifiers in the form of Bayesian networks that have been proposed in the literature, grouped by the number of the dependencies between predictor variables that they are able to take into account.

Classifiers based on Conditional Gaussian networks can be defined by the factorization $f(c,\mathbf{x}) = p(c)\prod_{i=1}^{n} f(x_i \mid \mathbf{pa}_{,i},C)$ where the class variable $\{C\} \subseteq \mathbf{pa}_i$ with $(i = 1,...,n)$ is a set of variables which are parents of X. We assume that the factorization of each continuous variable given its parents follows a Gaussian distribution, and therefore, since the conditional density function $f\left(x_i \middle| \mathbf{pa}_i, C\right)$ represents

Figure 1. Structures of Bayesian classifiers of different complexity and types that are revised in this Section

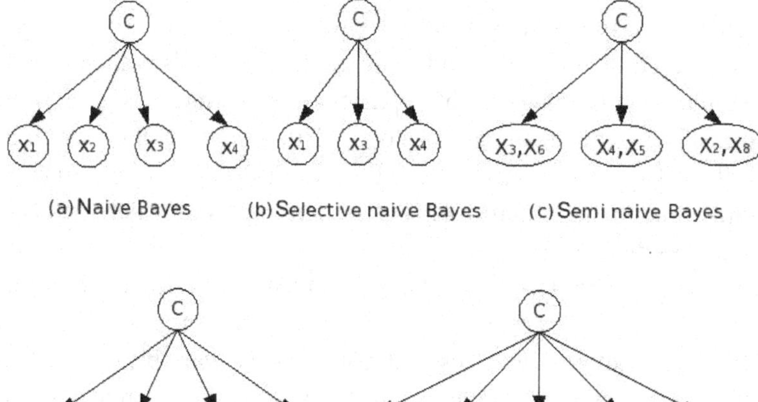

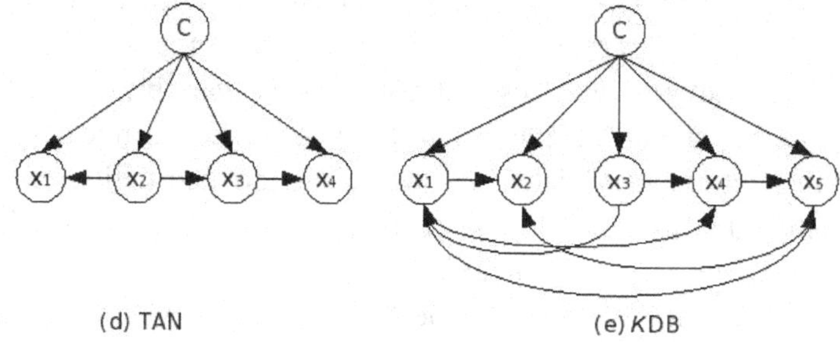

the probability of the predictor variable given its parents, we have that $f(x_i \mid \boldsymbol{pa}_i, c) \sim N(\mu_i^c, \sigma_i^c)$. The posteriori probability is computed as:

$$p(c \mid \boldsymbol{x}) \propto p(c, \boldsymbol{x}) \propto f(c, \boldsymbol{x}) = p(c) \prod_{i=1}^{n} f(x_i \mid \boldsymbol{pa}_i) \quad (3)$$

Filter Raking Naive Bayes

Filter ranking naive Bayes (FRankingNB) was introduced by Pérez et al. (2006), in which a mutual information measure is applied for each variable $(X_1,...,X_n)$ given the class— $I(X_i,C)$ —and then the probabilities are estimated from frequency counts. Essentially this is a filter ranking FSS applied to a naive Bayes classifier where a threshold τ is defined based on the fixed distribution of $I(X_i,C)$. Following this approach, a selection of the predictor variables is made by ranking these variables such that only the subset of variables whose surpasses $I(X_i,C) \geq \tau$ value is selected. Once this being done, a naive Bayes structure is created considering uniquely this subset of variables. This procedure aims at getting rid of irrelevant variables from the final naive Bayes classifier.

Selective Naive Bayes

In many real problem domains the information contribution is overlapped or repeated and FSS is applied to achieve a good predictive accuracy of learning algorithms. The *selective naive Bayes* algorithm (Kohavi & John, 1997) is a combination of FSS and the naive Bayes classifier. The main difference between selective naive Bayes and naive Bayes is that in the final model of the former structure some of the predictive variables can be removed.

Pérez et al. (2006) proposes an adaptation of the selective naive Bayes classifier to continuous domains.

Semi Naive Bayes

In most real problems relationships between variables exist and need to be considered for a good classification performance. The *semi naive Bayes* model (Kononenko, 1991) overcomes the conditional independence assumption imposed by naive Bayes and semi naive Bayes classifiers. The *semi naive Bayes* algorithm is able to take into account relationships between the predictor variables $(X_1,...,X_n)$ conditionally to the class variable C using special types of nodes: A joint node $\boldsymbol{y}_k$ is formed as the result of the cartesian product of a subset of variables (Pazzani, 1997). Each joint node represents a new variable that considers all the dependencies between the original variables that form it. If the joint variable is composed of multinomial random variables, the state of the joint variable is the cartesian product of the states of the multinomial random variables.

Pérez et al. (2006) proposed an adaptation of the semi naive Bayes algorithm to continuous domains with a Gaussian network model, based on a set of Gaussian variables that compose a *joint node* $\boldsymbol{y}_k$ that follows a multidimensional normal distribution. They propose the following joint density function:

$$f(\boldsymbol{y}_k|c)=(2\pi)^{-\frac{1}{2}m_k}|\Sigma_k^c|^{-\frac{1}{2}}\, e^{-\frac{1}{2}(\boldsymbol{y}_k-\boldsymbol{\mu}_k^c)^t(\Sigma_k^c)^{-1}(\boldsymbol{y}_k-\boldsymbol{\mu}_k^c)} \quad (4)$$

where m_k is the number of variables that comprise the join variable, the covariance matrix of $\boldsymbol{y}_k$ conditioned to a class value $C = c$ is represented by $\sum_k^c$, and $\boldsymbol{\mu}_k^c$ is the mean vector conditioned to the class value of the joint variable $\boldsymbol{y}_k$. The interested reader can find more information on this approach on Pérez et al. (2006).

Tree Augmented Naive Bayes

The *tree augmented naive Bayes* classifier (TAN) was introduced by Friedman, Geiger, and Goldsmidt (1997). The TAN classifier is another Bayesian network classifier that allows dependencies between variables. The main restriction on the dependencies that can be considered by this Bayesian classifier is that each predictive variable can have a maximum of two parents: the class variable C and one of the other predictive variables $(X_1,...,X_n)$.

In order to create the structure of a TAN classifier, Friedman, Geiger, and Goldsmidt (1997) propose to follow the general outline of the Chow and Liu (1968) procedure. Following this algorithm, the tree augmented naive Bayes structure is build in a two-phase procedure. Firstly, the dependencies between the different variables are learned. This algorithm applies a score based on the information theory, and the weight of an arc $(X_i - X_j)$ is defined by the mutual information measure conditioned to the class variable as:

$$I(X_i,X_j|C)=\sum_c\sum_{x_i}\sum_{x_j} p(x_i,x_j,c)\log\frac{p(x_i,x_j|c)}{p(x_i|c)p(x_j|c)} \quad (5)$$

Using the mutual information of each predictive variable and the class— $I(X_i,C)$ —as well as the conditional mutual information of each pair of domain variables given the class— $I(X_i,X_j \mid C)$ —the algorithm builds a tree structure by adding at each step the arc between two variables X_i and X_j which has the highest $I(X_i,X_j \mid C)$ without forming a loop. This procedure adds a total of $n-1$ arcs to the structure, forming a tree. In a second phase the structure is augmented to the naive Bayes paradigm.

As an extension, Pérez et al. (2006) propose a different approach to construct a tree augmented Bayesian classifier –the *wrapper tree augmented naive Bayes*– based on an adaptation of Keogh and Pazzani (1999) algorithm to the continuous domain. They used a hill climbing greedy search algorithm applied to the space of possible structures guided by an estimated accuracy as score. In order to adapt the TAN algorithm to continuous variables they propose a function to calculate the mutual information between every pair of predictor variables conditioned to the class variable. The mutual information between the joint density function of variable X_i and X_j conditioned to C is computed as:

$$I(X_i,X_j \mid C) = \frac{1}{2}\sum_{c=1}^{r} p(c) log(1-\rho_c^2(X_i,X_j)) \qquad (6)$$

k-Dependence Bayesian Classifier

The *k-dependence Bayesian classifier* (*k*DB) was introduced by Sahami (1996), and tries to overcome the restriction of TAN of having a maximum of two parent variables for each predictive variable, allowing every predictive variable to have up to *k* parents besides the class. The main characteristic of a *k*DB structure is the fact that it is the user who fixes the restrictive condition of the value of *k* which represents the maximum number of parents per variable.

The *k*DB structure is built using both mutual information and conditional mutual information – $I(X_i,X_j|C)$ – scores. The procedure starts by considering the class-node C in the structure. During each iteration, the algorithm selects the node not included in the structure with the highest $I(X_i \mid C)$, next the arc from C to X_i is added, and the value $I(X_i,X_j|C)$ is computed for all the possible new arcs from the X_j nodes already inserted in the structure. All these arcs are ordered, and the highest *k* nodes are added to the structure always respecting the limit of *k* parent-nodes apart from C. Pérez et al. (2006) propose an adaptation of this approach for the cases of the predictor continuous variables following a normal density.

GAUSSIAN-STACKED GENERALIZATION

In data mining one of the interesting research topics is to provide innovative methods to combine the predictions from multiple classifiers called *base-level classifiers*[3]. These are characterized by their different architectures or learning algorithms each providing complementary information, which is intended to be combined at meta-level to obtain a better estimate of the optimal decision boundary. This aims at improving the accuracy of the individual classification model (Dietterich, 1998). Nowadays, the usual approach is to normalize the class probability distribution of base-level classifiers with a subsequent loss of information. The application of a Gaussian network is an alternative to work with continuous variables that overrides this problem.

There are many combination methods to generate multiple versions of a number of base-level classifiers learned from different training data subsets that are repeatedly applied for predicting new cases. Examples of classical methods are bagging, boosting, cascading and stacked generalization. All of them are explained in Kuncheva (2004).

Stacked generalization —or simply *stacking*— is introduced by Wolpert (1992) as a scheme that combines multiple classification models that have been learned for supervised classification tasks. The configuration has two levels: at the base-level there are different learning algorithms and at meta-level one single learning algorithm is applied. First base-level classifiers are applied and their predictions are collected into a new data set called *meta-level data* by cross-validation. During this step, each of training data batch is applied to base-level classifiers and meta-level data is generated by a set of probability distributions of each base-level classifier, adding the true class.

On the stacking scheme a learning algorithm called *meta-level learning* or *meta-level classifier* is applied to obtain the final classification from meta-level data by cross-validation. There are many variants of the basic stacking algorithm. For instance, Merz (1999) introduces a variant of stacking adding correspondence analysis in order to detect correlations between the base-level classifiers whose dependencies are removed from the original meta-level data. This work makes use of the nearest neighbor method as meta-level classifier.

Another variant of stacking was proposed by Ting and Witten (1999) to combine the resultant probability distributions of base-level classifiers instead of concentrating on the single predicted nominal value of each classifier. The algorithm applies correspondence analysis to model the relationship between the learning examples and the way in which they are classified by base-level classifiers. At meta-level learning the multi-response linear regression (MLR) algorithm is applied, which is an adaptation of the linear regression algorithm, transforming a classification problem into different binary prediction problems. A linear equation is constructed for each class value, in which a value 1 is assigned if the class value is equal to the class under consideration or 0 otherwise.

Todorovski and Džeroski (2002) introduced a new learning method at meta-level into the stacking scheme. The proposed method applies Meta Decision Trees (MDTs) by replacing class-value predictions of its leaf nodes by the ones returned by base level-classifiers. Meta-level data has the probability distributions of each base-level classifier multiplied by the entropy and the maximum probability, reflecting the confidence of the different base-level classifiers.

Seewald (2003) suggests a modification of the stacking algorithm proposed by Ting & Witten (1999), creating meta-level data from each base-level classifier. Meta-level data is composed only with the probability values for the class under consideration and the class values are correct or incorrect. This stacking with MLR reduces the number of meta-level attributes independently of the number of classes. Each meta-level data should be used at meta-level to predict whether each base-level prediction is correct.

Džeroski and Ženko (2004) propose an extended meta-level data with class probability distributions, and additional features such as the entropy of the class probability distributions and the maximum probability returned by each classifier. A new induction of meta-level classifier was proposed, using the model tree induction at meta-level learning called stacking with multi-response model trees. Their work compares different approaches of stacking, and concludes that the stacking with multi-response model trees induction obtains more promising results than the stacking with MRL proposed by Seewald (2003).

All the cases described so far, are different stacking approaches with different meta-level learning algorithms, all of them applied to meta-level data with entropy of probability distribution, the maximum probability, or probability distributions of actual class. However, some of them require transforming meta-level data into binary format, leading to a loss of valuable information. We propose a new variant of stacking able to handle continuous data of prediction probabilities of every base-level classifier, capable to combine the whole information provided by those at meta-level through a Gaussian network.

Gaussian Networks Applied to Meta-Level Classification

Our approach for applying Gaussian networks as meta-level classifiers consists on constructing a Gaussian-stacking classifier based on a variant of the stacked scheme proposed by Ting and Witten (1999).

As ordinary Gaussian networks, in order to apply conditional Gaussian networks as meta-level classifiers the induction process contains three phases: preprocessing, structural learning and parametric learning. The preprocessing process consists on a transformation or reduction of variable space by FSS procedures –either filter or wrapper types–in order to improve the classification accuracy. However, the wrapper variable selection process is performed in parallel with the structural learning process.

The structural learning of Gaussian networks usually considers a search process. The search space for obtaining the best Gaussian network for a concrete problem is defined by all possible structures to construct the model, taking into account conditional dependencies among the variables. When searching for the most appropriate structures to construct the Gaussian network model, the structural learning procedure is guided by a scoring function that evaluates the dependencies between predictor variables. Examples of scoring functions are Bayesian information criterion (BIC), Bayesian Circlet equivalent (BDe) and edge exclusion test (EDGE).

Finally, the parametric learning consists in estimating parameters from the data, in order to model the dependence between predictor variables which are represented by the classifier structure. The conditional density function $f\left(x_i \mid \boldsymbol{pa}_i, C\right)$ represents the probability of the predictor variable given its parents. The posteriori probability defined in equation (3) is applied to the classification process.

In the context of supervised classification, the overfitting of an algorithm is the degree to which a case whose class is to be predicted is representative of the type of data that was used to build the classifier, since the lack of representative data for the training of the classifier leads on an incorrect classification of under-represented cases. In order to avoid overfitting on our stacked model, meta-level data is generated by k-fold cross validation (Stone, 1974) and its concatenation of probability distributions of each base-level classifier adding the true class. According to the k-fold cross validation method, each data set is partitioned into k folds such that each class is uniformly distributed among the k-folds. As a result in each fold, the class distribution is similar to such of the original data set. The classifier is trained and tested k times. In each case, one of folds is taken as test data set and remaining folds are added to form a training data set. The accuracy of each classifier has get by average of k test results. Figure 2 shows a stacking framework with Gaussian network at meta-level learning algorithm.

Our approach is not based on assuming that metadata coming from base-level classifiers has to follow a real normal distribution. On the contrary, the approach is based on the assumption that the function $f\left(x_i \mid \boldsymbol{pa}_i, C\right)$ is the one that follows a normal distribution which is founded on the assumption that predictor variables given their parents follow a Gaussian distribution. It is important to note that this function is not restricted to values between 0 and 1.

Figure 2. Stacking framework. The scheme shows the new meta-level data created through seven probability distributions of predictions for each instance adding the true class value.

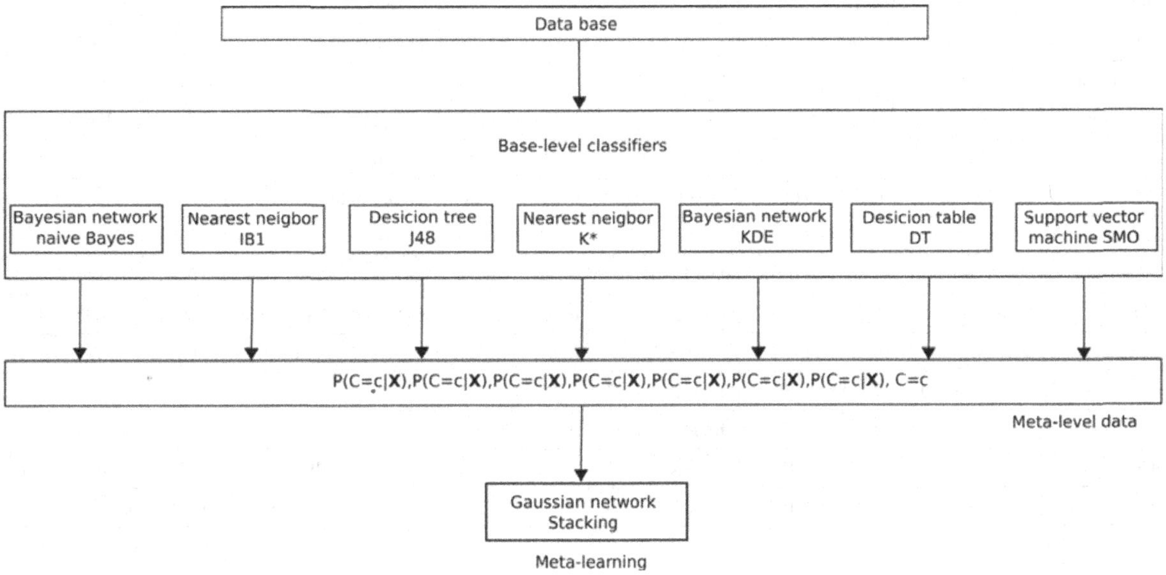

Data base

Base-level classifiers

Bayesian network naive Bayes
Nearest neigbor IB1
Desicion tree J48
Nearest neigbor K*
Bayesian network KDE
Desicion table DT
Support vector machine SMO

P(C=c|**X**),P(C=c|**X**),P(C=c|**X**),P(C=c|**X**),P(C=c|**X**),P(C=c|**X**),P(C=c|**X**), C=c

Meta-level data

Gaussian network Stacking

Meta-learning

Experimental Results of Gaussian-Stacking Applied to UCI Benchmark Databases

We introduced in the previous section some of the most representative classification paradigms in supervised learning applicable as base-level classifiers. All these are available in the Waikato Environment for Knowledge Analysis (Witten & Frank, 2005) –popularly known as WEKA– which is a workbench with a collection of state-of-the-art algorithms machine learning. One of the main advantages of this software package is the interface and the variety of tools for transforming datasets and for evaluating different classifiers statistically, including many learning models and algorithms widely applied in data mining such as paradigms described previously in this Chapter. WEKA is freely available at http://www.cs.waikato.ac.nz/ml/weka.

In order to measure the accuracy and performance of our Gaussian-stacking approach, we evaluated the classification performance of different classical classifiers separately: naive Bayes, IB1, J48, K*, naive Bayes KDE, Decision table and SMO algorithms. We apply them to a set of classical benchmarking classification problems from the UCI *Repository of machine learning data bases (*Asuncion & Newman, 2007), namely the following examples: breast-cancer, breast-W, diabetes, heart-statlog, hepatitis, ionosphere, iris, sonar, tic-tac-toe, vote, waveform and wine data bases.

In this experiment, in order to avoid overfitting problems of these classifiers, the accuracy was calculated by k-fold cross-validation with 10-fold for our case. Similarly, the accuracy of each Gaussian-stacking classifier type was determined by averaging k-fold test results. Default parameters of WEKA workbench were used for computing these values. All data bases were discretized by equal frequency in ten bins, this procedure discretized the continuous values of variables into nominal values.

Table 1 shows the accuracy and standard deviation per each classifier and classification problem. The classifier that obtained highest accuracy per each problem is highlighted in bold. This Table illus-

Table 1. Results of the classical classifiers applied to thirteen classification benchmark problems

Data Set	naive Bayes	IB1	J48	K*	naive Bayes -kDE	DT	SMO
balance	0.9040±0.0172	0.8656±0.0270	0.7664±0.0377	0.8848±0.0227	**0.9136±0.0137**	0.7456±0.0389	0.8768±0.0251
breast-cancer	0.7167±0.0790	0.7237±0.0948	**0.7552±0.0557**	0.7342±0.0930	0.7167±0.0790	0.7272±0.0757	0.6958±0.0754
breast-W	0.9599±0.0163	0.9513±0.0344	0.9456±0.0362	0.9542±0.0268	**0.9756±0.0179**	0.9542±0.0267	0.9699±0.0207
diabetes	0.7630±0.0552	0.7018±0.0469	0.7382±0.0566	0.6914±0.0262	0.7460±0.0638	0.7330±0.0363	**0.7734±0.0406**
heart-statlog	0.8370±0.0702	0.7518±0.0856	0.7666±0.0908	0.7518±0.0941	**0.8444±0.0455**	0.8296±0.0744	0.8407±0.0553
hepatitis	0.8451±0.0813	0.8064±0.0843	0.8387±0.0724	0.8193±0.0855	**0.8580±0.0798**	0.8129±0.1108	0.8516±0.0782
ionosphere	0.8262±0.0546	0.8632±0.0458	0.9145±0.0327	0.8461±0.0621	**0.9173±0.0205**	0.8945±0.0447	0.8860±0.0426
iris	0.9600±0.0466	0.9533±0.0548	0.9600±0.0562	0.9466±0.0525	**0.9666±0.0471**	0.9266±0.0583	0.9600±0.0466
sonar	0.6778±0.0929	**0.8653±0.0700**	0.7115±0.0710	0.8461±0.0785	0.7307±0.0944	0.7451±0.0817	0.7596±0.0779
tic-tac-toe	0.6962±0.0306	**0.9895±0.0098**	0.8455±0.0393	0.9686±0.0163	0.6962±0.0306	0.7828±0.0186	0.9832±0.0149
vote	0.9011±0.0455	0.9241±0.0353	**0.9632±0.0342**	0.9333±0.0434	0.9011±0.0455	0.9517±0.0508	0.9609±0.0340
waveform	0.7600±0.0149	0.7512±0.0113	0.7536±0.0225	0.7702±0.0112	0.8176±0.0149	0.7358±0.0284	**0.8618±0.0114**
wine	**0.9887±0.0234**	0.9831±0.0374	0.9382±0.0314	0.9831±0.0374	0.9887±0.0234	0.9662±0.0289	0.9831±0.0268

trates that the naive Bayes KDE classifier obtains the highest accuracy for several continuous databases –benchmarks– (balance, ionosphere, iris and wine) as well as for databases containing both continuous and discrete variables (statlog, hepatitis, and breast W). On other problems with continuous data (e.g. diabetes and waveform) the SMO algorithm achieves the highest accuracy, and the IB1 algorithm shows the highest accuracy the databases sonar and tic-tac-toe which contain continuous and discrete data respectively. The J48 algorithm performs best in accuracy for the discrete databases breast cancer and vote.

As a second phase of this experiment, we took the same classifiers of the first phase as base-level classifiers (naive Bayes, IB1, J48, K*, naive Bayes KDE, Decision table and SMO) to apply our stacking scheme. We concentrated again on the same set of thirteen problems of the previous experiment. Using the predictions of these base-level classifiers and the real class value for each case of database, we constructed meta-feature vectors. Finally, we built a meta-level database to be used for meta-level classification.

At meta-level, we applied the different Gaussian-stacking techniques introduced in previous section such as filter-ranking-naive Bayes, wrapper-selective naive Bayes, wrapper-semi naive Bayes, wrapper-tree augmented naive Bayes and wrapper-k-dependence Bayesian classifier adapted to continuous domain as proposed in Pérez et al. (2006).

In order to measure the comparative accuracy between the different combinations of our improvement of the Gaussian-stacking technique we compared the highest accuracy of each base-level classifier (naive Bayes, IB1, J48, K*, naive Bayes KDE, Decision Table and SMO) with results of five Gaussian-stacking classifiers. Table 2 shows in bold the highest accuracy among the five Gaussian-stacking classifiers. In all examples, Gaussian-stacking multiclassifiers obtain higher accuracy than each of the best base-level classifier for each domain presented in Table 1. These results are also according to the findings of Dietrich (1998) which reports the better performance of stacking approaches. For instance, if we take as an

Table 2. Results of Gaussian-stacking classifiers when applied with UCI data bases, showing the improvement in accuracy when combining base-level classifiers' outputs by dealing with probability distributions. The classifiers on Table 1 are the ones that have served as base-level classifiers on this experiment.

Data Set	filter-ranking naive Bayes	wrapper-selective naive Bayes	wrapper-semi naive Bayes	wrapper-TAN	wrapper-kDB
balance	0.9392±0.0171	**0.9568±0.0201**	0.9567±0.0298	0.9568±0.0328	0.9567±0.0161
breast-cancer	0.7551±0.0947	0.7546±0.0583	**0.7560±0.1099**	0.7549±0.0650	0.7550±0.0285
breast-W	0.9713±0.0239	0.9727±0.0175	0.9728±0.0185	**0.9728±0.0162**	0.9713±0.0143
diabetes	**0.7878±0.0449**	0.7825±0.0518	0.7826±0.0392	0.7812±0.0439	0.7825±0.0523
heart-statlog	0.8555±0.0730	**0.8555±0.0607**	0.8407±0.0469	0.8518±0.0682	0.8407±0.0952
hepatitis	0.8450±0.0812	0.8574±0.0833	0.8566±0.0717	**0.8712±0.0942**	0.85125±0.0585
ionosphere	0.9373±0.0398	**0.9400±0.0349**	0.9373±0.0523	0.9373±0.0437	0.9373±0.0457
iris	**0.9600±0.0442**	0.9600±0.0442	0.9466±0.0581	0.9600±0.0442	0.9600±0.0533
sonar	0.8707±0.0740	**0.8807±0.0882**	0.8747±0.0717	0.8747±0.0760	0.8754±0.0714
tic-tac-toe	0.9853±0.0095	0.9885±0.0127	**0.9958±0.0051**	0.9885±0.0098	0.9853±0.0106
vote	**0.9680±0.0354**	0.9655±0.0212	0.9632±0.0275	0.9678±0.0112	0.9676±0.0298
waveform	0.8450±0.0152	0.8469±0.0186	**0.8492±0.0138**	0.8459±0.0170	0.8468±0.0179
wine	0.9888±0.0222	**0.9944±0.0166**	0.9944±0.0166	0.9944±0.0166	0.9944±0.0166

example the diabetes database, for instance, SMO is the base-level classifier with highest accuracy in Table 1, having obtained 0.7734±0.0406, which is inferior of the accuracies obtained by all our Gaussian stacking classifiers, the filter-ranking naive Bayes classifier being the one that achieved the highest accuracy of 0.7878±0.0449 and wrapper-TAN the worst with an accuracy of 0.7812±0.0439.

These results evidence the validity of our approach and show that Gaussian-stacking classifiers are an adequate method to combine base-level classifiers outputs by dealing with probability distributions.

In the next sections of this chapter we apply our Gaussian network meta-classification approach to the complex real-problem of predicting the outcome of an embryo-batch based on computing for each IVF treatment the probability of implantation.

HUMAN EMBRYO CLASSIFICATION FOR IN-VITRO TREATMENTS

An important aspect to improve the success rates of in-vitro treatments is the selection of the embryo that will be most adequate to implant in order to ensure implantation. The precise examination of embryos on particular days after fertilization by human assisted reproduction methods facilitates the selection of the most promising embryos for transfer, and embryologists are familiar with non-invasive and precise techniques of embryo evaluation. Nonetheless, the procedures and methodologies that are applied in clinical practice vary from one country to another due to ethical and legislative reasons, which leads to different protocols of human embryo manipulation and different restrictions in aspects such as the period of time for the follow-up of promising embryos after fertilization.

Due to the complexity of this task, there is an increased interest in providing some kind of decision support system for embryologists. The recent literature shows examples of applying artificial intelligence methods to improve success rates of IVF programs. An important contribution of artificial intelligence to the embryo selection process is presented by Saith et al. (1998) and consists of the construction of a data mining model based on decision trees to investigate the relationship between the features of the embryo, oocyte and follicle. Another contribution on this research field is a case-based reasoning system proposed by Jurisica et al. (1998) in the form of an intelligent decision support system for IVF practitioners that, in some situations, is able to suggest possible treatments to improve the success rate. Trimarchi et al. (2003) provide a study of models based on data mining techniques, in particular the C5.0 algorithm, to infer classification trees. A pattern recognition algorithm to select embryos from images is introduced by Patrizi et al. (2004) to classify the objects given into a number of classes and to formulate from these a general rule. Another important contribution is made by Manna et al. (2004), comparing the precision in the recognition of viable embryos by a group of experts to that of a machine recognition procedure. Morales et al. (2008) introduce a novel approach to classify the embryo-batch problem on in-vitro treatment by Bayesian classifiers, and based on a subset feature selection process, conclude which are the most relevant features that should be taken into account by the classification process.

This chapter contributes to this research field by presenting a novel Gaussian meta-learning system that can assist on the selection of the most promising embryos-batch for implantation in IVF treatments.

Morphological Human Embryo Characterization on In-Vitro Treatment

Human assisted reproduction methods such as intra cytoplasmic sperm injection (ICSI) –in which sperm is injected into the oocyte– and in-vitro fertilization (IVF) –through insemination of oocyte and sperm– are widely applied to treat infertility. In order to obtain a sufficient number of oocytes, ovulatory stimulants are applied making pituitary increase secretion of follicle stimulating hormones. After extraction of these, embryos are formed outside the body and they are developed in a controlled atmosphere. Next, the embryologist chooses several embryos which seem the most promising regarding the likelihood of bringing forth a child. Since the morphology of pronuclear oocyte has been associated with the potential to implantation and development to the blastocyst stage, the embryo selection based on morphology assessment is known to be important to improve implantation and pregnancy rates (Giorgetti et al., 1995; Veek, 1999).

Routine embryo evaluation begins in early embryo development, 16-19 hours after oocyte fertilization (either in IVF or ICSI) where the embryologist catalogs zygotes according to a specific zygote scoring. Subsequent embryo evaluations are made in daily intervals, 40-48 hours and 64-68 hours, as well as 48 hours after fertilization being the most indicated time to catalog embryos according to an embryo scoring. The zygote and embryo analysis is performed under contrast-phase microscope with Hoffmann modulation contrast (HMC) or difference-interference contrast (DIC), enabling more precise assessment without fixing and staining. The aim of this analysis is to compare the embryos and to choose the one(s) to be transferred. Since an essential part of the embryo selection process requires measure to allow comparison between embryos, the literature provides several examples of scores for this purpose. Many of these scoring systems are based on combinations of several morphological parameters such as cleavage stage, embryonic fragmentation and blastomere uniformity, or the number and distribution of nucleoli precursor bodies in each pronucleus.

One of the most accepted zygote scores was proposed by Scott, Alvero and Leondires in 2000, which catalogs zygotes into the four following categories from the most promising to the least:

- **Z1:** Equal size of pronuclei. Equal size and number of nucleoli aligned in both pronuclei at the pronuclear junction.
- **Z2:** Equal size of pronuclei. Equal size and number of nucleoli scattered in both pronuclei.
- **Z3:** Equal size of pronuclei. Equal number of nucleoli and even or uneven size in each nucleolus aligned in one pronucleus at the pronuclear junction and scattered in the other pronucleus.
- **Z4:** Unequal or separated pronuclei.

From these, Z1 and Z2 are considered to be the promising zygotes to develop in suitable embryos for transfer. In general Z1 has a nucleoli range between three and seven.

The embryo evaluation in the second day after fertilization requires another score more suited for the characteristic of the embryo at this stage. As an example, Veek (1999) presents a score which categorizes embryos according to specific morphological parameters such as the number of cells, percentage of fragmentation, good cell-cell contact and the existence or not of multinucleated blastomeres. This morphological evaluation leads to the following embryo categorisation:

- **Type I:** Equal size of homogeneous blastomeres with no fragmentation.
- **Type II:** Equal size of homogeneous blastomeres with < 10% fragmentation.
- **Type III:** This type is usually divided in two subtypes:
  - *Type III-A:* Equal size of blastomeres with 10-25% fragmentation.
  - *Type III-B:* Unequal size blastomeres with 25-50% fragmentation.
- **Type IV:** Equal or unequal size of blastomeres with > 50% fragmentation.
- **Type V:** 100% fragmentation.

It must be noted that the literature provides many other zygote scoring systems to catalog embryos, in some of which other different criteria are taken into account rather than uniquely morphological characteristics.

IVF embryologist measure the quality of embryos following these zygote and embryo scoring systems on a specific day after fertilization and according to a systematized specific protocol.

Characterization of Clinical Cases and Morphological Embryo Features in a Database

The human embryo selection process is a complex biomedical problem due to the diverse legislative restrictions faced in different countries, often resulting in important procedural differences with direct implications in the design of embryologists' protocols. As an example, the law in Spain allows a maximum number of three embryos to be transferred in a same batch in order to reduce the incidence of multi-fetal pregnancies, but the number of oocytes that will be fecundated is left at the decision of the responsible biomedical team. This has obvious implications and differences in the procedures applies regarding other countries such as Sweden, in which it is not allowed that more than a single embryo is transferred in each IVF/ICSI treatment.

Embryologists assign a score to each embryo suitable for transfer following a score as described in the previous Section, and all available embryos are ranked accordingly from the highest to the lowest. Since it has been proved that implantation rate for each of the single embryos increases in the presence of other embryos (Matorras et al., 2005), in countries in which more than an embryo is allowed to be transferred at a time, usually decision is taken on transferring a batch of two or three embryos, although at the same time trying to reduce as much as possible the incidence of multiple pregnancies. The selected batch of embryos is afterwards transferred in the patient's uterus. As a result when a batch of embryos is transferred, and since in very rare cases will all the embryos manage to implant in the uterus, it is necessary to analyze the set of embryos transferred within the in embryo-batches as a whole from the data-mining perspective. This is the case because it is not possible to infer which of the embryos in the batch is the one implanted, although the general assumption in clinical practice is that the implanted embryo(s) will always be the one(s) that had the higher score within the batch.

In our experiment we worked with real data obtained from 63 clinical files at the IVF unit of Clínica del Pilar located in Donostia-San Sebastián (Spain), with information of treatments of the period from July 2003 through December 2005. These 63 cases were chosen from a total of 89 cycles of in-vitro treatment of patients aged 27-46, after discarding treatments that were not performed under comparable conditions. Within these 63 cases, a total of 189 embryos were transferred in batches of 3 embryos, and all patients age range is 30-40. Furthermore, we decided not to include in our study 26 cases of treatments consisting of two embryo-batches cases of women aged 27-29 and 41-46 due to the relative low number of cases present as well as the different characteristics of their clinical profiles that made clinicians not to opt for an embryo-batch of 3 embryos.

In all these clinical files the morphological characteristics of embryos at the 4-8 cell stage were taken 40-50 hours after fertilization and previously to transfer during the second or third day. Both fresh and frozen embryos were considered in this retrospective study, and a total of 18 treatments of the 63 ones were successful. Embryologists of the IVF unit of Clínica del Pilar catalog each zygote using Scott's score (Scott et al., 2000), and the embryo morphology evaluation is performed following Veek's score

Figure 3. Real zygote images of the database of Clínica del Pilar (Donostia-San Sebastian, Spain), cataloged according to Scott's score (Scott et al., 2000)

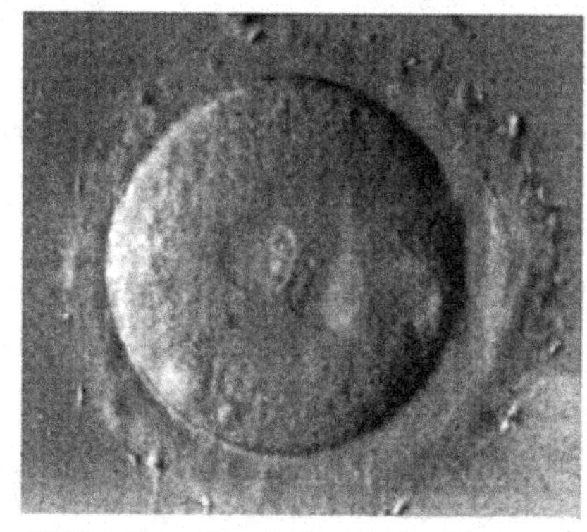

a) Z1 aligned, equal size and number of nucleoli

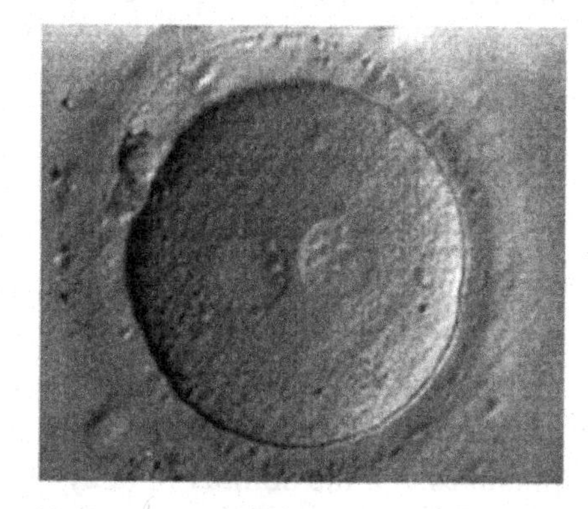

b) Z3 unequal aligment, number and size of nucleoli

(Veek, 1999). Figure 3 shows examples of real images dominated in the protocol of this clinic, in which the selection of embryos is based primarily on zygote score (Scott et al., 2000) and secondly in Veek's embryo catalog.

Apart from the morphological information of all the embryos, our database also contains other variables related to clinical parameters such as the patient's age, number of previous cycles of treatment, actual cycle, sperm quality, cause of female or male infertility, primary or secondary infertility[4], number of embryos transferred, whether embryos were frozen or not, quality of transference, and transference day. Table 3 shows the whole list of variables that contains the database with their respective value ranges.

If we would like to build a classifier considering all these parameters, a feature-vector can be constructed putting them together and later use it by any supervised classification method. Similarly, each embryo-batch of the database is assigned to a different class regarding its known clinical outcome of having led to pregnancy or not (e.g. we have two classes: implanted batch/ non implanted batch). Following this approach, the embryo selection problem is consequently transformed into a supervised classification problem. It must be noted that this characterization distinguishes only between implantation obtained or not, regardless of the number of embryos that managed to implant in case of pregnancy.

Once the information is structured in such a way, it is possible to transform the embryo selection problem into a supervised classification problem. This is done by building a classifier using a number of approaches in the literature. In our concrete problem of the selection of embryos, our feature vector

Table 3. Predictor features of the clinical database used for our experiment with real-data

Feature	*Range of values*
Number of actual cycle	Numerical
Number of previous cycles of treatment	Numerical
Age	Numerical
Donate	{Yes, No}
Sperm quality	{Good, Medium, Poor}
Cause female	{Yes, No}
Cause male	{Yes, No}
Primary infertility	{Yes, No}
Secondary infertility	{Yes, No}
Number of transferred embryos	Numerical
Number of frozen embryos	Numerical
Cell number	Numerical
Zygote score	{Z1, Z2, Z3, Z4}
Embryo categorization	{Type I, Type II, Type III, Type IV, Type V}
Blastomeres size	{Equal,Unequal, Defects of cytoplasm}
Fragmentation blastomeres	{0%,(0-10]%,(10-25]%, (25-50]%,(50-99]%,100%}
Thickness of zona pellucida	{None, Thick, Very Thick}
Multinuclear	{Yes, No}
Day of transference	Numerical
Quality of transference	{Good, Medium, Poor}

Table 4. Structure of the feature vector that is used to represent each case of IVF treatments of three embryo batches. The two values of the class variable are 1='implantation succeeded' and 0='no implantation'

Treatment	Embryo–related data 1	2	3	Clinical data of patient	Class
Batch 1	Emb 1	Emb 2	Emb 3	...	1
Batch 2	Emb 1	Emb 2	Emb 3	...	0
...	...	...	...	...	...
Batch n	Emb 1	Emb 2	Emb 3	...	1

Table 5. Results of Gaussian-stacking applied to the real problem of selecting embryo-batches of three embryos for IVF treatments

Gaussian-Stacking Classifier	Accuracy ± SD
filter-ranking naive Bayes	0.5809±0.2045
wrapper selective naive Bayes	0.7119±0.1552
wrapper semi naive Bayes	0.7166±0.1789
wrapper-TAN	0.7119±0.1465
wrapper-kDB	0.7119±0.1876

X is defined as a batch containing morphological characteristic of three embryos transferred on in-vitro treatment as well as the clinical information of the couple. We will only consider two classes, and therefore we will define $C = \{0,1\}$, where class 1 denotes the successful cases of at least one implantation occurred, and class 0 is assigned to the unsuccessful cases. Table 4 shows an example of feature vectors into embryo data base where we kept the embryologist's order of embryos in the batch following the Scott score –in such a way that Embl represents the most promising embryo and Emb3 represents the least promising one. As a result, our aim is to build a classifier in the form $\gamma : (x_1,\ldots,x_n) \rightarrow \{0,1\}$ that will allow us to predict the outcome of a new embryo-batch.

Experimental Results of Applying Gaussian-Stacking to the Selection of Embryo-Batches for In-Vitro Treatments

In order to test the applicability of our Gaussian-stacking method in a complex real medical problem, here we concentrate on the data of three embryo batches described in the previous Section. Again, the data applied at meta-level is obtained from the continuous predictions of seven base-level classifiers (naive Bayes, IB1, J48, K*, naive Bayes KDE, Decision table and SMO) adding the outcome of treatment as the class variable. In order to build this database of meta-level information, all base-level classifiers were fed with the database of 63 three embryo-batches. Leave-one-out validation was applied in order to avoid overfitting problems.

To build the Gaussian-stacking multiclassifier we apply at meta level learning the wrapper-TAN, wrapper-kDB, wrapper selective naive Bayes and wrapper semi naive Bayes algorithms, each classifier applied at one time.

The search for the best model is guided in all the cases following the estimated classification goodness measure. The only exception is filter-ranking naive Bayes, in which the search of possible graph structures for this model is guided by the mutual information criterion. Table 5 shows the accuracy and standard deviation obtained. The wrapper semi naive Bayes algorithm achieved the highest accuracy of 0.7166±0.1789, and filter-ranking naive Bayes reached the lowest accuracy with 0.5809±0.2045. Our results prove that Gaussian-stacking classifier can be used satisfactorily as a valid method for complex real medical problems such as artificial insemination treatments

As an additional test in order to compare the degree of agreement between base-level classifiers, we performed the Kappa statistic analysis over pairs of base-level classification models. Kappa statistic is a measure of inter-rater reliability (e.g. concordance), introduced by Cohen (1960). The Kappa statistic provides a measure of agreement between two classifiers to respectively classify N cases into K mutually exclusive categories of class variable C. In real problems where one class is much more common than the rest –as it is the case in our concrete problem– all reasonable classifiers tend to agree with one another; one way to surpass this is calculating the probability of agreement due to fortuity. The K statistics is defined as follows:

$$K = \frac{p(a) - p(b)}{1 - p(b)} \tag{7}$$

where $p(a)$ is an estimate of the probability that two classifiers agree, and $p(b)$ is the probability that agreement is random. K statistic is 1 when a pair of classifiers is in complete agreement, and negative values of K are obtained when less agreement is expected than kappa calculated at random.

In our experiment, the pair of base-level classifiers that obtained the highest Kappa were naive Bayes and SMO classifiers with a Kappa of 0.5414, and J48 and K* algorithms with a *kappa* of 0.5280. The pair of base-level classifiers that obtained the lowest Kappa is decision table and SMO algorithms with -0.0073. These Kappa measure based scales show a moderated grade of concordance between the pair of classifiers, and the negative value of Kappa shows that there is a systematic disagreement between these two classifiers.

CONCLUSION AND FUTURE WORK

This chapter presents a new approach for meta-level classification based on Gaussian networks. This method can serve for any complex real problem and could be the engine for a decision support system. This chapter shows the results of applying this technique to thirteen UCI benchmark databases, as well as to a real medical complex problem such as the selection of human embryo-batches for infertility treatments.

Different Gaussian-stacking multi-classifiers have been introduced and evaluated for their potential application to complex real medical decision problems. The results obtained with UCI databases showed a good performance of Gaussian-stacking classifiers as well as their appropriateness to combine several classification paradigms. Gaussian-stacking classifiers are able to handle the probability distributions provided by outputs of classifiers as continuous values, overcoming the need to perform a discretization step which is the case in many supervised classifiers.

When applied to our complex medical problem, Gaussian-stacking classifiers achieved very promising results and showed their validity to be used satisfactorily as a decision-support methodology in artificial insemination treatments to assist embryologists on their decision making. Furthermore, taking into account the lack of means for a systematic training of embryologists on the selection of embryos, this system could also serve as a training tool to improve the expertise of novel embryologists.

Our results confirm the positive behavior of stacking-based methods reported in the literature. Furthermore, this classification paradigm shows higher accuracy results than the filter selective naive Bayes, filter TAN and filter kDB classifiers on Morales et al. (2008) where the accuracies obtained were 68.25 %, 68.25 and 63.49% respectively.

In this work, we have not yet considered other methods for extraction of characteristics from images, neither have we increased the number of predictor variables that may improve the efficiency of Bayesian classifiers. This has been left for future work. Other future work trends in this direction include the acquisition of new data that includes morphological embryo features from human embryo images and clinical data of patient.

ACKNOWLEDGMENT

This work has been partially supported by the Saiotek and Research Groups 2007-2012 (IT-242-07) programs (Basque Government), TIN2008-06815-C02-01 and Consolider Ingenio 2010 - CSD2007-00018 projects (Spanish Ministry of Science and Innovation) and COMBIOMED network in computational biomedicine (Carlos III Health Institute).

The authors would also like to thank the staff of the Clínica del Pilar for their support and willingness to provide us with their data.

REFERENCES

Aha, D., & Kibler, D. (1991). Instance-based learning algorithms. *Machine Learning, 6*, 37-66.

Asuncion, A., & Newman, D. J. (2007). UCI Machine Learning Repository.

Cleary, J. G., & Trigg, L.E. (1995). K*: An instance- based learner using an entropic distance measure. *Proceedings of the 12th International Conference on Machine learning*, 108-114.

Chow, C., & Liu, C. (1968). Approximating discrete probability distributions with dependence trees. *IEEE Transactions on Information Theory, 14*, 462-467.

Cohen, J. (1960). A coefficient of agreement for nominal scales. *Educational and Psychological Measurement, 20*, 37-46.

Dietterich, T.G. (1998). Machine-learning research: Four current directions. *The AI Magazine, 18*(4), 97-136.

Duda, R., & Hart, P. (1973). *Pattern classification and scene analysis.* New York: John Wiley and Sons.

Džeroski, S., & Ženko, B. (2004). Is combining classifiers better than selecting the best one? *Machine Learning, 54*(3), 255-273.

ESHRE - European Society for Human Reproduction & Embryology (2007). High pregnancy rates achieved in ART through a personalised approach to ovarian stimulation treatment. In *The 23rd Annual Meeting of the European Society of Human Reproduction and Embryology*. Lyon, France.

Friedman, N., Geiger, D., & Goldsmidt, M. (1997). Bayesian network classifiers. *Machine Learning, 29*(2), 131-163.

Giorgetti, C., Terriou, P., Auquier, P., Hans, E., Spach, J. L., Salzmann, J., & Roulier, R. (1995). Embryo score to predict implantation after in-vitro fertilization: Based on 957 single embryo transfers. *Human Reproduction, 10*, 2427-2431.

John, G. H., & Langley, P. (1995). Estimating continuous distributions in Bayesian classifiers. *Proceedings of the Eleventh Conference on Uncertainty in Artificial Intelligence*, 338-345.

Jurisica, I., Mylopoulos, J., Glasgow, J., Shapiro, H., & Casper, R. (1998). Case-based reasoning in IVF: Prediction and knowledge mining. *Artificial Intelligence in Medicine, 12*(1), 1-24.

Keogh, E. J., & Pazzani, M. (1999). Learning augmented Bayesian classifiers: A comparison of distribution-based and classification-based approaches. *Uncertainty 99: The 7th International Workshop on Artificial Intelligence and Statistics*, 225-230.

Kohavi, R. (1995). The power of decision tables. In *Proceedings of 8th European Conference on Machine Learning*, 174-189.

Kohavi, R., & John, G. (1997). Wrappers for feature subset selection. *Artificial Intelligence, 97*(1-2), 273-324.

Kononenko, I. (1991). Semi-naive Bayesian classifiers. *Proceedings of the 6th European Working Session on Learning*, 206-219.

Kuncheva L. I. (2004). Combining *Pattern Classifiers. Methods and Algorithms.* Wiley.

Lauritzen, S. L. (1996). *Graphical models.* Clarendon Press, Oxford University.

Manna, C., Patrizi, G., Rahman, A., & Sallam, H. (2004). Experimental results on the recognition of embryos in human assisted reproduction. *Reproductive BioMedicine Online, 8*(4), 460-469.

Matorras, R., Matorras, F., Mendoza, R., Rodríguez, M., Remohí, J., Rodríguez-Escudero, F. J., & Simón, C. (2005). The implantation of every embryo facilitates the chances of the remaining embryos to implant in an IVF programme: a mathematical model to predict pregnancy and multiple pregnancy rates. *Human Reproduction, 20*, 2923-2931.

Merz, C. J. (1999). Using correspondence analysis to combine classifiers. *Machine Learning, 36*, 33-58.

Minsky, M. (1961). Steps toward artificial intelligence. *Transactions on Institute of Radio Engineers, 49*, 8-30.

Morales, D. A., Bengoetxea, E., Larrañaga, P., García, M., Franco, Y., Fresnada, M., & Merino, M. (2008). Bayesian classification for the selection of in-vitro human embryos using morphological and clinical data. *Computer Methods and Programs in Biomedicine, 90, 104-116.*

Patrizi, G., Manna, C., Moscatelli, C., & Nieddu, L. (2004). Pattern recognition methods in human-assisted reproduction. *International Transactions in Operational Research, 11*(4), 365-379.

Pazzani, M. (1997). Searching for dependencies in Bayesian classifiers. *Learning from Data: Artificial Intelligence and Statistics V*, 239-248.

Pérez, A., Larrañaga, P., & Inza, I. (2006). Supervised classification with conditional Gaussian Networks: Increasing the structure complexity from naive Bayes. *International Journal of Approximate Reasoning, 43*, 1-25.

Platt, J. C. (1999). Fast training of support vector machines using sequential minimal optimization. In Scholkopf, B., Burges, C., & Smola, A. J. (Eds.), *Advances in kernel methods - support vector learning (pp. 185-208).* MIT Press.

Puissant, F., Rysselberge, M. V., Barlow, P., Deweze, J., & Leroy, F. (1987). Embryo scoring as a prognostic tool in IVF treatment. *Human Reproduction, 2*, 705-708.

Quinlan, J. R. (1993). *C4.5: Programs for Machine Learning*: Morgan Kaufmann.

Sahami, M. (1996). Learning limited dependence Bayesian classifiers. *Proceedings of the 2nd International Conference on Knowledge Discovery and Data Mining*, 335-338.

Saith, R., Srinivasan, A., Michie, D., & Sargent, I. (1998). Relationships between the developmental potential of human in-vitro fertilization embryos and features describing the embryo, oocyte and follicle. *Human Reproduction Update, 4*(2), 121-134.

Seewald, A. (2003). *Towards understanding stacking.* Department of Informatics, Technical University of Wien.

Sierra, B., Serrano, N., Larrañaga, P., Plasencia E.J. Inza, I., Jiménez, J.J., Revuelta, P., & Mora M.L. (2001). Using Bayesian networks in the construction of a bi-level multi-classifier. A case study using intensive care unit patients data. *Artificial Intelligence in Medicine, 22*(3), 233-248.

Scott, L., Alvero, R., & Leondires, M. (2000). The morphology of human pronuclear embryos is positively related to blastocyst development and implantation. *Human Reproduction, 15*(11), 2394-2403.

Stone, M. (1974). Cross-validatory choice and assessment of statistical predictions. *Journal of the Royal Statistical Society Series B, 36*, 111-147.

Ting, k., & Witten, M. (1999). Issues in stacked generalization. *Journal of Artificial Intelligence Research (JAIR), 10*, 271-289.

Todorovski, L., & Džeroski, S. (2002). Combining classifiers with meta decision trees. *Machine Learning, 50*(3), 223-249.

Trimarchi, J. R., Goodside, J., Passmore, L., Silberstein, T., Hamel, L., & Gonzalez, L. (2003). Comparing data mining and logistic regression for predicting IVF outcome. *Fertility and Sterility, 80*(3), 100-100.

Vapnik, V. (1995). *The Nature of Statistical Learning Theory.* Springer-Verlag.

Veek, L. L. (1999). *An Atlas of Human Gametes and Conceptuses: An Illustrated Reference for Assisted Reproductive Technology*. Parthenon.

Witten, I. H., & Frank, E. (2005). *Data mining: Practical machine learning tools and techniques with java implementations*: Morgan Kaufmann Publishers.

Wolpert, D. H. (1992). Stacked generalization. *Neural Networks, 5*, 241-259.

KEY TERMS

Confusion Matrix: The matrix where are registered the outputs performance of classifier in terms of true positives, true negatives, false positives and false negatives.

Cost Matrix: The matrix who stored the cost of misclassification

Irrelevant Variables: In feature subset selection the irrelevant variables do not add extra information

Paradigms: In supervised classification are the algorithms that allow the classification task.

Predictor Variables: The features or characteristic of data.

Redundant Variables: Can be calculated taken into account the rest of variables.

Vector of Features: The batch of characteristics represented by predictor variables of each instance or case that conform de database.

ENDNOTES

1. In assisted reproduction the term *transfer* refers to the clinical procedure to insert embryos in the woman's uterus, while the term *implantation* relates to the success of achieving pregnancy (e.g. the embryo is implanted on the uterine wall).
2. Irrelevant variables are the ones that do not add extra information regarding the rest of features, leading to a loss of accuracy in the classification process if they are kept in the model, while redundant features are the ones that can be calculated given the rest of variables.
3. Base-level classifiers will be applied here to form a set of classifiers into the first level of staking scheme.
4. Primary infertility is defined as a couple that has never been able to conceive a pregnancy, after at least 1 year of unprotected intercourse. Secondary infertility is considered when a couple has previously succeeded in pregnancy at least once, but has not been able to achieve other pregnancies.

Chapter XVI
Mining Tuberculosis Data

Marisa A. Sánchez
Universidad Nacional del Sur, Argentina

Sonia Uremovich
Universidad Nacional del Sur, Argentina

Pablo Acrogliano
Hospital Interzonal Dr. José Penna, Argentina

ABSTRACT

This chapter reviews the current policies of tuberculosis control programs for the diagnosis of tuberculosis. The international standard for tuberculosis control is the World Health Organization's DOT (Direct Observation of Therapy) strategy that aims to reduce the transmission of the infection through prompt diagnosis and effective treatment of symptomatic tuberculosis patients who present at health care facilities. Physicians are concerned about the poor specificity of diagnostic methods and the increase in the notification of relapse cases. This works describes a data-mining project that uses DOT's data to analyze the relationship among different variables and the tuberculosis diagnostic category registered for each patient.

INTRODUCTION

Tuberculosis has been a major killer disease for several years. It is estimated that around 1.6 million people die each year from tuberculosis; and in 2005 figures indicate that approximately 8.8 million people developed the disease (World Health Organization, 2007b). The international standard for tuberculosis control is the World Health Organization's DOT (Direct Observation of Therapy) strategy that aims to reduce the transmission of the infection through prompt diagnosis and effective treatment of symptomatic tuberculosis patients who present at health care facilities. The treatment is based on the strict supervision of medicines intake. The supervision is possible thanks to the availability of an information system that records the individual patient data. These data can be used at the facility level to monitor treatment outcomes, at the district level to identify local problems as they arise, at provincial or national level to ensure consistently high-quality tuberculosis control across geographical areas (World Health Organization, 2007b). In Argentina, the Health Ministry gathers DOTS data since 1996.

Identification of individuals latently infected and effective treatment are important parts of tuberculosis control. The DOTS strategy recommends identification of infectious tuberculosis cases by microscopic examination of sputum smears. However, this function requires a strong laboratory network and high-quality sputum smear microscopy. In children, the diagnosis of pulmonary tuberculosis is difficult because collection of sufficient sputum for smear microscopy and culture is difficult. The HIV epidemic has led to huge rises in incidence of tuberculosis in the worst affected countries, with disproportionate increases in smear-negative pulmonary tuberculosis in children and adults (Getahun, 2007). Additionally, the use of chest radiography for diagnosis of pulmonary tuberculosis can be compromised by poor film quality, low specificity, and difficulties with interpretation (World Health Organization, 2004).

Physicians are concerned about the poor specificity of current methods. In particular, they want to analyze diagnosis of childhood tuberculosis. In addition, the notification rate of relapsed cases is slightly increasing so they are interested in finding patterns that can explain this trend. Thus, the purpose of this study is to review current policies of local tuberculosis control programmes for the diagnosis of tuberculosis.

Data analysis is vital for answering these questions. The availability of DOTS records gives an opportunity to use Data Mining techniques such as demographic clustering, or decision trees. In particular, decision trees have an immense prediction power and provide an explanation of the results. Decision trees are widely used in medicine (Jianxin, 2007; Prakash, 2006; Šprogar, 2002; Cios, 2002).

The chapter is further structured as follows: next section provides definitions of data mining concepts and tuberculosis terms. Then, we present our data mining project and highlight our key findings and the main issues and problems that have arisen during the project. Finally, we summarize the contributions of the chapter.

BACKGROUND

Technology evolution has promoted the increase in the volume and variety of data. The amount of data increases exponentially with time. As a consequence, the manual analysis of this data is complex and prone to errors. When the amount of data to be analyzed exploded in the mid-1990s, knowledge discovery emerged as an important analytical tool. The process of extracting useful knowledge from volumes of data is known as knowledge discovery in databases (Fayyad, 1996). Knowledge discovery's major objective is to identify valid, novel, potentially useful, and understandable patterns of data. Knowledge discovery is supported by three technologies: massive data collection, powerful multiprocessor computers, and data mining (Turban, 2005).

Data mining derives its name from the similarities between searching for valuable business information in a large database, and mining a mountain for a vein of valuable ore. Data mining can generate new business opportunities by providing automated prediction of trends and behaviors, and discovery of previously unknown patterns.

A data mining project compromises a multi-step, iterative process. CRISP-DM (CRoss-Industry Standard Process for Data Mining) was conceived in late 1996 by DaimlerChrysler, SPSS and NCR as an industry-, tool-, and application-neutral process model (Shearer, 2000). The CRISP-DM methodology is described in terms of a hierarchical process model, consisting of sets of tasks described at four levels of abstraction: phase, generic task, specialized task and process instance. In overview, the phases are:

- **Business understanding:** The initial phase focuses on understanding the project objectives and requirements from a business perspective. The business objectives drive the entire project and results will be evaluated against them.
- **Data understanding:** We should identify all internal and external sources of information that will be considered within the project. Data understanding tasks aim to discover first insights into the data. Also, data quality issues are addressed.
- **Data preparation:** Erroneous and missing data must be dealt with. The 60% of the time goes into preparing the data for mining (Cabena, 1997). The data must be converted into a single common format for processing; this may involve encoding data or reducing the number of variables with which to deal.
- **Modeling:** In this phase, various techniques for searching patterns in data are selected, applied, and their parameters are calibrated to optimal values. As the user gains insight into the problem, he may need to add or eliminate variables, or even to redefine his goals.
- **Evaluation:** The data mining results are evaluated in the business context. There is a review of the whole process and a description of next steps.
- **Deployment:** The purpose of this phase is to understand what actions need to be carried out in order to actually make use of the models and to incorporate this knowledge into the knowledge base.

Having defined the basic concepts, we now focus on a popular data mining method: decision trees.

Decision Trees

The decision tree representation is the most widely used logic method, and relatively small trees are easy to understand (Weiss, 1998). Decision trees classify instances by sorting them down the tree from the root to some leaf node, which provides the classification of the instance. Each node in the tree specifies a test of some attribute of the instance, and each branch descending from that node corresponds to one of the possible values for this attribute. An instance is classified by starting at the root node of the tree, testing the attribute specified by this node. Depending on the result of the test, the case is passed down the appropriate branch, and the process continues (Mitchell, 1997).

Using training data, the task is to determine the nodes in the tree and the tests associated with non-terminal nodes. Algorithms to perform this task are variations on a core algorithm that employs a top-down, greedy search through the space of possible decision trees. In this work, we consider Exhaustive CHAID (for **Chi**-squared **A**utomatic **I**nteraction **D**etection).

CHAID modeling is an exploratory data analysis method used to study the relationships between a dependent measure and a large series of possible predictor variables, that themselves may interact. The dependent measure may be a qualitative (nominal or ordinal) one or a quantitative indicator. For qualitative variables, a series of chi-square analyses are conducted between the dependent and predictor variables. For quantitative variables, analysis of variance methods are used where intervals (splits) are determined optimally for the independent variables to maximize the ability to explain a dependent measure in terms of variance components.

Exhaustive CHAID is an improvement over CHAID that does a more thorough job of examining all possible splits for each predictor but takes longer to compute (Biggs, 1991).

Validation and Risk Estimation

Once a tree has been built, we can assess its predictive value. For categorical targets, each node assigns a predicted category to all cases belonging to it. The risk estimate (or error) is the proportion of all cases incorrectly classified. For continuous targets, each node predicts the value as the mean value of cases in the node. The risk estimate is the within-node variance about each node's mean, averaged over all cases.

Partitioning and Cross-Validation are two different methods to estimate how well we can expect a tree to generalize new data. Partitioning requires setting aside part of the training sample. When the tree-growing process is complete, a risk estimate is computed based on classifying the held-out data with the tree (Brieman, 1984). Cross-Validation uses all the data to build the tree. The error is computed by partitioning the data into *k* separate groups or folders. Next, *k* tree are built. The first tree uses all groups except the first; the second tree uses all groups except the second, and so on, until each group has been excluded once. For each tree, a risk estimate is computed, and the cross-validated risk estimate is the average of these *k* risk estimates for the *k* trees, weighted by the number of cases in each fold.

Tuberculosis

In this section, we provide a brief overview of tuberculosis based on facts and definitions published by the World Health Organization.

Tuberculosis is a bacterial infection that causes more deaths in the world than any other infectious disease. The bacterium is called *Mycobacterium tuberculosis* and it usually affects the lungs. Pulmonary tuberculosis refers to disease involving the lung parenchyma. Extrapulmonary tuberculosis refers to tuberculosis of organs other than the lung, e.g. pleura, lymph nodes, abdomen, genitourinary tract, skin, joints and bones, meninges. Only people who have pulmonary tuberculosis are infectious. One-third of the world's population is currently infected and new infections are occurring at a rate of one per second (World Health Organization, 2007c).

Tuberculosis spreads from person to person through the air as a person with active tuberculosis coughs, sneezes, speaks, etc. However, not everyone infected with the bacteria becomes sick. After a person becomes infected, his immune system controls the tuberculosis bacteria. When the bacteria spread out of control, the infection becomes active.

A tuberculosis suspect is any person who presents a cough of long duration. A case is a patient in whom tuberculosis has been bacteriological confirmed or diagnosed by a clinician. A new patient has never had treatment for tuberculosis or has taken tuberculosis drugs for less than 1 month. A relapse is a patient previously treated for tuberculosis who has been declared cured or treatment completed, and is diagnosed with bacteriological positive tuberculosis.

The four determinants of case definition are site of tuberculosis disease; bacteriology (result of sputum smear); severity of disease; and history of previous treatment. The combination of these parameters provides a diagnostic classification (categories 1 through 4). The most severe cases are in category 1.

There are standardized treatment regimens for tuberculosis for each diagnostic category. The reasons for matching treatment to diagnostic category are (World Health Organization, 2003):

- To avoid under-treatment of previously treated cases and therefore to prevent acquired resistance
- To maximize cost-effective use of resources and to minimize side effects for patients by avoiding unnecessary over-treatment

Multidrug-resistant tuberculosis (MDR) is a form of tuberculosis that is resistant to at least two of the most powerful first-line anti-tuberculosis drugs. The WHO defines extensively drug resistant tuberculosis (XDR) as MDR plus resistance to any fluoroquinolone and at least one of three injectable second-line drugs. People who have active tuberculosis may develop MDR or XDR when they fail to fulfill their treatment. The best prevention of resistant drug tuberculosis is to ensure full compliance with treatment, and hence, DOT strategy is necessary.

CASE STUDY

Hospital Dr. José Penna (Bahía Blanca, Argentina) gathers data about tuberculosis patients from the south region of Buenos Aires province, an area with a population of over half a million. The Stop TB Programme in Argentina suggests the following algorithm for diagnosis (Ministerio de Salud, 2002):

1. Bacteriology
   a. Rapid direct test for confirming the presence of Mycobacterium tuberculosis.
   b. Sputum and blood culture is recommended selectively and is mainly used to confirm treatment failure and relapse; in pulmonary tuberculosis patients with repeated negative results and have chest radiographic findings suggestive of tuberculosis; in adult patients who are suspected of having extrapulmonary tuberculosis; and in symptomatic children with chest radiographic abnormalities consistent with tuberculosis.
2. Clinical peer review based on cough lasting two-three weeks or more.
3. Chest radiography as a complement to diagnostic since it may be misleading.
4. Tuberculin skin testing is selectively used as diagnostic criterion for tuberculosis because vaccination with bacillus Calmette-Guerin is universal.
5. Histopathological examination is recommended for patients suspected of having extrapulmonary tuberculosis.

Rapid diagnosis and treatment of tuberculosis is important for patients to receive adequate treatment and increase the chances of a successful outcome, but treatment of those without the disease should be avoided. Thus, the purpose of this study is to review current policies of local tuberculosis control programmes for the diagnosis of tuberculosis.

In what follows, we summarize the data understanding and preparation, modeling and evaluation phases of the data mining project. The project motivations have been discussed in the introduction of this chapter.

Data Understanding and Preparation

The project required close cooperation between data analysis experts and physicians not only to interpret results but also to prepare and transform data. Data belonged from different sources and a hard work was necessary to clean and consolidate data in a data warehouse.

We used 1655 records of patients from 1997 to 2006, described by 56 attributes. Data was manually recorded and there is a record for each patient. Some attributes are described in Table 1.

Males represent 56.52% of total cases and 14.8% are patients younger than 15 years. Notification rate for males aged 24-68 is higher compared with females.

There are 1358 cases (82%) of pulmonary tuberculosis and 286 (17.3%) of extrapulmonary disease. There are 11 cases with missing values.

Table 1. Some variables used in the study

Attributes	Description	Range of values
Category	Tuberculosis diagnostic category.	1..4
Plan	Therapeutic plan.	A string denoting any valid plan. There is a standard notation (Ministerio de Salud, 2002).
NMonth	Notification month.	dd/mm/yyyy
SDate	Date of start of treatment	dd/mm/yyyy
Age	Age of patient.	0..100
Weight	Weight.	0..150
Gender	Gender.	*Female, male.*
ReasonEx	Reason of examination.	*S* (Symptomatic), *C* (contact) and *E* (blood or radiographic exam), *E/S, S/C.*
Antecedents	Antecedents of previous treatments.	*O* (original), *R* (Relapse).
Pulmonary tuberculosis	Pulmonary radiography results.	*USC, UCC, BCC, BSC, Primaria, BCC-Miliar, BSC-Miliar, BCGITI* denote different types of pulmonary tuberculosis. *No* indicates no radiographic abnormalities.
Extrapulmonary tuberculosis	Extrapulmonary radiography results.	*Absceso perineal, osteoarticular, pleural,/osteoarticular, otra (utero), urogenital, cutanea, pleural, meningea, cerebral,peritoneal, digestive, meningea/miliar, otra (psoas), ganglionar/urogenital, ganglionar-digestiva, laringea, digestiva-peritoneal, ganglionar, digestive-peritoneal, digestiva-intestinal, ganglionar/otra.* *No* indicates no radiographic abnormalities.
Bacteriology result	Bacteriology or histopathological examination result.	*D* (direct test) , *C* (culture), *B* (biopsy), *ADA*. Examples of valid values are *D(+), D(-), D(++), D(+++), C(-), D(+)C (+), D(+)C (-), D(++)C (+),* and so on.
DDate	Date of death.	dd/mm/yyyy
HIV	HIV.	*Yes* (the patient has a HIV diagnostic), *blank* (not investigated).
MRR	Multidrug-resistant tuberculosis.	*Yes* (multidrug-resistant patient), *blank* (not investigated).
TDO	DOT compliance.	*Yes* (case observed in compliance with national DOTS programme). *No* (case not observed).

Data shows that 88.8% of diagnosed patients assist to a hospital because they have a cough lasting two weeks or more (symptomatic pulmonary patients); 9.2% have been in contact with infected individuals; 1% have abnormalities in blood and radiology exams; and 1% has missing values. Among them, 87.3% are new cases, while 12.2% are relapse illness (a patient previously treated for tuberculosis that has been declared cured or treatment completed, and is diagnosed with bacteriological positive tuberculosis). There are 0.5% of missing values. The notification rate of relapse cases is slightly increasing.

The tendency in the number of smear-positive or negative bacteriology results is fluctuating. However, the number of smear-negative results has been increasing in the last three years.

Modeling and Evaluation

In this study, we aimed to analyze the simultaneous relationship among the independent variables for tuberculosis diagnostic category. We set 0.05 as the level of significance. On the 56 variables that are entered in the Exhaustive CHAID method, the program for the decision tree automatically selects five, and 21 categories are created. The selected variables are *Antecedents*, *Bacteriology result*, *Age category*, *Pulmonary tuberculosis*, and *Extrapulmonary tuberculosis*.

The tree indicates that *Antecedents* is the most important determining factor (see Figures 1 and 2). This first-level split produces the two initial branches of the decision tree: original (O) and relapse (R) cases.

Original cases contain patients of categories 1 and 3 (Node 1). The best predictor for original cases is *Pulmonary tuberculosis*. The split based on *Pulmonary tuberculosis* produces four splits. The best predictor for pulmonary USC and "no" pulmonary tuberculosis (Node 3, Figure 2) is *Bacteriology result*. Smear-negative and positive cases are category 3 (Node 10). Smear-positive cases (Nodes 9 and 11) are category 1. Within these cases, the presence of severe extrapulmonary tuberculosis gives more evidence that the diagnostic tuberculosis category is 1, otherwise it is category 3 (Node 23). Node 11 contains only one smear-negative patient. The dominating class in node 12 is category 3. Further exploration of node 12 showed that the result of 58.7% of cases is not informed (value "NI") and among them, 69.56% are patients under 15 years.

The best split for more severe pulmonary tuberculosis (Node 4) is *Bacteriology result*: 99.2% of smear-positive results are category 1 (Node 13); smear-negative cases are category 1 (Node 14) but the absence of severe extrapulmonary tuberculosis gives more evidence that the diagnostic category maybe 3 (Node 15). Smear-negative cases with negative culture are treated as category 3 (Node 15).

Node 16 depicts severe pulmonary tuberculosis without bacteriological result. Further exploration of data within the node revealed that 37.20% are children less than 15 years without a bacteriology result.

The best split for non-pulmonary cases (Node 5) is *Extrapulmonary tuberculosis*: less severe diseases are category 3 while the rest are category 1. For non- pulmonary tuberculosis (Node 5), splitting on *Extrapulmonary tuberculosis* gives two branches that classify cases as category 3 or 1 according to the type of extrapulmonary disease.

Primary and BCGITI tuberculosis is treated as category 3 in original cases (Node 6).

Finally, relapse cases are category 2 if the bacteriology result is positive (Node 8). However, note that Node 19 is rather heterogeneous and some cases are treated as category 3.

The decision tree has 33 nodes, of which 21 are terminal nodes. Each node depicted in the tree can be expressed in terms of an "if-then" rule (see Table 2).

Figure 1. Exhaustive CHAID classification tree generated from tuberculosis data (N=1655)

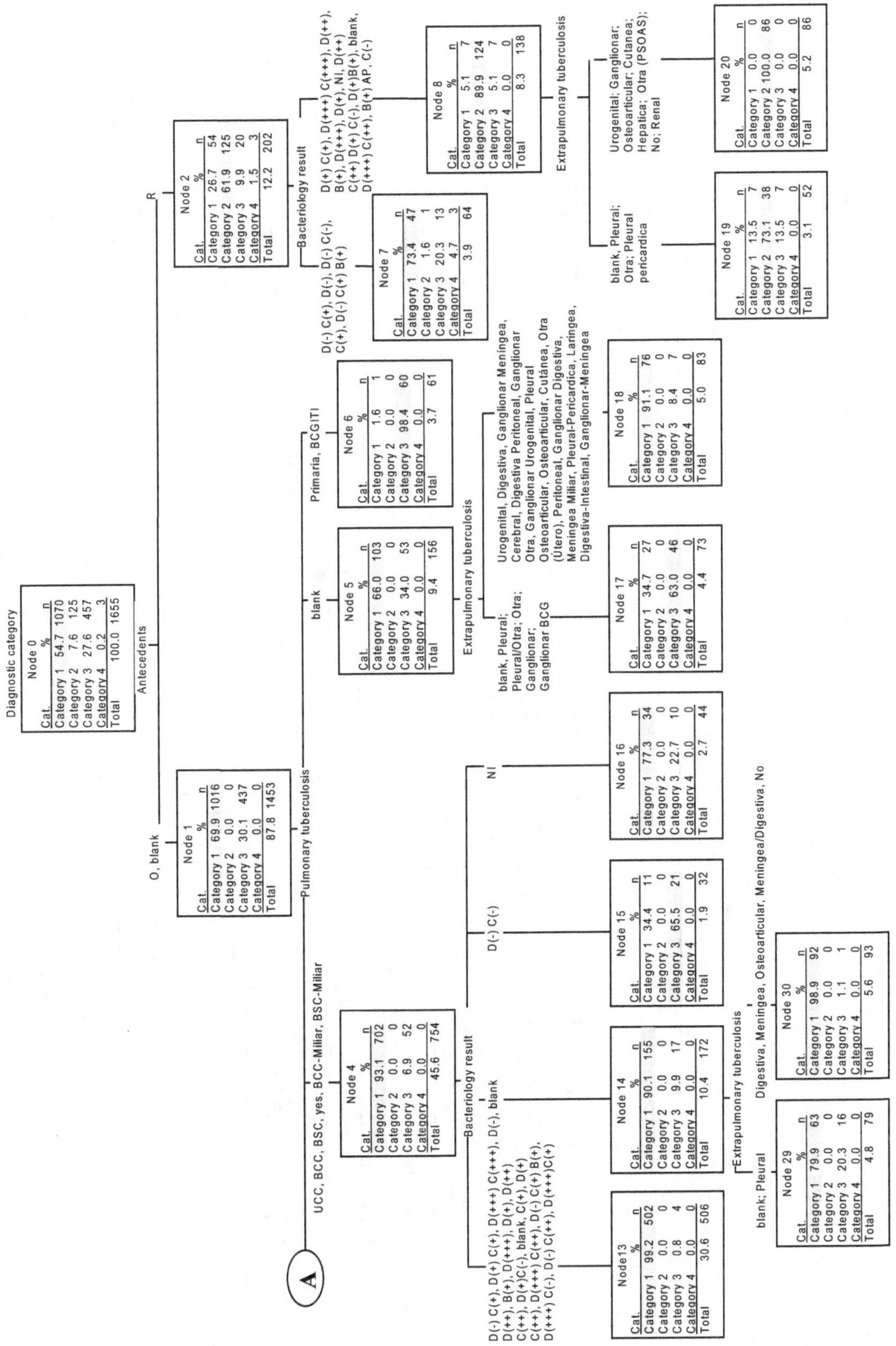

Diagnostic category

Node 0

Cat.	%	n
Category 1	54.7	1070
Category 2	7.6	125
Category 3	27.6	457
Category 4	0.2	3
Total	100.0	1655

Antecedents

O, blank

Node 1

Cat.	%	n
Category 1	69.9	1016
Category 2	0.0	0
Category 3	30.1	437
Category 4	0.0	0
Total	87.8	1453

R

Node 2

Cat.	%	n
Category 1	26.7	54
Category 2	61.9	125
Category 3	9.9	20
Category 4	1.5	3
Total	12.2	202

Pulmonary tuberculosis

A

UCC, BCC, BSC, yes, BCC-Miliar, BSC-Miliar

Node 4

Cat.	%	n
Category 1	93.1	702
Category 2	0.0	0
Category 3	6.9	52
Category 4	0.0	0
Total	45.6	754

blank

Node 5

Cat.	%	n
Category 1	66.0	103
Category 2	0.0	0
Category 3	34.0	53
Category 4	0.0	0
Total	9.4	156

Primaria, BCGITI

Node 6

Cat.	%	n
Category 1	1.6	1
Category 2	0.0	0
Category 3	98.4	60
Category 4	0.0	0
Total	3.7	61

Bacteriology result

D(-) C(+), D(-), D(-) C(-), C(+), D(-) C(+) B(+)

Node 7

Cat.	%	n
Category 1	73.4	47
Category 2	1.6	1
Category 3	20.3	13
Category 4	4.7	3
Total	3.9	64

D(+) C(+), D(+++) C(+++), D(++), B(+), D(+++), D(+), NI, D(++) C(++) D(+) C(-), D(+)B(+), blank, D(+++) C(++), B(+) AP, C(-)

Node 8

Cat.	%	n
Category 1	5.1	7
Category 2	89.9	124
Category 3	5.1	7
Category 4	0.0	0
Total	8.3	138

Bacteriology result

D(-) C(+), D(+) C(+), D(+++) C(+++), D(-), blank D(++), B(+), D(+++), D(+), D(++) C(++), D(+)C(-), blank, C(+), D(+) C(++), D(+++) C(++), D(-) C(+) B(+), D(+++) C(-), D(-) C(++), D(+++)C(+)

Node13

Cat.	%	n
Category 1	99.2	502
Category 2	0.0	0
Category 3	0.8	4
Category 4	0.0	0
Total	30.6	506

Node 14

Cat.	%	n
Category 1	90.1	155
Category 2	0.0	0
Category 3	9.9	17
Category 4	0.0	0
Total	10.4	172

D(-) C(-)

Node 15

Cat.	%	n
Category 1	34.4	11
Category 2	0.0	0
Category 3	65.5	21
Category 4	0.0	0
Total	1.9	32

NI

Node 16

Cat.	%	n
Category 1	77.3	34
Category 2	0.0	0
Category 3	22.7	10
Category 4	0.0	0
Total	2.7	44

Extrapulmonary tuberculosis

blank, Pleural; Pleural/Otra; Otra; Ganglionar; Ganglionar BCG

Node 17

Cat.	%	n
Category 1	34.7	27
Category 2	0.0	0
Category 3	63.0	46
Category 4	0.0	0
Total	4.4	73

Urogenital, Digestiva, Ganglionar Meníngea, Cerebral, Digestiva Peritoneal, Ganglionar Otra, Ganglionar Urogenital, Pleural Osteoarticular, Osteoarticular, Cutánea, Otra (Útero), Peritoneal, Ganglionar Digestiva, Meningea Miliar, Pleural-Pericardica, Laringea, Digestiva-Intestinal, Ganglionar-Meníngea

Node 18

Cat.	%	n
Category 1	91.1	76
Category 2	0.0	0
Category 3	8.4	7
Category 4	0.0	0
Total	5.0	83

Extrapulmonary tuberculosis

blank, Pleural; Otra; Pleural pericardica

Node 19

Cat.	%	n
Category 1	13.5	7
Category 2	73.1	38
Category 3	13.5	7
Category 4	0.0	0
Total	3.1	52

Urogenital; Ganglionar; Osteoarticular; Cutanea; Hepatica; Otra (PSOAS); No; Renal

Node 20

Cat.	%	n
Category 1	0.0	0
Category 2	100.0	86
Category 3	0.0	0
Category 4	0.0	0
Total	5.2	86

Extrapulmonary tuberculosis

blank; Pleural

Node 29

Cat.	%	n
Category 1	79.9	63
Category 2	0.0	0
Category 3	20.3	16
Category 4	0.0	0
Total	4.8	79

Digestiva, Meningea, Osteoarticular, Meningea/Digestiva, No

Node 30

Cat.	%	n
Category 1	98.9	92
Category 2	0.0	0
Category 3	1.1	1
Category 4	0.0	0
Total	5.6	93

Figure 2. Exhaustive CHAID classification tree generated from tuberculosis data (N=1655)

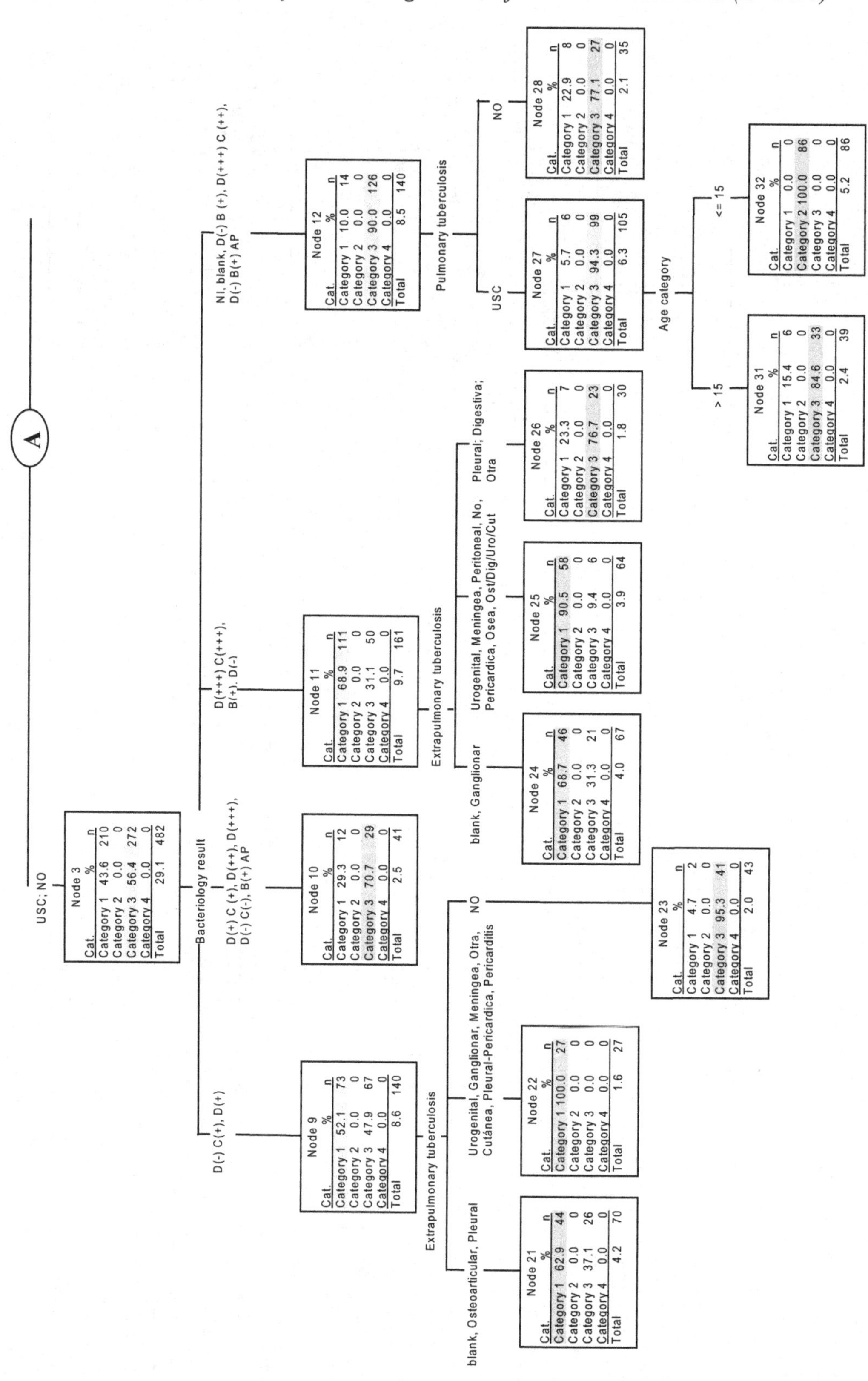

Table 2. Decision rules for prediction of diagnostic categories

Decision rules for the prediction of Diagnostic Category 1						
Node	*Antecedent*	*Pulmonary*	*Bacteriology result*	*Extrapulmonary tuberculosis*	*Age*	*%*
21	O, blank	USC, NO	D(-) C(+), D(+)	blank, Osteoarticular, Pleural	*	62.9
22	O, blank	USC, NO	D(-) C(+), D(+)	Urogenital, Ganglionar, Meningea, Otra, Cutánea, Pleural-Pericardica, Pericarditis	*	100.00
24	O, blank	USC, NO	D(+++) C(+++), B (+), D (-)	Ganglionar, blank	*	68.7
25	O, blank	USC, NO	D(+++) C(+++), B (+), D (-)	Urogenital, Meningea, Peritoneal, No, Pericardica, Osea, Ost/Dig/Uro/Cut	*	90.6
13	O, blank	Type 1	D(-) C(+), D(+) C(+), D(+++) C(+++), D(++), B(+), D(+++), D(+), D(++) C(++), D(+)C(-), blank, C(+), D(+) C(++), D(+++) C(++), D(-) C(+) B(+), D(+++) C(-), D(-) C(++), D(+++)C(+)	*	*	99.2
29	O, blank	Type 1	D(-), blank	blank, Pleural	*	79.7
30	O, blank	Type 1	D(-), blank	Digestiva, Meningea, Osteoarticular, Meningea/Digestiva, No	*	98.9
16	O, blank	Type 1	NI	*	*	77.3
18	O, blank	blank	*	Urogenital, Digestiva, Ganglionar Meníngea, Cerebral, Digestiva Peritoneal, Ganglionar Otra, Ganglionar Urogenital, Pleural Osteoarticular, Osteoarticular, Cutánea, Otra (Útero), Peritoneal, Ganglionar Digestiva, Meningea Miliar, Pleural-Pericardica, Laringea, Digestiva-Intestinal, Ganglionar-Meníngea	*	91.6
7	R	*	D(-) C(+), D(-), D(-) C(-), C(+), D(-) C(+) B(+)	*	*	73.4
Decision rules for the prediction of Diagnostic Category 2						
Node	*Antecedent*	*Pulmonary*	*Bacteriology result*	*Extrapulmonary tuberculosis*	*Age*	*%*
19	R	*	Result 1	Blank, Pleural, Otra, Pleural-pericardica	*	73.1
20	R	*	Result 1	Urogenital, Ganglionar, Osteoarticular, Cutanea, Otra (PSOAS), No, Hepatica, Renal	*	100.0
Decision rules for the prediction of Diagnostic Category 3						
Node	*Antecedent*	*Pulmonary*	*Result*	*Extrapulmonary*	*Age*	*%*
23	O, blank	USC, no	D(-) C(+), D(+)	no	*	95.3
10	O, blank	USC, no	D(+) C (+), D(++), D(+++), D(-) C(-), B(+) AP	*	*	70.7

continued on the following page

Table 2. (continued)

26	O, blank	USC, no	D(+++) C(+++), B(+), D(-)	Pleural, Digestiva, Otra	*	76.7
31	O, blank	USC, no	NI, blank, D(-) B (+), D(+++) C (++), D(-) B(+) AP	*	> 15	84.6
32	O, blank	USC, no	NI, blank, D(-) B (+), D(+++) C (++), D(-) B(+) AP	*	<= 15	100.0
28	O, blank	USC, no	NI, blank, D(-) B (+), D(+++) C (++), D(-) B(+) AP	*	*	77.1
15	O, blank	Type 2	D(-) C(-)	*	*	65.6
17	O, blank	blank	*	blank, Pleural, Pleural/Otra, Otra, Ganglionar, Ganglionar Bcg	*	63.0

*: *Non significant; Type 1: UCC, BCC, BSC, yes, BCC-Miliar, BSC-Miliar; Result 1: D(+) C(+), D(+++) C(+++), D(++), B(+), D(+++), D(+), NI, D(++) C(++) D(+) C(-), D(+)B(+), blank, D(+++) C(++), B(+) AP, C(-); Type 2: UCC, BCC, BSC, yes, BCC-MILIAR, BSC-MILIAR.*

Table 3. Confusion matrix (dependent variable: Diagnostic category)

Observed	**Predicted**				
	Category 1	**Category 2**	**Category 3**	**Category 4**	**Percent correct**
Category 1	989	7	74	0	92,4%
Category 2	1	124	0	0	99,2%
Category 3	104	7	346	0	75,7%
Category 4	3	0	0	0	,0%
Overall percentage	66,3%	8,3%	25,4%	,0%	88,2%

Model Assessment

To see how our tree does in classifying cases, we look at the risk summary to find out what proportion of cases is incorrectly classified. We used a 10-fold cross-validation to assess the models.

The risk summary shows that the current tree classifies almost 88.2% of the cases accurately (see Table 3). In addition, the confusion matrix shows exactly what types of errors are being made. The diagonal elements of the table represent the correct classifications. The off-diagonal elements represent the misclassifications.

For this tree, notice that in 104 cases where people were observed as category 3, we classify them as category 1.

Childhood Tuberculosis

The DOTS strategy is applicable to all patients with tuberculosis, including children. However, there are important differences between children and adults that may affect diagnostic.

Physicians were surprised because attribute *Age* had not appeared as a good predictor variable. Nevertheless, children under 15 years represent 14.8% of the data (245 patients). Hence, if some predictors split the set of child in different nodes, then splitting these nodes would probably not satisfy the stopping rules, and the nodes will not be split. To overcome this, we forced *Age* as the first predictor variable. The first-level split produced the two initial branches of the decision tree: ">15" and "<= 15; blank". The best predictor for patients older than 15 is *Antecedents* and the subtree with node 3 as root is quite similar to the first tree (see Figures 1 and 2).

The best predictor for children is *Pulmonary tuberculosis*, branches with USC, Primary, BCGITI or no radiology evidence are treated as category 3 (Nodes 5 and 7). Cases showing radiology abnormalities consistent with extensive pulmonary tuberculosis (Node 6) are classified as category 1. However, although *Bacteriology result* was the best predictor for *Pulmonary tuberculosis* (Nodes 5 and 6), branches labeled with all the variations of smear-positive results are missing. Compare this with nodes 12 and 20 in the same tree (see Figures 3 and 4). These supported previous findings revealing the poor specificity of direct tests in children (Siddiqi, 2003). Diagnosis based on positive sputum smears is rarely possible in children because they produce little sputum. Further analysis of data revealed that 48.57% of patients less than 15 years have a "not informed" result. This means that the direct test is not performed. The 20.81% of children is smear-negative, and only 19.60% of smear-negative cases has a culture or histopathological examination.

If we consider the whole database, there are 28.56% of negative direct tests, and only 23.55% of these are followed by another test. Microscopy for the detection of the bacilli is rapid and low cost. However, the diagnosis of tuberculosis may be missed initially and this error may incur delays in treatment of 12.5 weeks until the return of a positive culture result (in most cases, culture is not made). Until then, patients receive inadequate treatment and their chances of a successful outcome are reduced. This may contribute to the increasing trend in notification of relapse cases.

We explored 66 cases that are D(-) and C(-). Only 7.6% are cases of patients younger than 15 years. This suggests that the poor specificity of methods is not only due to age. Moreover, 94% of these patients have severe pulmonary tuberculosis. Notice that there are some relapse cases with negative output in the direct and culture tests. As reported by other studies, negative smear could be the result of poor quality smear microscopy (Getahun, 2007; Chintu, 2005).

This situation may have a great impact on children. Children are usually infected with tuberculosis by an adult or an older child with sputum smear-positive pulmonary tuberculosis. Less commonly, they may be infected by contact with smear-negative (often culture-positive) cases. The best way to prevent childhood tuberculosis is therefore by proper identification and treatment of infectious patients (World Health Organization, 2003).

Inconclusive Training Data

Data mining constitutes an important tool in the medical field. By identifying patterns within large volumes of data, data mining provides insight into diseases, shows new ways to classify an unseen case, and may guide a knowledge discovery process.

Decision trees have been already successfully used in medicine, but as in traditional statistics, some real world problems cannot be solved using the traditional way of induction. Decision trees have trouble dealing with inconclusive training data. In our study, the rules generated by the tree are consistent with the WHO tuberculosis diagnostic categories. However, the tree algorithm was unable to obtain a single classification at each leaf node. When we asked the physicians how they usually reach a decision about the right diagnostic category, they reported considerations absent in the database. Hence, the attributes

Figure 3. Exhaustive CHAID classification tree generated from tuberculosis data (N=1655, force Age as first variable)

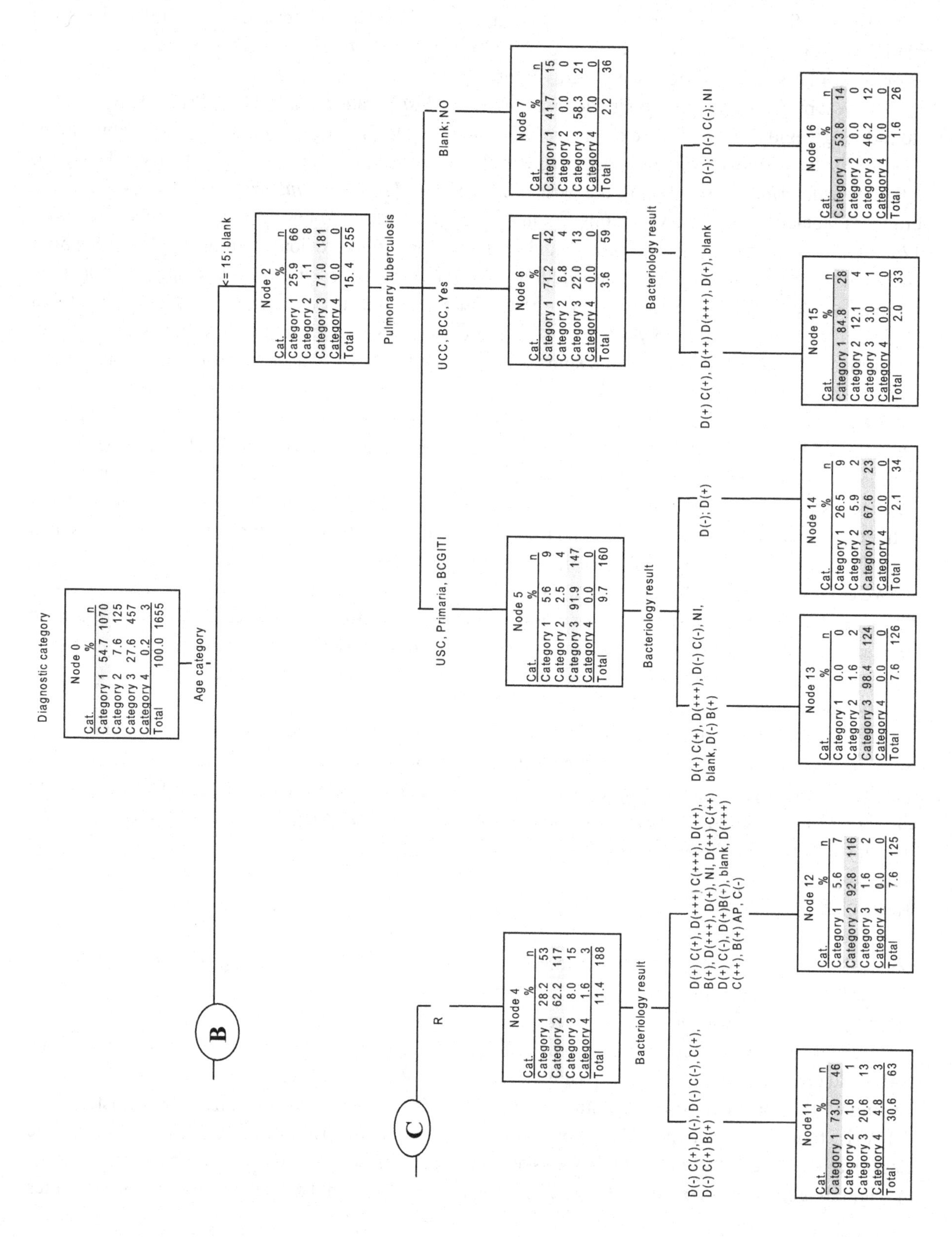

Figure 4. Exhaustive CHAID classification tree generated from tuberculosis data (N=1655, force Age as first variable)

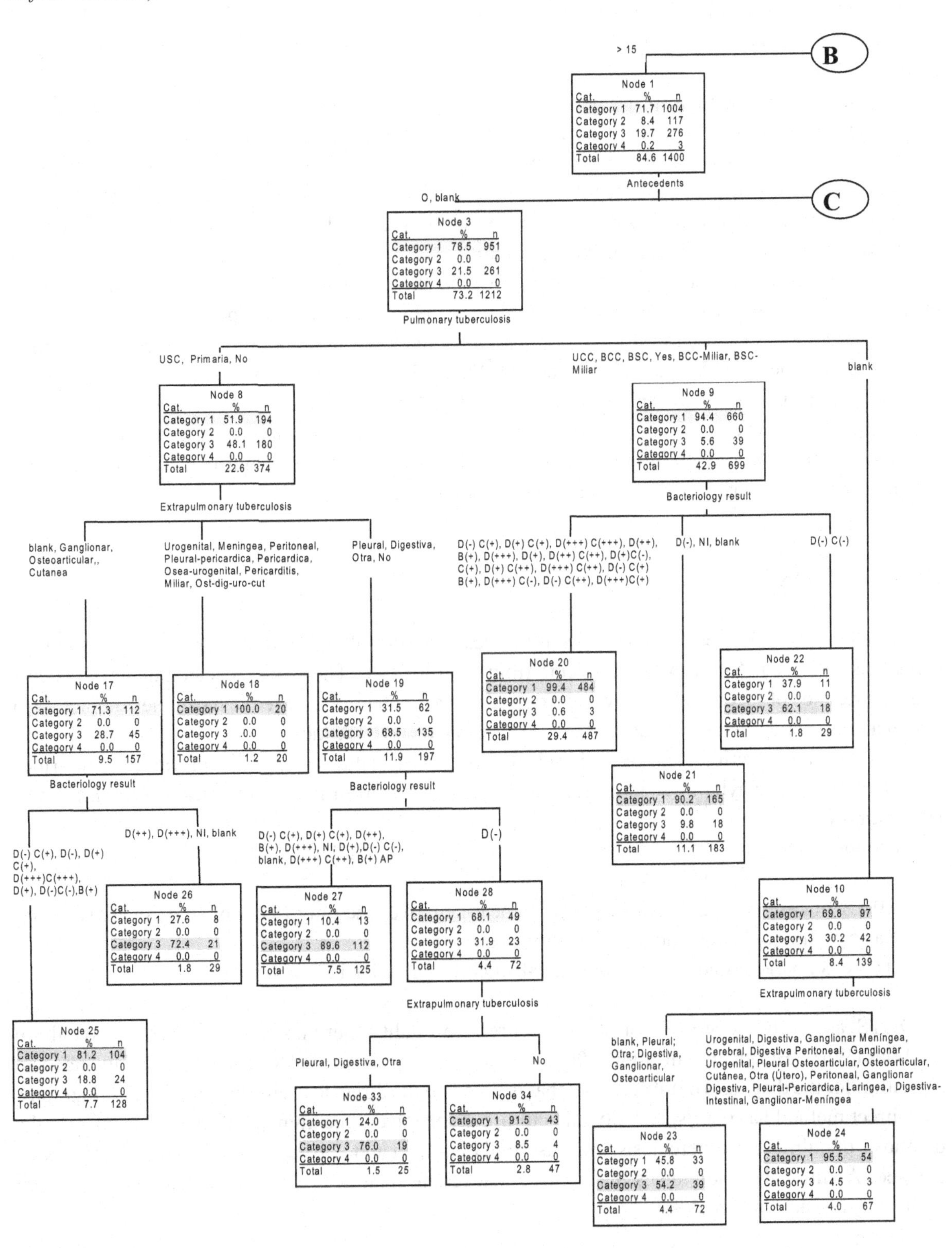

used in describing the examples are not sufficient to specify exactly one outcome for each example. Our attempts to produce a single classification at each leaf node did not work because we obtained overspecialized trees using irrelevant attributes. We used expert opinion to determine at what level the specialization should be stopped before reaching a single classification. Otherwise, the rules were unjustifiably narrow.

This problem is regarded in the literature as inconclusive data sets. Uthurusamy (1993) defines inconclusiveness as follows: given a learning problem expressed in terms of a fixed set of attributes and classes, a training set of examples that are known to be noise-free is inconclusive if there exists no set of rules that classifies all possible (observed and unobserved) examples perfectly using only given attributes. In this case, it is not correct to assume that there should be one class at each leaf node. So automatic pruning is not valid for inconclusive data.

At another facet of this problem, we acknowledge that the explanatory ability of decision trees guided the process of learning which attributes are used by the physician to classify patients.

Another issue arises when splitting is not possible without reaching the stopping rules (for example, the minimum node size). For example, in node 14 (Figure 3), the reason of examination (symptomatic o contact) would have been a good predictor of the diagnostic category (there are 11 symptomatic patients and 23 by contact). The physicians supported that the reason of examination is relevant information. In this case, we set 20 as the minimum node size, and this prevented further splitting. If we set a smaller value, we promote overfitting in another branches of the tree.

CONCLUSION

We aimed to review current policies of local tuberculosis control programmes for the diagnosis of tuberculosis. We used 1655 records of patients from 1997 to 2006. The model revealed that antecedents and the presence of severe pulmonary and extrapulmonary tuberculosis are the most relevant factors to assign a diagnostic category 1. Patients in this category receive the most powerful treatments.

Although the bacteriological result is selected by the algorithm as a predictor variable, the rules resemble that tests maybe misleading. The tree revealed a helpful insight in assessing the impact of late diagnostic.

The most important findings are summarized by the following facts:

- 20.8% of cases younger than 15 years is smear-negative, and only 19.6% of smear-negative cases has a culture or histopathological examination.
- There is no bacteriological test in 48.57% of children under 15 years.

DOTS, as part of the Stop TB Strategy, require high-quality sputum smear microscopy and culture facilities (World Health Organization, 2007b). Argentina adapted the WHO guidelines and included an algorithm for the diagnosis of tuberculosis that is based on the direct test, culture and chest radiography. The direct method has poor specificity and culture is selectively recommended. A longer delay in the diagnosis of pulmonary tuberculosis prevents rapid treatment and, the individual remains without been isolated. Additionally, individuals that receive inadequate treatment are more vulnerable to develop multidrug-resistant tuberculosis.

To summarize, the problem is twofold: (a) poor quality direct tests from inadequate sputum collection, storage, and staining, reading errors, or poor laboratory services; and (b) culture is selectively recommended. Sputum culture should be recommended as the national standard for the diagnosis of tuberculosis.

There were some limitations in this study. Although we included all the variables present in the database, our findings may still be affected by not including universal variables. The database was defined for the purpose of recording DOT data, which is different of knowledge data discovery. Future studies could expand on the variables taken into account. Data about multidrug-resistant cases and HIV is missing for some years. Finally, all cases in this study are collected from a regional database. The case notification rate in this region differs from others. Future work includes cross validating these results among different regions.

REFERENCES

Biggs, D., DeVille, B., & Suen, E. (1991). A Method of Choosing Multiway Partitions for Classification and Decision Trees. *Journal of Applied Statistics*, 18(1), 49–62.

Brieman, L., Friedman, J., Olshen, R., & Stone, C. (1984). *Classification and Regression Trees*. Belmont, CA: Wadsworth International Group.

Cabena, H., Stadler, V., & Zanasi (1997). *Discovering Data Mining. From Concept to Implementation*. Prentice Hall, Inc.

Cios, K., & Moore, G. (2002). Uniqueness of medical data mining. *Journal of Artificial Intelligence in Medicine*, *26*, 263-264.

Chintu C., & Mwaba, P. (2005). Tuberculosis in children with human immuno deficiency virus infection. *International Journal Tuberculosis Lung Disease*, *9*, 477-484.

Fayyad, U., Piatetsky-Shapiro, G., & Smyth, P. (1996). From data Mining to Knowledge Discovery: An Overview. In Fayyad U., Piatetsky-Shapiro G., Smyth P., & Uthurusamy R. (Ed.), *Advances in Knowledge Discovery and Data Mining*, (pp. 1-34). USA: AAAI Press.

Getahun, H., Harrington, M., O'Brien, R., & Nunn, P. (2007). Diagnosis of smear-negative pulmonary tuberculosis in peaple with HIV infection or AIDS in resource-constrained setting: informing urgent policy changes. *Lancet*, 369, 2042-2049.

Jianxin, C., Yanwei, X., Guangcheng, X., Jing, C., Jianqiang, Y., Dongbin, Z., & Jie,W. (2007). A Comparison of Four Data Mining Models: Bayes, Neural Network, SVM and Decision Trees in Identifying Syndromes in Coronary Heart Disease. Lecture Notes in Computer Science. *Advances in Neural Networks, 4491*, 1274-1279.

Mitchell T. (1997). *Machine Learning*. McGraw-Hill.

Prakash, O., & Ghosh, I. (2006). Developing an Antituberculosis Compounds Database and Data Mining in the Search of Motif Responsible for the Activity of a Diverse Class of Antituberculosis Agents. *Journal of Chemical Information and Modeling*, 46(1), 17-23.

Ministerio de Salud (2002). *Programa Nacional de Control de la Tuberculosis. Normas Técnicas 2002. Programa de Vigilancia de la Salud y Control de Enfermedades.* Ministerio de Salud, República Argentina: Imprenta Lux S.A.

Shearer, C. (2000). The CRISP-DM Model: The New Blueprint for Data Mining. *Journal of Data Warehousing, 4*(5), 13-21.

Siddiqi, K., Lambert, M., & Walley, J. (2003). Clinical diagnosis of smear-negative pulmonary tuberculosis in low-income countries: The current evidence. *Lancet, 3*, 288-296.

Šprogar, M., Lenič, M., & Alayon, S. (2002). Evolution in Medical Decision Making. *Journal of Medical Systems, 26*(5), 479-489.

Turban, E., Aronson, J., Ting-Peng, L., & McCarthy, R. (2005). *Decision support systems and intelligent systems.* 7a. ed. Upper Saddle River (N.Y.): Pearson Education.

Uthurusamy, R., Means, L., & Godden, K. (1993). Extracting Knowledge from Diagnostic Databases. *IEEE Expert, 8*(6), 27-38.

Weiss, S., & Indurkhya, N. (1998). *Predictive Data Mining. A Practical Guide.* San Francisco: Morgan Kaufmann Publishers, Inc.

World Health Organization (2003). *Treatment of Tuberculosis: Guidelines for National Programs.* Geneve: WHO. WHO document WHO/CDS/TB_2003.313.

World Health Organization (2004). *Toman's Tuberculosis: Case detection, treatment and monitoring-questions and answers.* Geneve: WHO. WHO document WHO/HTM/TB/2004.334.

World Health Organization (2006). *The World Health Organization Global Tuberculosis Program.* Available at http://www.who.int/tb/en

World Health Organization (2007a). *The five elements of DOTS.* Available at http://www.who.int/tb/dots/whatisdots/en

World Health Organization (2007b). *Global tuberculosis control: surveillance, planning, financing.* Geneve: WHO. WHO document WHO/HTM/TB/2007.376

World Health Organization (2007c). *Tuberculosis fact sheet N° 104.* Available at http://www.who.int/mediacentre/factsheets/fs104/en.

KEY TERMS

Attribute: A quantity describing an instance. An attribute has a domain defined by the attribute type (categorical, quantitative), which denotes the values that can be taken by an attribute.

Cross-Validation: A method for estimating the accuracy (or error) of an inducer by dividing the data into *k* mutually exclusive subsets (the "folds") of approximately equal size. The inducer is trained and tested *k* times. Each time it is trained on the data set minus a fold and tested on that fold. The accuracy estimate is the average accuracy for the *k* folds.

Contact: A person who has spent time with a person with infectious tuberculosis.

Culture: A test to see whether there are tuberculosis bacteria in your phlegm or other body fluids. This test can take 2 to 4 weeks in most laboratories.

DOTS: Directly Observed Therapy Strategy which aims to reduce the transmission of the infection through prompt diagnosis and effective treatment of symptomatic tuberculosis patients at health facilities.

CHAID Algorithm: (Chi square-Automatic-Interaction-Detection). An algorithm to build a decision tree based on the chi-square test of association.

Instance (case, record): A single object of the world from which a model will be learned, or on which a model will be used.

Multidrug-Resistant Tuberculosis: Active tuberculosis disease caused by bacteria resistant to two or more of the most important medicines.

Smear Test: A test to see whether there are tuberculosis bacteria in patient's phlegm. This test usually takes one day to get the results.

Tuberculosis: Tuberculosis is a bacterial infection caused by a germ called *Mycobacterium tuberculosis*. The bacteria usually attack the lungs, but they can also damage other parts of the body.

Chapter XVII
Knowledge-Based Induction of Clinical Prediction Rules

Mila Kwiatkowska
Thompson Rivers University, Canada

M. Stella Atkins
Simon Fraser University, Canada

Les Matthews
Thompson Rivers University, Canada

Najib T. Ayas
University of British Columbia, Canada

C. Frank Ryan
University of British Columbia, Canada

ABSTRACT

This chapter describes how to integrate medical knowledge with purely inductive (data-driven) methods for the creation of clinical prediction rules. It addresses three issues: representation of medical knowledge, secondary analysis of medical data, and evaluation of automatically induced predictive models in the context of existing knowledge. To address the complexity of the domain knowledge, the authors have introduced a semio-fuzzy framework, which has its theoretical foundations in semiotics and fuzzy logic. This integrative framework has been applied to the creation of clinical prediction rules for the diagnosis of obstructive sleep apnea, a serious and under-diagnosed respiratory disorder. The authors use a semio-fuzzy approach (1) to construct a knowledge base for the definition of diagnostic criteria, predictors, and existing prediction rules; (2) to describe and analyze data sets used in the data mining process; and (3) to interpret the induced models in terms of confirmation, contradiction, and contribution to existing knowledge.

INTRODUCTION

The ever-increasing number of electronic patients' records, specialized medical databases, and various computer-stored clinical files provides an unprecedented opportunity for automated and semi-automated discovery of patterns, trends, and associations in medical data. Data mining (DM) techniques combined with the fast and relatively easy access to large databases of patients' records can support clinical research and clinical care. One of the promising applications of DM techniques and secondary data analysis is the creation of clinical prediction rules (CPRs). The major functions of CPRs are to simplify the assessment process, to expedite diagnosis and treatment for serious cases, and to reduce the number of unnecessary tests for low-probability cases. However, before the rules can be used as formal guidelines in diagnosis, prognosis, and treatment, they must be validated on large and diversified populations and evaluated in clinical settings. This lengthy and costly process can be mitigated by automated rule induction from the existing data sources.

The secondary use of previously collected data for supporting the creation and evaluation of CPRs has several advantages: a significant reduction of data collection time and cost, availability of data from wide-ranging populations, access to large data sets, and access to rare cases. Moreover, DM techniques provide flexible and adaptable methods for the *exploratory* as well as the *confirmatory* data analyses. In exploratory analysis, DM techniques can be used to identify potential predictors and generate hypothetical rules. In confirmatory analysis, they can be used to evaluate a hypothesis by confirming, contradicting, or refining.

However, DM techniques alone are not sufficient to address problems concerning secondary analysis of medical data and the complexity of medical reasoning. Each step of the DM process requires integration of medical knowledge — from problem and data understanding, through to model induction, and finally to predictive model evaluation. To achieve this integration, the DM process needs an explicit knowledge representation which should be readable and verifiable by medical experts. Moreover, the models induced by DM techniques should be comprehensible, interpretable, and practical for clinical usage.

In this chapter, we concentrate on two major issues related to the applications of DM techniques in the creation of CPRs: (1) problems associated with the secondary use of medical data, which means that the data were originally collected for other purposes, so they may be only partially suitable for the new DM task; and (2) problems associated with the interpretation of the generated models in the context of existing knowledge. In order to address these two challenges, we have created a new knowledge representation framework, which combines a semiotic approach and a fuzzy logic approach, called by us, a *semio-fuzzy approach*. We have used this new framework to support medical knowledge representation in the diagnosis of obstructive sleep apnea (OSA) (Kwiatkowska & Atkins, 2004).

Our experience with medical DM is based on real clinical records. In our studies, we have used two types of data: patients' records from a specialized clinic and data collected for medical research. In the application of our framework, we focus on two DM phases: pre-processing and post-processing. First, we have constructed a knowledge base (KB) for OSA consisting of diagnostic criteria, known predictors, and existing CPRs. Then, in the pre-processing phase, we use the KB in the analysis of missing values, analysis of outliers, and analysis of the strength of predictors. Finally, in the post-processing phase, we utilize the KB to evaluate the induced models using three criteria: confirmation, contradiction, and contribution.

This chapter is organized as follows. The first section provides background information. The second section describes a new semio-fuzzy framework for medical knowledge representation. The third section shows the application of this framework in the creation of CPRs for OSA and discusses the pre-processing and post-processing DM phases. The final section presents conclusions and suggests directions for future research.

BACKGROUND

In this section, we briefly describe the etiology, diagnosis, and treatment of obstructive sleep apnea. Next, we discuss the role of clinical prediction rules in medicine and describe their creation process. Last, we discuss problems related to secondary use of medical data.

Obstructive Sleep Apnea

Obstructive sleep apnea (OSA) is a common and chronic respiratory disorder afflicting, according to conservative studies, 4% of men and 2% of women (Dement & Vaughan, 1999). This serious respiratory disorder is associated with significant risk for hypertension, congestive heart failure, coronary artery disease, stroke and arrhythmia. Patients with OSA have higher risk during and after anesthesia, since their upper airway may be obstructed as a consequence of sedation. As well, untreated OSA patients have higher rates of car accidents and accidents at work, since a typical symptom of OSA is daytime sleepiness. For these reasons patients should be diagnosed and treated as soon as possible.

OSA is caused by the recurrent collapsing of the upper airway during sleep ("apnea" means "without breath"). The soft tissue blocks the air passage, and the sleeping person literally stops breathing (apnea event) or experiences a partial obstruction (hypopnea event). The total number of apnea and hypopnea events per sleep hour is called the Apnea Hypopnea Index (AHI). An AHI > 15 is indicative of OSA.

Usually, patients are assessed by their family doctors and referred to specialized sleep disorder clinics. The initial assessment involves analysis of risk factors such as daytime sleepiness, snoring, high blood pressure, high body mass index (BMI), witnessed breathing pauses, morning headaches, age, and gender. The final diagnosis of OSA is based on the results from an overnight in-clinic polysomnography (PSG) combined with the results of a sleep questionnaire and the patient's medical history. PSG includes measurements and recordings of various signals during sleep, for example, electro-encephalogram, electro-cardiogram, electro-myogram, blood oxygenation from oximetry, thoraco-abdominal movement, and air flow. While PSG remains the gold standard for the diagnosis of OSA, it is also a costly and time-consuming procedure. Therefore, clinics in smaller centers (in locations lacking fast and easy access to PSG) use an alternative assessment process based on a combination of home-oximetry analysis and the application of CPRs (Mulgrew et al., 2007). This assessment process does not replace the standard in-clinic PSG; however, it can be used in the prioritization of patients awaiting PSG, in the initiation and evaluation of early treatment, and in the rapid screening for OSA in preoperative and postoperative care. While undiagnosed OSA poses risks for the patient, treatment is relatively simple and effective. The treatment of choice for moderate and severe OSA is a continuous positive airway pressure (CPAP), which prevents the upper airway from collapsing by creating a positive pressure in the pharynx during sleep.

Clinical Prediction Rules

Clinical prediction rules (CPRs) in various forms have been in use by medical practitioners for hundreds of years. However, recently, with the increasing acceptance of evidence-based medicine (EBM), CPRs play an even more important role in the clinical decision making process (Ebell, 2001; Knottnerus, 1995). In the authors' opinion, the EBM approach to the diagnosis must be carefully balanced with a casuistic (case-based) model of clinical decision-making. We must emphasize here that in a clinical practice the decisions are based on several factors: empirical evidence, clinical experience, pathophysiologic rationale, and patient values and preferences. Thus, CPRs are not meant to replace human medical experts. On the contrary, the rules are created and used to support and guide humans in making complex decisions to share specialized knowledge. Therefore, we adopt the following general definition of CPRs focusing on their role in medical decision making: "clinical prediction rules (CPRs) are tools designed to improve decision making in clinical practice by assisting practitioners in making a particular diagnosis, establishing a prognosis, or matching patients to optimal interventions based on a parsimonious subset of predictor variables from the history and physical examination" (Childs & Cleland, 2006). Furthermore, the authors view CPRs as a practical method of representing medical knowledge. The validated rules can be organized into useful repositories accessible by health professionals and automated computer procedures to identify patients at high risk.

CPRs have three components: *predictors*, a *calculation method*, and an *outcome*. Predictors are variables obtained from a patient's history, physical examination, and simple diagnostic tests. The calculation methods can be classified into three basic types: logistic scoring, recursive partitioning, and regression equations. The outcome, in most cases, is defined as a probability of a disorder or a specific score value.

We distinguish three approaches to CPR creation: *deductive*, *inductive*, and *integrative*.

1. The **deductive approach** (from hypotheses to data) leads from human-generated hypotheses to tests on data and is based on clinical experience and medical knowledge. This knowledge-driven approach to CPR creation uses mostly primary data sources, in the sense that first a medical hypothesis is formulated, and then the data are acquired to provide evidence or counter-evidence for the hypothesis.
2. The **inductive approach** (from data to hypotheses) generates hypotheses (rules) from clinical data. This data-driven approach is commonly based on DM techniques, which are used to generate predictive models from the *training* data and to evaluate them on the *test* data. The data-driven approach does not generally use existing expert knowledge.
3. The **integrative approach** combines a knowledge-driven approach and a data-driven approach to rule creation. This approach combines the power of the inductive methods with medical reasoning and existing medical knowledge. In this chapter, we describe a framework based on an integrative approach, and we use it for both exploratory and confirmatory purposes.

Secondary Analysis of Medical Data

Data sources can be described as primary or secondary. Primary data sources are data collected for a specific purpose and used for that intended purpose. Secondary data sources involve re-use of previously collected data for a purpose other than the one originally intended. Consequently, primary analysis uses primary data sources and secondary analysis uses secondary data sources.

Medical data are collected for three primary purposes: for individual patient care, for medical research, and for patient administration. For the patient's care, the data are successively obtained, stored, and used by the healthcare practitioners. Since the data acquisition method is driven by the diagnostic, prognostic, or treatment process, the data might be incomplete and exhibit varied granularity. For medical research, data are prospectively acquired through purposely designed clinical trials or epidemiological studies. For patient administration, data are collected and used for accounting and planning.

The secondary analysis of medical data has several advantages: a substantial reduction in data acquisition costs, an increased number of rare cases, and access to data from diversified populations. On the other hand, secondary analysis of data presents challenges related to the contextual nature and intrinsic complexity of medical data. We identify two types of problems: problems *at the data set level* and problems *at the record level.*

Problems at the data set level relate to the characteristics of the entire data set. We discuss two major problems:

1. **Sampling and method biases.** Clinical studies use diverse collection methods, inclusion criteria, sampling methods, sample sizes, types and numbers of measurements, and definitions of outcomes.
2. **Referral/selection and clinical spectrum biases.** In specialized clinics, patients are referred by the primary-care practitioners; therefore, the data represent a pre-selected group with high prevalence of OSA, higher severity of OSA, and co-occurrence of many medical problems (diabetes, hypertension).

Problems at the record level relate to the characteristics of the individual record. We limit our discussion to five major issues relevant to medical DM:

1. **Data heterogeneity.** Medical data originate from several sources. Each source has its own reliability and specific data type, such as numerical measurement, recorded biosignals, coded data, or narrative textual data.
2. **Varied granularity.** Medical data vary from very specific low level raw data (numerical values, biosignals) to information level (features and patterns).
3. **Imprecision.** Many medical concepts, for example, quality of life, sleepiness, and obesity arc difficult to define, measure, or quantify. Therefore, several measurements and their cutoff values are arbitrarily established to allow for decision making. For example, the value of BMI ≥ 30 kg/m^2 is established to indicate obesity; however, somebody with small muscle mass and a BMI = 28 may display higher fat content than somebody who is very muscular and whose BMI = 31.
4. **Incompleteness.** Medical decisions often are based on incomplete data. Clinical records may have missing values for the following reasons: logical exclusion of inapplicable data (data specific to female gender is omitted from a record of a male patient), intentional omission of sensitive data, unavailable information, discontinuation (drop-out) of study, and erroneous omission. Self-reported sensitive data are especially prone to intentional omissions, such as data on smoking habits, and the use of alcohol or recreational drugs.

5. **Corruption.** Medical data originate from multiple sources and various types of equipment; thus, data may display a measurement error, transmission error or data entry error.

A KNOWLEDGE-BASED FRAMEWORK FOR THE CREATION OF CLINICAL PREDICTION RULES

A framework for the creation of CPRs must address three issues: how to represent medical knowledge, how to analyze secondary data, and how to evaluate induced models in the context of existing knowledge. To address these challenges, we have introduced a new knowledge representation framework, a semio-fuzzy framework, which combines semiotic and fuzzy logic methods (Kwiatkowska & Atkins, 2004). In this section, we describe how our framework supports medical knowledge representation and integration into the DM process. First, we review the existing methods for domain knowledge integration within four main fields: data mining (DM), knowledge discovery in databases (KDD), machine learning (ML), and intelligent data analysis (IDA). Second, we introduce our new framework and we briefly describe essential concepts from semiotics and fuzzy logic. Last, we use a semio-fuzzy framework to define predictors and CPRs.

Existing Methods for the Integration of Domain Knowledge

We view data mining (DM) as a part of a larger process of knowledge discovery in databases (KDD). Thus, our discussion applies to both fields. The DM literature includes several discussions on the role of domain knowledge. Han and Kamber (2001) describe in detail concept hierarchy and measures, such as simplicity, certainty, support, and novelty. Witten and Frank (2000) discuss the significance of metadata for defining the attributes; however, they do not present a practical implementation of knowledge-based data analysis. Several methods are available for the integration of domain knowledge into DM in various applications, using different representation methods. For example, ontologies are used in the preprocessing phase to reduce dimensionality, in the mining phase to improve clustering and association rules, and in the post-processing phase to evaluate discovered patterns (Maedche et al., 2003).

Machine learning (ML) research includes several studies on the integration of prior knowledge into inductive learning. Mitchell (1997) describes three methods for combining inductive and analytical learning: knowledge utilization in hypothesis creation, goal alternation, and reduction of search steps. The three systems FOCL (First-Order Combined Learner), INLEN (Inference and Learning), and AVT-DTL (Attribute-Value Taxonomies Decision Tree Learning) represent a broad range of approaches to the integration of the domain knowledge. The FOCL system was created by Pazzani and Kibler (1992). FOCL uses domain theory in generation of candidate rules. Later, FOCL was extended to the FOCL-m system, which uses monotonicity constraints to promote rules consistent with the prior knowledge. The INLEN system was developed by Michalski and Kaufman (1998) for intelligent data exploration. INLEN uses background knowledge such as structured attributes, dependencies between attributes, and DM goals. The AVT-DTL system was developed by Zhang and Honavar (2003) to create decision trees with varied abstraction levels. In general, ML provides methods for knowledge integration into the learning algorithms; however, it does not address the entire DM process in the context of a specific application.

Intelligent data analysis (IDA) uses domain knowledge for the *atemporal* and *temporal* data abstractions (Lavrac et al., 2000). To illustrate atemporal abstractions, we use an example of a patient with BMI = 53 taking Prozac. The *qualitative* abstraction maps from quantitative data to qualitative data: "BMI > 50" is abstracted as "morbid obesity." The *generalization* abstraction maps an instance to a class: "Prozac" is mapped to "antidepressant medication"; and *definitional* abstraction maps from one conceptual category to another conceptual category: "patient is taking antidepressant medication" is mapped to "patient has depression." The focus of IDA is on generating useful information about a single patient. However, an interesting and not fully explored research direction is the use of data abstraction in medical DM.

A New Integrative Framework

The DM, KDD, ML, IDA fields have made significant progress in automated knowledge acquisition from data. Nevertheless, these fields have not fully addressed the main problem in medical DM: the integration of domain knowledge into each step of DM process. Furthermore, knowledge integration requires consolidation of the heterogeneous knowledge and reconciliation of the induced models. First, medical knowledge is not uniform; it originates from sources with different levels of certainty and completeness. Second, in a complex domain such as medicine, new models are not discovered in isolation; they are learned and evaluated in the context of the existing knowledge.

We use the new semio-fuzzy approach to define a consolidated medical knowledge base (KB) composed of facts, rules, and medical references, as shown in Figure 1.

Knowledge Integration into the Data Mining Process

We focus on two key DM phases: pre-processing and post-processing. Figure 2 shows the use of medical knowledge in these two phases. In the pre-processing phase, we concentrate on the data understanding and data preparation using descriptive and prescriptive data models. In the post-processing phase, we concentrate on comparing the generated models with existing CPRs. There are three expected results: *confirmation*, *contradiction*, and *contribution*.

Figure 1. The overall architecture of the knowledge-based data mining process

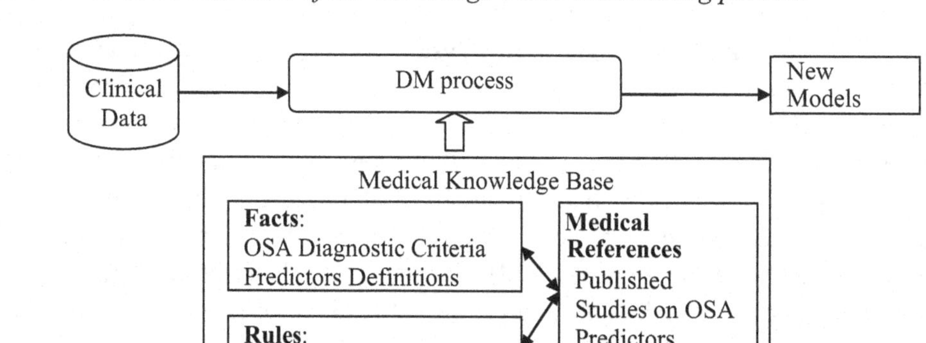

Figure 2. Integration of domain knowledge into the DM process

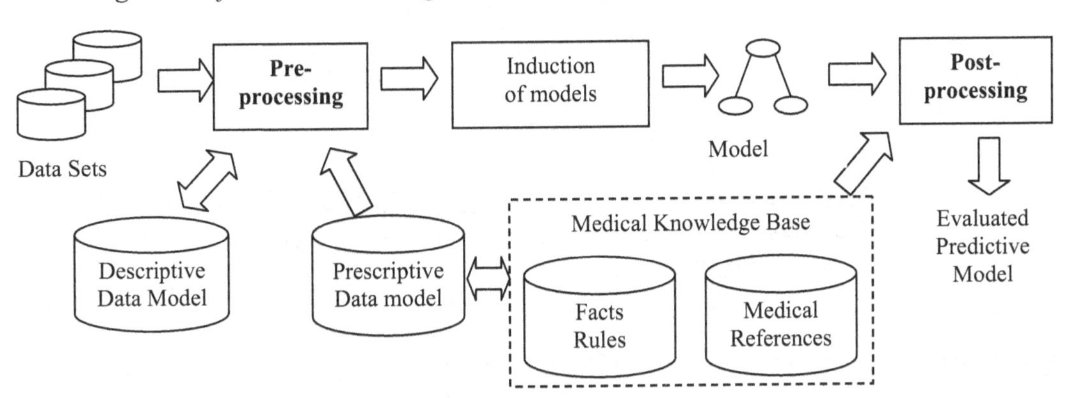

To support the secondary use of medical data in the creation of CPRs, we introduce two models: *descriptive data model* and *prescriptive data model*. The descriptive data model defines the characteristics of a particular data set used for DM: sampled population, sampling techniques, prevalence of disorder, and subgroups' characteristics. The prescriptive data model defines the typical characteristics of the medical data: ranges of possible values, typical values, and typical interdependencies between values.

A Semiotic Approach to Knowledge Representation

Originally, the term 'semiotics' (from the Greek word for sign 'semainon') was introduced in the second century by Galen, who classified semiotics (the contemporary symptomatology) as a branch of medicine (Sebeok, 1999). The use of the term semiotics to describe the study of signs was developed by Ferdinand de Saussure and Charles Sanders Peirce. Peirce defined 'sign' as any entity carrying some information and used in a communication process. Since signs and communication are present in all sciences, the semiotic approach has been used in almost all disciplines, from mathematics through literary studies to ethnography.

Peirce, and later Charles Morris, divided semiotics into three categories: *syntax* (the study of relations between signs), *semantics* (the study of relations between signs and the referred objects), and *pragmatics* (the study of relations between the signs and the agents who use the signs to refer to objects in the world). This triadic distinction is represented by Peirce's semiotic triangle: *concept* (object), *representation*, and *interpretation*.

We demonstrate the semiotic approach using an example of a strong predictor for OSA: obesity. Figure 3 shows the semiotic triangle for the concept (obesity), representation, and interpretation for specific subgroups.

A Fuzzy-Logic Approach to Knowledge Representation

Imprecision, missing or partial information and degrees of uncertainty are inherent in all medical data. Therefore, the traditional approaches of hard computing operating on precise numbers and using categorical approaches of true and false values must be replaced by computational models allowing for degrees of uncertainty, multi-valued logic, and non-monotonic reasoning. Fuzzy logic provides toler-

Figure 3. Semiotic representation for obesity

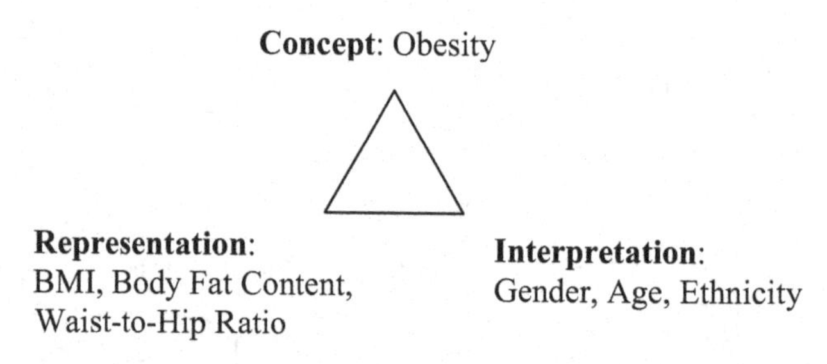

Figure 4. Membership functions (MFs) for BMI for females

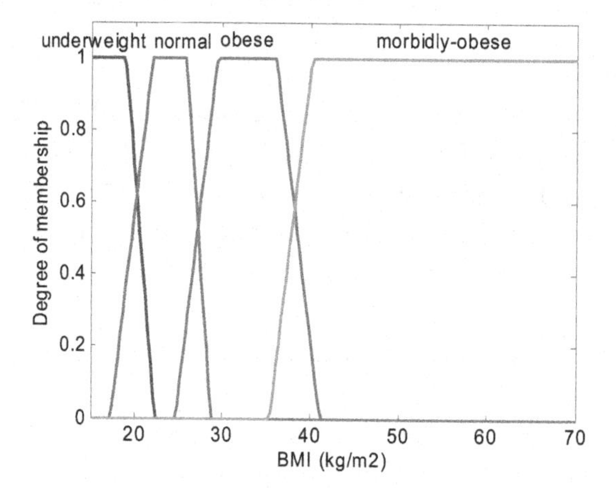

ance for errors, imprecision, and missing information. The history of fuzzy logic started in the 1920's, when Jan Łukasiewicz introduced multi-valued logic. Łukasiewicz extended the traditional two-valued logic {0,1} to a real interval [0,1] representing the possibility that a given value is true or false. While in traditional set theory, an element either belongs to a set or not, in fuzzy set theory, an element may belong to a set 'partially' with some degree of membership. In 1965, Lotfi Zadeh introduced the fuzzy set theory and created fuzzy logic as a new field of study (Zadeh, 1965). Since then, fuzzy logic has been used in several medical applications (Adlassnig, 1986).

We demonstrate the fuzzy-logic approach using again the example of obesity. The concept of obesity is represented by BMI, calculated as weight (kg) / height (m^2), and interpreted in a context of age, gender, and ethnicity. In a fuzzy system, BMI is defined by the linguistic variable $L_B = <X, T(X), U, M>$ where X is the name of the variable, $X =$ BMI, $T(X)$ is the set of possible terms, $T(BMI) =$ {*underweight*, *normal*, *obese*, *morbidly obese*}, U is the universe of discourse: the range of possible values for adults' BMI, U = [15, 70], M is a set of membership functions (MFs) defining the terms, $M = \{\mu_{underweight}, \mu_{normal}, \mu_{obese}, \mu_{morbidly\ obese}\}$. Figure 4 shows the four MFs for BMI. The X-axis corresponds to BMI values and Y-axis corresponds to the degree of membership. We have created the trapezoid MFs to reflect the standards for middle-aged white females. The underweight BMI is less than 19. The normal BMI is between 21 and 26. The BMI values between 19 and 21 are classified as partially underweight and partially normal. Obesity is defined as a BMI ≥ 30 and morbid obesity is defined as a BMI ≥ 40.

A Semio-Fuzzy Framework for the Creation of Clinical Prediction Rules

In this section, we formally define two concepts: predictors and clinical prediction rules, concepts we have already discussed informally.

Predictors

The semio-fuzzy framework addresses the imprecision of predictors and contextualization of the predictor interpretation in the diagnostic process. We define a predictor as an established or suspected symptom, sign, correlate, or co-morbid condition. Therefore, predictors may vary from quantitatively measurable ones such as neck circumference to qualitative predictors such as excessive daytime sleepiness. Our framework describes predictors at Morris' three levels: semantic (conceptualization), syntactic representation (operationalization), and pragmatic interpretation (utilization of measurements). The conceptualization level defines the medical concept (ontology) in terms of its general semantics. The representation level defines the measures of the medical concept. The interpretation level concerns a diagnostic value of the predictor and a practical utility of the predictor in clinical setting. We define a predictor as a quadruple: $P = < C, M, I, KB >$. The predictor conceptualization is represented by *C*, the set of applicable measures for the concept by *M*, and the set of possible interpretations by *I*. *KB* represents a knowledge base, which contains five types of facts: purpose, context, bias, agent, and view.

Clinical Prediction Rules

A clinical prediction rule (CPR) is specified by a rule statement, a certainty factor, and usability. We define a CPR as a triplet: $< RS, CF, U >$, where the rule statement, *RS*, represents the rule's syntax; the rule certainty factor, *CF*, is a part of the rule's semantics; and the usability, *U*, determines the rule's pragmatic value.

- **Rule Syntax**. We use an example to describe the syntax for IF-THEN rules. The rule "IF age > 65 AND gender = male AND hypertension = yes THEN OSA = yes" is comprised of two parts: a premise and a consequent. The premise uses predictors (age, gender, and hypertension) as variables in propositions. A proposition is a logical expression composed of a predictor variable, the relational operator $(<, \leq, >, \geq, =)$, and a value; for example, age > 65. The consequent of the rule specifies the outcome class, OSA = yes.
- **Rule Semantics**. The CPR is a hypothetical statement with two functions: descriptive and predictive. In the descriptive sense, rules characterize the subpopulations of patients with higher or lower risks for the disease. In the predictive sense, rules assess the probability of a new patient belonging to one of the classes. The hypothetical quality of the rule is defined by the certainty factor (CF), a degree of belief ranging from -1.0 (absolute disbelief) to +1.0 (absolute belief), assigned to the rule by medical experts based on their clinical experience.
- **Rule Pragmatics**. A rule's pragmatic value is determined by three criteria: internal validity, external validity, and clinical usability. Internal validity is based on specificity and sensitivity. The external validity is based on rule generality: transferability to a different data set. The clinical usability comprises interpretability, simplicity, and practicality. The rule interpretability and practicality are qualitatively determined by medical experts. The rule simplicity is measured, for example, by the number of predictors.

APPLICATION OF THE SEMIO-FUZZY FRAMEWORK: CONSTRUCTION OF THE KNOWLEDGE BASE FOR OSA

This section describes the application of the semio-fuzzy framework for the creation of a knowledge base (KB) for OSA. The KB includes the definition of OSA diagnostic criteria, the definitions of OSA predictors, and the description of published CPRs for OSA diagnosis.

Definition of OSA Diagnostic Criteria

We define three diagnostic criteria for OSA: AHI score, severity of OSA, and dichotomous approach to OSA diagnosis.

AHI score. The Apnea-Hypopnea Index (AHI) is calculated as the number of apnea and hypopnea events per hour of sleep (Douglas, 2002). An apnea event in an adult is defined as a complete cessation of air flow for at least 10 seconds. However, in some studies an apnea event additionally requires an oxygen desaturation of at least 4%. A hypopnea event is defined as an at least a 10 second event with reduced air flow by at least 50% and, additionally, one or both of two factors: oxygen desaturation drop of 4% or more and brief arousals from sleep. Figure 5 shows different scoring methods for apnea and hypopnea events. The use of diverse scoring criteria for AHI can result in significant differences in apnea diagnoses, especially for patients with low AHI scores.

Severity of OSA. The severity of OSA is established based on the AHI score alone or on a combination of AHI score and symptoms. In the diagnosis based solely on the AHI, apnea is classified as *mild* for AHI between 5 and 14.9, *moderate* for AHI between 15 and 29.9, and *severe* for AHI ≥ 30. The combination of AHI and symptoms is used, for example, by the International Classification of Sleep Disorders (Rosenberg & Mickelson, 2003). As shown in Table 1, the severity of OSA is defined in terms of the AHI, the degree of oxygen desaturation, and the severity of excessive daytime sleepiness (EDS).

A dichotomous approach to OSA diagnosis. The presence or absence of OSA is often established based on an arbitrary cutoff value for AHI. Many existing studies use the value AHI ≥ 15 as an indication of OSA. However, some studies use AHI ≥ 10 or even AHI ≥ 5 (Lam et al., 2005).

Definitions of OSA Predictors

In this subsection, we provide a classification of OSA predictors and describe an example of a KB for neck thickness, a well-known predictor of OSA.

Figure 5. AHI scoring methods

AHI = (# apnea event + # hypopnea event) / total hours of sleep
Apnea event = 100% air flow cessation ≥ 10 s
Apnea event = 100% air flow cessation ≥ 10 s AND Desaturation ≥ 4%
Hypopnea event = ≥ 50% air flow cessation ≥ 10 s
Hypopnea event = ≥ 50% air flow cessation ≥ 10 s AND (Desaturation ≥ 4% OR sleep arousal)

Table 1. Severity of OSA

OSA Severity	AHI	O_2 Desaturation	EDS
Mild	5-14	Mild	Mild
Moderate	15-29	Moderate	Moderate
Severe	≥ 30	Severe	Severe

Figure 6. KB for neck circumference

Purpose: Diagnostic Significance
KB1: A large neck is a characteristic sign of OSA [#3 – #10].
NC is correlated with AHI ($r^2 = 0.12$, $p < 0.005$) study of 169 male patients [#2]
NC > 43.2 cm for men and NC > 40.6 cm for women indicate risk for apnea [#11]

Context: Subpopulations
KB2 (Gender): In general, NC is significantly larger in men than in women [#1, 3, 6, 9, 10].
KB3 (Ethnicity): In general, Asians tend to have smaller necks than whites [#3].

Bias: Dependencies between Predictors
KB4 (BMI): People with higher BMI are expected to have larger NC. However, BMI appraises generalized obesity, while, the larger NC reflects the upper-body obesity, typical for men [#1]. NC was shown to be smaller in women despite a larger BMI [#7].

Agent: Patients and Health Professionals
Observation 1: Many patients do not know their NC (collar size).

View: Measurement Interpretation
KB5: NC for adults ranges 25-65 cm. Typical male NCs range 42-45 cm [#2]. Mean NC for women 36.5 ± 4.2 and 41.9 ± 3.8 for men [#1]. Male NCs can be described as small to normal (< 42), intermediate (42-45), and large (> 45) [#2].

We divide OSA predictors into six categories: (1) anatomical signs: obesity, large neck size, and craniofacial and upper airway abnormalities, (2) demographic factors: gender and age, (3) nocturnal symptoms: snoring, witnessed apnea (WA), breathing pauses, and choking, oxygen desaturation, (4) diurnal symptoms: excessive daytime sleepiness (EDS), (5) coexisting medical conditions: hypertension (HTN), depression, diabetes, and coronary artery disease; and (6) lifestyle factors: smoking habits and alcohol use.

In the OSA diagnostic process, neck thickness is operationalized as a neck circumference (NC). The NC can be (1) physically measured by a healthcare practitioner or (2) self-reported by a patient answering the question, "What is your collar size?"

We have created a KB for NC based on 11 published medical studies: #1 (Dancey et al., 2003); #2 (Ferguson et al., 1995); #3 (Lam et al., 2005); #4 (Millman et al., 1995); #5 (Ryan & Love, 1996); #6 (Rowley et al., 2000); #7 (Rowley et al., 2002); #8 (Jordan & McEvoy, 2003); #9 (Whittle et al., 1999); #10 (Young et al., 2002); #11(Woodson, 2003); and consultations with specialists from two respiratory clinics. Our findings are summarized in Figure 6.

Using a fuzzy-logic approach, the predictor NC is defined as a linguistic variable L_{NC} :

$$L_{NC} = \langle NC, \{small, normal, large, very\ large\}, [25, 60], \{\mu_{small}, \mu_{normal}, \mu_{large}, \mu_{very\ large}\} \rangle$$

where *NC* is the name of the variable. The terms {*small, normal, large, very large*} and the universe of discourse, the range 25-60 cm, have been created based on KB5. The four MFs define the degree of membership for specific NC values, as shown in Figure 7.

Figure 7. Membership functions (MFs) for neck circumference (NC) for females

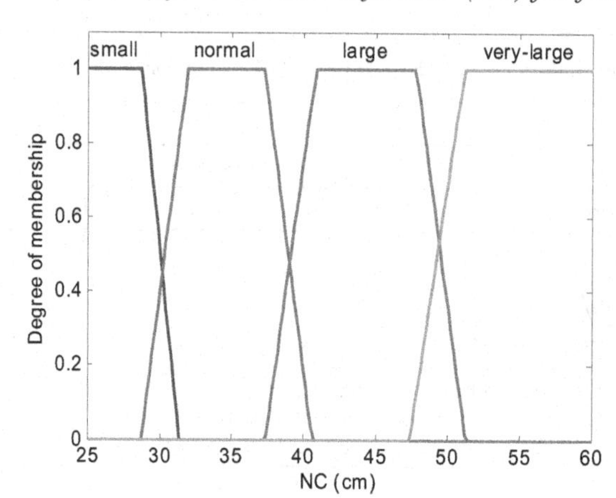

OSA Clinical Prediction Rules

Medical literature describes a wide range of CPRs for the diagnosis of OSA. We describe here seven representative models to exemplify the variability of the predictors, calculation methods, and outcomes:

- **Model #1** (Crocker et al., 1990) calculates P(OSA) = $e^x/(1+e^x)$ (AHI $\geq$ 15) using logistic function: x = -13.9 + 0.06 (Age) + 2.98 (WA) + 0.23 (BMI) + 1.35 (HTN), where WA (witnessed apnea) = 1 if present, 0 if absent; and HTN = 1 if present, 0 if absent.
- **Model #2** (Viner et al., 1991) calculates P(OSA) (AHI $\geq$ 10) using logistic function: x = -10.5132 + 0.9164 (gender) + 0.0470 (Age) + 0.1869 (BMI) + 1.932 (Snoring), where gender = 1 for male, 0 for female; and snoring = 1 if present, 0 if absent.
- **Model #3** (Maislin et al., 1995) calculates P(OSA) (AHI $\geq$ 10) using logistic function: x = -8.16 + 1.299 (Index) + 0.163 (BMI) – 0.025 (BMI*Index) + 0.032 (Age) + 1.278 (gender) where gender = 1 for male, 0 for female; Index = (sum of frequencies / number of symptoms present) of three nocturnal symptoms: (1) snorting/gasping, (2) loud snoring, (3) breath stopping/choking/struggling. The symptoms are measured on a scale from 0 to 4, where never = 0, rarely = 1, 1-2 times per week = 2, 3-4 times per week = 3, 5-7 times per week = 4.
- **Model #4** (Flemons et al., 1994) calculates a sleep apnea clinical score (SACS), which corresponds to the predicted value of AHI. SACS = 10^x + 1, where x = -2.132 + 0.069 (NC) + 0.31(HTN) + 0.206 (HS) + 0.224 (PR), where HTN = 1 if present, 0 if is absent; HS (habitual snorer) = 1 if yes, 0 if not; and PR = 1 if nocturnal choking/gasping is reported, 0 if not.
- **Model #5** (Roche et al., 2002) calculates P(OSA) (AHI $\geq$ 15) for obese symptomatic patients (BMI $\geq$ 25) using logistic function: x = -4.31 + 1.41(Gender) + 0.03(CT_{80}) + 0.78 (CS) where gender = 1 for male, 0 for female; and CT_{80} = cumulative time spent below 80% of arterial oxygen saturation; CS = clinical score which is a sum of four variables (score 0 or 1): habitual snoring, interrupted nocturnal breathing, EDS, and hypertension.
- **Model #6** (Roche et al., 2002) calculates the AHI for obese symptomatic patients (BMI $\geq$ 25), AHI = -7.24 + (7.04 * CS) + 0.38 * CT_{80}.

- **Model #7** (Sharma et al., 2004) uses a scoring equation to predict OSA ($AHI \geq 15$) for obese asymptomatic patients ($BMI \geq 25$): OSA score = 1.378(Gender) + 0.064(WHR) + 0.21(NC) where gender = 1 for male, 0 for female; WHR= waist-to-hip ratio. Score > 16.62 indicates OSA.

These models use three categories of outcomes: probability of OSA, calculated value for AHI, and a dichotomous outcome (OSA yes/no). Models #1, #2, #3, #5 use logistic regression to calculate a probability of OSA (defined as $AHI \geq 15$ or $AHI \geq 10$). Models #4 and #6 calculate the predicted value for AHI. Model #7 uses logistic scoring to provide binary outcome: OSA or non-OSA (defined as $AHI \geq 15$).

The analyzed models use 11 predictors summarized in Table 2.

APPLICATION OF THE SEMIO-FUZZY FRAMEWORK: INTEGRATION OF KNOWLEDGE IN THE PRE-PROCESSING PHASE

This section describes the application of the semio-fuzzy framework in the pre-processing phase of the DM process. First, we present construction of descriptive and prescriptive data models. Second, we discuss three examples of data analysis: analysis of missing data, analysis of outliers, and analysis of the strength of predictors within the context of specific population subgroups.

Construction of the Descriptive Data Model

Data sets characteristics. To develop CPRs for OSA diagnosis, we use two types of secondary data sources: data collected and used in research studies and patients' records. We use three data sets obtained from the Sleep Disorders Program, Vancouver Acute Hospitals:

- Data set *A* (795 records) had been collected and used in a clinical study of the correlation between OSA and periodic limb movements in sleep (PLMS). The results were published by Al-Alawi et al. (2006).

Table 2. OSA predictor category, predictors, and occurrence in CPR models

Category	Predictor	Occurrence
Anatomical Signs	Body Mass Index, BMI	Model #1 #2 #3
	Neck circumference, NC	#4 #7
	Waist to Hip Ratio, WHR	#7
Demographic Factors	Gender	#2 #3 #5 #7
	Age	#1 #2 #3
Nocturnal Symptoms	Snoring	#2 #3 #4 #5 #6
	Witnessed Apnea, WA	#1 #3 #5 #6
	Snorting/Gasping	#3 #4
	Desaturation (from Oximetry)	#5 #6
Diurnal Symptoms	Excessive Daytime Sleepiness	#5 #6
Coexisting Medical Conditions	Hypertension, HTN	#1 #4 #5 #6

- Data set *B* (239 records) had been collected and used in a clinical study of the correlation between OSA and craniofacial features. The results were published by Lam et al. (2004).
- Data set *C* (499 records) had been compiled from the patients' questionnaires and PSG results. The records from data set *C* were randomly split into a training set, C_{train}(n = 251), and a testing set, C_{test} (n = 248).

In the pre-processing phase, we analyze (1) the prevalence of OSA based on diagnostic criteria described in the KB and (2) the sampled population.

OSA Prevalence. Files *A*, *B*, and *C* use the AHI values obtained from PSG, as the diagnostic standard for OSA. In our data analysis, we apply the dichotomous diagnostic approach. To analyze the prevalence of OSA, we use three cutoff criteria: AHI ≥ 5, AHI ≥ 10, and AHI ≥ 15. The results, shown in Table 3, demonstrate significant differences in prevalence of OSA for each of the cutoff values.

Sampled Population. The clinical data sets *A*, *B*, and *C* are based on the records of patients referred to the specialized clinics by their primary care physicians. Using the data of patients who have been referred increases the prevalence of OSA.

Construction of the Prescriptive Data Model

The prescriptive model uses anatomical typicality measure (ATM) to evaluate each data instance relative to predefined biomedical rules (Kwiatkowska et al., 2007). A fuzzy inference system calculates the ATM (ranging from 0 to 1) based on a NC, BMI, and Gender (knowledge fact KB4). For example, an adult female patient, who is underweight (BMI = 18), and has a large neck (NC = 43 cm) would be considered anatomically atypical (ATM < 0.5).

Analysis of Missing Values

In this subsection, we describe how the knowledge-based approach is used for analysis of missing values. We use the data on smoking habits to illustrate analysis of sensitive data with a large proportion of missing data. Smoking habits are operationalized as a self-reported variable used in the OSA questionnaires. In general, smoking can be reported as "history of smoking" and "currently smoking." Furthermore, smoking can be represented by a categorical variable (yes/no) or a continuous variable indicating the number of cigarettes smoked per day, week, or year.

In data set *A*, smoking habits are reported as a "currently smoking" (yes/no). The variable has the following distribution of values: "no" = 495 (52 %), "yes" = 118 (15 %), and "missing values" = 182 (23 %). Interestingly, the missing values have a higher rate than the answer "yes." We conclude that the

Table 3. Prevalence of OSA using three cutoff criteria

Data Set	Prevalence of OSA based on AHI cutoff values		
	AHI ≥ 5	AHI ≥ 10	AHI ≥ 15
A (N = 795)	92 % (731)	79 % (625)	66 % (523)
B (N = 233)	84 % (195)	70 % (162)	59 % (137)
C_{train} (N = 251)	83 % (207)	68 % (170)	52 % (130)

"currently smoking" variable cannot be used as a predictor for two reasons. First, 23% of the patients did not answer the question "Do you currently smoke?" Second, many patients with serious respiratory problems quit smoking and will answer "no" for that question.

Analysis of Outliers

Outlier detection is an important subject studied in statistics and, recently, in the context of the DM process. The statistical methods have been successfully used for the detection of univariate and multivariate outliers in homogeneous samples. However, these quantitative methods are sensitive to non-homogeneous samples with multiple subgroups displaying different patterns. Medical DM uses data sets from heterogeneous groups, often with skewed distributions. Thus, we have used the prescriptive data model, and we have calculated an ATM for all instances from data set *B*. Using the ATM, we have identified two medical outliers which we define as instances with ATM < 0.5: outlier *O1* (gender = female, ethnicity = Asian, weight = 86 kg, height = 161 cm, BMI = 33.18, NC = 43 cm) and outlier *O2* (gender = male, ethnicity = white, weight = 70 kg, height = 176 cm, BMI = 22.6, NC = 30.8 cm). Both outliers were not detected by a simple univariate outlier analysis; however, they were detected after dividing the data sets into gender groups and further splitting them into ethnicity subgroups based on KB2 and KB3.

Analysis of the Strength of a Predictor

We use data set *B* to study NC as a predictor for AHI, because this variable is based on the clinically measured NC. Interestingly, in data set *C*, NC is based on self-reported NC and it has 41 % missing values (this confirms Observation 1 from the KB). We study the correlation between NC and AHI based on KB1. Table 4 shows values for the Pearson's correlation r and the coefficient of determination r^2 for the specific subgroups created based on the KB2 and KB3.

Pearson's correlation r is noticeably different for each of the subgroups. However, these differences are not statistically significant (two-tailed z-test at 95% confidence). There are several possible reasons for not achieving statistical significance, for example, a low ratio of females to males 40:193. Furthermore, the r^2 for all males ($r^2 = 0.04$) is noticeably lower than the r^2 reported in KB1 ($r^2 = 0.12$). We observe that the strength of the predictor changes within each specific subgroup. Therefore, medical knowledge is necessary to identify subgroups in mixed populations.

Table 4. Pearson's correlations and linear regression between NC and AHI for data set B

Data set *B* (*N = 233*)	Pearson's r	r^2
All Patients (N = 233)	0.29(**)	0.08
Women (n = 40)	0.37(*)	0.14
Men (n = 193)	0.19 (**)	0.04
Asian (n = 161)	0.27 (**)	0.08
white (n = 72)	0.41 (**)	0.16

** *Correlation is significant at the 0.01 level (two-tailed)*
* *Correlation is significant at the 0.02 level (two-tailed)*

APPLICATION OF THE SEMIO-FUZZY FRAMEWORK: INTEGRATION OF KNOWLEDGE IN THE POST-PROCESSING PHASE

In this section, we describe knowledge-based interpretation of the induced models in terms of *confirmation*, *contradiction*, and *contribution*. We have concentrated on two types of predictive models: logistic regression (LR) and decision tree (DT). For all models, we use AHI $\geq$ 15 as a cutoff value for OSA.

Logistic Regression Model

We have used a logistic regression (LR) model for two reasons: (1) the existing CPRs (Models #1, #2, #3, and #5) use LR and (2) LR can be used for explanation of prediction. We have induced LR1 model from data set C_{train} using a logistic model tree algorithm provided by the open-source Weka repository (Witten & Frank, 2005). The LR1 model calculates P(OSA) = $e^x/(1+ e^x)$, where x = -5.03 + 0.28(Gender) + 0.07(BMI) - 0.19(Depression) + 0.24(HTN) - 1.49(Diabetes) + 0.02(Age) + 0.4(Snoring). The variables are listed in Table 5. In data set C, snoring is reported using a Likert scale from 1 to 5, as 1 = never, 2 = rarely, 3 = sometimes (1-2 nights/week), 4 = frequently (3-4 nights/week), and 5 = almost always.

Decision Tree Model

We have used a decision tree (DT) model for three reasons: (1) it is easily comprehensible by humans, (2) it is easily convertible into a set of rules, and (3) it provides intuitive graphical representation supporting explanations of predictions. We have generated three models from files *A*, *B*, and *Ctrain* using the decision tree learner J48 (based on C4.5) provided by the Weka repository (Witten & Frank, 2005). Model DT1 generated from data set *A*, model DT2 generated from data set *B* and model DT3 generated from data set *Ctrain* are shown in Figure 8, Figure 9, and Figure 10. In the three figures, the leaves (rectangles) indicate the prevailing class, the total number of instances in a specific branch, and the total number of instances erroneously classified. For example, in Model DT1, the right most branch represents a rule: "IF BMI > 26.8 AND HTN = yes THEN OSA = yes." The corresponding leaf specifies OSA (200.0/47.0), which means that 200 records have BMI > 26.8 and htn = yes. However, out of 200 records, 47 instances

Table 5. Variables, their coding, and ORs

Variables	Coding for LR	Odds Ratio
Gender	0-female, 1-male	1.32
BMI	continuous	0.93
Depression	0-no, 1-yes	1.21
HTN	0-no, 1-yes	0.79
Diabetes	0-absent, 1-present	4.44
Age	continuous	0.98
Snoring	1, 2, 3, 4, 5	0.67

Figure 8. Decision tree induced from data set A (N = 795), Model DT1

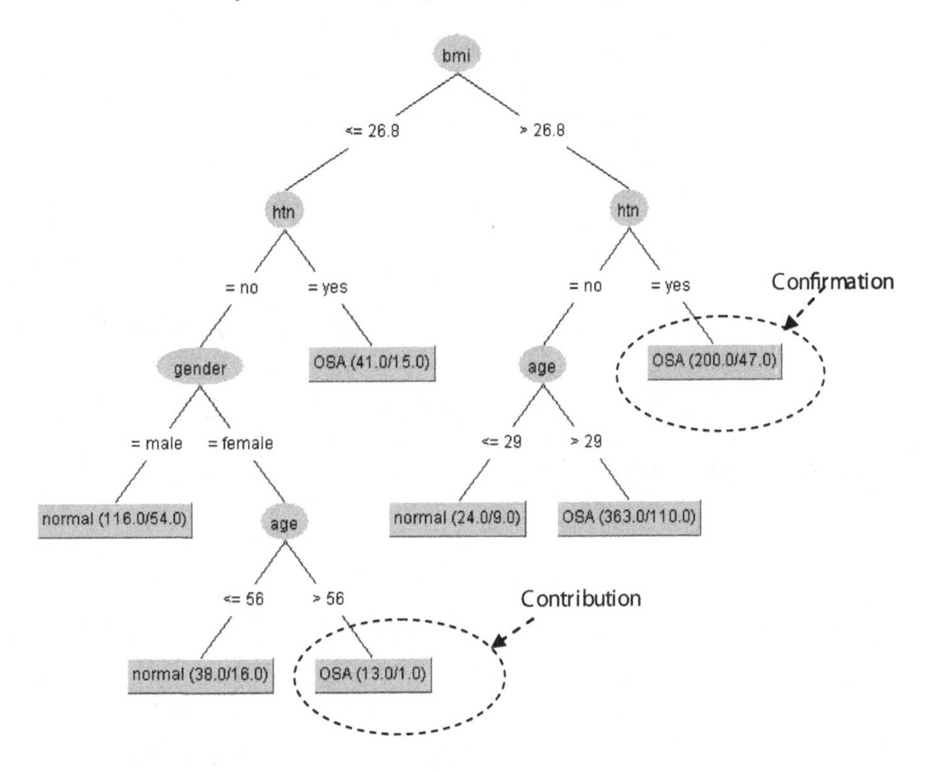

Figure 9. Decision tree induced from data set B (N = 239), Model DT2

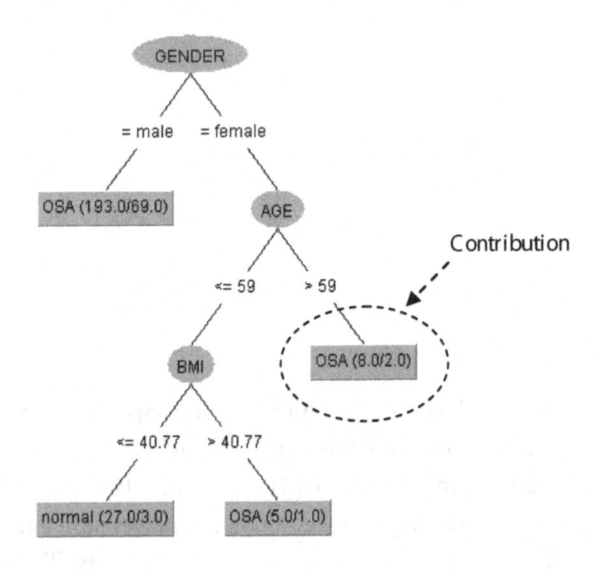

Figure 10. Decision tree induced from training data set C_{train} (N = 251), Model DT3

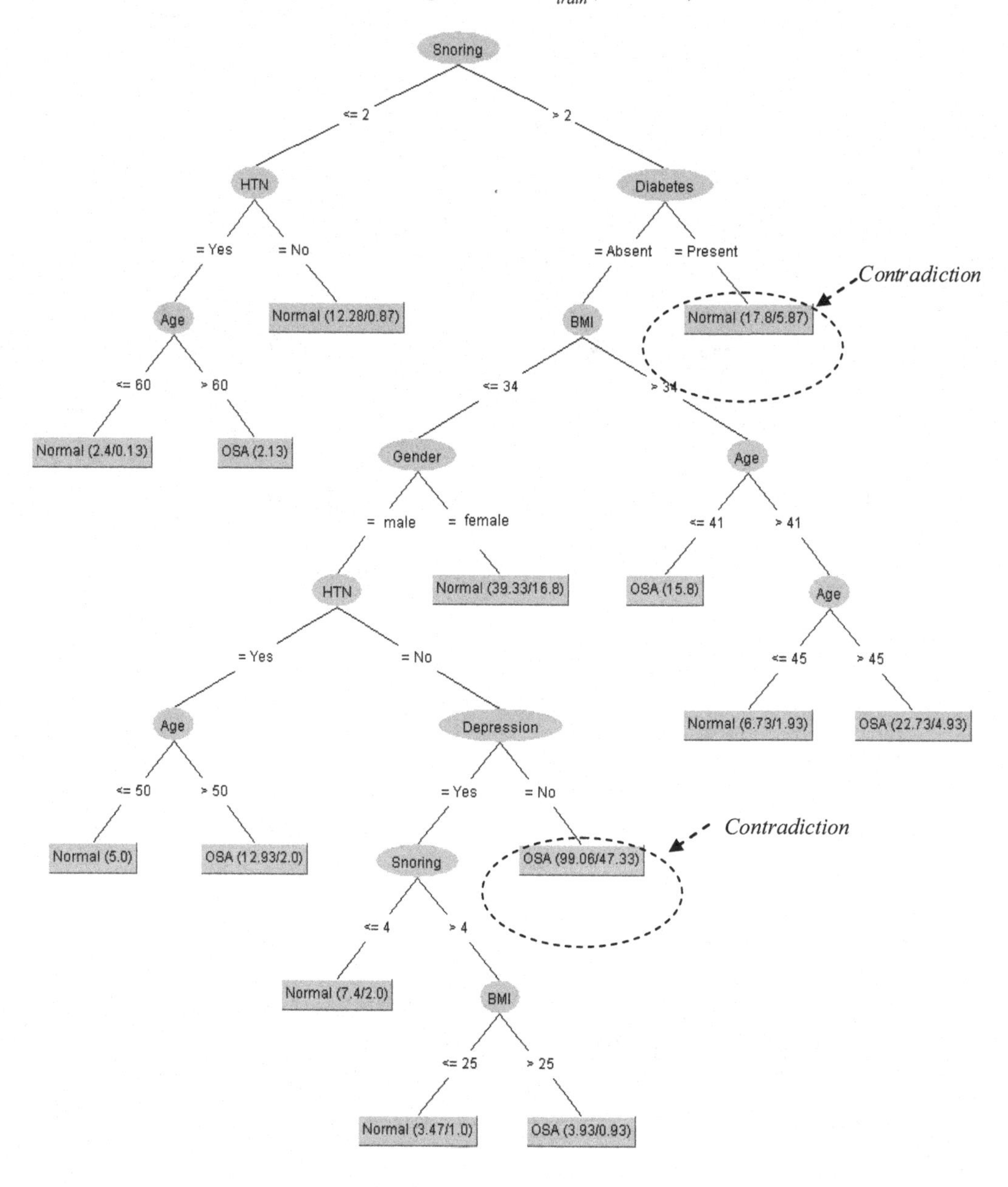

do not have OSA. Thus, the rule has 25.2 % (200/795) support and 76.5 % (153/200) accuracy. Also, using the same figures, we have indicated examples of confirmation, contradiction, and contribution. In DT1, we have marked the right most node (BMI > 26.8 and HTN = yes) as **confirmation,** since the corresponding rule confirms the existing knowledge that hypertension and higher BMI are good predictors of OSA. In DT3, we have marked two nodes as **contradictions**. These two contradictions will be discussed in detail in the subsection on evaluation of induced models. In DT1 and DT2, we have marked two nodes as **contributions**, since they provide a new insight. Interestingly, they divide female patients into particular age groups (age > 56 in DT1 and age > 59 in DT2). This specific age-based division for females can be associated with an increased risk of OSA among postmenopausal women.

Evaluation of the Induced Models

After generation of models from the data, we perform two steps. In step 1, we interpret LR and DT models for individual predictors to examine how the models confirm each other, provide contradictory examples, or identify new insights. In step 2, we compare the induced models with the existing prediction rules stored in the KB. We use two models, LR1 and DT3, to demonstrate the knowledge-based interpretation. Both models were generated from the training set (n = 251) and tested on a separate testing set (n = 248). The overall sensitivity and specificity of these models are low. For example, DT3 model tested on the test set has sensitivity = 59% and specificity = 56%. However, we must point out that the OSA assessment process is not based on the CPRs alone, but on a combination of home-oximetry and the rules (Mulgrew et al., 2007).

Step 1: Interpretation of Single Predictors from LR1 and DT3

We interpret separately each of the predictors using two models, LR1 and DT3, derived from the same data set *Ctrain*. The odds ratios and coding for each variable are shown in Table 5. The odds ratio is defined as the probability of occurrence over probability of non-occurrence of OSA.

- **Gender.** In the LR1 model, gender has an odds ratio, OR = 1.32, which means that if the gender of an instance is changed from female to male (leaving the values of other predictors the same), the odds of having OSA increase by 1.32. In the DT3, gender is used in one node at the fourth level. The rule, "Snoring > 2 AND Diabetes = Absent AND BMI ≤ 34 AND gender = female THEN outcome = normal" classifies instances as non-OSA.
- **BMI.** In the LR1, BMI has an odds ratio, OR = 0.93, which means that for each increase of BMI by 1 unit, the odds of having OSA increase by 0.93. In the DT3, BMI is used in two nodes: splitting cases between BMI ≤ 34 and BMI > 34, and BMI ≤ 25 and BMI > 25. The interesting insight is that the tree automatically splits on BMI = 25, which is the generally accepted upper limit of normal BMI.
- **Depression.** In the LR1, depression has an odds ratio, OR = 1.21, and a negative coefficient, which means that for a single change from depression "no" to depression "yes", the odds of having OSA decrease by 1.21. This is an unusual finding, since many studies indicate strong co-occurrence and, even, correlation between depression and OSA (Schroder & O'Hara, 2005). To discuss our finding, we have to define the term "depression." In general, this predictor may be defined as a previously diagnosed depressive disorder or depressive symptoms (measured by psychological scales). In data set *C*, depression is self-reported as being previously diagnosed with a "major mood disorder." Furthermore, we have found that many patients were referred to the Respiratory Clinic and sent for PSG studies after being diagnosed with clinical depression to exclude possible OSA.
- **HTN.** In the LR1, HTN has an odds ratio, OR = 0.79, which means that if the value for HTN is changed from "no" to "yes," the odds of having OSA increase by 0.79. In the DT3 model, HTN is used in two nodes.
- **Diabetes.** In the LR1, diabetes has an odds ratio, OR = 4.44, and negative coefficient, which means that if the value for diabetes is changed from absent to present, the odds of having OSA decrease by 4.44. In the DT3, diabetes is used in rule, "IF Snoring > 2 AND Diabetes = Present THEN outcome = Normal." Although, this rule has an accuracy of 72%, it has a small support of

6.8%. This is an unusual finding, since several medical studies demonstrate association between OSA and diabetes mellitus (Punjabi & Beamer, 2005). Thus, we have to analyze the two different measurements: (1) diabetes as a self-reported, physician-diagnosed "diabetes mellitus" and (2) a clinical test such as fasting glucose test. The values for the diabetes variable in data set C had been collected based on self-reported previously diagnosed diabetes.

- **Age.** In the LR1 model, age has an odds ratio, OR = 0.98, which means that if the value for age is increased by one year, the odds of having OSA increase by 0.98. In the DT3, age is used in three nodes and splits the data by 41, 45, 50, and 60. In two cases, lower age values correspond to a higher ratio of "Normal" values. However, in one node, the tree divides 43 cases into three groups with age ≤ 41, age in range (41,45), and age > 45, and the prevailing values are "OSA" for age ≤ 41, "Normal" for range 41–45, and "OSA" for age > 45.
- **Snoring.** In the LR1, snoring has an odds ratio, OR = 0.67, which means that if the value for snoring is increased by one unit, the odds of having OSA increase by 0.67. In the DT3, snoring is used as a root node and, again, at the seventh level to differentiate between a habitual snorer (value 4) and people who snore less often.

Step 2: Convergence of the Induced Models with Clinical Prediction Rules for OSA

We compare our LR1 model with three existing predictive models from the KB: Model #1, #2, and #3. All logistic regression models calculate the probability of OSA based on the LR equation: $P(OSA) = e^x/(1+e^x)$. Model #1 uses the same predictors as the LR1 (gender, BMI, and HTN), with the exception of witnessed apnea (WA). The direction of changes is positive in both models. Model #2 uses all four predictors, and the directions of changes are the same as those in Model LR1. Model #3 uses BMI and age and an index for nocturnal symptoms. The direction for age and BMI are the same as the direction in the Model LR1.

CONCLUSION AND FUTURE WORK

In this chapter, we show that purely data-driven techniques are insufficient for medical data mining. Using an empirical approach, we demonstrate how knowledge can be integrated into each step of the DM process. We concentrate on two crucial phases for the successful application of DM in medicine: pre-processing and post-processing. We present a new integrative framework, a semio-fuzzy framework, for building a knowledge repository containing OSA diagnostic criteria, definitions for predictors, and published CPRs for OSA diagnosis. We address issues related to a representational framework for OSA predictors and predictive rules. We use three clinical data sets to study the prevalence of OSA, to analyze the missing values, to detect medical outliers, to analyze the strength of a predictor, to induce new models, and to evaluate the induced models in the context of existing knowledge.

We demonstrate that the semiotic approach to the definition of predictors provides a tool to compare variables from different data sets. Without such a tool, a data-driven approach does not differentiate between subjective and objective measurements, and sensitive and neutral data. We used two examples to illustrate the significance of medical knowledge in data analysis: neck circumference and smoking behavior. There are two measures for NC: the clinical measure and the self-reported collar size. For the reported collar size, 41% of the values are missing (interestingly, the number of missing values for "collar size" for females is 82%). This situation excludes the data for collar size from analysis. Furthermore, the imprecision of self-reported "collar size," as opposed to a clinically measured value, excludes the comparison of the results with other data sets containing the exact measurements. For the self-reported smoking value, 23% of the values are missing, which also excludes this variable from analysis. We observe that the data analysis must investigate the reasons for missing values.

These two cases illustrate the need for a precise definition of the medical predictors and their interpretation. The purely data-driven approach treats values for subjective, objective, or sensitive medical data with equal scrutiny and combines them into a uniform model. However in order to meaningfully interpret the resulting models, we must not only capture the actual numeric data (syntax), but also the meaning of the variables (semantics) and the usage of the variables (pragmatics).

We demonstrate that a straightforward application of statistical methods for outlier detection will miss a large number of outliers because of the masking effect by other values. This situation is evident in our study of NC outliers, where the values of NC come from a mixed population of females, males, whites and Asians. The traditional statistical methods apply to primary data analysis; therefore, identification of outliers in various data sets from mixed populations requires a prescriptive model. Consequently, we introduce an anatomical typicality measure and a knowledge-driven approach to identification of outliers.

We show that that the automatically induced models and patterns must be carefully interpreted in the context of existing knowledge. In the case of secondary analysis of medical data, the induced models may include structural artifacts resulting from the sampling and referral biases. In post-processing, we identify two contradictory findings: the presence of depression decreases the likelihood of OSA and the presence of diabetes decreases the likelihood of OSA. We examine these findings from two perspectives: semiotic definition of these predictors and comparison with the published studies. We note important differences between the definitions of depression as "self-reported, physician-diagnosed depression," as opposed to "feelings of depression measured on psychological scales." Similarly, diabetes can be measured as "self-reported physician-diagnosed diabetes" or by a "clinical test of fasting glucose level." Since, many published studies use the clinical measurements, as opposed to self-reporting of "being previously diagnosed," we observe that these findings cannot be compared with the existing medical knowledge. We conclude that the classification model and patterns automatically induced from data must be examined for the definition of predictors and compared with existing knowledge.

Research presented in this chapter has motivated projects in two domains, computational and medical. From the computational perspective, this research will span further studies in applying the knowledge representational framework based on semiotics and fuzzy logic. Further studies are needed for fuzzy rule-based typicality measures, data ambiguity measures, and model interpretation. Further applications of the semio-fuzzy framework to other disorders, such as depression and asthma, have been already planned.

From the medical perspective, this research evokes interest in the application of comprehensible computational models and intelligent data analysis. Furthermore, from a strictly practical perspective, some questions presented in this chapter have initiated further clinical studies. For example, a pilot clinical study has commenced at Thompson Rivers University. This study evaluates the CPAP treatment and measures several predictors before and after treatment, among them excessive daytime sleepiness and depressive feelings.

ACKNOWLEDGMENT

The research presented in this chapter was partially supported by a grant from the Natural Sciences and Engineering Research Council of Canada (NSERC grant #327545-06). The authors would like to thank Linda McMillan for her help with the manuscript.

REFERENCES

Adlassnig, K. P. (1986). Fuzzy set theory in medical diagnosis. *IEEE Transactions on Systems, Man, and Cybernetics, SMC-16*, 260-265.

Al-Alawi, A., Mulgrew, A., Tench, E., & Ryan, C. F. (2006, July). Prevalence, Risk Factors and Impact of Daytime Sleepiness and Hypertension of Periodic Leg Movements with Arousals in Patients with Obstructive Sleep Apnea. *Journal of Clinical Sleep Medicine*, 2(3), 281-7.

Childs, J. D., & Cleland, J. A. (2006). Development and application of clinical prediction rules to improve decision making in physical therapist practice. *Physical Therapy, 86*(1), 122-131.

Crocker, B. D., Olson, L. G., & Saunders, N. A. (1990). Estimation of the probability of distributed breathing during sleep before a sleep study. *American Review of Respiratory Disease, 142*, 14-18.

Dancey, D. R., Hanly, P. J., Soong, C., Lee, B., Shepard, J., & Hoffstein, V. (2003). Gender differences in sleep apnea: The role of neck circumference, *Chest, 123*, 1544-1550.

Douglas, N. J. (2002). *Clinicians' Guide to Sleep Medicine*. London: Arnold.

Ebell, M. H. (2001). *Evidence-based Diagnosis: A handbook of Clinical Prediction Rules*. New York: Springer.

Ferguson, K. A., Ono, T., Lowe, A. A., Ryan, C. F., & Fleetham, J. A. (1995). The Relationship Between Obesity and Craniofacial Structure in Obstructive Sleep Apnea. *Chest, 108*(2), 375-381.

Flemons, W. W., Whitelaw, W. W., & Remmers, J. E. (1994). Likelihood ratios for a sleep apnea clinical prediction rule. *American Journal of Respiratory and Critical Care Medicine, 150*, 1279-1285.

Han, J., & Kamber, M. (2001). *Data Mining: Concepts and Techniques*. San Francisco: Morgan Kaufmann.

Jordan, A. S., & McEvoy, R. D. (2003). Gender differences in sleep apnea: Epidemiology, clinical presentation and pathogenic mechanisms. *Sleep Medicine Reviews, 7*(5), 377-389.

Knottnerus, J. A. (1995). Diagnostic prediction rules: principles, requirements and pitfalls. *Medical Decision Making, 22*(2), 341-360.

Kwiatkowska, M., & Atkins, M. S. (2004). A Semio-Fuzzy Approach to Information Fusion in the Diagnosis of Obstructive Sleep Apnea. *Proceedings of the NAFIPS*. Banff, Canada, 55-60.

Kwiatkowska, M., Atkins, M. S., Ayas, N. T., & Ryan, C. F. (2007). Knowledge-Based Data Analysis: First Step Toward the Creation of Clinical Prediction Rules Using a New Typicality Measure. *IEEE Transactions on Information Technology in Biomedicine, 11*(6), 651-660.

Lam, B., Ip, M. S. M., Tench, E., & Ryan, C. F. (2005). Craniofacial profile in Asian and white subjects with obstructive sleep apnea. *Thorax, 60*(6), 504-510.

Lavrac, N., Keravnou, E. & Zupan, B. (2000). Intelligent Data Analysis in Medicine. In A. Kent (Ed.), *Encyclopedia of Computer Science and Technology* (pp. 113-157). New York: Dekker.

Maislin, G., Pack, A. I., Kribbs, N. B., Smith, P., Schwartz, A., Kline, L., Schwab, R., Dinges, D. & et al. (1995). A survey screen for prediction of apnea. *Sleep, 18*, 158-166.

Maedche, A., Motik, B., Stojanovic, L., Studer, R., & Volz, R. (2003). Ontologies for enterprise knowledge management. *IEEE Intelligent Systems, 18*(2), 26-33.

Michalski, R. S., & Kaufman, K. A. (1998). Data Mining and Knowledge Discovery: A Review of Issues and a Multistrategy Approach. In R. S. Michalski, I. Bratko & M. Kubat (Eds.), *Machine Learning and Data Mining: Methods and Applications* (pp. 71-112). Chichester: John Wiley & Sons Ltd.

Millman, R. P., Carlisle, C. C., McGarvey, S. T., Eveloff, S. E., & Levinson, P. D. (1995). Body fat distribution and sleep apnea severity in women. *Chest, 107*(2), 362-366.

Mitchell, T. M. (1997). *Machine Learning.* Boston: McGraw-Hill.

Mulgrew, A. T., Fox, N., Ayas, N. T., & Ryan, C. F. (2007). Diagnosis and Initial Management of Obstructive Sleep Apnea without Polysomnography: A Randomized Validation Study. *Annals of Internal Medicine, 146*, 157-166.

Pazzani, M. J., & Kibler, D. (1992). The utility of knowledge in inductive learning. *Machine Learning,* 9(1), 57-97.

Punjabi, N. M., & Beamer, B. A. (2005). Sleep Apnea and Metabolic Dysfunction. In *Principles and Practice of Sleep Medicine* (Fourth Edition ed., pp. 1034-1042): Elsevier Saunders.

Roche, N., Herer, B., Roig, C., & Huchon, G. (2002). Prospective Testing of Two Models Based on Clinical and Oximetric Variables for Prediction of Obstructive Sleep Apnea. *Chest, 121*(3), 747-752.

Rosenberg, R., & Mickelson, S. A. (2003). Obstructive sleep apnea: Evaluation by history and polysomnography. In D. N. F. Fairbanks, S. A. Mickelson & B. T. Woodson (Eds.), *Snoring and Obstructive Sleep Apnea* (Third ed.). Philadelphia: Lippincott Williams & Wilkins.

Rowley, J. A., Aboussouan, L. S., & Badr, M. S. (2000). The use of clinical prediction formulas in the evaluation of obstructive sleep apnea. *Sleep, 23*(7), 929-938.

Rowley, J. A., Sanders, C. S., Zahn, B. R. & Badr, M. S. (2002). Gender differences in upper airway compliance during NREM sleep: role of neck circumference. *Journal of Applied Physiology, 92*, 2535-2541.

Ryan, C. F., & Love, L. L. (1996). Mechanical properties of the velopharynx in obese patients with obstructive sleep apnea. *American Journal of Respiratory and Critical Care Medicine, 154*(3), 806-812.

Sebeok, T. A. (1999). *Signs: An Introduction to Semiotics*: University of Toronto Press.

Sharma, S. K., Kurian, S., Malik, V., Mohan, A., Banga, A., Pandey, R. M., Handa, K. K., & Mukhopadhyay, S. (2004). A stepped approach for prediction of obstructive sleep apnea in overtly asymptomatic obese subjects: a hospital based study. *Sleep Medicine, 5*, 451-357.

Schroder, C. M., & O'Hara, R. (2005). Depression and Obstructive Sleep Apnea (OSA). *Annals of General Psychiatry, 4*(13).

Viner, S., Szalai, J. P., & Hoffstein, V. (1991). Are history and physical examination a good screening test for sleep apnea? *Annals of Internal Medicine, 115*, 356-359.

Whittle, A. T., Marshall, I., Mortimore, I. 1., Wraith, P. K., Sellar, R. J. & Douglas, N. J. (1999). Neck soft tissue and fat distribution comparison between normal men and women by magnetic resonance imaging. *Thorax, 54*, 323-328.

Witten, I. H., & Frank, E. (2005). *Data Mining: Practical Machine Learning Tools and Technologies* (Second ed.). Amsterdam: Morgan Kaufmann.

Woodson, B. T. (2003). Obstructive sleep apnea: Evaluation by physical examination and special studies. In D. N. F. Fairbanks, S. A. Mickelson & B. T. Woodson (Eds.), *Snoring and Obstructive Sleep Apnea* (third ed., pp. 51-67). Philadelphia: Lippincott Williams & Wilkins.

Young, T., Peppard, P. E., & Gottlieb, D. J. (2002). Epidemiology of Obstructive Sleep Apnea: A Population Health Perspective. *American Journal of Respiratory and Critical Care Medicine, 165*(9), 1217-1239.

Zadeh, L. (1965). Fuzzy Sets. *Information and Control, 8*(3), 338-353.

Zhang, J., & Honavar, V. (2003). Learning decision tree classifiers from attribute value taxonomies and partially specified data. *Proceedings of the Twentieth International Conference on Machine Learning (ICML 2003)*. Washington, DC, 880-887.

KEY TERMS

AHI – Apnea/Hypopnea Index: The number of apneas and hypopneas per hour of sleep.

Apnea: The cessation of airflow at the nostrils and mouth for at least 10 seconds (British spelling: apnoea).

BMI – Body Mass Index: Weight in kg/(height in meters)^2.

CPAP – Continuous Positive Airway Pressure: A method of respiratory ventilation used primary in the treatment of sleep apnea.

Fuzzy Logic: A type of logic that recognizes more than simple true and false values. With fuzzy logic, propositions can be represented with degrees of truthfulness.

Hypopnea: Reduction of the ventilation by at least 50% (but not a total cessation of airflow) from the previous baseline during sleep.

Obstructive Apnea: The cessation of airflow (at least 10 seconds) in the presence of continued inspiratory effort.

Oxygen Desturation: Less than normal amount of oxygen carried by haemoglobin in the blood; values below 90% are considered abnormal.

Oximetry: Continuous monitoring of oxygen saturation of arterial blood from a pulse oximeter; the sensor is usually attached to the finger.

OSA – Obstructive Sleep Apnea: A disorder caused by repetitive upper airway obstruction during sleep.

PSG – Polysomnogram: Continuous and simultaneous recording of physiological variables during sleep. The study involves several parameters: electro-encephalogram (EEG), electro-oculogram (EOG), chin electro-myogram (EMG), nasal/oral airflow, thoracic movement, abdominal movement, blood oxygen saturation (SaO2), electro-cardiogram (ECG), leg electro-myogram, snoring sounds, and body positions recording.

Semiotics: The study of signs, sign systems and their meanings.

Chapter XVIII
Data Mining in Atherosclerosis Risk Factor Data

Petr Berka
University of Economics, Prague, Czech Republic;
Academy of Sciences of the Czech Republic, Prague, Czech Republic

Jan Rauch
University of Economics, Prague, Czech Republic;
Academy of Sciences of the Czech Republic, Prague, Czech Republic

Marie Tomečková
Academy of Sciences of the Czech Republic, Prague, Czech Republic

ABSTRACT

The aim of this chapter is to describe goals, current results, and further plans of long-time activity concerning application of data mining and machine learning methods to the complex medical data set. The analyzed data set concerns a longitudinal study of atherosclerosis risk factors. The structure and main features of this data set, as well as methodology of observation of risk factors, are introduced. The important first steps of analysis of atherosclerosis data are described in details together with a large set of analytical questions defined on the basis of first results. Experience in solving these tasks is summarized and further directions of analysis are outlined.

INTRODUCTION

Atherosclerosis is a slow, complex disease that typically starts in childhood and often progresses when people grow older. In some people it progresses rapidly, even in their third decade. Many scientists think it begins with damage to the innermost layer of the artery. Atherosclerosis involves the slow buildup of deposits of fatty substances, cholesterol, body cellular waste products, calcium, and fibrin (a clotting material in the blood) in the inside lining of an artery. The buildup (referred as a plaque) with the formation of the blood clot (thrombus) on the surface of the plaque can partially or totally block the flow of blood through the artery. If either of these events occurs and blocks the entire artery, a heart attack or stroke or other life-threatening events may result.

People with a family history of premature cardiovascular disease (CVD) and with other risk factors of atherosclerosis have an increased risk of the complications of atherosclerosis. Research shows the benefits of reducing the controllable risk factors for atherosclerosis: high blood cholesterol, cigarette smoking and exposure to tobacco smoke, high blood pressure, diabetes mellitus, obesity, physical inactivity.

Atherosclerosis-related diseases are a leading cause of death and impairment in the United States, affecting over 60 million people. Additionally, 50% of Americans have levels of cholesterol that place them at high risk for developing coronary artery disease. Similar situation can be observed in other countries. So the education of patients about prevention of atherosclerosis is very important.

In the early seventies of the twentieth century, a project of extensive epidemiological study of atherosclerosis primary prevention was developed under the name National Preventive Multifactorial Study of Hard Attacks and Strokes in the former Czechoslovakia. The aims of the study were:

- Identify atherosclerosis risk factors prevalence in a population generally considered to be the most endangered by possible atherosclerosis complications, i.e. middle aged men.
- Follow the development of these risk factors and their impact on the examined men health, especially with respect to atherosclerotic cardiovascular diseases.
- Study the impact of complex risk factors intervention on their development and cardiovascular morbidity and mortality.
- 10–12 years into the study, compare risk factors profile and health of the selected men, who originally did not show any atherosclerosis risk factors with a group of men showing risk factors from the beginning of the study.

Men born between 1926 and 1937 living in centre of the capital of the Czechoslovakia -Prague - were selected from election lists in year 1975. The invitation for examination included a short explanation of the first examination purpose, procedure and later observations and asked for co-operation. At that time, no informed signature of the respondent was required. Entry examinations were performed in the years 1976–1979 and 1,419 out of 2,370 invited men came for the first examination and risk factors of atherosclerosis were classified according to the well defined methodology. The primary data covers both entry and control examination. 244 attributes have been surveyed with each patient at entry examination and there are 219 attributes, which values are codes or results of size measurements of different variables. 10,610 control examination were further made, each examination concerns 66 attributes. Some additional irregular data collections concerning these men were performed. Study is named STULONG – LONGitudinal STUdy - and continues for twenty years.

The observation resulted into data set consisting of four data matrices that are suitable for application of both classical statistical data analysis method and for application of data mining and machine learning. The project to analyze these data by methods of data mining started by setting large set of analytical questions. The goal of this chapter is to describe first steps in application of data mining and machine learning methods to the STULONG data. We also summarize the additional analyzes inspired by set of analytical questions and we introduce further planned work.

The chapter is organized as follows: Methodology of the examination of patients is introduced in section *Methodology*. The data set resulting from the observation is described in section *STULONG Data Set*. We applied three GUHA procedures as well as the machine learning procedure KEX, all these procedures are implemented in the LISp-Miner system, see http://lispminer.vse.cz/. Their applications are described in sections *Applying GUHA Method* and *Applying KEX*. The additional analyses are summarized in section *Additional Analyses*. Further plans are described in section *Further Work*.

METHODOLOGY

The methodology covers definition of risk factors, first examination, men classification for long-term observation, long-term observation and intervention of atherosclerosis risk factors. Main features of all this parts of methodology are described in the following subsections.

Risk Factors Definition

The following risk factors were defined:

- *Arterial hypertension*: Blood pressure (BP) ≥ 160/95 mm Hg, men with the risk of hypertension were also those, who at the time of the first examination had both blood pressure values within the standard limits, who however were treated by medicaments
- *Hypercholesterolemia*: Cholesterol level ≥ 260mg% (6,7 mmol/l)
- *Hypertriglyceridemia*: Triglycerides level ≥ 200mg% (2,2 mmol/l)
- *Smoking*: ≥ 15 cig./day currently or smoking of the same number of cigarettes within 1 year prior to the study commencement (pipe or cigar smokers were considered non-smokers),
- *Overweight*: Brocca index > 115 % (Brocca index: height in cm minus 100 = 100 %),
- *Positive family case history*: Death of father or mother from ischemic heart disease, heart or vascular stroke before reaching 65 years of age.

Later, additional risk factors based on laboratory examinations were added:

- *Blood sugar* level ≥ than 6,3 and > 8 mmol/l = disturbed gluc. tolerance, blood sugar level ≥ 8 mmol/l = diabetes mellitus,
- *HDL cholesterol* (cholesterol ester of high density): Normal level over 1,2 mmol/l,
- *LDL cholesterol* (cholesterol ester of low density): Normal level up to 4,0 mmol/l,
- *Uric Acid*: Normal level up to 420 micromol/l.

First Examination Methodology

Initial examination started through an interview and a form completion by a doctor. The form included all general administrative data on the examined man, the level of education reached, data on function and responsibility at the workplace, general habits –physical activity in the lessure time, smoking habits, alcohol drinking. Data on family and personal history focused around cardiovascular diseases, chest or legs pain and breathlessness stating its level. Of course, the initial examination included also general physical investigation including blood pressure measuring, basic anthropometric examination – weight, height, skin folds over the triceps and subscapular muscles, registration of ECG and blood and urine laboratory tests. Further tests were performed, e.g. stress test to identify chest pain, when necessary. 244 attributes were identified for each man.

Men Classification for Long-Term Observation

All men were divided according to the presence of risk factors (RF), global health conditions and ECG result into following groups:

- **NG** = Group of men showing no RF defined above, without manifestation of cardio-vascular diseases or other serious illness making their ten-year-long observation impossible and without and ECG alteration.
- **RG** = Group of men with at least one RF defined above, without manifestation of cardiovascular diseases or other serious illness making their ten-year-long observation impossible and without and ECG alteration.
- **PG** = Group of men with a manifested cardiovascular disease or other serious disease making their ten-year-long observation impossible (e.g. malignancy, advanced failure of liver or kidneys, serious nerve or psychological complaints). The pathologic group included also men with diabetes treated by peroral antidiabetics or by insulin and men with pathologic ECG.

Long-Term Observation Methodology

Long-term observation of patients was based on their division into the groups stated above:

- The risk group **RG** was randomly divided into two sub-groups designated as **RGI** (intervened risk group) and **RGC** (control risk group). The patients in the **RGI** group were invited for check up minimum twice in year. Following pharmacological intervention, they were invited as necessary. The patients in the **RGC** group received a short written notice including their laboratory results and ECG description and a recommendation to deliver these results to their physician; possible intervention of RF consists in the decision of these physicians. At the first examination, no significant difference in age, socio-economic factors or RF occurrence was demonstrated between the RGI and RGC groups.
- 10 % of men in the **NG** group was examined minimum 1 time per year just as the risk group – (they are denoted **NGS**). In this group of men, similarly to the risk group, intervention was initiated as the RF was identified and confirmed (hyperlipoproteinemia, arterial hypertension). The remaining men of the **NG** were invited for a control examination 10–12 years later.
- Men from the **PG** group were excluded from further observation.

Intervention of Atherosclerosis Risk Factors

Intervention was the key problem of the study. We tried to optimize and modify affectable risk factors. Intervention was based on non-pharmacological influence. Pharmacological intervention may be mostly used only in the last years of the study.

- *Non-pharmacological intervention:* Interviews on lifestyle, i.e. diet, physical activity, suitability or necessity to stop smoking and reduce weight. The interviews were repeated during each visit and except for general instructions, they focused also toward specific RF of a given man.
- *Pharmacological intervention:* Treatment of arterial hypertension and hyperlipoproteinemia– was very limited in the initial stages of the study. Pharmacological therapy was recommended with respect to the overall risk of a given man and his possible other diseases.

The regular visits at a doctor themselves could represent an intervention, provided the patient again the reason of the visit, parameters to be followed and desirable parameter values.

STULONG DATA SET

The study (STULONG) was realized at the 2nd Department of Medicine, 1st Faculty of Medicine of Charles University and Charles University Hospital, U nemocnice 2, Prague 2 (head. Prof. M. Aschermann, MD, SDr, FESC), under the supervision of Prof. F. Boudík, MD, ScD, with collaboration of M. Tomečková, MD, PhD and Ass. Prof. J. Bultas, MD, PhD. The data were transferred to the electronic form by the European Centre of Medical Informatics, Statistics and Epidemiology of Charles University and Academy of Sciences (head. Prof. RNDr. J. Zvárová, DrSc). The data resource is on the web pages http://euromise.vse.cz/challenge2003. Data resulting from the longitudinal study of the risk factors of the atherosclerosis is in the form of four data matrices. Part of this data is at http://euromise.vse.cz/challenge2004/.

1. **Data Matrix ENTRY:** Data matrix ENTRY contains results of entry examinations. 244 attributes were identified for each man. Data matrix ENTRY has 1417 rows and 219 columns. Each row corresponds to one patient (2 men were excluded) and each column corresponds to one of 219 values of which are codes or results of size measurements. Attributes can be divided into groups according to the Table 1.
2. **Data Matrix CONTROL:** Data matrix CONTROL contains results of long-term observation. of risk factors and clinical demonstration of atherosclerosis. Values of 66 attributes have been recorded for each of 10 610 control examinations. Rows of data matrix CONTROL correspond to particular control examinations, columns correspond to particular attributes. Attributes can be divided into groups according to the Table 1.
3. **Data Matrix LETTER:** Additional information about health status of 403 men was collected by the postal questionnaire at the end of the study. Values of 62 attributes were result of this action. Results are stored in the data matrix LETTER with 403 rows corresponding to men and 60 columns corresponding to attributes. Attributes can be divided into groups according to the Table 1.
4. **Data Matrix DEATH:** There is also data concerning death of 389 patients. Data describes date of death of each of these patients and a numerical code of death. Data are in the form of simple data matrix, see also section *Applying 4ft-Miner.*

Table 1. Groups of attributes of the data tables

Data table	Group of attributes	# of attributes
ENTRY	Identification data	2
ENTRY	Social characteristics	6
ENTRY	Physical activity	4
ENTRY	Smoking	3
ENTRY	Drinking of alcohol	9
ENTRY	Sugar, coffee, tea	3
ENTRY	Personal history	18
ENTRY	Family history	160
ENTRY	Questionnaire A_2 (diseases and difficulties)	3
ENTRY	Physical examination	8
ENTRY	Biochemical examination	3
CONTROL	identification data	4
CONTROL	patients changes since the last examination	8
CONTROL	experiences sicknesses	6
CONTROL	Questionnaire A_2 (diseases and difficulties)	28
CONTROL	physical examination	10
CONTROL	biochemical examination	10
LETTER	identification data	3
LETTER	the assessment of the health status	12
LETTER	answers of patients – diseases	19
LETTER	answers of patients – dyspnea	7
LETTER	answers of patients – smoking	8
LETTER	answers of patients – physical activity	4
LETTER	answers of patients – diet	5
LETTER	answers of patients – weight	2

PROBLEM DESCRIPTION

The STULONG data were analyzed using some statistical methods: descriptive statistics, logistic regression and survival analysis. The domain experts were curious about applying data mining methods to these data. Therefore they asked some questions concerning some uncovered relations hidden in the data.

The listed analytic questions (possible tasks), which have not been subjected to study yet, can be divided into four groups:

1. Analytic questions related to the entry examination:
   - What are the relations between social factors and some of (physical activity, smoking, alcohol consumption, BMI, blood pressure, cholesterol, triglycerides) for men in the respective groups?

- What are the relations between physical activity and some of (smoking, alcohol consumption, BMI, blood pressure, cholesterol, triglycerides) for men in the respective groups?
- What are the relations between alcohol consumption and some of (smoking, BMI, blood pressure, cholesterol, triglycerides) for men in the respective groups?
- Is there a correlation between the skin folds and BMI in the particular basic groups of patients?

2. Analytic questions related to the long-term observation:
   - Are there any differences in the entry examination between men of the risk group, who came down with the observed cardiovascular diseases and those who stayed healthy w.r.t. social factors, physical activity, smoking, alcohol consumption, BMI, blood pressure, cholesterol?
   - Are there any differences between men of the two risk subgroups RGI, RGC, who came down with the observed cardiovascular diseases in the course of 20 years and those who stayed healthy?
   - Are there any differences in the development of risk factors and other characteristics between men of the risk group, who came down with the observed cardiovascular diseases and those who stayed healthy w.r.t change of job, change of physical activity, change of smoking, change of diet, change of BMI, change of blood pressure?
3. Analytic questions concerning postal questionnaire
4. Analytic questions concerning entry examination, long-term observation and death

According these questions, various data mining tasks can be formulated. The descriptive tasks - associations or segmentation (subgroup discovery), are used if the main purpose of the data mining is to find some relation between attributes or examples. As the analytic questions suggest to focus on mining for descriptive models, the results of most analyzes were different forms of association rules . Classification (and regression) tasks can be used if the main purpose of the data mining is to build a model for decision or decision support. The classification tasks performed on STULONG data can deal either with classifying patients into the three predefined groups normal, risk or pathological or with classifying them into classes derived from the data. The classification problem can be eventually turned into a regression problem; a real-valued risk estimate for an individual can be calculated.

We will show how some of these tasks have been solved using GUHA method and KEX.

APPLYING GUHA METHOD

GUHA Principle

We used GUHA method to start the analysis of STULONG data. GUHA is an original Czech method of exploratory data analysis developed since 1960s (Hájek & Havránek, 1978). Its principle is to offer all interesting facts following from the given data to the given problem. It is realized by GUHA procedures. The GUHA-procedure is a computer program the input of which consists of the analyzed data and of a few parameters defining a very large set of potentially interesting patterns. The output of the GUHA procedure is a list of all prime patterns. The pattern is prime if both it is true in the analyzed data and it does not immediately follow from other output patterns.

The most known GUHA procedure is the procedure ASSOC (Hájek & Havránek, 1978) mining for association rules corresponding to various relations of two Boolean attributes. These rules have much stronger expression power than „classical“ association rules using confidence and support; see e.g. (Aggraval et al., 1996). The procedure ASSOC was several time implemented, see e.g. (Hájek, 1981; Hájek, Sochorová & Zvárová, 1995). Its last and contemporary most used implementation is the procedure 4ft-Miner (Rauch & Šimůnek, 2005). It is important that implementation of the procedure ASSOC does not use the well known a-priori algorithm but it is based on representation of analyzed data by suitable strings of bits. This approach proved to be very efficient to compute various contingency tables. It led to implementation of five additional GUHA procedures mining various patterns verified using one or two contingency tables. All these procedures are included in the academic software system LISp-Miner (Rauch & Šimůnek, 2005), see also http://lispminer.vse.cz. Important feature of these procedures are also very fine tools to define sets of patterns to be verified.

We show examples of applications of three of these procedures to STULONG data. The applications prove that the methods of data mining can find patterns interesting from the point of view of data owner. They led to formulation of a set of analytical questions for additional data mining activity.

Applying 4ft-Miner

An example of application of 4ft-Miner procedure concerns analysis of death causes. The relative frequencies of particular death causes are in Table 2.

We are interested if under some conditions described in the data matrices ENTRY and CONTROL, the relative frequency differ from the relative frequency given in Table 2. This is a very complex task; we show an example how the procedure 4ft-Miner can contribute to its solution. We solve the analytical question “*Under which combinations of Boolean characteristics of physical examination, biochemical examination and of patients lifestyle factors is the relative frequency of the causes of death much higher than the relative frequency given in Table 2?*”. Symbolically we can write this question as:

$$Physical(?) \wedge Biochemical(?) \wedge Vices(?) \rightarrow^{+} Cause\_of\_Death(?)$$

Table 2. Relative frequencies of particular death causes

Cause of death	# of patients	%
myocardial infarction	80	20.6
coronary heart disease	33	8.5
stroke	30	7.7
general atherosclerosis	22	5.7
sudden death	23	5.9
tumorous diseases	114	29.3
other causes	79	20.3
cause of the death unknown	8	2.0
Total	**389**	**100.0**

This question concerns only attributes of data matrix ENTRY. Here *Physical*(?) denotes a Boolean attribute derived from attributes of the group *Physical examination*, see Table 1. Similarly *Biochemical*(?) denotes a Boolean attribute derived from attributes of the group *Biochemical examination* and *Lifestyle*(?) denotes a Boolean attribute derived from suitable additional attributes describing patient's lifestyle behavior. The expression *Cause_of_Death*(?) denotes Boolean attributes derived from particular causes of death. An example is the Boolean attribute *Cause_of_Death* (*myocardial infarction*) that is true for a patient if and only if the cause of death of this patient was myocardial infarction.

We use rich possibilities of 4ft-Miner procedure to define a set of relevant association rules to answer this analytical question. We describe it here very informally; the precise description is out of range of this chapter, for more details see (Rauch & Šimůnek, 2005). The procedure 4ft-Miner mines for association rules $\varphi \approx \psi$. Here φ and ψ are Boolean attributes derived from input attributes – columns of analyzed data matrix. Symbol $\approx$ is called 4ft-quantifier. It defines a relation of φ and ψ in analyzed data matrix. Boolean attribute φ is called *antecedent*, ψ is called *succedent*. There are various 4ft-quantifiers. A condition concerning a contingency table of φ and ψ is assigned to each 4ft-quantifier. Contingency table of φ and ψ in data matrix $\mathcal{M}$ is denoted as 4ft($\varphi,\psi,\mathcal{M}$). It is a quadruple $\langle a,b,c,d \rangle$ of integer numbers, a is number of rows of $\mathcal{M}$ satisfying both φ and ψ, b is number of rows of $\mathcal{M}$ satisfying φ and not satisfying ψ etc., see Table 3.

The association rule $\varphi \approx \psi$ is true in data matrix $\mathcal{M}$ if the condition associated to $\approx$ is satisfied in 4ft($\varphi,\psi,\mathcal{M}$). We use 4ft-quantifier $\Rightarrow^{+}_{p,Base}$ called AA-quantifier (above average) with parameters $p > 0$ and $Base \geq 1$. It is defined by condition:

$$\frac{a}{a+b} \geq (1+p)\frac{a+c}{a+b+c+d} \wedge a \geq Base$$

If the rule $\varphi \Rightarrow^{+}_{p,Base} \psi$ is true in data matrix $\mathcal{M}$ then both relative frequency of rows of $\mathcal{M}$ satisfying ψ among rows satisfying φ is at least 100p percent greater than relative frequency of rows satisfying ψ among all rows of $\mathcal{M}$ and there are at least *Base* rows of $\mathcal{M}$ satisfying both φ and ψ.

We use the AA quantifier $\Rightarrow^{+}_{1.0,15}$ with parameters $p = 1.0$ and $Base = 15$ to solve our analytical question *Physical*(?) $\wedge$ *Biochemical*(?) $\wedge$ *Vices*(?) $\rightarrow^{+}$ *Cause_of_Death*(?). Thus we search Boolean attributes *Physical*(?) $\wedge$ *Biochemical*(?) $\wedge$ *Vices*(?) and *Cause_of_Death*(?) such that both among patients satisfying *Physical*(?) $\wedge$ *Biochemical*(?) $\wedge$ *Vices*(?). There is at least 100 percent higher relative frequency of patients with a particular cause of death than in the whole data matrix DEATH, and there are at least 15 patients satisfying *Physical*(?) $\wedge$ *Biochemical*(?) $\wedge$ *Vices*(?) $\wedge$ *Cause_of_Death*(?).

Note that we have to enhance data matrix DEATH by attributes of ENTRY used to derive Boolean attributes *Physical*(?), *Biochemical*(?), and *Lifestyle*(?). This enhanced data matrix will be used as an input of the 4ft-Miner procedure. An additional part of input of the procedure 4ft-Miner are the specifications

Table 3. Contingency table 4ft($\varphi,\psi,\mathcal{M}$) of φ and ψ in data matrix $\mathcal{M}$

$\mathcal{M}$	ψ	$\neg\psi$
φ	a	b
$\neg\varphi$	c	d

of the set of relevant antecedent and set of relevant succedents which are automatically derived. Set of all succedents will be specified as a set of all possible Boolean attributes *Cause_of_Death*(?). There are however lot of possibilities how to define set of all possible antecedents *Physical*(?) $\wedge$ *Biochemical*(?) $\wedge$ *Lifestyle*(?), we show one of them. We use attributes *Weight*, *Height* and *Subscapular* to specify *Physical*(?); we use attributes *Triglycerides* and *Cholesterol* to specify *Biochemical*(?), and we use attributes *Smoking*, *Coffee*, *Beer*, *Vine*, and *Liquors* to specify *Lifestyle*(?). There are again lot of possibilities how to specify these particular Boolean attributes, we use specification shown in Figure 1.

It means that *Physical*(?) is defined as *partial antecedent Physical* that is conjunction of 0 - 3 Boolean attributes derived from *Weight*, *Height* and *Subscapular*, see expression "*Physical* 0 – 3" in Figure 1. Similarly for *Biochemical*(?) and *Vices*(?). Note that empty conjunction is identically true. Boolean attributes to be automatically derived from the attribute *Weight* are specified by the expression "*Weight*(*int*), 10 – 10 *B*, *pos*". We explain here only "*Weight*(*int*), 10 – 10", for explanation of additional details see (Rauch & Šimůnek, 2005).

The attribute *Weight* has values (i.e. categories) 52 – 133, it means weight of the patient in kg. The expression "*Weight*(*int*), 10 – 10" denotes that Boolean attributes *Weight*⟨52;61⟩, *Weight*⟨53;62⟩, …, *Weight*⟨124;133⟩ are automatically generated. Note that coefficients ⟨52;61⟩, ⟨53;62⟩, …, ⟨124;133⟩ of these Boolean attributes are intervals of categories. Both minimal and maximal length of these coefficients is 10 (see "*Weight*(*int*), 10 – 10"). This way 72 Boolean attributes are derived from the attribute *Weight*.

Boolean attributes derived from attributes *Height*, *Subscapular*, *Triglycerides* and *Cholesterol* are defined analogously. The attribute *Height* means height of patient in cm, it has values 158 - 194. The attribute *Subscapular* means skinfold above musculus subscapularis measured in mm, it has values from the interval 4 – 70. The attribute *Triglycerides* means triglycerides in mg%, its original values ranges from 28 to 670. New categories were defined as intervals (0;100⟩, (100;150⟩, (150;200⟩, …, (350;400⟩, > 400 . The attribute *Cholesterol* denotes cholesterol in mg%, it has 157 distinct values in interval 131 – 530.

The attribute *Smoking* has four distinct categories expressing various levels of intensity of smoking, analogously for attributes *Coffee*, *Beer*, *Vine*, and *Liquors* that have three distinct categories expressing various levels of consumption. The Boolean attributes to be derived from these attributes are specified by

Figure 1. Example of specification of the set of relevant antecedents

ANTECEDENT	
Physical	0 - 3
» Weight (int), 10 - 10	B, pos
» Height (int), 10 - 10	R, pos
» Subscapular (int), 5 - 5	B, pos
Biochemical	0 - 2
» Triglycerides (int), 1 - 3	B, pos
» Cholesterol (int), 20 - 25	B, pos
Vices	0 - 5
» Smoking (subset), 1 - 1	B, pos
» Coffee (subset), 1 - 1	R, pos
» Beer (subset), 1 - 1	R, pos
» Vine (subset), 1 - 1	R, pos
» Liquors (subset), 1 - 1	R, pos

the expression "(subset), 1 – 1", see Figure 1. It means that subsets containing exactly one category from the set of corresponding categories will be used. Examples of such Boolean attributes are *Smoking(non smoker)* and *Coffee(≥3 cups/day)*.

Tens of millions of association rules in the form of:

$$Physical(?) \wedge Biochemical(?) \wedge Lifestyle(?) \Rightarrow^{+}_{1.0,15} Cause\_of\_Death(?)$$

are defined by this way. Procedure 4ft-Miner generates and verifies them in 313 sec (on PC with 1.66 GHz and 2 GB RAM), only 4.3 $*10^6$ of rules were actually verified because of various optimizations. There are 36 rules satisfying given conditions. The strongest one (i.e. the rule with the highest $|\frac{a}{a+b} - \frac{a+c}{a+b+c+d}|$) is the rule:

$$Height\langle 174;183\rangle \wedge Triglycerides(150;200\rangle \Rightarrow^{+}_{1.21,15} Myocardial\ infarction$$

with contingency table, Table 4. Here we write only *Infarction* instead of *Cause_of_Death* (*Myocardial infarction*).

It means that relative frequency of patients who died from infarction among patients satisfying *Height*⟨174;183⟩ ∧ *Triglycerides*(150;200⟩ (i.e. 15/(15+18) = 0.454) is 121 per cent higher than relative frequency of patients who died from infarction among all 389 patients recorded in the data matrix DEATH (i.e. (15+65) / 389 = 0.206).

The second strongest one is the rule:

$$Cholesterol\ \langle 247;273\rangle \wedge Coffee\ (\geq 3\ cups/day) \Rightarrow^{+}_{1.18,16} Tumorous\ disease$$

with contingency table, Table 5.

It means that relative frequency of patients who died from tumorous diseases among patients satisfying *Cholesterol* ⟨247;273⟩ ∧ *Coffee* (≥ 3 *cups/day*) (i.e. 16/(16+9) = 0.64) is 118 per cent higher than relative frequency of patients who died from infarction among all 389 patients recorded in the data matrix DEATH (i.e. (16+98) / 389 = 0.293).

Table 4. Contingency table of Height⟨174;183⟩ ∧ Triglycerides(150;200⟩ and Infarction

Enhanced data matrix DEATH	*Infarction*	¬ *Infarction*
Height⟨174;183⟩ ∧ *Triglycerides*(150;200⟩	15	18
¬ (*Height*⟨174;183⟩ ∧ *Triglycerides*(150;200⟩)	65	291

Table 5. Contingency table of Cholesterol ⟨247;273⟩ ∧ Coffee (≥ 3cups/day) and Tumorous disease

Enhanced data matrix DEATH	*Tumorous disease*	¬ *Tumorous disease*
Cholesterol ⟨247;273⟩ ∧ *Coffee* (>=3 *cups/day*)	16	9
¬ (*Cholesterol* ⟨247;273⟩ ∧ *Coffee* (>=3 *cups/day*))	98	266

Let us note that the results say nothing about possibility to generalize these relations to additional data sets. Results only say that there are some interesting patterns in the data set STULONG.

Applying SD4ft-Miner

An example of application of SD4ft-Miner procedure concerns analysis of ENTRY data matrix. We solve the analytical question *Are there any strong differences between normal and risk patients what concerns confidence of association rule:*

Physical(?) $\wedge$ *Lifestyle*(?) $\rightarrow$ *Blood_pressure*(?) ?

where *Physical*(?) and *Lifestyle*(?) are Boolean attributes defined in the previous section *Applying 4ft-Miner.* Moreover, *Blood_pressure*(?) is a Boolean attribute derived from the attributes *Systolic* and *Diastolic* describing patient's blood pressure. This question can be symbolically written as:

normal x *risk*: *Physical*(?) $\wedge$ *Lifestyle*(?) $\rightarrow$ *Blood_pressure*(?) ?

We use a simplified version of the GUHA procedure SD4ft-Miner (Rauch & Šimůnek, 2005). It mines for SD4ft-patterns - i.e. expressions of the form α x β: $\varphi \approx \psi$. This pattern means that the subsets given by Boolean attributes α and β differ in what concerns the relation of Boolean attributes φ and ψ. The difference is defined by the symbol $\approx$ that is here called SD4ft-quantifier. The SD4ft-quantifier corresponds to a condition concerning two contingency tables, see Figure 2.

The first one is the table 4ft(φ,ψ, $\mathcal{M}/\alpha$) of φ and ψ on $\mathcal{M}/\alpha$. It concerns data matrix $\mathcal{M}/\alpha$ that consists of all rows of data matrix $\mathcal{M}$ satisfying α. Term a_α denotes the number of rows of data matrix $\mathcal{M}/\alpha$ satisfying both φ and ψ etc. The second 4ft-table is 4ft(φ,ψ, $\mathcal{M}/\beta$) of φ and ψ on $\mathcal{M}/\beta$, see Figure 2. It is defined in an analogous manner.

The SD4ft pattern α x β: $\varphi \approx \psi$ is true in the data matrix $\mathcal{M}$ if the condition corresponding to SD4ft-quantifier $\approx$ is satisfied for contingency tables 4ft(φ,ψ, $\mathcal{M}/\alpha$) and 4ft(φ,ψ, $\mathcal{M}/\beta$). An example of SD4ft-quantifier is the SD4ft-quantifier $\Rightarrow^{D}_{0.4,40,40}$. It corresponds to the condition:

$$\left|\frac{a_\alpha}{a_\alpha + b_\alpha} - \frac{a_\beta}{a_\beta + b_\beta}\right| \geq 0.4 \wedge a_\alpha \geq 40 \wedge a_\beta \geq 40$$

Thus, if the pattern α x β: $\varphi \Rightarrow^{D}_{0.4,40,40} \psi$ is true in data matrix $\mathcal{M}$ then the confidence of association rule $\varphi \rightarrow \psi$ on $\mathcal{M}/\alpha$ differs from its confidence on $\mathcal{M}/\beta$ at least 0.4 and moreover there are at least 40 rows of $\mathcal{M}/\alpha$ satisfying $\varphi \wedge \psi$ and there are at least 40 rows of $\mathcal{M}/\beta$ satisfying $\varphi \wedge \psi$.

Figure 2. Contingency tables 4ft(φ,ψ, $\mathcal{M}/\alpha$) and 4ft(φ,ψ, $\mathcal{M}/\beta$)

$\mathcal{M}/\alpha$	ψ	$\neg\psi$
φ	a_α	b_α
$\neg\varphi$	c_α	d_α

$\mathcal{M}/\beta$	ψ	$\neg\psi$
φ	a_β	b_β
$\neg\varphi$	c_β	d_β

The input parameters of the SD4ft-Miner procedure define the set of Boolean attributes to be used as the condition α defining a subset of rows of analyzed data matrix, the set of Boolean attributes to be used as the condition β, the set of possible antecedents φ, set of possible succedents ψ, and the SD4ft-quantifier $\approx$. We use the following parameters to solve our question:

normal × *risk*: *Physical*(?) ∧ *Vices*(?) → *Blood_pressure*(?)

- The set of Boolean attributes to be used as a condition α has only one element - *Group(NG)* i.e. the Boolean defining the set of normal patients, see section *Men Classification for Long-Term Observation.*
- The set of Boolean attributes to be used as a condition β has only one element - *Group(RG)* i.e. the Boolean defining the set of risk patients.
- The partial antecedents *Physical*(?) and *Vices*(?) to define the set of antecedents, see Figure 1.
- The set of Boolean attributes *Blood_pressure*(?) defined as a conjunction of length 1-2 of Boolean attributes *Systolic*(?) and *Diastolic*(?), see below.

The Boolean attributes *Systolic*(?) are derived from the attribute *Systolic* with values ⟨90;100⟩, …, ⟨220;230⟩. We use coefficients – intervals of length 1-3 to derive Boolean attributes *Systolic*(?). It means that the Boolean attributes *Systolic*⟨90;100), *Systolic*⟨90;110), *Systolic*⟨90;120), …, *Systolic*⟨210;220), *Systolic*⟨210;230), *Systolic*⟨220;230) are defined. The Boolean attributes *Diastolic*(?) are derived analogously from the attribute *Diastolic* with values ⟨50;60), …, ⟨140;150).

The procedure SD4ft-Miner generated and tested all about $22*10^6$ patterns of the form:

Group(*NG*) x *Group*(*RG*): *Physical*(?) ∧ *Vices*(?) $\Rightarrow^{D}_{0.4,40,40}$ *Blood_pressure*(?)

in 12 minutes (the same PC as for 4ft-Miner). Only two patterns satisfy given conditions. The stronger (i.e. the pattern with greatest difference of confidences of $\varphi \rightarrow \psi$) one is the pattern:

NG x *RG*: *Non-smoker* ∧ *Beer*(≤ *1*) $\Rightarrow^{D}_{0.44,67,42}$ *Diastolic*⟨60;90)

where we write *NG* instead of *Group*(*NG*), *RG* instead of *Group*(*RG*) and *Beer*(≤ *1*) instead of *Beer*(*up to 1 litre / day*). This pattern concerns the association rule:

Non-smoker ∧ *Beer*(≤ *1*) → *Diastolic*⟨60;90)

and it says that the confidence of this rule on the set of normal patients is 0.44 greater than its confidence on the set of risk patients, see corresponding contingency tables in Figure 3 where we write only *NS* ∧ *Beer*(≤ *1*) → *Ds*⟨60;90) and also graphical output in Figure 4.

This pattern shows strong difference between normal and risk patients that must be carefully interpreted with respect to the methodology described in section *Men Classification for Long-Term Observation*, see above.

Figure 3. Association rule $NS \wedge Beer(\leq 1) \rightarrow Ds\langle 60;90)$ on groups of normal and risk patients

Group(NG)	$Ds\langle 60;90)$	$\neg Ds\langle 60;90)$
$NS \wedge Beer(\leq 1)$	67	12
$\neg (NS \wedge Beer(\leq 1))$	160	37

Confidence = 67/(67 + 12) = 0.85

Group(NG)	$Ds\langle 60;90)$	$\neg Ds\langle 60;90)$
$NS \wedge Beer(\leq 1)$	42	61
$\neg (NS \wedge Beer(\leq 1))$	460	296

Confidence = 42/(42+61) = 0.41

Figure 4. Example of graphical output of the SD4ft-Miner procedure

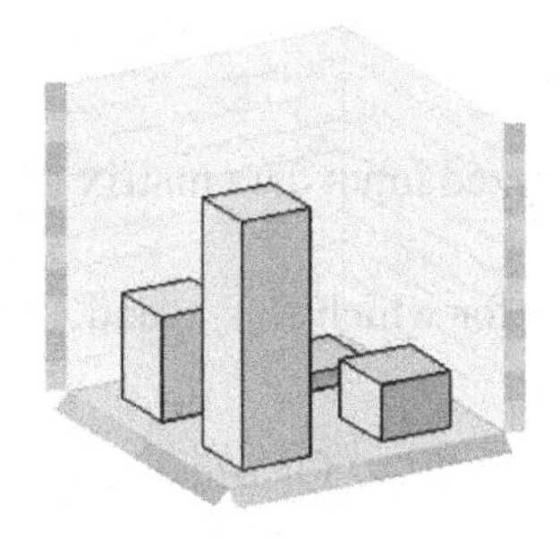

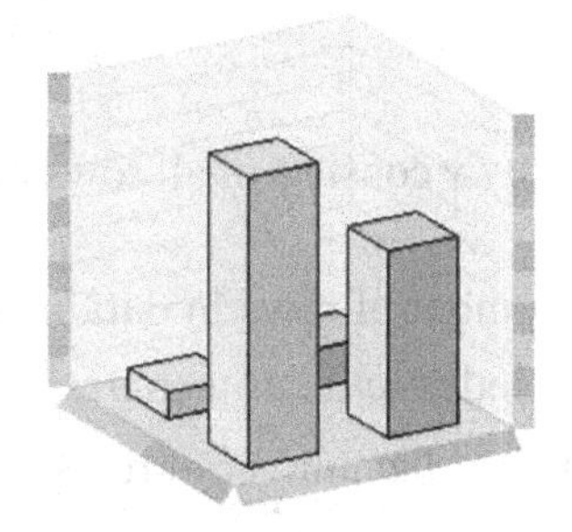

Applying KL-Miner

An example of application of KL-Miner procedure concerns also analysis of ENTRY data matrix. We solve the analytical question *Are there any strong ordinal dependencies among attributes describing physical examination, biochemical examination and blood pressure in the set of all patients or in some subgroups of patients described by lifestyle?* Symbolically we can write this question as:

ORDINAL DEPENDENCIES(*Physical, Biochemical, Blood pressure*) / *Lifestyle*(?)

We use the same attributes as in the previous examples. It means that physical examination is described by attributes *Weight, Height* and *Subscapular*, biochemical examination is described by attributes *Triglycerides* and *Cholesterol*, and blood pressure is described by *Systolic* and *Diastolic*. Further, we consider vices *Smoking, Coffee, Beer, Vine* and *Liquors*.

An example of such ordinal dependency is "If values of attribute *Triglycerides* increase then values of *Cholesterol* increase too". Additional example is "For the patients drinking more than 3 cups of coffee daily, there is a strong dependency: if systolic blood pressure increases, then diastolic blood pressure increases too".

We use the KL-Miner procedure (Rauch, Šimůnek & Lín, 2005) that mines for patterns of the form $R \approx C / \gamma$. Here R and C are categorial attributes. The attribute R has categories (possible values) $r_1, \ldots, r_K$, the attribute C has categories $c_1, \ldots, c_L$. The KL-Miner procedure deals with data matrices. We suppose that R and C correspond to columns of the analyzed data matrix and that the Boolean attribute γ is derived from the other columns of the analyzed data matrix.

The expression $R \approx C / \gamma$ means that the attributes R and C are related in the way given by the symbol $\approx$ when the condition given by the derived Boolean attribute γ is satisfied. We call the symbol $\approx$

KL-quantifier. The expression $R \approx S / \gamma$ is called *KL-hypothesis* or *KL-pattern*. The KL-pattern R and C is true in the data analyzed data matrix $\mathcal{M}$ if the condition corresponding to the KL-quantifier $\approx$ is satisfied for the contingency table of R and C on the data matrix $\mathcal{M} / \gamma$:

M / γ	c_1	$\cdots$	c_L	Σ_l
r_1	$n_{1,1}$	$\cdots$	$n_{1,L}$	$n_{1,*}$
$\vdots$	$\vdots$	$\ddots$	$\vdots$	$\vdots$
r_K	$n_{K,1}$	$\cdots$	$n_{K,L}$	$n_{K,*}$
Σ_k	$n_{*,1}$	$\cdots$	$n_{*,L}$	n

Here:

- The data matrix $\mathcal{M} / \gamma$ consists of all rows of the analyzed input data matrix $\mathcal{M}$ satisfying the condition γ
- $n_{k,l}$ denotes the number of rows in data matrix $\mathcal{M} / \gamma$ for which $R = r_k$ and $C = c_l$ (from now on, k will be used as a row index and l as a column index
- $n_{k,*} = \sum_l n_{k,l}$ denotes the number of rows in data matrix $\mathcal{M} / \gamma$ for which $R = r_k$
- $n_{*,l} = \sum_k n_{k,l}$ denotes the number rows in data matrix $\mathcal{M} / \gamma$ for which $C = c_l$
- $n_{*,l} = \sum_l \sum_k n_{k,l}$ denotes the number of all rows in data matrix $\mathcal{M} / \gamma$.

There are various possibilities how to define KL-quantifier $\approx$. One possibility is to set lower or upper threshold values for simple aggregate functions $\min_{k,l}\{n_{k,l}\}$, $\max_{k,l}\{n_{k,l}\}$, $\sum_{k,l} n_{k,l}$, $\frac{1}{KL}\sum_{k,l} n_{k,l}$. It is also possible to apply lower or upper threshold values to additional statistical and information theoretic functions, e.g. to conditional entropy, information dependence, Pearson χ^2 statistic or to mutual information.

We use Kendall's coefficient τ_b that is defined as:

$$\tau_b = \frac{2(P - Q)}{\sqrt{(n^2 - \sum_k n_{k,*}^2)(n^2 - \sum_l n_{*,l}^2)}}$$

where $P = \sum_{k,l} n_{k,l} \sum_{i>k} \sum_{j>l} n_{i,j}$ and $Q = \sum_{k,l} n_{k,l} \sum_{i>k} \sum_{j<l} n_{i,j}$. The Kendall's coefficient τ_b takes values from $\langle -1; 1 \rangle$ with the following interpretation:

- $\tau_b > 0$ indicates positive ordinal dependence (i.e. high values of C often coincide with high values of R and low values of C often coincide with low values of R
- $\tau_b < 0$ indicates negative ordinal dependence,
- $\tau_b = 0$ indicates ordinal independence
- $|\tau_b = 1|$ indicates that C is a function of R.

Note that the KL-quantifier can be also a conjunction of several particular applications of threshold values.

Input of the KL-Miner procedure consists of the analyzed data matrix $\mathcal{M}$, a set R = $\{R_1,\ldots,R_u\}$ of row attributes, a set C = $\{C_1,\ldots,C_v\}$ of column attributes, specification of the KL-quantifier $\approx$ and definition of the set Γ relevant conditions γ. The KL-Miner procedure automatically generates all relevant patterns $R \approx C / \gamma$ satisfying $R \in$ R, $C \in$ C and $\gamma \in \Gamma$ and verifies them in the data matrix M.

We used KL-Miner procedure with the following parameters to solve our analytical question ORDINAL DEPENDENCIES(*Physical, Biochemical, Blood pressure*) / *Lifestyle*(?):

- We used the ENTRY data matrix.
- The set R of row attributes was defined as R = {*Weight, Height, Subscapular, Triglycerides, Cholesterol, Systolic, Diastolic*}.
- The set C of column attributes was defined in the same way, i.e. C = {*Weight, Height, Subscapular, Triglycerides, Cholesterol, Systolic, Diastolic*}.
- The KL-quantifier was defined as the conjunction $\tau_b > 0.6 \wedge \sum_{k,l} n_{k,l} \geq 30$ where the condition $\sum_{k,l} n_{k,l} \geq 30$ means that there are at least 30 rows satisfying the condition γ.
- the set of relevant conditions γ was defined as the set of Boolean attributes, see Figure 1.

The procedure KL-Miner generated and tested all about 31 710 patterns of the given form, (various optimization techniques are used). The output consists of 470 patterns. Note that the KL-patterns with KL-quantifier defined as $\tau_b > 0.6 \wedge \sum_{k,l} n_{k,l} \geq 30$ are symmetrical, thus the output contains e.g. both *Systolic* $\approx$ *Diastolic* / γ and *Diastolic* $\approx$ *Systolic* / γ. The structure of the output set of 470 patterns is as follows.

There are 462 patterns of the form *Systolic* $\approx$ *Diastolic* / γ or *Diastolic* $\approx$ *Systolic* / γ, the strongest pair of patterns is for γ defined by the conjunction:

Coffe(1-2 *cups / day*) $\wedge$ *Beer* ($\geq$ *1 litre / day*) $\wedge$ *Vine* (*not drink*) $\wedge$ *Liquors*(*not drink*)

There are 44 patients satisfying this condition and the value of the Kendall's coefficient τ_b is 0.819.

There are 6 patterns of the form *Weight* $\approx$ *Height* / γ or *Height* $\approx$ *Weight* / γ, the strongest pair of patterns is for γ defined by the conjunction:

Smoking(*15–20 cig. / day*) $\wedge$ *Coffe*(*not drink*) $\wedge$ *Beer* ($\leq$ *1 litre /day*) $\wedge$ *Vine* ($\leq$ 1/2 litre / *day*)

There are 30 patients satisfying this condition and the value of the Kendall's coefficient τ_b is 0.65.

There are 2 patterns *Triglicerides* $\approx$ *Cholesterol* / γ and *Cholesterol* $\approx$ *Triglicerides* / γ with the condition γ defined by the conjunction:

Smoking($\geq$ *21 cig . /day*) $\wedge$ *Coffe*($\geq$ 3 *cups / day*) $\wedge$ *Vine* ($\leq$ 1/2 litre./*day*)

There are 39 patients satisfying this condition and the value of the Kendall's coefficient τ_b is 0.64.

These patterns show interesting relations concerning ENTRY data matrix that however again require careful interpretation that induce additional application of particular analytical procedures.

APPLYING KEX

KEX

The procedure KEX (Rauch & Berka, 1997) was designed to perform symbolic empirical multiple concept learning from examples, where the induced concept description is represented as weighted decision rules in the form:

`Ant ⇒ C(w)`

`Ant` is a conjunction of attribute-value pairs, `C` is a single category (class), and weight `w` from the interval [0,1] expresses the uncertainty of the rule.

The basic idea of the algorithm is to incrementally build from data a knowledge base of an expert system by adding new rule when the knowledge base becomes inconsistent with the training examples (Berka & Ivánek, 1994).

The pseudo-code of the KEX algorithm is shown in Figure 5. KEX works in an iterative way, in each iteration testing and expanding an implication `Ant ⇒ C`. This process starts with an "empty rule" weighted with the relative frequency of the class `C` and stops after testing all implications created according to the user defined criteria.

During testing, the validity (i.e. the conditional probability $P(C \mid Ant)$ of an implication is computed. If this validity significantly differs from the composed weight (value obtained when composing weights of all sub-rules of the implication `Ant ⇒ C)`, then this implication is added to the knowledge base. To test the difference between validity and composed weight, we use the chi-square goodness-of-fit test. The weight of this new rule is computed from the validity and from the composed weight using inverse composing function. For composing weights we use a pseudobayesian (Prospector-like) combination function:

Figure 5. Simplified sketch of the KEX algorithm

KEX algorithm

Initialization

1. for all category (attribute-value pair) A add $A \Rightarrow C$ to *OPEN* so that *OPEN* remains ordered according to decreasing frequency of A
2. add empty rule $\varnothing \Rightarrow C$ to the rule set *KB*

Main loop

while *OPEN* is not empty do

1. **select** the first implication $Ant \Rightarrow C$ from *OPEN*
2. **test** if this implication significantly improves the set of rules *KB* build so far (we test using the χ^2 test the difference between the rule validity and the result of classification of an example covered by *Ant*) then add $Ant \Rightarrow C$ as a new rule to *KB*
3. for all possible categories A
   - **(a)** **expand** the implication $Ant \Rightarrow C$ by adding A to *Ant*
   - **(b)** **add** $Ant \wedge A \Rightarrow C$ to *OPEN* so that *OPEN* remains ordered according to decreasing frequency of the condition of rules
4. **remove** $A \Rightarrow C$ from *OPEN*

$$x \oplus y = \frac{xy}{xy + (1-x)(1-y)}$$

When expanding, new implications are created by adding single attribute-value pairs to *Ant*. New implications are stored according to frequencies of *Ant* in an ordered list. Thus, for any implication in question during testing, all its sub-implications have been already tested.

We will clarify the step 2 of the KEX algorithm using the following simple example. Let the implication in question be `7a11a` $\Rightarrow$ `1+` with the validity computed from a contingency table as $a/(a + b)$ being 11/(11+14) = 0.44. Suppose further, there are the following rules in the KB, which are applicable for the *Ant* combination:

```
     ⇒ 1+ (0.6800)
11a  ⇒ 1+ (0.2720)
 7a  ⇒ 1+ (0.3052)
```

From these three rules, we can compute the composed weight:

$$cw = 0.6800 \oplus 0.2720 \oplus 0.3052 = 0.2586$$

Since this composed weight significantly (according to chi-square test) differs from the validity, we must add the implication `7a11a` $\Rightarrow$ `1+` into KB with weight w such, that:

$$w \oplus 0.2586 = 0.44$$

Unlike divide-and-conquer or set covering algorithms, KEX doesn't remove covered examples from the data. So, one example can be covered with more rules. During consultation for a particular case, all applicable rules (e.g. rules whose `Ant` parts correspond to characteristics of the case) are fired and their weights are combined using $\oplus$. An unseen example is assigned to the class with the highest composed weight.

KEX Applied to the STULONG Study

Using KEX we analyzed the data concerning examination of patients when entering the STULONG study. These data contain the information about lifestyle, personal history, family history, some laboratory tests and about classification w.r.t atherosclerosis risk (non risk group, risk group, pathological group).

The goal of this analysis was to identify characteristics, other than those used to define the risk factors, that can classify the patients into normal, risk, or pathological group. We performed several analyses for different subsets S1 - S4 of input attributes:

- **S1:** Classification based only on already known risk factors (this rule base should confirm the classification of patients in the analyzed data)
- **S2:** Classification based on attributes concerning lifestyle, personal and family history (but without special laboratory tests)

- **S3:** Classification based on attributes concerning lifestyle and family history
- **S4:** Classification based only on attributes concerning lifestyle

The classification accuracies (computed using 10 fold cross-validation) of the rule bases resulting from these analyses are summarized in Table 6. The classification accuracy is defined as:

(# patients correctly classified to class C) / (# patients classified to class C)

As a final output we selected the rule base S2. The reason for this choice was twofold: the rules have reasonable high classification accuracy and they do not use any "special" attributes concerning laboratory tests. These rules have been used to build a rule-based consultation system AtherEx. This system, freely accessible at http://www.euromise.cz, can help a non-expert user to evaluate her atherosclerosis risk (Berka et al., 2005).

ADDITIONAL ANALYSES

The STULONG data have been used during the Discovery Challenge workshops organized at the ECML conferences 2002, 2003 and 2004. About 25 different analyses, reported at these workshops, covered a variety of data mining tasks: segmentation, subgroup discovery, mining for association rules of different types, mining for sequential and episode rules, classification, regression. The workshop papers can be found at http://lisp.vse.cz/challenge. The general lessons learned can be summarized as follows (Berka et al, 2007):

- **Cooperate with domain experts:** The well known problem with expert systems is the so called knowledge acquisition bottleneck. This is the nickname for the necessity to involve the domain expert in the time consuming and tedious process of knowledge elicitation. Machine learning methods were understood as a way how to eliminate this problem. Nevertheless, in real-world data mining, we can observe similar problem we can call "data acquisition bottleneck". The most difficult steps of the KDD process are data understanding and data preparation. In real-world problems, we need experts who help with understanding the domain, with understanding the problem, with understanding the data.
- **Use external data if possible:** There are many external factors that are not directly collected for the data mining task, but that can have a large impact on the data analysis.

Table 6. Rule bases created from the data

Rule base	#.rules	total accuracy	accuracy for normal group	accuracy for other groups
S1	19	0.87	0.83	0.88
S2	**39**	**0.84**	**0.74**	**0.87**
S3	32	0.77	0.63	0.83
S4	27	0.73	0.48	0.83

- **Use powerful preprocessing methods:** Typical preprocessing actions are joining tables, aggregation, discretization and grouping, handling missing values, creating new attributes. Very often, theses operations are performed domain independent. More background knowledge should be used in these transformations.
- **Look for simple models first:** One of the common sources of misunderstanding between domain experts and data mining experts is that data mining experts are interested in applying their sophisticated algorithms and domain experts are interested in simple results. Sometimes even "simple" reporting and summarization gives acceptable results.
- **Make the results understandable and/or acceptable:** The crucial point for success of a data mining application on real-world problem is the acceptance of results by the domain experts and potential users. The best solution is worthless if it is not used. Understandability of results is the keyword for this lesson. Domain experts are not interested in tables showing improvement of accuracy of 2.47 % or in lists of thousands of rules. They want to know the strengths and limitations of the classifiers or insight into found patterns. So explanation of the results, post-processing or visualization is of the great importance.
- **Show some preliminary results soon:** To convince the domain experts (and the managers as well) about the usefulness of data mining methods, some preliminary results should be delivered in the early stage of the project. Even an initial data exploration can be highly appreciated.

CONCLUSION AND FURTHER WORK

The analysis like that described in sections *Applying GUHA method* and *Applying KEX* had shown that data mining methods can find interesting patterns hidden in the STULONG data and that this knowledge can be used in a reasonable way. They started lot of additional analyses that are summarized in the previous section. One of important conclusions is that the crucial point for the success of a data mining application on real-world problem is the acceptance of results by the domain experts and potential users. Understandability of results is the keyword and thus the explanation of the results is very important.

The explanation can be done e.g. by arranging results of data mining into an analytical report structured both according to the analyzed problem and to the user's needs. A possibility to produce such analytical report automatically is described in (Matheus et al., 1996), see also (Rauch, 1997). Thus we started research the goal of which is to develop a software system supporting automatic creation of reasonable analytical reports (Rauch & Šimůnek, 2007). Its first stage is intended to store relevant background knowledge, to use it to semi-automatically formulate reasonable analytical questions, to solve the formulated questions by GUHA procedures implemented in the LISp-Miner system and to assist in arranging results into well structured analytical report.

ACKNOWLEDGMENT

The work described here has been supported by Grant No. 201/08/0802 of the Czech Science Foundation and by Grant No. 1M06014 of Ministry of Education, Youth and Sports, of the Czech Republic.

REFERENCES

Aggraval, R. et al. (1996). Fast Discovery of Association Rules. In U.M Fayyad, G. Piatetsky-Shapiro, P. Smyth & R.S. Uthurasamy (Eds.) *Advances in Knowledge Discovery and Data Mining.* AAAI Press.

Berka, P., & Ivánek, J. (1994). Automated Knowledge Acquisition for PROSPECTOR-like Expert Systems. In. L. Bergadano, L. deRaedt (Eds.) *Proc. European Conference on Machine Learning,* (pp. 339 – 342). Berlin, Springer.

Berka, P., Laš, V., & Tomečková, M. (2005). AtherEx: an Expert System for Atherosclerosis Risk Assessment. In S. Miksch, J. Hunter & E. Keravnou (Eds.) *Proc. 10th Conference on Artificial Intelligence in Medicine* (pp. 79-88). Berlin, Springer.

Berka, P., Rauch, J., & Tomečková, M. (2007). Lessons Learned from the ECML/PKDD Discovery Challenge on the Atherosclerosis Risk Factors Data. *Computing and Informatics*, 26(3), 1001-1016.

Kohavi, R., Mason, L., Parekh, R., & Zheng, Z. (2004). Lessons and Challenges from Mining Retail E-commerce Data. *Machine Learning*, 57(1/2), 83-114.

Hájek, P., & Havránek (1978). *Mechanizing Hypothesis Formation (Mathematical Foundations for a General Theory),* Springer-Verlag, Berlin.

Hájek, P. (guest editor) (1981)..*International Journal of Man-Machine Studies*, second special issue on GUHA, 15.

Hájek ,P., Sochorová, A., & Zvárová J. (1995). GUHA for personal computers. *Computational Statistics & Data Analysis* 19, 149 - 153.

Matheus, J. et al. (1996). Selecting and Reporting What is Interesting: The KEFIR Application to Healthcare Data. In U.M Fayyad, G. Piatetsky-Shapiro, P. Smyth & R.S. Uthurasamy (Eds.) *Advances in Knowledge Discovery and Data Mining* (pp 495-515). AAAI Press.

Rauch, J. (1997). Logical Calculi for Knowledge Discovery in Databases. In J. Komorowski, J. Zytkow (Eds.) *Proc. European Conference on Principles of Data Mining and Knowledge Discovery.* (pp. 47 – 57). Berlin, Springer Verlag.

Rauch, J., & Berka, P. (1997). Knowledge Discovery in Financial Data - a Case Study. *Neural Network World,* 4-5(7).

Rauch, J., & Šimůnek, M. (2005). An Alternative Approach to Mining Association Rules. In T.Y. Lin, (Ed.) *Proc. Data Mining: Foundations, Methods, and Applications* (pp. 219-238). Springer-Verlag.

Rauch, J., & Šimůnek, M. (2005). GUHA Method and Granular Computing. In X. Hu, (Ed.). *Proceedings of IEEE conference Granular Computing* (pp. 630—635).

Rauch, J., Šimůnek, M., & Lín, V. (2005). Mining for Patterns Based on Contingency Tables by KL-Miner – First Experience. In T.Y. Lin (Ed.) *Foundations and Novel Approaches in Data Mining* (pp. 155-167) Berlin, Springer Verlag.

Rauch, J., & Šimůnek, M. (2007). Semantic Web Presentation of Analytical Reports from Data Mining – Preliminary Considerations. In Proc. *Web Intelligence* (pp. 3–7). IEEE Computer Society.

KEY TERMS

Association Rules: Relation between two Boolean attributes, It is defined by a condition concerning contingency table of these attributes. Usually, this condition is given by lower thresholds for confidence and support.

Atherosclerosis: Involves the slow buildup of deposits of fatty substances, cholesterol, body cellular waste products, calcium, and fibrin in the inside lining of an artery. It is a slow, complex disease that typically starts in childhood and often progresses when people grow older.

Decision Rules: If-then rules that are used to classify new examples.

GUHA method: Original Czech method of exploratory data analysis developed since 1960s. Its principle is to offer all interesting facts following from the given data to the given problem.

Hypertension: Blood pressure (BP) ≥ 160/95 mm Hg.

Hypercholesterolemia: Cholesterol level ≥ 260mg% (6,7 mmol/l).

Hypertriglyceridemia: Triglycerides level ≥ 200mg% (2,2 mmol/l).

KL-Pattern: Pattern expressing a relation between two many-valued attributes. The relation is defined by a condition concerning contingency table of two attributes in question.

Overweight: Brocca index > 115 % (Brocca index: height in cm minus 100 = 100 %).

SD4ft-Pattern: Pattern expressing a fact that two sets of observed objects differs what concerns quality of relation of two Boolean attributes when a given condition is satisfied. Both sets as-well as the condition are defined by suitable Boolean attributes.

Compilation of References

Aamodt, A. (2004). Knowledge-Intensive Case-Based Reasoning in CREEK. In: Funk, P., Gonzalez Calero, P.A. (eds.): *Proceedings European Conference on Case-Based Reasoning*, ECCBR 2004, Springer-Verlag, Berlin 5- 15.

Acharya, U.R., Suri, J.S., Spaan, J., & Krishnan, S.M. (2007). *Advances in Cardiac Signal Processing*. Springer Berlin Heidelberg.

Adams, N. M., & Hand, D. J. (1999). Comparing classifiers when the misallocation costs are uncertain. *Pattern Recognition*, *32*(7), 1139-1147.

Addison, P.S. (2005). Wavelet transforms and the ECG: A review. *Physiological Measurement* 26 (pp. 155-199), Institute of Physics Publishing.

Adlassnig, K. P. (1986). Fuzzy set theory in medical diagnosis. *IEEE Transactions on Systems, Man, and Cybernetics, SMC-16*, 260-265.

Agarwal, R., Gotman, J., Flanagan, D., & Rosenblatt, B. (1998). Automatic EEG analysis during long-term monitoring in the ICU. *Electroenceph. clin. Neurophysiol*, 10744-58

Aggraval, R. et al. (1996). Fast Discovery of Association Rules. In U.M Fayyad, G. Piatetsky-Shapiro, P. Smyth & R.S. Uthurasamy (Eds.) *Advances in Knowledge Discovery and Data Mining*. AAAI Press.

AGREE, Appraisal of Guidelines Research and Evaluation (AGREE), 2004. Available Online at: http://www.agreecollaboration.org/instrument/

Aha, D. (2003). Workshop – Mixed-Initiative Case-Based Reasoning. In McGinty, L. (ed.): *ICCBR'03 Workshop Proceedings*, Trondheim 127-209.

Aha, D., & Kibler, D. (1991). Instance-based learning algorithms. *Machine Learning, 6*, 37-66.

Aikins, J. S. (1983). Prototypal Knowledge in Expert Systems. *Artificial Intelligence, 20*(2),163-210.

Alacorn, R. D., Glover, S., Boyer, W., & Balon, R. (2000). Proposing an algorithm for the pharmacological treatment of posttraumatic stress disorder. *Ann Clin Psychiatry, 12*(4) 239-246.

Al-Alawi, A., Mulgrew, A., Tench, E., & Ryan, C. F. (2006, July). Prevalence, Risk Factors and Impact of Daytime Sleepiness and Hypertension of Periodic Leg Movements with Arousals in Patients with Obstructive Sleep Apnea. *Journal of Clinical Sleep Medicine*, 2(3), 281-7.

Alkan, A., Koklukaya, E., & Subasi, A. (2005). Automatic seizure detection in EEG using logistic regression and artificial neural network. *Journal of Neuroscience Methods, 148*, 167–176.

American Heart Association (2006). *Heart and stroke statistical update*. Http://www.american heart.org

Anderberg M.R. (1974). *Cluster Analysis for Applications*. Academic Press, New York

Armitage, P., & Berry, G. (1994). *Statistical Methods in Medical Research*, Oxford: Blackwell Science.

Arnt, A., & Zilberstein, S. (2004). Attribute measurement policies for time and cost sensitive Classification.

In *Proceedings of the 4th IEEE International Conference on Data Mining* (ICDM'04), (pp. 323-326).

Arshadi, N., & Jurisica, I. (2005). Data Mining for Case-based Reasoning in high-dimensional biological domains. *IEEE Transactions on Knowledge and Data Engineering, 17*(8), 1127-1137.

Asuncion, A., & Newman, D. J. (2007). *UCI Machine Learning Repository* [http://www.ics.uci.edu/~mlearn/MLRepository.html]. Irvine, CA: University of California, Department of Information and Computer Science.

Audette, M., Ferrie, F., & Peters, T. (2000). An algorithm overview of surface registration techniques for medical imaging. *Medical Image Analysis*, 4(4), 201-217.

Azuaje, F. (1998). Knowledge discovery in electrocardiographic data based on neural clustering algorithms. In *Proceedings Medicon '98 of the International Federation for Medical & Biological Engineering.*

Baeza-Yates, R. A., & Ribeiro-Neto, B. A. (1999). *Modern Information Retrieval*. ACM Press / Addison-Wesley.

Baguley, D. M. (2006). What progress have we made with tinnitus? In *Acta Oto-Laryngologica*, 126(5).

Bailey, J., Manoukian, T., & Ramamohanarao, K. (2002). Fast algorithms for mining emerging patterns. *Proceedings of the Sixth European Conference on Principles Data Mining and Knowledge Discovery (PKDD'02)* (pp. 39-50). Helsinki, Finland: Springer.

Bajcsy, R., & Kovacic, S. (1989). Multiresolution elastic matching. *Comp Vision Graphics Image Processing, 46*, 1–21, April 1989

Baneyx, A., Malaisé, V., Charlet, J., Zweigenbaum, P., & Bachimont, B. Synergie entre analyse distributionnelle et patrons lexico-syntaxiques pour la construction d'ontologies différentielles. *In Actes Conférence TIA-2005* (pp. 31-42). Rouen.

Barro, S., Ruiz, R., Cabello, D., & Mira, J. (1989). Algorithmic sequential decision-making in the frequency domain for life threatening ventricular arrhythmias and imitative artefacts: A diagnostic system. *Journal of Biomedical Engineering*, 11, 320–328.

Bayardo, R. J. (2005). The hows, whys, and whens of constraints in itemset and rule discovery. *Proceedings of the workshop on Inductive Databases and Constraint Based Mining* (pp. 1-13) Springer.

Becquet, C., Blachon, S., Jeudy, B., Boulicaut, J. F. & Gandrillon O. (2002). Strong Association Rule Mining for Large Gene Expression Data Analysis: A Case Study on Human SAGE Data. *Genome Biology*, 3(12):531-537.

Bellazzi, R., & Zupan, B. (2008). Predictive data mining in clinical medicine: Current issues and guidelines. *International Journal of Medical Informatics, 77*(2), 81-97.

Berka, P., & Ivánek, J. (1994). Automated Knowledge Acquisition for PROSPECTOR-like Expert Systems. In. L. Bergadano, L. deRaedt (Eds.) *Proc. European Conference on Machine Learning*, (pp. 339 – 342). Berlin, Springer.

Berka, P., Laš, V., & Tomečková, M. (2005). AtherEx: an Expert System for Atherosclerosis Risk Assessment. In S. Miksch, J. Hunter & E. Keravnou (Eds.) *Proc. 10th Conference on Artificial Intelligence in Medicine* (pp. 79-88). Berlin, Springer.

Berka, P., Rauch, J., & Tomečková, M. (2007). Lessons Learned from the ECML/PKDD Discovery Challenge on the Atherosclerosis Risk Factors Data. *Computing and Informatics*, 26(3), 1001-1016.

Berners-Lee, T., Hendler, J., & Lassila, O. (2001). The Semantic Web. *Scientific American*, May 2001.

Besl, P. J., & MaKey, N. D. (1992). A method for registration of 3-D shapes. *IEEE Trans. PAMI*, 14(2), 239-256.

Bichindaritz, I. (1994). A case-based assistant for clinical psychiatry expertise. *Journal of the American Medical Informatics Association*, Symposium Supplement, 673-677.

Bichindaritz, I., & Montani, S. (2007). Workshop – Case-Based Reasoning in the Health Science. In Wilson, D.C., Khemani, D. (eds.): *ICCBR- Workshop Proceedings*, Belfast 257-368.

Bichindaritz, I., Kansu, E., & Sullivan, K. M. (1998). Case-based Reasoning in Care-Partner. In: Smyth, B., Cunningham, P. (eds.): *Proceedings European Workshop on Case-based Reasong*, EWCBR-98, Springer-Verlag, Berlin, 334-345.

Biebow, B., & Szulman, S. (1999). Terminae: A linguistic-based tool for the building of a domain ontology. *In proceedings of the 11th European Workshop, Knowledge Acquisition, Modeling and Management (EKAW' 99)* (pp. 49-66). Dagstuhl Castle, Germany.

Biggs, D., DeVille, B., & Suen, E. (1991). A Method of Choosing Multiway Partitions for Classification and Decision Trees. *Journal of Applied Statistics*, 18(1), 49–62.

Bishop, C. M. (2006). *Pattern Recognition and Machine Learning*. Springer.

Bishop, C. M. (1996). *Neural Networks for Pattern Recognition*. Oxford, Oxford University Press.

Blachon, S., Pensa, R. G., Besson, J., Robardet, C., Boulicaut, J.-F., & Gandrillon, O. (2007). Clustering formal concepts to discover biologically relevant knowledge from gene expression data. *Silico Biology, 7.*

Blanco-Velasco, M., Weng, B., & Barner, K. E. (2007). ECG signal denoising and baseline wander correction based on the empirical mode decomposition. *Computers in Biology and Medicine.*

Bodenstein, G. & Praetorius, H.M. (1977). Feature extraction from the electroencephalogram by adaptive segmentation. In *Proc. IEEE*, 65, 642-652

Bonchi, F., & Lucchese, C. (2006). On condensed representations of constrained frequent patterns. *Knowledge and Information Systems, 9*, 180-201.

Bonet, B., & Geffner, H. (1998). Learning sorting and decision trees with POMDPs. In *Proceedings of the 15th International Conference on Machine Learning* (ICML), (pp. 73-81).

Bonnevay, S., & Lamure, M. (2003). Bases de connaissances anatomo-fonctionnelles : application au cerveau et au cœur. *Santé et Systémique*, 7(3), 47-75, Hermès.

Borgefors, G. (1988). Hierarchical Chamfer Matching: A Parametric Edge Matching Algorithm. *IEEE Transactions on Pattern Analysis and Machine Intelligence, 10*, 849-865.

Bortolan, G. & Pedrycz, W. (2002). An interactive framework for an analysis of ECG signals. *Artificial Intelligence in Medicine, 24* 109-132.

Bortolan, G., et al. (1991). ECG classification with neural networks and cluster analysis. *Computers in Cardiology, 20, 177-180.* IEEE Computer Soc. Press.

Bottaci, L., & Drew, P. J. (1997). Artificial Neural Networks Applied to Outcome Prediction for Colorectal Cancer Patients in Separate Institutions. *Lancet, 350*(16), 469-473.

Boulicaut, J.-F., Bykowski, A., & Rigotti, C. (2003). Free-sets: A condensed representation of boolean data for the approximation of frequency queries. *Data Mining and Knowledge Discovery journal, 7*, 5-22. Kluwer Academics Publishers.

Brachman, R. J., & Schmolze, J. G. (1985). An overview of the KL-ONE knowledge representation system. *Cognitive Science 9*(2), 171-216.

Bradie, B. (1996). *Wavelet Packed-Based Compression of Single Lead ECG. IEEE Trans. Biomed. Eng.,* 43, 493-501.

Braga, F., Caiani, E. G., Locati, E., & Cerutti, S. (2004). Automated QT/RR Analysis Based on Selective Beat Averaging Applied to Electrocardiographic Holter 24 H. *Computers in Cardiology 31.* IEEE Computer Soc. Press.

Bratko, I., Mozetic, I. & Lavrac, N. (1989). *Kardio: A study in deep and qualitative knowledge for expert systems.* MIT Press.

Breiman, L. (2001) Random Forests. *Machine Learning,* 45(1), 5–32.

Breiman, L., Freidman, J. H., Olshen, R. A., & Stone, C. J. (1984). *Classification and regression trees*, Belmont, California: Wadsworth.

Bresson, C., Keime, C., Faure, C., Letrillard, Y., Barbado, M., Sanfilippo, S., Benhra, N., Gandrillon, O., & Gonin-Giraud, S. (2007). Large-scale analysis by sage reveals new mechanisms of v-erba oncogene action. *BMC Genomics, 8*.

Brieman, L., Friedman, J., Olshen, R., & Stone, C. (1984). *Classification and Regression Trees*. Belmont, CA: Wadsworth International Group.

Brigelius-Flohe, R. (2006). Glutathione peroxidases and redox-regulated transcription factors. *Biol Chem, 387*, 1329-1335.

Brown, L. G. (1992). A survey of image registration techniques. *ACM Computing Surveys, 24*(4), 325-376.

Buchanan, B. G., & Shortliffe, E. H. (Eds.). (1984). *Rule-Based Expert Systems: The MYCIN Experiments of the Stanford Heuristic Programming Project*. Reading, MA: Addison-Wesley

Buitelaar, P., Olejnik, D., & Sintek., M. (2003). OntoLT: A protégé plug-in for ontology extraction from text. *In Proceedings of the International Semantic Web Conference (ISWC)*.

Burges, C. J. C: (1998). A Tutorial on Support Vector Machines for Pattern Recognition. *Data Mining and Knowledge Discovery*, 2, 121-167.

Cabena, H., Stadler, V., & Zanasi (1997). *Discovering Data Mining. From Concept to Implementation*. Prentice Hall, Inc.

Calders, T., Rigotti, C., & Boulicaut, J.-F. (2005). A survey on condensed representations for frequent sets. *Constraint-Based Mining and Inductive Databases* (pp. 64-80). Springer.

Camastra, F., & Verri, A. (2005). A novel Kernel Method for Clustering. *IEEE Transaction on Pattern Analysis and Machine Intelligence (PAMI), 27(5)*, 801-805.

Carmona-Saez, P., Chagoyen, M., Rodriguez, A., Trelles, O., Carazo, J. M., & Pascual-Montano, A. (2006). Integrated analysis of gene expression by association rules discovery. BMC *Bioinformatics, 7*, 54.

Carnap, R. (1937). *The Logical Syntax of Language*. New York: Harcourt.

Carnap, R. (1950). *Logical Foundation of Probability*. Chicago: University of Chicago Press.

Casale, P. N., Devereux, R. B., Alonso, D., Campo, E., & Kligfield, P. (1987). Improved sex-specific criteria of left ventricular hypertrophy for clinical and computer interpretation of electrocardiograms: validation with autopsy findings. *Circulation, 75*, 565-572.

Chai, X., Deng, L., Yang, Q., & Ling, C. X. (2004). Test-cost sensitive naive Bayes classification. In *Proceedings of the 4th IEEE International Conference on Data Mining* (ICDM'2004).

Chaussabel, D., & Sher, A. (2002). Mining microarray expression data by literature profiling. *Genome Biology, 3*.

Chen, C., Pellizari, C. A., Chen, G. T. Y., Cooper, M. D., & Levin, D. N. (1987). Image analysis of PET data with the aid of CT and MR images. *Information processing in medical imaging*, 601-611.

Chen, D., Chang, R., Kuo, W., Chen, M., & Huang, Y. (2002). Diagnosis of breast tumors with sonographic texture analysis using wavelet transform and neural networks. *Ultrasound in Medicine & Biology, 28*(10), 1301-1310.

Chen, H. (2001). *Knowledge Management Systems: A Text Mining Perspective*. Tucson, AZ: The University of Arizona.

Childs, J. D., & Cleland, J. A. (2006). Development and application of clinical prediction rules to improve decision making in physical therapist practice. *Physical Therapy, 86*(1), 122-131.

Chintu C., & Mwaba, P. (2005). Tuberculosis in children with human immuno deficiency virus infection. *International Journal Tuberculosis Lung Disease, 9*, 477-484.

Chow, C., & Liu, C. (1968). Approximating discrete probability distributions with dependence trees. *IEEE Transactions on Information Theory, 14*, 462-467.

Christov, I., & Bortolan, G. (2004). Ranking of pattern recognition parameters for premature ventricular contractions classification by neural networks. *Physiogical Measurement* 25, 1281–1290) .

Christov, I., Herrero, G., Krasteva, V., Jekova, I., Grotchev, A., & Egiazarian, K. (2006). Comparative Study of Morphological and Time-Frequency ECG Descriptors for Heartbeat Classification. *Medical Engineering & Physics*, 28, 876 – 887. Elsevier.

Chudáček, V., Lhotská, L., & Huptych, M. (2006). Feature Selection in Body Surface Potential Mapping. In *IEEE ITAB International Special Topics Conference on Information Technology in Biomedicine,* Piscataway: IEEE.

Cimiano, P., & Vorlker, J. (2005). Text2Onto – A Framework for Ontology Learning and Data-driven Change Discovery. In Andres Montoyo, Rafael Munoz, Elisabeth Metais (Ed.), *the 10th International Conference on Applications of Natural Language to Information Systems (NLDB), Lecture Notes in Computer Science. Springer: 3513.* (pp. 227-238). Alicante, Spain.

Cios, K., & Moore, G. (2002). Uniqueness of medical data mining. *Journal of Artificial Intelligence in Medicine, 26*, 263-264.

Clark, P., & Niblett, T. (1989). The CN2 induction algorithm. *Machine Learning*, 261–283.

Cleary, J. G., & Trigg, L.E. (1995). K*: An instance- based learner using an entropic distance measure. *Proceedings of the 12th International Conference on Machine learning*, 108-114.

Clifford, G. D., Azuaje, F., & McSharry, P. E. (2006). *Advanced Methods and Tools for ECG Data Analysis*. Artech House, Inc., Norwood, MA.

Cohen, A. (1986). *Biomedical Signal Processing*. CRC Press, Boca Raton, Florida,USA.

Cohen, I., & Cohen, I. (1993, November). Finite-element methods for active contour models and balloons for 2-D and 3-D images. *IEEE Pattern Anal. Machine Intelligence*, 15, 1131-1147.

Cohen, J. (1960). A coefficient of agreement for nominal scales. *Educational and Psychological Measurement, 20*, 37-46.

Colens, M. F. (1986). Origins of medical informatics. *Western Journal of Medicine,* 145, 778-785.

Collignon, A., Maes, F., Delaere, D., Vandermeulen, D., Suetens, P., & Marchal, G. (1995). Automated multimodality image registration based on information theory. In *Proc. 14th International Conference of Information Processing in Medical Imaging 1995,* vol.3, (Bizais, Y., Barillot, C. and Di Paola, R. eds.), Ile Berder, France, pp. 263–274, June 1995.

Copeland, G. P. (2002). The POSSUM system of surgical audit. *Archives of Surgery, 137*, 15-19.

Coppini, G., Diciotti, S., Falchini, M., Villari, N., & Valli, G. (2003). Neural networks for computer-aided diagnosis: detection of lung nodules in chest radiograms. *IEEE Transactions on Information Technology in Biomedicine, 7*(4), 344-357.

Corchado, J. M., Corchado, E. S., Aiken, J., Fyfe, C., Fernandez, F., & Gonzalez, M. (2003). Maximum likelihood Hebbian learning based retrieval method for CBR systems. In Ashley, K. D., Bridge, D. G. (eds.): *Proceedings International Conference on Case-based Reasoning*, ICCBR 2003, Springer-Verlag, Berlin 107-121.

Corcho, O., Lopez, M. F., & Perez, A. G. (2003). Methodologies, tools and languages for building ontologies. Where is their meeting point? *Data & Knowledge Engineering, 46*(1), 41-64.

Cover, T., & Thomas, J. (1991). *The Elements of Information Theory*. NewYork: Plenum Press.

Crémilleux, B., & Boulicaut, J.-F. (2002). Simplest rules characterizing classes generated by delta-free sets. *Proceedings 22nd Int. Conf. on Knowledge Based Systems and Applied Artificial Intelligence* (pp. 33-46). Cambridge, UK.

Cremilleux, B., Soulet, A., Klema, J., Hebert, C., & Gandrillon, O. (2009). Discovering Knowledge from Local Patterns in SAGE data. In P. Berka, J. Rauch and

D. J. Zighed (Eds.), *Data mining and medical knowledge management: Cases and applications*. Hershey, PA: IGI Global.

Crocker, B. D., Olson, L. G., & Saunders, N. A. (1990). Estimation of the probability of distributed breathing during sleep before a sleep study. *American Review of Respiratory Disease, 142*, 14-18.

Cuesta-Frau, D., Perez-Cortes, J. C., & Andreu-Garcıa, G. (2003). Clustering of electrocardiograph signals in computer-aided Holter analysis. *Computer Methods and Programs in Biomedicine* 72,179-196.

Cuffel, B. J. (2003). Remission, residual symptoms, and nonresponse in the usual treatment of major depression in managed clinical practice. *J Clin Psychiatry, 64*(4) 397-402.

Curro, V., Buonuomo, P. S., Onesimo, R., Vituzzi, A., di Tanna, G. L., & D'Atri, A. (2004). A quality evaluation methodology of health web-pages for non-professionals. *Med Inform Internet Med,* 29(2), 95-107.

Cybenko, G. (1988). *Continuous valued neural networks with two hidden layers are sufficient* (Technical Report). Department of Computer Science, Medford, Tufts University.

Cybenko, G. (1989). Approximation by superpositions of a sigmoidal function. *Mathematics of Control, Signals and Systems, 2*, 303-314.

Dancey, D. R., Hanly, P. J., Soong, C., Lee, B., Shepard, J., & Hoffstein, V. (2003). Gender differences in sleep apnea: The role of neck circumference, *Chest, 123*, 1544-1550.

Daqrouq, K. (2005). ECG Baseline Wandering Reduction Using Discrete Wavelet Transform. *Asian Journal of Information Technology 4*, 989-995.

Dash, M., & Liu, H. (1997). Feature selection for classification. *Intelligent Data Analysis, 1(3).*

Daube, J. R. (2002). *Clinical Neurophysiology Second Edition*. Mayo Foundation for Medical Education and Research, New York.

Daubechies, I. (1992). Ten lectures on Wavelets. CBMS-NSF, *SIAM*, 61, Philadelphia, Pennsylvania, USA.

Davidson, A. M., Cameron, J. S., & Grünfeld, J.-P. (eds.) (2005). *Oxford Textbook of Nephrology, 3*. Oxford University Press

Davidson, R. J. (1991). Cerebral asymmetry and affective disorders: A developmentalperspective. In: Cicchetti, D., Toth, S.L. (eds.) *Internalizing and externalizing expressions of dysfunction*. Rochester Symp. on Developmental Psychopathology 2, Hillsdale 123-133.

Davies, M., & Owen, K. (1990). Complex uncertain decisions: medical diagnosis. Case Study 10 in *Expert System Opportunities from the DTI's Research Technology Initiative*, HMSO.

de Chazal, P., & Reilly, R. (2004). Automatic classification of heart beats using ECG morphology and heart beat interval features. *Journal of Electrocardiology,* 32, 58–66.

De Groot, M. H. (1962). Uncertainty, information and sequential experiments. *Annals of Mathematical Statistics,* 33, 404-419.

De Raedt, L., & Zimmermann, A. (2007). Constraint-based pattern set mining. *Proceedings of the Seventh SIAM International Conference on Data Mining*. Minneapolis, Minnesota, USA: SIAM.

De Raedt, L., Jäger, M., Lee, S. D., & Mannila, H. (2002). A theory of inductive query answering. *Proceedings of the IEEE Conference on Data Mining* (ICDM'02) (pp. 123-130). Maebashi, Japan.

DeGroot, L. J. (1994). Thyroid Physiology and Hypothyroidsm. In Besser, G.M., Turner, M. (eds.) *Clinical endocrinilogy*. Wolfe, London Chapter 15.

Dejing, D., & Paea, L. (2006). Ontology-based Integration for Relational Databases. *In Proceedings of the 2006 ACM symposium on Applied computing* (pp. 461-466). Dijon, France.

DeRisi, J., Iyer, V., & Brown, P. (1997). Exploring the metabolic and genetic control of gene expression on a genomic scale. *Science, 278*, 680-686.

Diaz, J. A., Griffith, R. A., Ng, J. J., Reinert, S. E., Friedmann, P. D., & Moulton, A. W. (2002). Patients'use of the Internet for medical Information. *J Gen Intern Med,* 17(3), 180-5.

Diaz-Uriarte, R., & Alvarez de Andres, S. (2006). Gene selection and classification of microarray data using random forest. *BMC Bioinformatics*, *7*(3).

Dietterich, T.G. (1998). Machine-learning research: Four current directions. *The AI Magazine, 18*(4), 97-136.

DISCERN (2008). *DISCERN: Quality criteria for consumer health information.* Retrieved from http://www.discern.org.uk/.

Domingos, P. (1999). MetaCost: A general method for making classifiers cost-sensitive. In *Proceedings of the 5th ACM SIGKDD International Conference on Knowledge Discovery and Data Mining* (KDD-99), (pp. 155-164).

Dong, G., & Li, J. (1999). Efficient mining of emerging patterns: discovering trends and differences. *Proceedings of the Fifth International Conference on Knowledge Discovery and Data Mining (ACM SIGKDD'99)* (pp. 43-52). San Diego, CA: ACM Press.

Dony, R. D. & Haykin, S. (1995). Neural Network Approaches to Image Compression. In *Proc. IEEE,* 83, 288-303.

Douglas, N. J. (2002). *Clinicians' Guide to Sleep Medicine.* London: Arnold.

Drummond, C., & Holte, R. C. (2000). Exploiting the cost (in)sensitivity of decision tree splitting criteria. In *Proceedings of the 17th International Conference on Machine Learning* (ICML), (pp. 239-246).

Drummond, C., & Holte, R. C. (2006). Cost curves: An improved method for visualizing classifier performance. *Machine Learning, 65*, 95-130.

Duda, R. O., Hart, P. E., & Stork, D. G (2001). *Pattern Classification*, New York: John Wiley & Sons.

Duda, R., & Hart, P. (1973). *Pattern classification and scene analysis.* New York: John Wiley and Sons.

Džeroski, S., & Ženko, B. (2004). Is combining classifiers better than selecting the best one? *Machine Learning, 54*(3), 255-273.

Ebell, M. H. (2001). *Evidence-based Diagnosis: A handbook of Clinical Prediction Rules.* New York: Springer.

Eberhart, R. C., Dobbins, R. W. & Webber,W. R. S.(1989). EEG Analysis using CaseNet. In *Proceedings of the IEEE-EMBS 11th Annual Conference*, Seattle, WA, 2046-2047.

Eccles, M., & Mason, J. (2001). How to develop cost-conscious guidelines. *Health Technology Assessment, 5*(16), 1-69.

Eklund, P. (1994). Network size versus preprocessing, In R.R. Yager and L.A. Zadeh (Ed.), *Fuzzy Sets, Neural Networks and Soft Computing*, (pp 250-264). New York: Van Nostrand Reinhold.

Eklund, P., & Forsström, J. (1995). Computational intelligence for laboratory information systems, *Scandinavian Journal of Clinical and Laboratory Investigation, 55(Suppl. 222*), 75-82.

Eklund, P., Riissanen, T., & Virtanen, H. (1991). On the fuzzy logic nature of neural Nets. In *Neural Networks \& their Applications: Proceedings of Neuro-Nimes '91* (pp293-300), Nimes, France, November 4-8.

Elkan, C. (2001). The foundations of cost-sensitive learning. In *Proceedings of the 17th International Joint Conference on Artificial Intelligence* (IJCAI'01), (pp. 973-978).

Ellenius, J., Groth, T., Lindahl, B., & Wallentin, A. (1997). Early Assessment of Patients with Suspected Acute Myocardial Infarction by Biochemical Monitoring and Neural Network Analysis. *Clinical Chemistry, 43*, 1919-1925.

Elter, M., Schulz-Wendtland, & Wittenberg, T. (2007). The prediction of breast cancer biopsy outcomes using two CAD approaches that both emphasize an intelligible decision process. *Medical Physics*, *34*(11), 4164-4172.

ESHRE - European Society for Human Reproduction & Embryology (2007). High pregnancy rates achieved in ART through a personalised approach to ovarian stimulation treatment. In *The 23rd Annual Meeting of the European Society of Human Reproduction and Embryology.* Lyon, France.

European Commission. (2002). *eEurope 2002: Quality Criteria for Health related Websites.* Retrieved from http://europa.eu.int/information_society/eeurope/ehealth/ doc/communication_acte_en_fin.pdf.

Euzenat, J., Barrasa, J., Bouquet, P., Bo, J.D., et al. (2004). State of the Art on Ontology Alignment. *Knowledge Web, Statistical Research Division, Room 3000-4, Bureau of the Census, Washington, DC, 20233-9100 USA,* deliverable 2.2.3.

Everitt, B. S. (1994). *Cluster Analysis,* 3rd ed. John Wiley & Son, New York.

Eysenbach, G. (2000). Consumer health informatics. *BMJ,* 320 (4), 1713-16.

Eysenbach, G. (2003). The Semantic Web and healthcare consumers: A new challenge and opportunity on the horizon? *J Health Techn Manag,* 5, 194-212.

Faure, D., & Nedellec, C. (1998). A corpus-based conceptual clustering method for verb frames and ontology. *In Proceedings of the LREC Workshop on Adapting lexical and corpus resources to sublanguages and applications.*

Fawcett, T. (2004). *ROC graphs: Notes and practical considerations for researchers.* Technical report, HP Laboratories, Palo Alto.

Fawcett, T., & Provost, F. (1999). Activity monitoring: Noticing interesting changes in behavior. In *Proceedings of the 5th ACM SIGKDD International Conference on Knowledge Discovery and Data Mining* (KDD-99), (pp. 53-62).

Fayyad, U., Piatetsky-Shapiro, G., & Smyth, P. (1996). From data Mining to Knowledge Discovery: An Overview. In Fayyad U., Piatetsky-Shapiro G., Smyth P., & Uthurusamy R. (Ed.), *Advances in Knowledge Discovery and Data Mining,* (pp. 1-34). USA: AAAI Press.

Feinstein, A. (1958). *Foundation of Information Theory.* Mc Graw Hill, New York.

Ferguson, K. A., Ono, T., Lowe, A. A., Ryan, C. F., & Fleetham, J. A. (1995). The Relationship Between Obesity and Craniofacial Structure in Obstructive Sleep Apnea. *Chest, 108*(2), 375-381.

Ferrara, E., & Widrow, B. (1981). The time-sequenced adaptive filter. *IEEE Trans. 28,* 519-523.

Fitzpatrick, J.M., Hill, D.L.G. & Maurer, C.R. (2000). *Handbook of medical imaging,* (pp. 375-435). Bellingham, WA: SPIE Press.

Flemons, W. W., Whitelaw, W. W., & Remmers, J. E. (1994). Likelihood ratios for a sleep apnea clinical prediction rule. *American Journal of Respiratory and Critical Care Medicine, 150,* 1279-1285.

Freitas, J. A. (2007). *Uso de Técnicas de Data Mining para Análise de Bases de Dados Hospitalares com Finalidades de Gestão.* Unpublished doctoral dissertation, University of Porto, Portugal.

Freitas, J. A., Costa-Pereira, A., & Brazdil, P. (2007). Cost-sensitive decision trees applied to medical data. In: I. Y. Song, J. Eder, & T. M. Nguyen (Eds.): *9th International Conference on Data Warehousing and Knowledge Discovery (DaWaK 2007), LNCS, 4654,* 303-312, Springer-Verlag Berlin Heidelberg.

Friedman, N., Geiger, D., & Goldsmidt, M. (1997). Bayesian network classifiers. *Machine Learning, 29*(2), 131-163.

Furey, T.S., Cristianini, N., Duffy, N., Bednarski, D.W., Schummer, M. & Haussler, D. (2000). Support vector machine classifcation and validation of cancer tissue samples using microarray expression data. *Bioinformatics, 16,* 906–914.

Gamper, J., Nejdl, W., & Wolpers, M. (1999). Combining ontologies and terminologies in information systems. *In Proc. 5th International Congress on Terminology and knowledge Engineering.* Innsbruck, Austria.

Gant, V., Rodway, S., & Wyatt, J. (2001). Artificial neural networks: Practical considerations for clinical applications. In V. Gant, R. Dybowski (Eds.), *Clinical applications of artificial neural networks* (pp. 329-356). Cambridge, Cambridge University Press.

Gargasas, L., Ruseckas, R. & Jurkoniene, R., (1999). An expert system for diagnosis of coronary heart disease (CHD) with analysis of multicardiosignals. *Medical & Biological Engineering Computing 37(Supplement 2)*, 734-735.

Gelder, M. G., Lopez-Ibor, U., & Andeasen, N.C. (eds.) (2000). *New Oxford Textbook of Psychiatry.* Oxford University Press, Oxford.

Georgii, E., Richter, L., Ruckert, U., & Kramer S. (2005) Analyzing Microarray Data Using Quantitative Association Rules. *Bioinformatics*, 21(Suppl. 2), ii123–ii129.

Getahun, H., Harrington, M., O'Brien, R., & Nunn, P. (2007). Diagnosis of smear-negative pulmonary tuberculosis in peaple with HIV infection or AIDS in resource-constrained setting: informing urgent policy changes. *Lancet*, 369, 2042-2049.

Giorgetti, C., Terriou, P., Auquier, P., Hans, E., Spach, J. L., Salzmann, J., & Roulier, R. (1995). Embryo score to predict implantation after in-vitro fertilization: Based on 957 single embryo transfers. *Human Reproduction, 10*, 2427-2431.

Glenisson, P., Mathys, J., & Moor, B. D. (2003) Meta-clustering of gene expression data and literature-based information. *SIGKDD Explor. Newsl.* 5(2), 101–112.

Gletsos, M., Mougiakakou, S. G., Matsopoulos, G. K., Nikita, K. S., Nikita, A. S., & Kelekis, D. (2003). A computer-aided diagnostic system to characterize CT focal liver lesions: Design and optimization of a neural network classifier. *IEEE Transaction on Information Technology in Biomedicine, 7*(3), 153-162.

Glover, J., Ktonas, P., Raghavan, N., Urnuela, J., Velamuri, S., & Reilly, E.(1986). A multichannel signal processor for the detection of epileptogenic sharp transients in the EEG. *IEEE Trans. Biomed. Eng., 33*(12), 1121-1128.

Goldberger, A. L., Amaral, L., Glass, L., Hausdorf, J. M., Ivanov, P. C., Moody, G., Peng, C. K., & Stanley, H. E. (2000). PhysioBank, PhysioToolkit, and PhysioNet: Components of a New Research Resource for Complex Physiologic Signals. *Circulation*, 101(23), 215-220.

Golub, T., Slonim, D., Tamayo, P., Huard, C., Gaasenbeek, M., Mesirov, J., Coller, H., Loh, M., Downing, J., Caligiuri, M., Bloomfield, C., & Lander, E. (1999). Molecular classification of cancer: Class discovery and class prediction by gene expression monitoring. *Science*, 531–537.

Gotman, J. (1981). Quantitative EEG-Principles and Problems. *Electroenceph. Clin. Neurophysiol., 52*, 626-639.

Gower, J. C. (1988). Classification, geometry and data analysis. In H.H. Bock, (Ed.), *Classification and Related Methods of Data Analysis. Elsevier*, North-Holland, Amsterdam.

Gramatikov, B., Brinker, J., Yi-Chun, S., & Thakor, N. V. (2000) Wavelet Analysis and Time-Frequency Distribution of the Body Surface ECG Before and After Angioplasty. *Computer Methods and Programs in Biomedicine* (pp. 87-98). Elsevier Science Ireland Ltd.

Greiner, R., Grove, A. J., & Roth, D. (2002). Learning cost-sensitive active classifiers. *Artificial Intelligence, 139*(2), 137-174.

Gremy, F. (1989). Crisis of meaning and medical informatics education: A burden and/or a relief? *Methods of Information in Medicine,* 28,189-195.

Griffiths, K. M., Tang, T. T., Hawking, D., & Christensen, H. (2005) Automated assessment of the quality of depression Web sites. *J Med Internet Res.*,7(5), e59.

Groselj, C. (2002). Data Mining Problems in Medicine. *15th IEEE Symposium on Computer-Based Medical Systems (CBMS'02).* Maribor, Slovenia.

Gruber, T. R. (1991). The Role of Common Ontology in Achieving Sharable, Reusable Knowledge Base. In J. Allen, Fikes and E. Sandewall, Eds. *Principles of knowledge representations and reasoning,* Cambridge, MA, Morgan Kaufmann.

Gruber, T. R. (1993). A translation approach to portable ontology specification. *Knowledge Acquisition,* 5(2), Special issue: Current issues in knowledge modeling, 199-220.

Guarino, N., Carrara, M., & Giaretta, P. (1995). Ontologies and knowledge bases: towards a terminological clarification. In N. Mars (Ed.), *Towards Very Large Knowledge Bases, Knowledge Building and Knowledge Sharing* (pp. 25-32). IOS Press, Amsterdam.

Gupta, K. M., Aha, D. W., & Sandhu, N. (2002). Exploiting Taxonomic and Causal Realations in Conversational Case Retrieval. In Craw, S., Preeece, A. (eds.): *Proceedings European Conference on Case-Based Reasoning,* ECCBR 2002, Springer-Verlag, Berlin 133-147.

Guyatt, G. H., Feeny, D. H., & Patrick, D. L. (1993). Measuring health-related quality of life. *Annals of Internal Medicine, 118*(8), 622-629.

Hai, G. A. (2002). Logic of diagnostic and decision making in clinical medicine. Politheknica publishing, St. Petersburg.

Hájek ,P., Sochorová, A., & Zvárová J. (1995). GUHA for personal computers. *Computational Statistics & Data Analysis* 19, 149 - 153.

Hájek, P. (guest editor) (1981). *International Journal of Man-Machine Studies*, second special issue on GUHA, 15.

Hájek, P., & Havránek (1978). *Mechanizing Hypothesis Formation (Mathematical Foundations for a General Theory),* Springer-Verlag, Berlin.

Halkiotis, S., Botsis, T., & Rangoussi, M. (2007). Automatic detection of clustered microcalcifications in digital mammograms using mathematical morphology and neural networks. *Signal Processing, 87*(3), 1559-1568.

Halliwell, B. (2007). Biochemistry of oxidative stress. *Biochem Soc Trans, 35*, 1147-1150.

Hamamoto, I., Okada, S., Hashimoto, T., Wakabayashi, H., Maeba, T., & Maeta, H. (1995). Predictions of the early prognosis of the hepatectomized patient with hepatocellular carcinoma with a neural network. *Comput Biol Med, 25*(1), 49-59.

Han, J., & Kamber, M. (2001). *Data Mining: Concepts and Techniques.* San Francisco: Morgan Kaufmann.

Hanczar, B., Courtine, M., Benis, A., Hennegar, C., Clement, C. & Zucker, J. D. (2003). Improving classification of microarray data using prototype-based feature selection. *SIGKDD Explor. Newsl.*, *5*(2), 23--30. ACM, NY, USA.

Hand, D. J. (2002*). ESF exploratory workshop on pattern detection and discovery in data mining, 2447 of Lecture Notes in Computer Science.* Chapter Pattern detection and discovery, 1-12. Springer.

Hand, D. J., & Till, R. J. (2001). A simple generalisation of the area under the ROC curve for multiple class classification problems. *Machine Learning, 45*, 171-186.

Hanley, J. A., & McNeil, B. J. (1982). The meaning and use of the area under a receiver operating characteristic (ROC) curve. *Radiology, 143*(1), 29-36.

Haux, R. (1997). Aims and tasks of medical informatics. *International Journal of Medical Informatics,* 44, 3-10.

Haykin, S. (1994). *Neural networks. A comprehensive foundation.* Macmillan, New York.

Haykin, S. (1999). *Neural networks: A comprehensive foundation*, 2nd ed. Macmillan College Publishing Company, Inc.

Hearst, M. A. (1999). Untangling Text Data Mining. In Proceedings of ACL'99: *the 37th Annual Meeting of the Association for Computational Linguistics* (pp. 20-26). Maryland.

Hébert, C., Blachon, S., & Crémilleux, B. (2005). Mining delta-strong characterization rules in large sage data. *ECML/PKDD'05 Discovery Challenge on gene expression data co-located with the 9th European Conference on Principles and Practice of Knowledge Discovery in Databases (PKDD'05)* (pp. 90-101). Porto, Portugal.

Heller, M. F., & Bergman, M. (1953). Tinnitus in normally hearing persons. In *Ann. Otol.*

Henry, J. A., Jastreboff, M. M., Jastreboff, P. J., Schechter, M. A., & Fausti, S. (2003). Guide to conducting tinnitus retraining therapy initial and follow-up interviews. In *Journal of Rehabilitation Research and Development*, 40(2),159-160.

Hirschfeld, R. M. (2002). Partial response and nonresponse to antidepressant therapy: Current approaches and treatment options. *J Clin Psychiatry, 63*(9) 826-37.

Hollmén, J., Skubacz, M., & Taniguchi, M. (2000). Input dependent misclassification costs for cost-sensitive classifiers. In *Proceedings of the 2nd International Conference on Data Mining*, (pp. 495-503).

Holter, N.J. (1961). New methods for heart studies. *Science 134,* 1214.

HON, Health on the Net Foundation (2001). *HONCode*. Retrieved from http://www.hon.ch

HON, Health on the Net Foundation. (2005). *Analysis of 9th HON Survey of Health and Medical Internet Users Winter 2004-2005.* Retrieved from http://www.hon.ch/Survey/Survey2005/res.html

Hornero, R., Espino, P., Alonso, A. & Lopez, M. (1999). Estimating Complexity from EEG Background Activity of Epileptic Patients. *IEEE Engineering in Medicine and Biology*, Nov./Dec. 1999, 73-79.

Hornik, M., Stinchcombe, M., & White, H. (1989). Multilayer feedforward networks are universal approximators. *Neural Networks*, 2, 359-366.

Hotho, A., Staab, S., & Stumme, G. (2003). Ontologies improve text document clustering. *In Proceedings of the 3rd IEEE conference on Data Mining* (pp. 541-544). Melbourne, FL.

Huan, Z. (1998). Extensions to the K-Means Algorithm for Clustering Large Data Sets with Categorical Values. *Data Mining and Knowledge Discovery, 2(3).* Kluwer Academic Publishers

Huptych, M., Burša, M., & Lhotská, L. (2006). A Software Tool for ECG Signals Analysis and Body Surface Potential Mapping. In *IEEE ITAB International Special Topics Conference on Information Technology in Biomedicine*. Piscataway: IEEE.

Jager, F., Moody, G. B., Divjak, S., & Mark, R.G. (1994). Assessing the robustness of algorithms for detecting transient ischemic ST segment changes. *Computers in Cardiology* (pp. 229–232).

Jain, A. K. (1999). Data clustering: A review. *ACM Computing Surveys, 31(3).*

Jalaleddine, S. M. S. , Hutchens, Ch. G. , Strattan, R. D. & Coberly, W. A.(1990). ECG Data Compression Techniques - A Unified Approach. *IEEE Trans.Biomed. Eng., 37,* 329-343.

Janet, F. (1997). Artificial Neural Networks Improve Diagnosis of Acute Myocardial Infarction. *Lancet, 350(9082)*, 935.

Japkowicz, N., & Stephen, S. (2002). The class imbalance problem: A systematic study. *Intelligent Data Analysis, 6*(5), 429-449.

Jasper, H. H. (1958). Report of the Committee on Methods of Clinical Examination in Electroencephalography. *Electroenceph. Clin. Neurophysiol, 10*, 370-1.

Jastreboff, M. M., Payne, L., & Jastreboff, P. J. (1999). *Effectiveness of tinnitus retraining therapy in clinical practice.* (Presentation).

Jastreboff, M. M., Payne, L., & Jastreboff, P. J. (2003). Tinnitus and hyperacusis. In *Ballenger's Otorhinolaryngology Head and Neck Surgery* (Eds. Snow Jr, J.B., Ballenger, J.J.), BC Decker Inc., pp. 456-475.

Jastreboff, P. J. (1995). Tinnitus as a phantom perception: theories and clinical implications, in *Mechanisms of Tinnitus,* Vernon, J. and Moller, A.R. (Eds), Boston, MA, Allyn & Bacon., pp. 73-94.

Jastreboff, P. J., & Hazell, J. W. (2004). *Tinnitus retraining therapy,* Cambridge, United Kingdom, Cambridge University Press.

Jeff, S. (1987). *Concept acquisition through representational adjustment.* Doctoral dissertation, Department of Information and Computer Science, University of California, Irvine, CA

Jeras, M., Magjarević, R., & Paćelat, E. (2001). Real time P-wave detection in surface ECG. *Proceedings Medicon 2001 of the International Federation for Medical & Biological Engineering.*

Jianxin, C., Yanwei, X., Guangcheng, X., Jing, C., Jianqiang, Y., Dongbin, Z., & Jie,W. (2007). A Comparison of Four Data Mining Models: Bayes, Neural Network, SVM and Decision Trees in Identifying Syndromes in Coronary Heart Disease. Lecture Notes in Computer Science. *Advances in Neural Networks, 4491,* 1274-1279.

John, G. H., & Langley, P. (1995). Estimating continuous distributions in Bayesian classifiers. *Proceedings of the Eleventh Conference on Uncertainty in Artificial Intelligence,* 338-345.

Jollife, I.T. (2002). *Principal Component Analysis.* Springer.

Jordan, A. S., & McEvoy, R. D. (2003). Gender differences in sleep apnea: Epidemiology, clinical presentation and pathogenic mechanisms. *Sleep Medicine Reviews, 7*(5), 377-389.

Jurisica, I., Mylopoulos, J., Glasgow, J., Shapiro, H., & Casper, R. (1998). Case-based reasoning in IVF: Prediction and knowledge mining. *Artificial Intelligence in Medicine, 12*(1), 1-24.

Kadambe, S., Murray, R., & Boudreaux-Bartels, G. F. (1999). Wavelet transformed-based QRS complex detector. *IEEE Trans. Biomed. Eng.* 46, 838–848.

Kalinowsky, L., & Hippius, H. (1969). *Pharmacolological, convulsive and other somatic treatments in psychiatry.* Grunee&Stratton, New York London.

Kallin, L. , Räty, R., Selén, G., & Spencer, K. (1998). A Comparison of Numerical Risk Computational Techniques in Screening for Down's Syndrome. In P. Gallinari and F. Fogelman Soulie, (Eds.), *Industrial Applications of Neural Networks* (pp.425-432). Singapore: World Scientific.

Kanungo, T., Mount, D. M., Netanyahu, N., Piatko, C., Silverman, R. & Wu, A. Y. (2002). An efficient K-Means clustering algorithm: Analysis and implementation. *IEEE Trans. Pattern Analysis and Machine Intelligence, 24,* 881-892.

Karel, F. (2006) Quantitative and ordinal association rules mining (QAR mining). In *Knowledge-Based Intelligent Information and Engineering Systems*, 4251, 195–202. Springer LNAI.

Karel, F., & Klema, J. (2007). Quantitative Association Rule Mining in Genomics Using Apriori Knowledge. In Berendt, B., Svatek, V. Zelezny, F. (eds.), Proc. of The *ECML/PKDD Workshop On Prior Conceptual Knowledge in Machine Learning and Data Mining.* University of Warsaw, Poland, (pp. 53-64).

Karkaletsis, V., Spyropoulos, C. D., Grover, C., Pazienza, M. T., Coch, J., & Souflis, D. (2004) A Platform for Crosslingual, Domain and User Adaptive Web Information Extraction. In *Proceedings of the European Conference in Artificial Intelligence* (ECAI), Valencia, Spain; p. 725-9.

Karoui, L., Aufaure, M.A., & Bennacer, N. (2006). Context-based Hierarchical Clustering for the Ontology Learning. *The 2006 IEEE/WIC/ACM International Conference on Web Intelligence (WI-06) jointly with the 2006 IEEE/WIC/ACM International Conference on Data Mining (ICDM-06)* (pp. 420-427). Hong-Kong.

Kasabov, N. (1996), *Neural Networks, Fuzzy Systems and Knowledge Engineering.* USA:MIT Press.

Kass, M., Witkin, A., & Terzopoulos, D. (1988). Snakes: active contour models. *International Journal of Computer Vision*, pp.321-331.

Kaufman, L., & Rousseeuw, P. J. (1990). *Finding Groups in Data—An Introduction to Cluster Analysis.* Wiley.

Keime, C., Damiola, F., Mouchiroud, D., Duret, L. & Gandrillon, O. (2004). Identitag, a relational database for SAGE tag identification and interspecies comparison of SAGE libraries. *BMC Bioinformatics, 5*(143).

Kendall, M. G., & Stuart, A. (1979). *The advanced theory of statistics.* 4 ed. New York: Macmillan publishing, New York.

Keogh, E. J., & Pazzani, M. (1999). Learning augmented Bayesian classifiers: A comparison of distribution-based and classification-based approaches. *Uncertainty 99: The 7th International Workshop on Artificial Intelligence and Statistics*, 225-230.

Khan, M. G. (2003). *Rapid ECG Interpretation.* Elsevier Inc. New York

Kjaer, M., Krogsgaard, M., & Magnusson, P., et al. (2003). *Textbook of sports medicine.* Oxford: Blackwell Publishing.

Kléma, J., & Zelezny, F. In P. Berka, J. Rauch and D. J. Zighed (Eds.), *Data mining and medical knowledge management: Cases and applications, chapter Gene Expression Data Mining Guided by Genomic Background Knowledge.* IGI Global.

Kléma, J., Blachon, S., Soulet, A., Crémilleux, B., & Gandrillon, O. (2008). Constraint-based knowledge discovery from sage data. *Silico Biology, 8*(0014).

Kléma, J., Soulet, A., Cremilleux, B., Blachon, S., & Gandrilon, O. (2006). Mining Plausible Patterns from Genomic Data. *Proceedings of Nineteenth IEEE International Symposium on Computer-Based Medical Systems*, Los Alamitos: IEEE Computer Society Press, 183-188.

Knobbe, A., & Ho, E. (2006). Pattern teams. *Proceedings of the 10th European Conference on Principles and Practice of Knowledge Discovery in Databases (PKDD'06)* (pp. 577-584). Berlin, Germany: Springer-Verlag.

Knottnerus, J. A. (1995). Diagnostic prediction rules: principles, requirements and pitfalls. *Medical Decision Making, 22*(2), 341-360.

Kohavi, R. (1995). The power of decision tables. In *Proceedings of 8th European Conference on Machine Learning*, 174-189.

Kohavi, R., & John, G. (1997). Wrappers for feature subset selection. *Artificial Intelligence, 97*(1-2), 273-324.

Kohavi, R., & Provost, F. (1998). Glossary of Terms. *Machine Learning, 30(2/3)*, 271-274.

Kohavi, R., Mason, L., Parekh, R., & Zheng, Z. (2004). Lessons and Challenges from Mining Retail E-commerce Data. *Machine Learning*, 57(1/2), 83-114.

Kohler, C., Darmoni, S. D., Mayer, M. A., Roth-Berghofer, T., Fiene, M., & Eysenbach, G. (2002). MedCIRCLE – The Collaboration for Internet Rating, Certification, Labelling, and Evaluation of Health Information. Technology and Health Care, Special Issue: Quality e-Health. *Technol Health Care, 10*(6), 515.

Kohonen, T. (1995). *Self-Organizing Maps.* Springer, Berlin, Heidelberg.

Kókai, G., Alexin, Z., & Gyimóthy, T., (1997). Application of inductive logic programming for learning ECG waveforms. *Proceedings of AIME97,* 1211,126-129.

Kononenko, I. (1991). Semi-naive Bayesian classifiers. *Proceedings of the 6th European Working Session on Learning*, 206-219.

Kononenko, I. (2001). Machine Learning for Medical Diagnosis: History, State of the Art and Perspective. *Artificial Intelligent Medicine. 23(1)*, 89-109.

Kononenko, I., & Kukar, M. (2007). *Machine Learning and Data Mining.* Horwood Publishing Ltd.

Kordík, P. (2006). *Fully Automated Knowledge Extraction using Group of Adaptive Models Evolution.* Doctoral thesis, Czech Technical University in Prague.

Kornreich, F. (1997). Appropriate electrode placement in evaluating varied cardiac pathology. In Liebman J. (ed) *Electrocardiology '96. From the cell to the body surface.* Publ.World Scientific 1997.

Korotkina, R. N., Matskevich, G. N., Devlikanova, A. S., Vishnevskii, A. A., Kunitsyn, A. G., & Karelin, A. A. (2002). Activity of glutathione-metabolizing and antioxidant enzymes in malignant and benign tumors of human lungs. *Bulletin of Experimental Biology and Medicine, 133*, 606-608.

Kraemer, H. C. (1992), *Evaluating Medical Tests*. Newbury Park, CA: Sage Publications.

Krajča, V., & Petránek, S. (1992). Automatic epileptic spike detection by median filtering and simple arithmetic sharp transient detector: a clinical evaluation. In *Proc. VI Mediterranean Conference on Medical and Biological Engineering*, 1, 209-212. Capri, Italy.

Krajča, V., Matoušek, M., Petránek, S., Grießbach, G., Ivanova, G., & Vršecká, M.(1997). Feature extraction from the EEG of comatose patients by global adaptive segmentation, *42. Internationales wissenschaftliches Kolloquium* TU Ilmenau, Band 2, pp.156-161.

Krajča, V., Petránek, S., Patáková, I., & Värri A. (1991). Automatic identificaton of significant graphoelements in multichannel EEG recordings by adaptive segmentation and fuzzy clustering. *Int. J. Biomed. Comput.*, 28, 71-89.

Krajča, V., Principe, J. C., Petránek, S., & Vyšata, O. (1996). Use of time-delayed self-organized principal components analysis for feature extraction from the EEG. *Third International Hans Berger Congress*, Jena, p. 50.

Krajča, V., Principe, J.C. & Petránek S.. (1997). Dimensionality reduction and reconstruction of the EEG signal by self-organized principal components analysis. *First European Conference on Signal Analysis and Prediction*, Prague.

Ktonas, P. Y. (1983). Automated analysis of abnormal electroencephalograms, *CRC Crit. Rev. Bioeng.*, 9., 39-97.

Kuhan, G., Gadiner, E. D., Abidia, A. F., Chetter, I. C., Renwick, P. M., Johnson, B. F., Wilkinson, A. R., & McCollum, P. T. (2001). Risk Modelling study for carotid endatorectomy. *British Journal of Surgery, 88*, 1590-1594.

Kukar, M. & al. (1999). Analysing and improving the diagnosis of ischaemic heart disease with machine learning. *Artificial Intelligence in Medicine,* 16, 25-50.

Kullback, S., & Leibler, R. (1951). On information and sufficiency. *Annals of Mathematical Statistics,* 22, 79-86.

Kuncheva L. I. (2004). Combining *Pattern Classifiers. Methods and Algorithms.* Wiley.

Kundu, M., Nasipuri, M. & Basu, D.K., (1998). A knowledge based approach to ECG interpretation using fuzzy logic. *IEEE Trans. System, Man and Cybernetics, 28*,237-243.

Kwiatkowska, M., & Atkins, M. S. (2004). A Semio-Fuzzy Approach to Information Fusion in the Diagnosis of Obstructive Sleep Apnea. *Proceedings of the NAFIPS*. Banff, Canada, 55-60.

Kwiatkowska, M., Atkins, M. S., Ayas, N. T., & Ryan, C. F. (2007). Knowledge-Based Data Analysis: First Step Toward the Creation of Clinical Prediction Rules Using a New Typicality Measure. *IEEE Transactions on Information Technology in Biomedicine, 11*(6), 651-660.

Labsky, M., & Svatek, V. (2006, June) Information Extraction with Presentation Ontologies. In: ESWC'06 *Workhshop on Mastering the Gap: From Information Extraction to Semantic Representation*, Budva, Montenegro.

Labsky, M., Svatek, V., Nekvasil, M., & Rak D. (2007). The Ex Project: Web Information Extraction using Extraction Ontologies. In: *Proc. PriCKL'07, ECML/PKDD Workshop on Prior Conceptual Knowledge in Machine Learning and Knowledge Discovery.* Warsaw, Poland, October 2007.

Lagerholm, M., & al. (2000). Clustering ECG complexes using Hermite functions and self-organizing maps. *IEEE Transaction on Biomedical Engineering, 47*(7), 838-848.

Lähdevirta, J. (1971). Nephropathia epidemica in Finland: A clinical, histological and epidemiological study. *Annals of clinical research, 3(Suppl 8)*, 1-154.

Lam, B., Ip, M. S. M., Tench, E., & Ryan, C. F. (2005). Craniofacial profile in Asian and white subjects with obstructive sleep apnea. *Thorax, 60*(6), 504-510.

Lauritzen, S. L. (1996). *Graphical models.* Clarendon Press, Oxford University.

Lavrac, N. (1999). Selected techniques for data mining in medicine. *Artificial Intelligence in Medicine, 16*, 3-23.

Lavrač, N., & Zupan, B. (2005). Data Mining in Medicine. In O. Maimon & L. Rokach (Eds.). *Data Mining and Knowledge Discovery Handbook*, Springer US.

Lavrac, N., Gamberger, D., & Turney, P. (1996). Preprocessing by a cost-sensitive literal reduction algorithm: REDUCE. In *Proceedings of the Workshop Mathematical and Statistical Methods, at the International School for the Synthesis of Expert Knowledge* (ISSEK'96), (pp. 179-196).

Lavrac, N., Keravnou, E. & Zupan, B. (2000). Intelligent Data Analysis in Medicine. In A. Kent (Ed.), *Encyclopedia of Computer Science and Technology* (pp. 113-157). New York: Dekker.

Lavrac, N., Zelezny, F., & Flach, P. (2002). RSD: Relational subgroup discovery through first-order feature construction. In *Proceedings of the 12th International Conference on Inductive Logic Programming*, 149–165.

Lee, J. W., Lee, J. B., Park, M., & Song, S. H. (2005). An extensive evaluation of recent classification tools applied to microarray data. *Computation Statistics and Data Analysis, 48*, 869-885.

Lee, Y., & Lee, Ch. K. (2003) Classification of Multiple Cancer Types by Multicategory Support Vector Machines Using Gene Expression Data. *Bioinformatics, 19*(9), 1132-1139.

Lehman, D., Ozaki, H., & Pal I. (1987). EEG alpha map series: brain micro states by space oriented adaptive segmentation. *Electroenceph. clin. Neurophysiol., 67*, 271-288

Lehmann, T. M., Gönner, C., & Spitzer, K. (1999). Survey: Interpolation methods in medical image processing. *IEEE Transactions on Medical Imaging, 18*(11), 1049-1075.

Li, C., Zheng, C., & Tai, C.(1995). Detection of ECG Characteristic Points Using Wavelet Transforms. *IEEE Transaction on Biomedical Engineering*, 42, 21-28.

Li, J., Liu, G., & Wong, L. (2007). Mining statistically important equivalence classes and delta-discriminative emerging patterns. *Proceedings of the 13th ACM SIGKDD international conference on Knowledge discovery and data mining (KDD'07)* (pp. 430-439). New York, NY, USA: ACM.

Liese, F., Vajda, I. (2006). On divergences and information in statistics and information theory. *IEEE Transactions on Information Theory,* 52, 4394-4412.

Lindahl, D., Palmer, J., Ohlsson, M., Peterson, C., Lundin, A., & Edenbrand, L. (1997). Automated interpretation of myocardial SPECT perfusion images using artificial neural networks. *J Nucl Med, 38*, 1870-1875.

Ling, C. X., Sheng, V. S., & Yang, Q. (2006). Test strategies for cost-sensitive decision trees. *IEEE Transactions on Knowledge and Data Engineering, 18*(8), 1055-1067.

Ling, C. X., Yang, Q., Wang, J., & Zhang, S. (2004). Decision trees with minimal costs. In *Proceedings of the 21st International Conference on Machine Learning* (ICML).

Lisboa, P. J. G. (2002). A review of evidence of health benefit from artificial neural networks in medical intervention. *Neural Network, 15*, 11-39.

Liu, H., & Motoda, H. (1998). *Feature Selection for Knowledge Discovery and Data Mining.* Kluwer Academic, Norwell, MA USA.

Lizotte, D. J., Madani, O. & Greiner, R. (2003). Budgeted learning of naiveBayes classifiers. In *Proceedings of the 19th Conference in Uncertainty in Artificial Intelligence* (UAI'03), (pp. 378-385).

Lopes da Silva, F., Dijk, A., & Smits, H. (1975). Detection of nonstationarities in EEGs using the autoregressive model - An application to EEGs of epileptics. In *CEAN-Computerized EEG analysis*, G.Dolce, H.Kunkel Eds., Stuttgart, Germany, G. Fischer Verlag, pp.180-199.

Lux, R.L (1982): Electrocardiographic body surface potential mapping CRC. *Crit. Rev. Biomed. Eng.*, 8, 253 – 279.

Ma, J., & Knight, B. A. (2003). Framework for Historical Case-Based Reasoning. In 5th *International Conference on Case-Based Reasoning,* Springer Berlin 246-260.

Maccabee, P. J., & Hassan, N. F. (1992). Digital filtering: basic concepts and application to evoked potentials. *Muscle Nerve,* 15, 865-875.

Madeira, S. C., & Oliveira, A. L. (2004). Biclustering algorithms for biological data analysis: A survey. IEEE/ACM Trans. Comput. *Biology Bioinform., 1,* 24-45.

Maedche, A., & Staab, S. (2004). Ontology learning. In S. Staab and R. Studer (Ed.), *Handbook on Ontologies* (pp. 173-189). Springer.

Maedche, A., Motik, B., Stojanovic, L., Studer, R., & Volz, R. (2003). Ontologies for enterprise knowledge management. *IEEE Intelligent Systems, 18*(2), 26-33.

Maintz, J. B. A. & Viergever, M. A. (1998). A Survey of Medical Image Registration. *Medical Image Analysis, 2*(1), 1-36.

Maintz, J. B. A., van den Elsen, P. A. & Viergever, M. A. (1996). Evaluation of ridge seeking operators for multimodality medical image registration. *IEEE Trans. PAMI, 18*(4), 353-365.

Maislin, G., Pack, A. I., Kribbs, N. B., Smith, P., Schwartz, A., Kline, L., Schwab, R., Dinges, D. & et al. (1995). A survey screen for prediction of apnea. *Sleep, 18,* 158-166.

Malik, M., & Camm, A. J. (1995). *Heart rate variability.* New York, 52-60, 533-539.

Mallat, S. (1992). Characterization of Signals from Multi-scale Edges. *IEEE Trans. Pattern Anal. Machine Intelligence*, 14, 710-732.

Manna, C., Patrizi, G., Rahman, A., & Sallam, H. (2004). Experimental results on the recognition of embryos in human assisted reproduction. *Reproductive BioMedicine Online, 8*(4), 460-469.

Mannila, H., & Toivonen, H. (1997). Levelwise search and borders of theories in knowledge discovery. *Data Mining and Knowledge Discovery, 1,* 241-258.

Margineantu, D. D., & Dietterich, T. G. (2000). Bootstrap methods for the cost-sensitive evaluation of classifiers. In *Proceedings of the 17th International Conference on Machine Learning* (ICML-2000), (pp. 583-590).

Marling, C., & Whitehouse, P. (2001). Case-Based Reasoning in the care of Alzheimer's disease patients. In: Aha, D.W., Watson, I. (eds.): *Case-Based Reasoning Research and Development,* Springer Berlin, 702-715.

Martin, D., Brun, C., Remy, E., Mouren, P., Thieffry, D., & Jacq, B. (2004). GOToolBox: functional investigation of gene datasets based on Gene Ontology. *Genome Biology 5*(12), R101.

Matheus, J. et al. (1996). Selecting and Reporting What is Interesting: The KEFIR Application to Healthcare Data. In U.M Fayyad, G. Piatetsky-Shapiro, P. Smyth & R.S. Uthurasamy (Eds.) *Advances in Knowledge Discovery and Data Mining* (pp 495-515). AAAI Press.

Matorras, R., Matorras, F., Mendoza, R., Rodríguez, M., Remohí, J., Rodríguez-Escudero, F. J., & Simón, C. (2005). The implantation of every embryo facilitates the chances of the remaining embryos to implant in an IVF programme: a mathematical model to predict pregnancy and multiple pregnancy rates. *Human Reproduction, 20,* 2923-2931.

Mattes, D., Haynor, D. R., Vesselle, H., Lewellen, T. K., & Eubank, W. (2003) PET-CT image registration in the chest using free-form deformations. *IEEE Transactions on Medical Imaging,* 23(1), 120-128.

Mayer, M. A., Leis, A., Sarrias, R., & Ruíz, P. (2005). Web Mèdica Acreditada Guidelines: realiability and quality of health information on Spanish-Language websites. In Engelbrecht R et al. (ed.). *Connecting Medical Informatics and Bioinformatics.* Proc of MIE2005, 1287-92.

McCray, A. T., & Tse, T. (2003). Understanding search failures in consumer health information systems. *Proc AMIA Symp* (pp. 430-434).

McCulloch, W. S., & Pitts, W. (1943). A logical calculus of the ideas immanent in neurons activity. *Bulletin of Mathematical Biophysics,* 5, 115-133.

McSherry, D. (2001). Interactive Case-Based Reasoning in Sequential Diagnosis. *Applied Intelligence* 14, 65-76.

McSherry, D. (2007). Hypothetico-Deductive Case-Based Reasoning. In: (Bichindaritz, Montani, 2007) 315-324.

Melville, P., Saar-Tsechansky, M., Provost, F., & Mooney, R. (2004). Active feature-value acquisition for classifier induction. In *Proceedings of the 4th IEEE International Conference on Data Mining* (ICDM'04), (pp. 483-486).

Mendelsson, E. (1997). *Introduction to Mathematical Logic.* London: Chapman & Hall.

Merz, C. J. & Murphy, P. (1996). UCI *Repository of Machine Learning Database.* Available: http://www.ics.uci.edu/~mlearn/MLRepository.html

Merz, C. J. (1999). Using correspondence analysis to combine classifiers. *Machine Learning, 36*, 33-58.

Messai, R., Zeng, Q., Mousseau, M., & Simonet, M. (2006). Building a Bilingual French-English Patient-Oriented Terminology for Breast Cancer. *In proceedings of MedNet 2006, Internet and Medicine.* Toronto, Canada.

Michalski, R. S. & Chilausky, R. L. (1980). Learning by Being Told and Learning from Examples: An Experimental Comparison of the Two Methods of Knowledge Acquisition in the Context of Developing an Expert System for Soy- bean Disease Diagnosis. *International Journal of Policy Analysis and Information Systems, 4(2)*, 125-161.

Michalski, R. S., & Kaufman, K. A. (1998). Data Mining and Knowledge Discovery: A Review of Issues and a Multistrategy Approach. In R. S. Michalski, I. Bratko & M. Kubat (Eds.), *Machine Learning and Data Mining: Methods and Applications* (pp. 71-112). Chichester: John Wiley & Sons Ltd.

Michie, D., Spiegelhalter, D. J., & Taylor, C. C. (1994) (eds). *Machine learning, neural and statistical classification*, Ellis Horwood Series in Artificial Intelligence, Prentice Hall.

Millman, R. P., Carlisle, C. C., McGarvey, S. T., Eveloff, S. E., & Levinson, P. D. (1995). Body fat distribution and sleep apnea severity in women. *Chest, 107*(2), 362-366.

Ministerio de Salud (2002). *Programa Nacional de Control de la Tuberculosis. Normas Técnicas 2002. Programa de Vigilancia de la Salud y Control de Enfermedades.* Ministerio de Salud, República Argentina: Imprenta Lux S.A.

Minsky, M. (1961). Steps toward artificial intelligence. *Transactions on Institute of Radio Engineers, 49*, 8-30.

Minsky, M. (1975). A Framework for Representing Knowledge. In The Psychology of Computer Vision (Ed.), *P.H. Winston, McGraw-Hill* (pp. 211-277). New York.

Mitchell, T. M. (1997). *Machine Learning.* New York: McGraw-Hill.

Mobley, B., Leasure, R., & Davidson, L. (1995). Artificial neural network predictions of lengths of stay on a post-coronary care unit. *Heart Lung, 24*(3), 251-256.

Moehr, J. R. (1989). Teaching medical informatics: Teaching on the seams of disciplines, cultures, traditions. *Methods of Information in Medicine,* 28, 273-280.

Morales, D. A., Bengoetxea, E., Larrañaga, P., García, M., Franco, Y., Fresnada, M., & Merino, M. (2008). Bayesian classification for the selection of in-vitro human embryos using morphological and clinical data. *Computer Methods and Programs in Biomedicine, 90, 104-116.*

Morik, K., Boulicaut, J.-F., & (eds.), A. S. (Eds.). (2005). *Local pattern detection, 3539* of *LNAI.* Springer-Verlag.

Mothe, J., & Hernandez, N. (2007). TtoO: Mining thesaurus and texts to build and update a domain ontology. In H. O. Nigro, S. G. Císaro, and D.Xodo. Idea Group Inc (Ed.), *Data Mining with Ontologies: Implementations, Findings, and Frameworks.*

Mugler, D. H., & Clary, S. (2000). Discrete Hermite Functions. *Proceedings of the Int'l Conf. on Scientific Computing and Mathematical Modeling, IMACS.*

Mulgrew, A. T., Fox, N., Ayas, N. T., & Ryan, C. F. (2007). Diagnosis and Initial Management of Obstructive Sleep Apnea without Polysomnography: A Randomized Validation Study. *Annals of Internal Medicine, 146*, 157-166.

Murtagh, F. (1999) *Multivariate Data Analysis with Fortran, C and Java Code*. Queen's University Belfast and Astronomical Observatory Strasbourg.

Murtagh, F., Heck A. (1987). *Multivariate Data Analysis*. Kluwer Academic Publishers, Dordrecht

Nardi, D., & Brachman, R. J. (2003). An introduction to description logics. In F. Baader, D. Calvanese, D.L. McGuinness, D. Nardi, P.F. Patel-Schneider (Ed.), *the Description Logic Handbook* (pp. 5-44). Cambridge University Press.

Nasr, M., Fedele, M., Esser, K., & A, D. (2004). GPx-1 modulates akt and p70s6k phosphorylation and gadd45 levels in mcf-7 cells. *Free Radical Biology and Medicine, 37*, 187-195.

Nave, G. & Cohen, A. (1990). *ECG Compression Using Long-Term Prediction*. IEEE Trans. Biomed.Eng., *40*, 877-885.

Neches, R., Fikes, R.E., Finin, T., Gruber, T.R., Senator, T., & Swartout, T. (1991). Enabling technology for knowledge sharing. *AI Magazine 12*(3), 36-56.

Negnevitsky, M. (2004). Design of a hybrid neuro-fuzzy decision-support system with a heterogeneous structure. *Proceedings IEEE International Conference on Fuzzy Systems, 2,* 1049-1052.

Nestor, P. J., Scheltens, P., & Hodges, J. R. (2004, July). Advances in the early detection of Alzheimer's disease. *Nature Reviews Neuroscience, 5*(Supplement), S34-S41.

Ng, R. T., Lakshmanan, V. S., Han, J., & Pang, A. (1998). Exploratory mining and pruning optimizations of constrained associations rules. *Proceedings of ACM SIGMOD'98* (pp. 13-24). ACM Press.

Nicoletti, D.W., & Onaral, B. (1991). The Application of Delta Modulation to EEG Waveforms for Database Reduction and Real-time Signal Processing. *Annals of Biomedical Engineering, 19*, 1-14.

Nieminen, A., & Neuvo, Y. (1987). EEG spike detection based on median type filters. In *Proc. of Int. Conf. on Digital Signal Processing*, Florence, Italy, 559-563.

Nigro, H. O., Gonzalez Cisaro, S. E., & Xodo, D. H. (Ed.). (2007). *Data Mining with ontologies – Implementations, findings and frameworks.* Information Science Reference, IGI Gobal.

Nilsson, N. (1980). *Principles of artificial intelligence*, Palo Alto: Tioga Publishing Co.

Nunes, J.C., & Nait Ali, A. (2005). Hilbert Transform-Based ECG Modeling. *Biomedical Engineering, 39(3).* New York: Springer.

Núñez, M. (1991). The use of background knowledge in decision tree induction. *Machine Learning, 6*, 231-250.

O'Connor, M. A., & Walley, W. J. (2000). An information theoretic self-organising map with disaggregation of output classes. *2nd Int. Conf. on Environmental Information systems, Stafford, UK.* 108-115. ISBN 9 72980 501 6.

Ohn, M. S., Van-Nam, H., & Yoshiteru, N. (2004). An alternative extension of the K-means algorithm for clustering categorical data. *International Journal Mathematic Computer Science, 14(2),* 241-247.

Oja, E. (1982). A simplified neuron model as a principal component analyzer. *J.Math.Biol., 15*, 267-273.

Osser, D. N., & Patterson, R. D. (1998). Algorithms for the pharmacotherapy of depression, parts one and two. *Directions in Psychiatry,* 18, 303-334.

Palakal, M., Mukhopadhyay, S., & Stephens, M. (2005). Identification of Biological Relationships from Text Documents. *Book Series: Integrated Series In Information Systems. Book: Medical Informatics, 8*, 449-489.

Pan, F., Cong, G., Tung, A. K. H., Yang, Y., & Zaki, M. J. (2003). CARPENTER: finding closed patterns in long biological datasets. *Proceedings of the 9th ACM SIGKDD international conference on Knowledge discovery and data mining (KDD'03)* (pp. 637-642). Washington, DC, USA: ACM Press.

Patrizi, G., Manna, C., Moscatelli, C., & Nieddu, L. (2004). Pattern recognition methods in human-assisted reproduction. *International Transactions in Operational Research, 11*(4), 365-379.

Pazzani, M. (1997). Searching for dependencies in Bayesian classifiers. *Learning from Data: Artificial Intelligence and Statistics V*, 239-248.

Pazzani, M. J., & Kibler, D. (1992). The utility of knowledge in inductive learning. *Machine Learning*, 9(1), 57-97.

Pensa, R., Robardet, C., & Boulicaut, J.-F. (2005). A bi-clustering framework for categorical data. *Proceedings of the 9th European Conference on Principles and Practice of Knowledge Discovery in Databases (PKDD'05)* (pp. 643-650). Porto, Portugal.

Pérez, A., Larrañaga, P., & Inza, I. (2006). Supervised classification with conditional Gaussian Networks: Increasing the structure complexity from naive Bayes. *International Journal of Approximate Reasoning, 43*, 1-25.

Pham, M.H., Bernhard, D., Diallo, G., Messai, R., & Simonet, M. (2007). SOM-based Clustering of Multi-lingual Documents Using an Ontology. In H. O. Nigro, S. G. Císaro, and D.Xodo. Idea Group Inc (Ed.), *Data Mining with Ontologies: Implementations, Findings, and Frameworks.*

Platt, J. C. (1999). Fast training of support vector machines using sequential minimal optimization. In Scholkopf, B., Burges, C., & Smola, A. J. (Eds.), *Advances in kernel methods - support vector learning (pp. 185-208).* MIT Press.

Pluim, J. P., Maintz, J. B. A., & Viergever, M. A. (2003, August) Mutual-information-based registration of medical images: a survey. *IEEE Transactions on Medical Imaging*, 22(8), 986-1004.

Poli, R., Cagnoni, S., & Valli, G., (1994). *A genetic algorithm approach to the design of optimum QRS detectors.* University of Florence Technical Report No. 940201, Florence, Italy.

Povinelli, R. J., & Feng, X. (1998). Temporal pattern identification of time series data using pattern wavelets and genetic algorithms, in *Artificial Neural Networks in Engineering*, Proceedings, pp. 691-696.

Powell, M. J. D. (1964). An efficient method for finding the minimum of a function of several variables without calculating derivatives. *Comput. J., 7*, 155-163.

Powers, D., & Xie, Y. (2007). *Statistical methods for categorical data analysis*, Elsevier.

Prakash, O., & Ghosh, I. (2006). Developing an Antituberculosis Compounds Database and Data Mining in the Search of Motif Responsible for the Activity of a Diverse Class of Antituberculosis Agents. *Journal of Chemical Information and Modeling*, 46(1), 17-23.

Prank, K., Jurgens, C., Muhlen, A., & Brabant, G. (1998). Predictive Neural Networks for Learning the Time Course of Blood Glucose levels from the Complex Interaction of Counterregulatory Hormones. *Neural Computation, 10*(4), 941-954.

Prentzas, J., & Hatzilgeroudis, I. (2002). Integrating Hybrid Rule-Based with Case-Based Reasoning. In Craw, S., Preeece, A. (eds.): *Proceedings European Conference on Case-Based Reasoning,* ECCBR 2002, Springer-Verlag, Berlin, 336-349.

Press, W. H., Teukolsky, S. A., Vetterling, W. T., & Flannery, B. P. (1992). *Numerical Recipes in C.* Cambridge Univ. Press, Cambridge, U.K.

Provost, F., & Fawcett, T. (2001). Robust classification for imprecise environments. *Machine Learning, 42*(3), 203-231.

Prytherch, D. R., Sutton, G. L., & Boyle, J. R. (2001). Portsmouth POSSUM models for abdominal aortic aneurysm surgery. *British Journal of Surgery, 88(7),* 958-63.

Puissant, F., Rysselberge, M. V., Barlow, P., Deweze, J., & Leroy, F. (1987). Embryo scoring as a prognostic tool in IVF treatment. *Human Reproduction, 2*, 705-708.

Punjabi, N. M., & Beamer, B. A. (2005). Sleep Apnea and Metabolic Dysfunction. In *Principles and Practice of Sleep Medicine* (Fourth Edition ed., pp. 1034-1042): Elsevier Saunders.

Qian, J., Barlow, J. S., & Beddoes, M. P. (1988). A simplified arithmetic detector for EEG sharp transients - preliminary results. *IEEE Trans. Biomed. Eng.*, *35*(1), 11-17.

Quinlan, J. R. (1993). *C4.5: Programs for Machine Learning.* Morgan Kaufmann.

Quinlan, J.R. (1986) Induction of decision trees. *Machine Learning, 1,* 81-106.

Rainbow, University of Economics Prague, Knowledge Engineering Group. (2005). *Reusable Architecture for Intelligent Brokering Of Web information access (Rainbow).* Retrieved from: http://rainbow.vse.cz/descr.html

Rauch, J. (1997). Logical Calculi for Knowledge Discovery in Databases. In J. Komorowski, J. Zytkow (Eds.) *Proc. European Conference on Principles of Data Mining and Knowledge Discovery.* (pp. 47 – 57). Berlin, Springer Verlag.

Rauch, J., & Berka, P. (1997). Knowledge Discovery in Financial Data - a Case Study. *Neural Network World,* 4-5(7).

Rauch, J., & Šimůnek, M. (2005). An Alternative Approach to Mining Association Rules. In T.Y. Lin, (Ed.) *Proc. Data Mining: Foundations, Methods, and Applications* (pp. 219-238). Springer-Verlag.

Rauch, J., & Šimůnek, M. (2005). GUHA Method and Granular Computing. In X. Hu, (Ed.). *Proceedings of IEEE conference Granular Computing* (pp. 630—635).

Rauch, J., & Šimůnek, M. (2007). Semantic Web Presentation of Analytical Reports from Data Mining – Preliminary Considerations. In Proc. *Web Intelligence* (pp. 3–7). IEEE Computer Society.

Rauch, J., Šimůnek, M., & Lín, V. (2005). Mining for Patterns Based on Contingency Tables by KL-Miner – First Experience. In T.Y. Lin (Ed.) *Foundations and Novel Approaches in Data Mining* (pp. 155-167) Berlin, Springer Verlag.

Rector, A. L., & Nowlan, W. A. (1993). The GALEN Project. *Computer Methods and Programs in Biomedicine, 45,* 75-78.

Rezvani, S., & Prasad, G. (2003). A hybrid system with multivariate data validation and Case-based Reasoning for an efficient and realistic product formulation. In Ashley, K.D., Bridge, D.G. (eds.): *Proceedings International Conference on Case-based Reasoning,* ICCBR 2003, Springer-Verlag, Berlin 465-478.

Rhode, K. S., Sermesant, M., Brogan, D., Hegde, S., Hipwell, J., Lambiase, P., Rosenthsal, E., bucknall, C., Qureshi, S. A., Gill, J.S., Razavi, R., & Hill, D. L.G. (2005, November). A system for real-time XMR guided cardiovascular intervention. *IEEE Transactions on Medical Imaging,* 24(11), 1428-1440.

Rieger, J., Lhotská, L., Krajča, V., & Matoušek, M. (2004). Application of Quantitative Methods of Signal Processing to Automatic Classification of Long-Term EEG Records. In *Biological and Medical Data Analysis.* Springer Verlag, 2004, 333-343.

Ringland, G. A., & Duce, D. A. (1987). *Approaches in Knowledge Representation: An Introduction.* John Wiley& Sons.

Rioult, F., Boulicaut, J.-F., Crémilleux, B., & J., B. (2003). Using transposition for pattern discovery from microarray data. *Proceedings of the 8th ACM SIGMOD Workshop on Research Issues in Data Mining and Knowledge Discovery (DMKD'03)* (pp. 73-79). San Diego, CA.

Roche, C. (2003). *The Differentia Principle: a Cornerstone for Ontology.* Knowledge Management and Philosophy Workshop in WM 2003 Conference, Luzern.

Roche, C. (2005). Terminologie et ontologie. *LAROUSSE – Revue, 157,* 1-11.

Roche, N., Herer, B., Roig, C., & Huchon, G. (2002). Prospective Testing of Two Models Based on Clinical and Oximetric Variables for Prediction of Obstructive Sleep Apnea. *Chest, 121*(3), 747-752.

Rosenberg, R., & Mickelson, S. A. (2003). Obstructive sleep apnea: Evaluation by history and polysomnography. In D. N. F. Fairbanks, S. A. Mickelson & B. T. Woodson (Eds.), *Snoring and Obstructive Sleep Apnea* (Third ed.). Philadelphia: Lippincott Williams & Wilkins.

Rosse, C., & Mejino, J. L. V. (2003). Reference ontology for bioinformatics: the Foundational Model of Anatomy. *J Biomed Inform, 36*(6), 478-500.

Rowan, K. M., Kerr, J. H., Major, E., McPherson, K., Short, A., & Vessey, M. P. (1994). Intensive Care Society's Acute Physiology and Chronic Health Evaluation (APACHE II) study in Britain and Ireland: a prospective, multicenter, cohort study comparing two methods for predicting outcome for adult intensive care patients. *Critical Care Medicine, 22*, 1392-1401.

Rowley, J. A., Aboussouan, L. S., & Badr, M. S. (2000). The use of clinical prediction formulas in the evaluation of obstructive sleep apnea. *Sleep, 23*(7), 929-938.

Rowley, J. A., Sanders, C. S., Zahn, B. R. & Badr, M. S. (2002). Gender differences in upper airway compliance during NREM sleep: role of neck circumference. *Journal of Applied Physiology, 92*, 2535-2541.

Rueckert, D., Hayes, C., Studholme, C., Summers, P., Leach, M., & Hawkes, D. J. (1998). Non-rigid registration of breast MR images using mutual information. *MICCAI'98 lecture notes in computer science*, Cambridge, pp.1144-1152.

Ryan, C. F., & Love, L. L. (1996). Mechanical properties of the velopharynx in obese patients with obstructive sleep apnea. *American Journal of Respiratory and Critical Care Medicine, 154*(3), 806-812.

Sahami, M. (1996). Learning limited dependence Bayesian classifiers. *Proceedings of the 2nd International Conference on Knowledge Discovery and Data Mining*, 335-338.

Saith, R., Srinivasan, A., Michie, D., & Sargent, I. (1998). Relationships between the developmental potential of human in-vitro fertilization embryos and features describing the embryo, oocyte and follicle. *Human Reproduction Update, 4*(2), 121-134.

Salton, G., & Buckley, C. (1988). Term-weighting approaches in automatic text retrieval. *Information Processing Management, 24*(5), 513–523.

Salzberg, B. & Heath, R. (1971). The detection of surface EEG correlates of deep brain spiking in schizophrenic patients using matched digital filters. *Electroenceph. Clin.Neurophysiol., 38*, 550.

Sanger, S (ed.) (2004). *Check-In.* Retrieved from http://www.patienten-information.de/content/ informationsqualitaet/informationsqualitaet/images/check_in.pdf

Sanger, T. D. (1989). Optimal unsupervised learning in a single-layer linear feedforward neural network. *Neural Networks,* 12, 459-473.

Sartori, M. A., & Antsaklis, P. J. (1991). A Simple Method to Derive Bounds on the Size and to Train Multilayer Neural Networks. *IEEE Transactions on Neural Networks,* 4*(2),* 467-471.

Scahill, R. I. Frost, C., Jenkins, R., Whitwell, J. L., Rossor, M. N., & Fox, N.C. (2003, July). A longitudinal study of brain volume changes in normal aging using serial registered magnetic resonance imaging. *Archives of Neurology*, 60(7), 989-994.

Scarfone, C., Lavely, W. C., Cmelak, A. J., Delbeke, D., Martin, W. H., Billheimer, D., & Hallahan, D. E. (2004). Prospective feasibility trial of radiotherapy target definition for head and neck cancer using 3-dimensional PET and CT imaging. *Journal of Nuclear Medicine*, 45(4), 543-552, Apr 2004.

Scheffer, T., & Wrobel, S. (2002). Text Classification Beyond the Bag-of-Words Representation. Proceedings of the *International Conference on Machine Learning (ICML) Workshop on Text Learning.*

Schmidt, R., & Gierl, L. (2001). Case-based Reasoning for Antibiotics Therapy Advice: An Investigation of Retrieval Algorithms and Prototypes. *Artificial Intelligence in Medicine,* 23 (2), 171-186.

Schmidt, R., & Vorobieva, O. (2006). Case-Based Reasoning Investigation of Therapy Inefficacy. *Knowledge-Based Systems,* 19(5), 333-340.

Schroder, C. M., & O'Hara, R. (2005). Depression and Obstructive Sleep Apnea (OSA). *Annals of General Psychiatry, 4*(13).

Scott, L., Alvero, R., & Leondires, M. (2000). The morphology of human pronuclear embryos is positively related to blastocyst development and implantation. *Human Reproduction, 15*(11), 2394-2403.

Sebeok, T. A. (1999). *Signs: An Introduction to Semiotics*: University of Toronto Press.

Seewald, A. (2003). *Towards understanding stacking.* Department of Informatics, Technical University of Wien.

Sevon, P., Eronen, L., Hintsanen, P., Kulovesi, K., & Toivonen, H. (2006). Link discovery in graphs derived from biological databases. In *3rd International Workshop on Data Integration in the Life Sciences* (DILS'06), Hinxton, UK.

Shannon, C. E. (1948). A mathematical theory of communication. *Bell System Technical Journal, 27*, 379-423 and 623-656.

Sharma, S. K., Kurian, S., Malik, V., Mohan, A., Banga, A., Pandey, R. M., Handa, K. K., & Mukhopadhyay, S. (2004). A stepped approach for prediction of obstructive sleep apnea in overtly asymptomatic obese subjects: a hospital based study. *Sleep Medicine, 5*, 451-357.

Shearer, C. (2000). The CRISP-DM Model: The New Blueprint for Data Mining. *Journal of Data Warehousing, 4*(5), 13-21.

Shehroz, S. K., & Shri, K. (2007). Computation of initial modes for K-modes clustering algorithm using evidence accumulation. *20th International Joint Confference on Artificial Intelligence (IJCAI-07)*, India.

Sheng, S., & Ling, C. X. (2005). Hybrid cost-sensitive decision tree. In *Proceedings of the 9th European Conference on Principles and Practice of Knowledge Discovery in Databases* (PKDD).

Sheng, S., Ling, C. X., & Yang, Q. (2005). Simple test strategies for cost-sensitive decision trees. In *Proceedings of the 16th European Conference on Machine Learning* (ECML), (pp. 365-376).

Shortliffe, E. H. (1990). Clinical decision-support systems. In Shortliffe, E.H., Perreault, L. E.,Wiederhold, G., & Fagan, L. M. (Eds.). *Medical informatics - Computer Applications in Health Care*, Addison-Wesley, Reading, M.A.

Shuguang, L., Qing, J., & George, C. (2000). Combining case-based and model-based reasoning: a formal specification. In *Seventh Asia-Pacific Software Engineering Conference*, APSEC'00 416.

Siddiqi, K., Lambert, M., & Walley, J. (2003). Clinical diagnosis of smear-negative pulmonary tuberculosis in low-income countries: The current evidence. *Lancet, 3*, 288-296.

Siebes, A., Vreeken, J., & Van Leeuwen, M. (2006). Item sets that compress. *Proceedings of the Sixth SIAM International Conference on Data Mining.* Bethesda, MD, USA: SIAM.

Siegwart, D. K., Tarassenko, L., Roberts, S. J., Stradling, J.R. & Parlett J. (1995). Sleep apnoea analysis from neural network post-processing. *Artificial Neural Networks*, 26-28 June 1995.Conference Publication No. 409, IEE pp. 427-437.

Sierra, B., Serrano, N., Larrañaga, P., Plasencia E.J. Inza, I., Jiménez, J.J., Revuelta, P., & Mora M.L. (2001). Using Bayesian networks in the construction of a bi-level multi-classifier. A case study using intensive care unit patients data. *Artificial Intelligence in Medicine, 22*(3), 233-248.

Silipo, R., & Marchesi, C. (1998). Artificial Neural Networks for automatic ECG analysis. *IEEE Transactions on Signal Processing, 46*(5), 1417-1425.

Simonet, M., Patriarche, R., Bernhard, D., Diallo, G., Ferriol, S., & Palmer, P. (2006). Multilingual Ontology Enrichment for Semantic Annotation and Retrieval of Medical Information. *MEDNET'2006*, Toronto - Canada.

Smith, B. (2003). Ontology. Chapter in L. Floridi (ed.), *Blackwell Guide to the Philosophy of Computing and Information* (pp. 155-166). Oxford, Blackwell.

Smith, B., Ashburner, M., Rosse, C., Bard, J., Bug, W., Ceusters, W., Goldberg, L. J., Eilbeck, K., Ireland, A., Mungall, C. J., Leontis, N., Rocca-Serra, P., Ruttenberg, A., Sansone, S., Scheuermann, R. H., Shah, N., Whetzel, P. L., & Lewis, S. (2007). The OBO Foundry: coordinated evolution of ontologies to support biomedical data integration. *Nat Biotech,* 25(11), 1251-1255.

Smith, S. W. (1997). *Digital Signal Processing.* California Technical Publishing, San Diego, CA, USA.

Solberg, H. E. (1987). Approved recommendation (1986) of the theory of reference values, Part I. The Concept of reference values. *Journal of Clinical Chemistry & Clinical Biochemistry, 25*, 337-342.

Soong, A. C. K. & Koles, Z. (1995). Principal component localisation of the sources of the background EEG. *IEEE Trans. Biomed.Eng.*, 42, 59-67.

Soualmia, L. F, Darmoni, S. J., Douyère, M., & Thirion, B. (2003). Modelisation of Consumer Health Information in a Quality-Controled gateway. In Baud R et al. (ed.). *The New Navigators: from Professionals to Patients.* Proc of MIE2003, 701-706.

Soulet, A. (2007). Résumer les contrastes par l'extraction récursive de motifs. Conférence *sur l'Apprentissage Automatique (CAp'07)* (pp. 339-354). Grenoble, France: Cépaduès Edition.

Soulet, A., & Crémilleux, B. (2008). Mining constraint-based patterns using automatic relaxation. *Intelligent Data Analysis, 13*(1). IOS Press. To appear.

Soulet, A., & Crémilleux, B. (2005). An efficient framework for mining flexible constraints *Proceedings 9th Pacific-Asia Conference on Knowledge Discovery and Data Mining (PAKDD'05)* (pp. 661-671). Hanoi, Vietnam: Springer.

Soulet, A., Crémilleux, B., & Rioult, F. (2004). Condensed representation of emerging patterns. *Proceedings 8th Pacific-Asia Conference on Knowledge Discovery and Data Mining (PAKDD'04)* (pp. 127-132). Sydney, Australia: Springer-Verlag.

Soulet, A., Klema J., & Cremilleux, B. (2007). Efficient Mining Under Rich Constraints Derived from Various Datasets. In Džeroski, S., Struyf, J. (eds.), *Knowledge Discovery in Inductive Databases*, LNCS,4747, 223-239. Springer Berlin / Heidelberg.

Soulet, A., Kléma, J., & Crémilleux, B. (2007). *Post-proceedings of the 5th international workshop on knowledge discovery in inductive databases in conjunction with ECML/PKDD 2006 (KDID'06), 4747 of Lecture Notes in Computer Science, chapter Efficient Mining under Rich Constraints Derived from Various Datasets,* 223-239. Springer.

Spencer, K., Coombes, E. J., Mallard, A. S., & Ward A. M. (1992). Free beta human choriogonadotropin in Down's syndrome screening: a multicentre study of its role compared with other biochemical markers. *Annals of clinical biochemistry, 29(Suppl 216),* 506-518.

Šprogar, M., Lenič, M., & Alayon, S. (2002). Evolution in Medical Decision Making. *Journal of Medical Systems, 26*(5), 479-489.

Stamatakis, K., Chandrinos, K., Karkaletsis, V., Mayer, M. A, Gonzales, D. V, Labsky, D.V, Amigó, E., & Pöllä, M. (2007) AQUA, a system assisting labelling experts assess health Web resources. In *Proceedings of the 12th International Symposium for Health Information Management Research* (iSHIMR 2007), Sheffield, UK, 18-20 July, 75-84.

Stamatakis, K., Metsis, V., Karkaletsis, V., Ruzicka, M., Svátek, V., Amigó, E., & Pöllä, M. (2007). Content collection for the labelling of health-related web content. In *Proceedings of the 11th Conference on Artificial Intelligence in Medicine* (AIME 07), LNAI 4594, Amsterdam, 7-11 July, 341-345.

Starmark, J. E., Stalhammar, D., & Holmgren, E. (1998). The Reaction Level Scale (RLS85). Manual and Guidelines. *Acta Neurochirurgica, 91*(1), 12-20.

Stein, M. B. (2003). Attending to anxiety disorders in primary care. *J Clin Psychiatry,* 64(suppl 15), 35-39.

Stone, M. (1974). Cross-validatory choice and assessment of statistical predictions. *Journal of the Royal Statistical Society Series B, 36*, 111-147.

Strzodka, R., Droske, M., & Rumpf, M. (2004) Image registration by a regularized gradient flow - a streaming implementation in DX9 graphics hardware. *Computing, 73*(4), 373–389.

Studholme, C., Hill, D. L. G., & Hawkes, D. J. (1999) An overlap invariant entropy measure of 3D medical image alignment. *Pattern Recognition, 32*, 71–86.

Subsol, G., Thirion, J. P., & Ayache, N. (1998). A scheme for automatically building three dimensional morphometric anatomical atlases: application to a skull atlas. *Medical Image Analysis*, 2(1), 37-60.

Suzuki, K., Feng Li, Sone, S., & Doi, K. (2005). Computer-aided diagnostic scheme for distinction between benign and malignant nodules in thoracic low-dose CT by use of massive training artificial neural network. *IEEE Transactions on Medical Imaging, 24*(9), 1138 – 1150.

Swets, J. (1988). Measuring the accuracy of diagnostic systems. *Science, 240*, 1285-1293.

Swets, J. A., Dawes, R. M., & Monahan, J. (2000). Better decisions through science. *Scientific American, 283*(4), 82-87.

Taccardi, B. (1963). Distribution of heart potentials on the thoracic surface of normal human subjects. *Circ. Res.*, 12, 341-52.

Taktak, A. F. G., Fisher, A. C., & Damato, B. (2004). Modelling survival after treatment of intraocular melanoma using artificial neural networks and Bayes theorem. *Physics in Medicine and Biology, 49*(1), 87-98.

Teasdale, G., & Jennet, B. (1974). Assessment of coma and impaired consciousness. A practical scale. *The Lancet*, ii, 81-84.

Thakor, N. V., & Yi-Sheng, Z. (1991). Application of Adaptive Filtering to ECG Analysis noise cancellation and arrhythmia detection. *IEEE Transaction on Biomedical Engineering,* 38,785-94.

Thévenaz, P., & Unser, M. (2000). Optimization of mutual information for multiresolution registration. *IEEE Transaction on Image Processing*, 9(12), 2083-2099.

Tibshirani, R., Hastie, T., Narasimhan, B., & Chu, G. (2002). Diagnosis of multiple cancer types by shrunken centroids of gene expression. Proc. *Natl Acad. Sci.*, 99(10), 6567-6572.

Ting, K. M. (2002). An Instance-Weighting Method to Induce Cost-Sensitive Trees. *IEEE Transactions on Knowledge and Data Engineering, 14*(3), 659-665.

Ting, K., & Witten, M. (1999). Issues in stacked generalization. *Journal of Artificial Intelligence Research (JAIR), 10*, 271-289.

Todorovski, L., & Džeroski, S. (2002). Combining classifiers with meta decision trees. *Machine Learning, 50*(3), 223-249.

Toga, A. W., & Thompson P. M. (2001, September) The role of image registration in brain mapping. *Image and Vision Computing Journal*, 19, 3–24.

Tom, F. (2006). An introduction to ROC analysis. *Pattern Recognition Letters, 27.* Science Direct, Elsevier.

Townsend, D. W., Beyer, T., & Blodgett, T. M. (2003). PET/CT Scanners: A Hardware Approach to Image Fusion. *Semin Nucl Med* XXXIII(3), 193-204.

Trajkovski, I., Zelezny, F., Lavrac, N., & Tolar, J. (in press). Learning Relational Descriptions of Differentially Expressed Gene Groups. *IEEE Trans. Sys Man Cyb C, spec. issue on Intelligent Computation for Bioinformatics.*

Trajkovski, I., Zelezny, F., Tolar, J., & Lavrac, N. (2006) Relational Subgroup Discovery for Descriptive Analysis of Microarray Data. In *Procs 2nd Int Sympos on Computational Life Science*, Cambridge, UK 9/06. Springer Lecture Notes on Bioinformatics / LNCS.

Tresp, V., Briegel, T., & Moody, J. (1999). Neural-network models for the blood glucose metabolism of adiabetic. *IEEE Transactions on Neural Networks, 10*(5), 1204-1213.

Trimarchi, J. R., Goodside, J., Passmore, L., Silberstein, T., Hamel, L., & Gonzalez, L. (2003). Comparing data mining and logistic regression for predicting IVF outcome. *Fertility and Sterility, 80*(3), 100-100.

Trna, M. (2007) *Klasifikace s apriorni znalosti.* CTU Bachelor's Thesis, In Czech.

Troncy, R., & Isaac, A. (2002). DOE: une mise en œuvre d'une méthode de structuration différentielle pour les ontologies. *In Actes 13e journées francophones sur Ingénierie des Connaissances (IC)* (pp. 63-74).

Turban, E., Aronson, J., Ting-Peng, L., & McCarthy, R. (2005). *Decision support systems and intelligent systems.* 7a. ed. Upper Saddle River (N.Y.): Pearson Education.

Turney, P. (1995). Cost-sensitive classification: empirical evaluation of a hybrid genetic decision tree induction algorithm. *Journal of Artificial Intelligence Research, 2*, 369-409.

Turney, P. (2000). Types of cost in inductive concept learning. In *Proceedings of the Workshop on Cost-Sensitive Learning at the 17th International Conference on Machine Learning* (WCSL at ICML-2000), (pp. 15-21).

Tusher, V.G., Tibshirani, R. & Chu G. (2001) Significance analysis of microarrays applied to the ionizing radiation response. Proc. *Natl Acad. Sci.*, 98(9). 5116–5121.

Tversky, A. (1977). Features of similarity. *Psychological review,* 84, 327-352.

UCI Machine Learning Repository, University of California, Irvine. Retrieved November 15, 2007, from http://mlearn.ics.uci.edu/ MLRepository.html.

Unser, M., & Aldroubi, A. (1993, November). A multiresolution image registration procedure using spline pyramids. Proc. of SPIE 2034, 160-170, Wavelet Applications in Signal and Image Processing, ed. Laine, A. F.

Uschold, M., & Jasper, R. (1999). A Framework for Understanding and Classifying Ontology Applications. *In: Proc.IJCAI99 Workshop on Ontologies and Problem-Solving Methods.* Stockholm.

Uschold, M., & King, M. (1995). *Towards a methodology for building ontologies.* Workshop on Basic Ontological Issues in Knowledge Sharing, held in conduction with IJCAI-95.

Uthurusamy, R., Means, L., & Godden, K. (1993). Extracting Knowledge from Diagnostic Databases. *IEEE Expert, 8*(6), 27-38.

Vaarala, M. H., Porvari, K. S., Kyllonen, A. P., Mustonen, M. V., Lukkarinen, O., & Vihko, P. T. (1998). Several genes encoding ribosomal proteins are over-expressed in prostate-cancer cell lines: confirmation of l7a and l37 over-expression in prostate-cancer tissue samples. *Int. J. Cancer, 78*, 27-32.

Vajda, I., Veselý, A., & Zvárová, J. (2005). On the amount of information resulting from empirical and theoretical knowledge. *Revista Matematica Complutense,* 18, 275-283.

van Bemmel, J. H., & McCray, A. T. *eds.* (1995). *Yearbook of Medical Informatics.* Stuttgart: Schattauer Verlagsgesellschaft.

Van den Elsen, P. A., Maintz, J. B. A., Pol, E. -J. D., & Viergever, M. A. (1995, June). Automatic registration of CT and MR brain images using correlation of geometrical features. *IEEE Transactions on Medical Imaging, 14*(2), 384 – 396.

Vapnik, V. (1995). *The Nature of Statistical Learning Theory.* Springer-Verlag.

Veek, L. L. (1999). *An Atlas of Human Gametes and Conceptuses: An Illustrated Reference for Assisted Reproductive Technology.* Parthenon.

Velardi, P., Navigli, R., Cuchiarelli, A., & Neri, F. (2005). Evaluation of Ontolearn, a methodology for automatic population of domain ontologies. In P. Buitelaar, P. Cimiano, and B. Magnini (Eds), *Ontology Learning from Text: Methods, Applications and Evaluation.* IOS Press.

Velculescu, V., Zhang, L., Vogelstein, B. & Kinzler, K. (1995). Serial Analysis of Gene Expression. *Science, 270*, 484–7.

Velculescu, V., Zhang, L., Vogelstein, B., & Kinzler, K. (1995). Serial analysis of gene expression. *Science, 270*, 484-487.

Viner, S., Szalai, J. P., & Hoffstein, V. (1991). Are history and physical examination a good screening test for sleep apnea? *Annals of Internal Medicine, 115*, 356-359.

Viola, P. A., & Wells, W. M. (1995, June) Alignment by maximization of mutual information. In *Proc. 5th International Conference of Computer Vision*, Cambridge, MA, 16-23.

Vorobieva, O., Rumyantsev, A., & Schmidt, R. (2006). Incremental Development of an Explanation Model for Exceptional Dialysis Patients. In Bichindaritz, I., Montani, S. (Eds.) *Workshop on CBR in the Health Sciences*, ECCBR'06 Workshop Proceedings, University of Trier Press, 170-178.

W3C. (2004). *Resource Description Framework (RDF)*. Retrieved from http:// www.w3.org/TR/rdf-schema/

W3C. (2005). *RDF-Content Labels (RDF-CL)*. Retrieved from http://www.w3.org/ 2004/12/q/doc/content-labels-schema.htm

W3C. (2007). *Protocol for Web Description Resources (POWDER)*. Retrieved from http://www.w3.org/2007/powder/

Wackermann, J., Lehmann, D., Michel, C. M., & Strik, W. K. (1993). Adaptive Segmentation of Spontaneous EEG Map Series into Spatially Defined Microstates. *International Journal of Psychophysiology*, 14(3), 269-283.

Walczak, S., & Nowack, W.J. (2001). An artificial neural network to diagnosing epilepsy using lateralized burst of theta EEGs. *Journal of Medical Systems, 25*(1), 9–20.

Walczak, S., Pofahl, W. E., & Scorpio, R. J. (2003). A decision support tool for allocating hospital bed resources and determining required acuity of care. *Decision Support Systems, 34*(4), 445-456.

Waldon, M.G. (2004). Estimation of average stream velocity. In *Journal of Hydrologic Engineering, 130*(11), 1119-1122.

Wang, F., Quinion, R., Carrault, G., & Cordier, M. O. (2001). Learning structural knowledge from the ECG. in: J. Crespo, V. Maojo, F. Martin, eds., *Medical Data Analysis - Second International Symposium*, LNCS 2199. *ISMDA 2001.* Springer Verlag.

Wang, X., & Feng, D. (2005). Active Contour Based Efficient Registration for Biomedical Brain Images. *Journal of Cerebral Blood Flow & Metabolism, 25*(Suppl), S623.

Wang, X., & Feng, D. (2005). Biomedical Image Registration for Diagnostic Decision Making and Treatment Monitoring. Chapter 9 in R. K. Bali (Ed.) *Clinical Knowledge Management: Opportunities and Challenges*, pp.159-181, Idea Group Publishing

Wang, X., S. Eberl, Fulham, M., Som, S., & Feng, D. (2007) Data Registration and Fusion, Chapter 8 in D. Feng (Ed.) *Biomedical Information Technology*, pp.187-210, Elsevier Publishing

Wang, Y., & Liu, Z. (2006, May 31). Automatic detecting indicators for quality of health information on the Web. *Int J. Med Inform.*

Wei Ji, Naguib, R. N. G., Macall, J., Petrovic, D., Gaura, E., & Ghoneim, M. (2003). Prognostic prediction of bilharziasis-related bladder cancer by neuro-fuzzy classifier. *Information Technology Applications in Biomedicine*, 181-183.

Weiss, S., & Indurkhya, N. (1998). *Predictive Data Mining. A Practical Guide.* San Francisco: Morgan Kaufmann Publishers, Inc.

Whittle, A. T., Marshall, I., Mortimore, I. l., Wraith, P. K., Sellar, R. J. & Douglas, N. J. (1999). Neck soft tissue and fat distribution comparison between normal men and women by magnetic resonance imaging. *Thorax, 54*, 323-328.

Wiener, N. (1948). *Cybernetics: On the Control and Communication in the Animal and the Machine*. Cambridge, MA: MIT Press

Winker, M. A., Flanagan, A., Chi-Lum, B. (2000). Guidelines for Medical and Health Information Sites on the

Internet: principles governing AMA Web sites. American Medical Association. *JAMA, 283*(12), 1600-1606.

Witten, I. H., & Frank, E. (2005). *Data mining: Practical machine learning tools and techniques with java implementations*: Morgan Kaufmann Publishers.

Witten, I. H., & Frank, E. (2005). *Data Mining: Practical Machine Learning Tools and Technologies* (Second ed.). Amsterdam: Morgan Kaufmann.

Wolpert, D. H. (1992). Stacked generalization. *Neural Networks, 5*, 241-259.

Woodson, B. T. (2003). Obstructive sleep apnea: Evaluation by physical examination and special studies. In D. N. F. Fairbanks, S. A. Mickelson & B. T. Woodson (Eds.), *Snoring and Obstructive Sleep Apnea* (third ed., pp. 51-67). Philadelphia: Lippincott Williams & Wilkins.

Working group for paediatric endocrinology of the German society for endocrinology and of the German society for children and youth medicine (1998) 1-15.

World Health Organization (2003). *Treatment of Tuberculosis: Guidelines for National Programs*. Geneve: WHO. WHO document WHO/CDS/TB_2003.313.

World Health Organization (2004). *Toman's Tuberculosis: Case detection, treatment and monitoring-questions and answers*. Geneve: WHO. WHO document WHO/HTM/TB/2004.334.

World Health Organization (2006). *The World Health Organization Global Tuberculosis Program*. Available at http://www.who.int/tb/en

World Health Organization (2007). *The five elements of DOTS*. Available at http://www.who.int/tb/dots/whatisdots/en

World Health Organization (2007). *Global tuberculosis control: surveillance, planning, financing*. Geneve: WHO. WHO document WHO/HTM/TB/2007.376

World Health Organization (2007). *Tuberculosis fact sheet N° 104*. Available at http://www.who.int/mediacentre/factsheets/fs104/en.

Xu, C., & Prince, J. L. (1998, March). Snakes, shapes, and gradient vector flow. *IEEE Trans. Image Processing, 7*, 359-369.

Yan Sun, Jianming Lu, & Yahagi, T. (2005). Ultrasonographic classification of cirrhosis based on pyramid neural network. *Canadian Conference on Electrical and Computer Engineering*, 1678-1681.

Yang, Y. (1999). An evaluation of statistical approaches to text categorization. *Information Retrieval, 1*(1-2), 69-90.

Yii, M. K., & Ng, K. J. (2002). Risk-adjusted surgical audit with the POSSUM scoring system in a developing country. *British Journal of Surgery, 89*, 110-113.

Young, T., Peppard, P. E., & Gottlieb, D. J. (2002). Epidemiology of Obstructive Sleep Apnea: A Population Health Perspective. *American Journal of Respiratory and Critical Care Medicine, 165*(9), 1217-1239.

Zadeh, L. (1965). Fuzzy Sets. *Information and Control, 8*(3), 338-353.

Zadeh, L. A., (1965). *Fuzzy sets*. Inform. Control (pp. 338–353).

Zadrozny, B., Langford, J., & Abe, N. (2003). Cost-sensitive learning by cost-proportionate example weighting. In *Proceedings of the 3rd IEEE International Conference on Data Mining* (ICDM'03).

Zelezny, F., & Lavrac, N. (2006) Propositionalization-Based Relational Subgroup Discovery with RSD. *Machine Learning, 62*(1-2), 33-63.

Zengyou, H., Xiaofei, X., & Shengchun, D. (2005). TC-SOM: Clustering Transactions Using Self-Organizing Map. *Neural Processing Letters, 22*, 249–262.

Zhang, J., & Honavar, V. (2003). Learning decision tree classifiers from attribute value taxonomies and partially specified data. *Proceedings of the Twentieth International Conference on Machine Learning (ICML 2003)*. Washington, DC, 880-887.

Zhang, S., Qin, Z., Ling, C. X., & Sheng, S. (2005). "Missing is useful": Missing values in cost-sensitive decision trees. *IEEE Transactions on Knowledge and Data Engineering. 17*(12), 1689-1693.

Zhang, X., & Ras, Z. W. (2006). Differentiated harmonic feature analysis on music information retrieval for instrument recognition, in *Proceedings of IEEE International Conference on Granular Computing (IEEE GrC 2006)*, IEEE, pp. 578-581.

Zubek, V. B., & Dietterich, T. G. (2002). Pruning improves heuristic search for cost-sensitive learning. In *Proceedings of the 19th International Conference of Machine Learning* (ICML), (pp. 27-35).

Zvárová, J. (1997). On the medical informatics structure. *International Journal of Medical Informatics,* 44, 75-82.

Zvárová, J., & Studený, M. (1997). Information theoretical approach to constitution and reduction of medical data. *International Journal of Medical Informatics,* 44, 65-74.

About the Contributors

Petr Berka is a full professor at the Dept. of Information and Knowledge Engineering, University of Economics and also works in the Centre of Biomedical Informatics, Institute of Computer Science, Academy of Sciences of the Czech Republic. His main research interests are machine learning, data mining and knowledge-based systems.

Jan Rauch is an associate professor at the Dept. of Information and Knowledge Engineering, University of Economics and also works in the Centre of Biomedical Informatics, Institute of Computer Science, Academy of Sciences of the Czech Republic. His main research interest is data mining.

Djamel Abdelkader Zighed received his Master's in computer and automatic science in 1982 and his PhD in computer science in 1985 – both from university Lyon 1. He was a assistant professor at University Lyon 1 in 1984-1987. In 1987, he joined the University Lyon 2 where he worked as lecturer (1987-1991), professor (1991-2000) and 1st class professor (2000 -). He is interested in data mining (including mining complex data), machine learning and knowledge engineering. He is the founder and was director (1995-2002) of the ERIC laboratory (laboratory for development of methods and software for knowledge engineering, and more specifically automatic knowledge discovery in databases).

* * *

Pablo Luis Acrogliano received the degree of doctor in medicine from Universidad de Buenos Aires. He is a staff at the Neumology Service Dr. Raul H. Catá at Hospital Dr. José Penna in Bahía Blanca, Argentina. He is working as a doctor specialized in Neumology, as regional supervisor of the Regional Tuberculosis Control Program, and as teaching instructor of epidemiology in Dirección de Capacitación de Profesionales de la Salud in Buenos Aires province.

M. Stella Atkins received the BSc degree in chemistry from Nottingham University in 1966 and the PhD degree in computer science from the University of British Columbia in 1985. She is a professor in the School of Computing Science at Simon Fraser University (SFU), and director of the Medical Computing Lab at SFU. Her research interests include medical image display and analysis, telehealth, and computers in medicine. This includes medical image display, denoising and enhancement, segmentation, image registration, and radiology workstation design. Additionally, she is interested in the use of eyegaze trackers, which provide a new imaging modality for seeing inside the brain.

Najib T. Ayas is an associate professor of medicine, University of British Columbia. His research is focused on the health, economic, and safety effects of sleep deprivation and sleep apnea. He is author or co-author of over 40 peer-reviewed publications, and his work has been published in a number of high impact journals including the New England Journal of Medicine, JAMA, and Annals of Internal Medicine.

Endika Bengoetxea received his B.Sc. in Computer Studies from the University of the Basque in 1994, his M.Sc. in Medical Imaging (Medical Physics) from the University of Aberdeen in 1999, and his Ph.D. in Signal and Image Treatment from the French Ecole Nationale Supérieure des Télécommunications in 2002. He joined the University of the Basque Country in 1996 where he is currently professor of the Computer Engineering Faculty, and member of the research group Intelligent Systems Group. His research interests are on the application of Bayesian networks for optimization or classification problems applied to biomedical problems.

Pavel Brazdil got his PhD degree from the University of Edinburgh in 1981. Since 1998 he is full professor at Faculty of Economics. Currently he is the coordinator of R&D Unit LIAAD (earlier known as group NIAAD of LIAAC) founded in 1988. Pavel Brazdil is known for his activities in machine learning, data mining, metalearning, economic modeling, text mining and applications in medicine and bioinformatics. He has participated in two international projects, was a technical coordinator of one of them (METAL) and participated in various international research networks. He has organized more than 10 international conferences or workshops and participated in many program committees (including 14 different editions of ECML). He has (co-)edited 5 books published by major publisher and published more than 120 articles.

Enrique Amigó Cabrera, PhD in computer science (UNED,/Universidad Nacional de Educación a Distancia/, 2006), BsD in computer science (UPM, Universidad Politécnica de Madrid, 2000). /Teacher assistant in the department LSI of UNED. His research is focused on information synthesis tasks and the evaluation of summarization, translation and clustering systems. His work has been also focused on interactive information access systems. He has participated in several national and international research projects (HERMES, MEDIEQ, QUEAVIS)

Václav Chudáček received his Master's degree in biomedical engineering at the Faculty of Electrical Engineering of the Czech Technical University in Prague, Czech Republic in 2003. He is currently working towards the PhD degree in Biomedical Signal and Data Processing group (BioDat) at the Department of Cybernetics, Faculty of Electrical Engineering of the Czech Technical University in Prague. His main research interests are in applications of artificial intelligence methods for analysis of ECG and CTG signals.

Altamiro Costa-Pereira got the PhD degree from the University of Dundee in 1993. Currently he is full professor at FMUP and director of the Department of Biostatistics and Medical Informatics. He is also coordinator of the research unit CINTESIS and director of two master programs (Master's in medical informatics, Master's in evidence and decision making in healthcare) and one PhD program (doctoral program in clinical and health services research). Since 1999, he has been an independent expert, acting as evaluator, at the European Commission. He is author of more than two hundred publications, including fifty indexed by the ISI, which attracted more the 300 citations.

Bruno Crémilleux is professor in computer science at GREYC laboratory (CNRS UMR 6072), University of Caen, France. He is currently heading the data mining research group. He received his PhD in 1991 from the University of Grenoble, France and a habilitation degree in 2004 from the University of Caen. His current research interests include knowledge discovery in databases, machine learning, text mining and their applications notably in bioinformatics and medicine.

Darryl N. Davis, director of research candidate in the Department of Computer Science, the University of Hull, UK. His PhD came from the Faculty of Medicine, University of Manchester. He has worked in data mining and intelligent systems in medicine since 1988. Medical domains include urology, orthodontics, cervical cancer, neuroanatomy, colorectal cancer and cardiovascular medicine.

Gayo Diallo is member of the City eHealth Research Centre at City University of London, where he is working on the EU funded project SeaLife (Semantic Web Browser for the Life Science). Prior to joining City University, Gayo Diallo completed in 2006 his PhD thesis in computer science at University of Joseph Fourier Grenoble 1 within the TIMC-IMAG Laboratory (Osiris Group). He was also a part time lecturer at University Pierre Mendes-France Grenoble 2 from 2001 to 2006. His research interests include DB&IR integration, Semantic Web technologies and ontologies, knowledge representation and reasoning, information contextualisation and adaptation.

Patrik Eklund, professor in computer science, is involved in research both on the theoretical as well the applied side. Research is carried in algebra and logic for computer science application, intelligent computing and medical informatics. Medical and health informatics research involves information infrastructures and platforms, including various patient record systems and repositories. The overall scope and motivation is to enhance methodological issues to support effective and efficient development of guidelines and workflows.

Dagan Feng received his ME in electrical engineering & computing science (EECS) from Shanghai Jiao Tong University in 1982, MSc and PhD in computer science / biocybernetics from the University of California, Los Angeles (UCLA) in 1985 and 1988 respectively. He joined the University of Sydney at the end of 1988, as lecturer, senior lecturer, reader, professor and head of Department of Computer Science / School of Information Technologies. He is currently associate dean of Faculty of Science at the University of Sydney, chair-professor of information technology, Hong Kong Polytechnic University and advisory or guest professor at several universities in China. His research area is biomedical & multimedia information technology (BMIT). He is the Founder and Director the BMIT Research Group. He has published over 500 scholarly research papers, pioneered several new research directions, and received the Crump Prize for Excellence in Medical Engineering from UCLA. He is a fellow of Australian Academy of Technological Sciences and Engineering, ACS, HKIE, IET, and IEEE, special area editor of IEEE Transactions on Information Technology in Biomedicine, and is the current chairman of International Federation of Automatic Control (IFAC) Technical Committee on Biological and Medical Systems.

Alberto Freitas received the MSc and PhD degrees from the University of Porto (Portugal) in 1998 and 2007, respectively. He is member of the Faculty of Medicine of University of Porto (FMUP), in the Department of Biostatistics and Medical Informatics. He is also member of CINTESIS (Centre for

Research in Health Technologies and Information Systems), a research unit recognized and supported by the Portuguese Foundation for Science and Technology (FCT) [POCTI/0753/2004] and hosted by FMUP. His research interests include health information systems and data mining.

Olivier Gandrillon is a researcher at the Centre National de La Recherche Scientifique (CNRS). He is heading a research group in Lyon that is interested in defining the molecular basis for self-renewal, as well as pathological modifications of this process. For this, the group used the SAGE technique extensively. He has been involved for years in transdisciplinary efforts together with computer scientists to make sense of the huge amount of data generated by this transcriptomic approach.

Václav Gerla received his Master's degree in biomedical engineering at the Faculty of Electrical Engineering of the Czech Technical University in Prague, Czech Republic in 2005. He is currently working toward his PhD degree in artificial intelligence and biocybernetics at the Czech Technical University. His research interests are in biomedical signal processing, pattern recognition and biomedical informatics. He is working on automated classification of sleep and the EEG signals of newborns.

Dagmar Villarroel Gonzales is a medical doctor from the Universidad del Rosario in Bogota, Colombia; in October 2005 received her Master's in public health from the Hannover Medical School. She joined the German Agency for Quality in Medicine (Joint Institution of The German Medical Association and the National Association of the Statutory Health Insurance Physicians) in 2004, where she works on appraisal of medical information for patients in internet and development of medical guidelines.

Céline Hébert received her PhD in data mining in 2007 from the University of Caen, France. Her fields of interest include data mining (especially pattern discovery and interestingness measures) and hypergraph theory.

Michal Huptych received his Master's degree in biomedical engineering at the Faculty of Electrical Engineering of the Czech Technical University in Prague, Czech Republic in 2005. He is currently working towards the PhD degree in Biomedical Signal and Data Processing group (BioDat) at the Department of Cybernetics, Faculty of Electrical Engineering of the Czech Technical University in Prague. His main research interests are in applications of signal processing and artificial intelligence methods for biomedical signals analysis.

Pawel Jastreboff is a professor and director of Emory Tinnitus & Hyperacusis Center at the Emory University School of Medicine since January 1999. His previous affiliations include University of Maryland and Yale University. He received his PhD and DSc degrees in neuroscience from the Polish Academy of Science. He did his postdoctoral training at the University of Tokyo, Japan. Dr. Jastreboff holds visiting professor appointment at Yale University School of Medicine, the University College of London, and Middlesex Hospital in London, England. In 1988, on the basis of his research on the physiological mechanisms of tinnitus he proposed a neuro-physiological model of tinnitus and Tinnitus Retraining Therapy (TRT). He also created an animal model of tinnitus, and his present research is aimed at delineating the mechanisms of tinnitus and designing new methods of tinnitus and hyperacusis alleviation.

Wenxin Jiang is a PhD student in the Computer Science Department at the University of North Carolina at Charlotte. His research interest includes knowledge discovery and data mining, music information retrieval, and flexible query answering systems. He is an author of 6 research papers, including one journal publication. His research is supported by NSF.

Lena Kallin-Westin, senior lecturer in computer science, carried out her PhD studies within the field of intelligent computing and medical informatics. The special area of interest has been the preprocessing perceptron and its applications. In recent years, her focus of research interest has moved from intelligent computing to another field concerning learning and knowledge representation; computer science didactics. Within that area, she is currently working with assessment and quality measurements of examination.

Pythagoras Karampiperis holds a Diploma (2000) and MSc on electronics and computer engineering (2002) and an MSc on operational research (2002), all from the Technical University of Crete, Greece. His main scientific interests are in the areas of technology-enhanced learning, next generation service-based learning systems and Semantic Web technologies. He is the co-author of more than 45 publications in scientific books, journals and conferences with at least 50 citations.

Filip Karel is a PhD student at the Department of Cybernetics, CTU. Currently he is working on his doctoral thesis focused on quantitative association rule mining. His main research interests are association rules, medical data mining and usage of e-learning.

Vangelis Karkaletsis is a research director at NCSR "Demokritos". He holds a PhD in artificial intelligence from the University of Athens. He has substantial experience in the field of language and knowledge engineering, especially Web content analysis, ontology evolution, adaptive information filtering and extraction. He is currently coordinating the EC-funded project MedIEQ on quality labeling of health related web content. He is also technical manager of the EC-funded project QUATRO Plus on web content labeling and social networking, and leads the text information extraction and ontology evolution tasks in the BOEMIE project. He is the local chair of the European Conference on Computational Linguistics (EACL-09) and vice chair of the Hellenic Artificial Intelligence Society (EETN).

Jiří Kléma is an assistant professor in artificial intelligence (AI) at the Department of Cybernetics, Czech Technical University in Prague (CTU). He received his PhD in AI and biocybernetics from CTU and carried out post-doctoral training at the University of Caen, France. His main research interest is data mining and its applications in industry, medicine and bioinformatics.

Vladimír Krajča received his Master's degree in control engineering at the Faculty of Electrical Engineering of the Czech Technical University in Prague, Czech Republic in 1979, and his PhD degree in biomedical engineering at the Czech Technical University in Prague in 1985. He is the head of the Electrophysiological Laboratories at the Department of Neurology, Faculty Hospital Na Bulovce in Prague. His research interests are: digital signal processing, adaptive segmentation of stochastic signals, cluster analysis, pattern recognition and artificial intelligence, fuzzy sets and neural networks for signal processing, principal component analysis, independent component analysis.

Mila Kwiatkowska received the MA degree in interdisciplinary studies of Polish philology and informatics from the University of Wroclaw in 1979, the MSc degree in computing science from the University of Alberta in 1991, and the PhD degree in computing science from Simon Fraser University in 2006. She is currently an assistant professor in the Computing Science Department at Thompson Rivers University (TRU). Her research interests include medical data mining, medical decision systems, clinical prediction rules, knowledge representation, fuzzy logic, semiotics, and case-based reasoning.

Martin Labský received his MSc in information technologies from the University of Economics in Prague (2002). Currently he is a PhD student at the Department of Knowledge Engineering at the UEP, with statistical methods for information extraction as thesis topic. His research interests include machine learning methods, knowledge representation and natural language processing. (Co-)author of more than 10 reviewed papers.

Pedro Larrañaga received his MSc degree in mathematics from the University of Valladolid, in Spain, in 1981, and his PhD in computer science from the University of the Basque Country, in Spain, in 1995. He is professor at the Department of Artificial Intelligence of the Technical University of Madrid. His research topics include Bayesian networks and evolutionary computation with applications in medicine and bioinformatics.

Lenka Lhotská received her Master's degree in cybernetics at the Faculty of Electrical Engineering of the Czech Technical University in Prague, Czech Republic in 1984, and her PhD degree in cybernetics at the Czech Technical University in Prague in 1989. Currently she is head of the biomedical signal and data processing group (BioDat) at the Department of Cybernetics, Faculty of Electrical Engineering of the Czech Technical University in Prague. Her research interests are in artificial intelligence methods and their applications in medicine.

Les Matthews is a respiratory therapist with a Diploma in Adult Education from University of British Columbia and a Master's degree in education from Gonzaga University. With 30 years of experience in education and clinical practice he is an assistant professor of respiratory therapy and the supervisor of the Obstructive Sleep Apnea clinic at Thompson Rivers University. His research interests include ambulatory monitoring, auto titration CPAP, patient mentoring and clinical simulation

Miquel Angel Mayer MD and PhD in health and life sciences is a Specialist of Family and Community Medicine. He is the Director of Web Médica Acreditada (WMA) of the Medical Association of Barcelona, the first Spanish trust mark and e-health initiative. He participated in several international semantic web projects as MedCIRCLE and QUATRO and currently he is involved in the EU project MedIEQ and QUATRO Plus for the implementation of semantic web vocabularies and technologies helping users to get the best health information on the Internet.

Radja Messai was trained in computer science (bachelor of science from the University of Batna - Algeria in 2003) and is currently a PhD student at the UJF University in Grenoble. She is working on health-related ontology and terminology services for patients and citizens.

Jitka Mohylová received her Master's degree in radioelectronics, specialization medical electronics at the Faculty of Electrical Engineering of the Brno University of Technology, Czech Republic in 1983, and her PhD degree in cybernetics at the Czech Technical University in Prague in 1999. Since 1990 she has been with the Department of General Electrical Engineering, Faculty of Electrical Engineering and Computer Science of the VŠB – Technical University of Ostrava. Currently she is also lecturing at the University of Zilina, Slovakia. Her research interests are in signal processing and electronics and their applications in medicine.

Dinora A. Morales received her BA and MSc degree in computer science from Technological Institute of Querétaro, México in 1999, and MSc in neurobiology from Institute of Neurobiology, National University of México in 2003. Since October, 2005 she is a member of Intelligent Systems Group of the University of the Basque Country where she has been working for her PhD. She is interested in learning from data within machine learning, artificial intelligence, and statistics. In particular, she is interested in learning probabilistic graphical models such as Bayesian networks. Actually her work concentrates in developing algorithms for supervised classification from human embryo selection in assisted reproduction techniques data.

Thuy T.T. Nguyen received the BSc degree in mathematics from Hanoi 1 University of Pedagogy in 1993. She received the MSc in computer science from Hanoi Nation University in Vietnam in 1999. She is now a PhD candidate in the Department of Computer Science, the University of Hull, UK. Her project is on the use of pattern recognition and data mining techniques to predict cardiovascular risk. She has published four papers from this research with specific focus on the use of neural nets and unsupervised clustering techniques.

Svojmil Petránek received his Master's degree in radioelectronics, specialization Medical Electronics at the Faculty of Electrical Engineering of the Czech Technical University in Prague, Czech Republic in 1971, MD at the School of Medicine, Charles University, Prague, Czech Republic in 1977 and his PhD degree in medicine at Charles University in Prague in 1983. He is the head of the Department of Neurology, Faculty Hospital Na Bulovce in Prague. His research interests are: neurophysiology, EEG processing, automated classification of EEG.

Matti Pöllä received his MSc(Tech) degree in electrical and communications engineering in 2005 from Helsinki University of Technology (TKK), Finland. Presently he works as a researcher at the Adaptive Informatics Research Centre at TKK. His current research interests include text data mining using bio-inspired algorithms.

Zbigniew W. Ras is a professor of computer science in the College of Computing and Informatics at the University of North Carolina, Charlotte. Also, he is a professor and member of the senate at the Polish-Japanese Institute of Information Technology in Warsaw, Poland. His previous affiliations include: University of Florida (Gainesville), Columbia University (New York), University of Tennessee (Knoxville), and Lockheed Research Lab (Palo Alto). He received his PhD degree from the University of Warsaw (Poland) and DSc degree (habilitation) from the Polish Academy of Sciences. He is the editor-in-chief of the Journal of Intelligent Information Systems (Springer) and the deputy editor-in-chief of Fundamenta Informaticae Journal. He is the editor/co-editor of 32 books and the author of more than 200 papers all in the area of intelligent information systems.

Marek Růžička is part-time software engineer at the Department of Information and Knowledge Engineering, University of Economics, Prague. He has long-term experience in the development of software tools for semantic annotation, knowledge management and information search, in the framework of projects undertaken at University of Economics, Prague (MGT, M-CAST, MedIEQ) as well as at INRIA - Sophia-Antipolis, France (LifeLine, Corese).

C. Frank Ryan graduated from the National University of Ireland (Galway) in 1979. He completed his post-graduate clinical training in Internal Medicine and Respiratory Medicine in Dublin at the Royal College of Surgeons in Ireland. After pursuing a post-doctoral research fellowship in respiratory sleep disorders at the University of British Columbia in Vancouver, he joined the Faculty of Medicine at UBC and the active staff at Vancouver Coastal Health in 1990 . He is a professor of medicine at UBC and a consultant in internal medicine, respiratory medicine and sleep disorders medicine at Vancouver Coastal Health. Dr. Ryan's clinical and research interests include respiratory sleep and neuromuscular diseases, and pleural diseases.

Marisa A. Sánchez received a PhD in computer science from Universidad Nacional del Sur in Bahía Blanca, Argentina. She is currently a professor of graduate and post-graduate courses at Department of Management Sciences at Universidad Nacional del Sur. From 1994 to 2004 she had been on the faculty at Departments of Computer Science and Electrical Engineering. She has been a fellow at the International Institute for Software Technologies of the United Nations University, Macao, and at Politécnico de Milano, Italy. Her research interests include data warehousing, knowledge discovery, and data mining. She is also interested in business process modeling.

Rainer Schmidt studied social science and computer science (both with MSc) and received a PhD in medical informatics. After working on explanation-based learning (EBL) at the University of Dortmund, in 1993 he moved to Munich, where he started working on case-based reasoning for medical applications. Since 1996 he is working at the University of Rostock still in the same research area – only interrupted by working at the Robert Gordon University in Aberdeen, Scotland, in 1998.

Arnaud Soulet is an associate professor in computer science at LI laboratory, University of Tours François Rabelais, France. He received his PhD in 2006 from the University of Caen, France. His main research interests include data mining and machine learning (especially applied in bioinformatics and medicine).

Ana Simonet is an assistant professor in computer science at the University Pierre Mendès-France in Grenoble. Both her teaching and her research work are oriented towards conceptual modeling. She has developed a novel approach to database design, based on an initial ontological schema that is automatically transformed into a database schema optimized for a given set of queries. She is an active member of the TIMC group working on data and knowledge modeling and representation. Besides her interest in the design of information systems she is also involved in the integration of heterogeneous databases, following an ontology-based approach.

Michel Simonet is the head of the knowledge base and database team of the TIMC laboratory at the Joseph Fourier University of Grenoble. His group works on the design and the implementation of knowledge bases and databases, using an ontology-based approach, and currently on the integration of Information Systems by using the tools and methodologies they have developed. They work on two main projects: a database and knowledge base management system, named OSIRIS, and a system for database conception and reverse engineering based on original concepts and a new methodology. In the recent years Michel Simonet has managed the European ASIA-ITC GENNERE with China and has been responsible of ontology enrichment in the European IP project Noesis, a platform for wide-scale integration and visual representation of medical intelligence.

Konstantinos Stamatakis has experience in the area of information discovery and extraction from online resources. Being a research associate in NCSR "Demokritos" during the last years he has worked in several national and European RTD projects and has developed methods and tools for Web crawling and spidering and an information discovery platform incorporating several applications involved in information identification and extraction from the Web (ontologies, formation of corpora, training, crawling, spidering, extraction of information, data storage and representation). He is currently involved in the MedIEQ project being responsible for the web content collection tools to be developed in the project.

Vojtěch Svátek is associate professor at the Department of Information and Knowledge Engineering, University of Economics, Prague. His main areas of research are knowledge modeling and knowledge discovery from databases and texts. Local contact person of EU projects K-Space and MedIEQ, organizer of numerous events (e.g. Co-Chair of the EKAW conference in 2006), author of about 80 papers.

Pamela L. Thompson is a doctoral student in the department of computer science at the University of North Carolina at Charlotte. She received her undergraduate degree in management information systems and her MBA from James Madison University in Harrisonburg, Virginia. She is an associate professor at Catawba College in Salisbury, NC. Her research is focusing on the development of a decision support system for diagnosis and treatment of tinnitus.

Jakub Tolar received his MD from Charles University in Prague, Czech Republic, and his PhD in molecular, cellular, developmental biology and genetics from the University of Minnesota. He has been interested in the use of hematopoietic transplantation for bone marrow failure (e.g., aplastic anemia and dyskeratosis congenita) and metabolic disorders (e.g., mucopolysaccharidosis type I and adrenoleukodystrophy). His research focuses on the use of bone marrow derived stem cells and Sleeping Beauty transposon gene therapy for correction of genetic diseases and improving outcome of blood and marrow transplantation.

Marie Tomečková is a physician working at the Dept. of Medical Informatics and in the Centre of Biomedical Informatics, Institute of Computer Science, Academy of Sciences of the Czech Republic. Her specialization is non-invasive cardiology, namely epidemiology of atherosclerosis.

Igor Trajkovski is a researcher at the Department of Knowledge Technologies of the Jožef Stefan Institute in Ljubljana, Slovenia. He received a MSc in computer science from the Saarland University and Max Plank Institute for Informatics in Germany and is now a PhD student at the Jožef Stefan International Postgraduate School in Ljubljana. His research interests are in machine learning, microarray data analysis, common sense knowledge representation and reasoning.

Sonia Uremovich received a Bachelor's in business administration from Universidad Nacional del Sur in Bahía Blanca, Argentina. She is teaching assistant at Department of Management Sciences at Universidad Nacional del Sur, and at a Technical High School. Her research interests include decision support systems in management.

Igor Vajda was born in Martin, Czechoslovakia, in 1942. He graduated in mathematics from the Czech Technical University, Prague, in 1965. He received the PhD degree in probability and statistics from the Charles University, Prague, in 1968, and the DrSc degree in mathematical informatics from the same university in 1990. From 1965 he served as a research assistant, from 1966 as a researcher, and from 1990 as a principal researcher at the Institute of Information Theory and Automation, Czech Academy of Sciences, Prague. During 1966 -2007 he was visiting scientist or visiting professor at various universities and research institutes in Europe, Russia and USA. His research interests include information theory, asymptotic statistics and statistical decisions. Dr. Vajda is fellow of IEEE, associate editor of several international scientific journals and chairs or vice-chairs various committees at the Czech Technical University. He was awarded several prizes for outstanding results of research.

Arnošt Veselý graduated at Faculty of Technical and Nuclear Physics of Czech Technical University in Prague. Scientific degree in logic he received in 1990 at Philosophical Faculty of Charles University. From 1992 he is a member of Department of Information Engineering of Czech University of Life Sciences in Prague and from 2001 he is associate professor in information management. He reads lectures in operating systems and artificial intelligence. From 2001 he is a member of Department of Medical Informatics at Institute of Computer Science of the Academy of Sciences of the Czech Republic. His main interests are neural networks and formalization of knowledge mainly with regard to their applications in medicine.

Xiu Ying Wang received her PhD in computer science from The University, of Sydney in 2005. Currently she is working in the School of Information Technologies, The University of Sydney. She is a member of IFAC and executive secretary of IFAC TC on BioMed. Her research interests include image registration for applications in biomedicine and multimedia, and computer graphics.

Xin Zhang received her PhD in information technology degree from the University of North Carolina at Charlotte in December, 2007. Beginning Fall of 2008, she will join the University of North Carolina at Pembroke as an assistant professor in the Department of Mathematics and Computer Science. Her research interest includes knowledge discovery and data mining, music information retrieval, and flexible query answering systems. She is an author of 12 research papers, including two journal publications. Her PhD research was supported by NSF.

Jana Zvárová graduated in 1965 at Charles University in Prague, Faculty of Mathematics and Physics. She received PhD scientific degree in 1978 at Charles University in Prague. She passed the habilitation for Doc. (associated professor) in 1991 and became Prof. (full professor) at Charles University in Prague in 1999. Since 1994 she is the principal researcher at the Institute of Computer Science, Academy of

Sciences of the Czech Republic, head of the Department of Medical Informatics and the director of the European Center of Medical Informatics, Statistics and Epidemiology (EuroMISE Center). She has been the representative of the Czech Republic in the International Medical Informatics Association (IMIA) and European Federation for Medical Informatics (EFMI). She is chairing the board of biomedical informatics of the PhD studies of Charles University and Academy of Sciences of the Czech Republic. She has been a member of the editorial boards of national and international journals, she has served as the expert in the field for the EC and Czech governmental institutions. She has published more then 200 of papers in national and international literature, received several medals for her work.

Filip Železný is the head of the Intelligent Data Analysis research group at GL. He received his PhD in AI and biocybernetics from CTU and carried out post-doctoral training at the University of Wisconsin in Madison. He was a visiting professor at the State University of New York in Binghamton. Currently he is a grantee of the Czech Academy of Sciences and the European Commission. His main research interest is relational machine learning and its applications in bioinformatics.

Index

S

T

U

W